OXFORD MEDICAL PUBLICATIONS

Oxford Handbook of
Surgical Nursing

Published and forthcoming Oxford Handbooks in Nursing

Oxford Handbook of Adult Nursing
George Castledine and Ann Close

Oxford Handbook of Cancer Nursing
Edited by Mike Tadman and Dave Roberts

Oxford Handbook of Cardiac Nursing, 2e
Edited by Kate Olson

Oxford Handbook of Children's and Young People's Nursing, 2e
Edited by Edward Alan Glasper, Gillian McEwing, and Jim Richardson

Oxford Handbook of Clinical Skills for Children's and Young People's Nursing
Paula Dawson, Louise Cook, Laura-Jane Holliday, and Helen Reddy

Oxford Handbook of Clinical Skills in Adult Nursing
Jacqueline Randle, Frank Coffey, and Martyn Bradbury

Oxford Handbook of Critical Care Nursing
Sheila Adam and Sue Osborne

Oxford Handbook of Dental Nursing
Elizabeth Boon, Rebecca Parr, Dayananda Samarawickrama, and Kevin Seymour

Oxford Handbook of Diabetes Nursing
Lorraine Avery and Sue Beckwith

Oxford Handbook of Emergency Nursing, 2e
Edited by Robert Crouch, Alan Charters, Mary Dawood, and Paula Bennett

Oxford Handbook of Gastrointestinal Nursing
Edited by Christine Norton, Julia Williams, Claire Taylor, Annmarie Nunwa, and Kathy Whayman

Oxford Handbook of Learning and Intellectual Disability Nursing
Edited by Bob Gates and Owen Barr

Oxford Handbook of Mental Health Nursing, 2e
Edited by Patrick Callaghan and Catherine Gamble

Oxford Handbook of Midwifery, 2e
Janet Medforth, Susan Battersby, Maggie Evans, Beverley Marsh, and Angela Walker

Oxford Handbook of Musculoskeletal Nursing
Edited by Susan Oliver

Oxford Handbook of Neuroscience Nursing
Edited by Sue Woodward and Catheryne Waterhouse

Oxford Handbook of Nursing Older People
Beverley Tabernacle, Marie Barnes, and Annette Jinks

Oxford Handbook of Orthopaedic and Trauma Nursing
Rebecca Jester, Julie Santy, and Jean Rogers

Oxford Handbook of Perioperative Practice
Suzanne Hughes and Andy Mardell

Oxford Handbook of Prescribing for Nurses and Allied Health Professionals
Sue Beckwith and Penny Franklin

Oxford Handbook of Primary Care and Community Nursing, 2e
Edited by Vari Drennan and Claire Goodman

Oxford Handbook of Renal Nursing
Edited by Althea Mahon, Karen Jenkins, and Lisa Burnapp

Oxford Handbook of Respiratory Nursing
Terry Robinson and Jane Scullion

Oxford Handbook of Surgical Nursing
Edited by Alison Smith, Maria Kisiel, and Mark Radford

Oxford Handbook of Women's Health Nursing
Edited by Sunanda Gupta, Debra Holloway, and Ali Kubba

Oxford Handbook of
Surgical Nursing

Edited by

Alison Smith
Lecturer,
University of Birmingham, UK

Maria Kisiel
Formerly Head of Department of Adult
and Critical Care Nursing,
Birmingham City University, UK

Mark Radford
Chief Nursing Officer,
University Hospitals Coventry
and Warwickshire NHS Trust,
and Professor,
Birmingham City University, UK

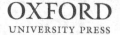

OXFORD
UNIVERSITY PRESS

Great Clarendon Street, Oxford, OX2 6DP,
United Kingdom

Oxford University Press is a department of the University of Oxford.
It furthers the University's objective of excellence in research, scholarship,
and education by publishing worldwide. Oxford is a registered trade mark of
Oxford University Press in the UK and in certain other countries

Published in the United States of America by Oxford University Press
198 Madison Avenue, New York, NY 10016, United States of America

British Library Cataloguing in Publication Data

Data available

Library of Congress Control Number: 2015942566

ISBN 978–0–19–964266–3

Printed and bound in Great Britain by
Ashford Colour Press Ltd

Foreword

Florence Nightingale stated that 'Apprehension, uncertainty, waiting, expectation, fear of surprise, do a patient more harm than any exertion.' The prospect of surgery can and does generate these emotions. This Handbook offers nurses with an interest in and passion for surgical nursing a holistic perspective that can help to address not only these emotions but also the physical and practical elements of practice.

The pace, scale, and sophistication of new treatments and technologies make surgery one of the fastest changing and exciting specialties. The ability to perform surgery on patients with complex medical problems and chronic illness means that the skills required to provide competent and compassionate care for these patients must extend well beyond the fundamentals of pre- and post-operative care. Surgical nurses require both a broad and deep knowledge and the necessary skills if they are to be able to confidently assess patients' needs and pre-empt potential complications. This is more important than ever now that many nurses are also undertaking more advanced procedures as part of the multidisciplinary team.

This Handbook will both act as an aide-memoire and help to build a knowledge base that will enable surgical nurses to understand their core role and their contribution to the modern surgical team. It will be of benefit to nurses and allied health professionals working on surgical wards and also in the many settings in which surgical care is delivered, including day-surgery, high-dependency, outpatient, and pre-operative assessment clinics. It can be used by clinicians at different stages in their professional development, including pre- and post-registration, as well as those undertaking specialist and advanced practice.

This evidence-based, easily accessible, concise Handbook, which can be used at the bedside, offers practical advice on how to effectively assess, plan, implement, and evaluate surgical care. It also explains the wider role of the surgical nurse in effective ward management and leadership, and the implications for patient care.

Patients and their families deserve and expect a high-quality, dignified, and safe experience when they have surgery. This requires skilled, compassionate, and competent surgical clinicians who strive to continue to enhance and develop their knowledge, skills, and practice. This Handbook without doubt supports the attainment of this. It is packed with a wealth of information, and has the benefit of being written and edited by credible, respected, and experienced clinicians and academics, all of whom understand the challenges that face nurses and allied health professionals working today in this dynamic and fast-moving field.

Janice Stevens CBE MA RGN
Director for Midlands and East
Health Education England

Preface

Contributing to the writing and editing of this book has been both challenging and rewarding, and the end result is a product of the passion and expertise of the many contributors for improving the care of the surgical patient. It is hoped that, by using this key resource, the reader will gain an insight into the diverse nature of surgical nursing and develop confidence in their clinical practice. Each chapter has been written by healthcare professionals with a passion for and expertise in their subject area. The key references and suggestions for further reading at the end of each section provide the reader with opportunities to supplement their knowledge further.

Surgery is a complex and varied specialty that has seen significant changes and technical advances in recent years. Central to this has been the skill and support of the surgical nurse in ensuring improved outcomes and compassionate care for patients. From the operating theatre to the hospital bed, the surgical nursing specialty has developed and diversified to keep pace with the many advances and improvements in surgery. Many textbooks in this subject area provide comprehensive information in an attempt 'to cover all bases', which often means that these textbooks are large and not easily transportable to the bedside.

In developing the *Oxford Handbook of Surgical Nursing*, the editors have aimed to adhere to the Oxford Handbook philosophy of providing high-quality, quick-reference, pocket-sized resources that enable nurses to easily check key clinical facts. It is hoped that this Handbook will also complement and build upon other publications, while enabling nurses and other allied healthcare professionals to quickly access concise relevant information to support their clinical practice.

Alison Smith
Maria Kisiel
Mark Radford
2016

Contents

Contributors

Debra Adams
(*Chapter 14*)
Head of Infection Prevention and
Control (Midlands and East)
NHS Trust Development
Authority, UK

Ann-Marie Cannaby
(*Chapter 2*)
Executive Director of Nursing
Hamad Medical
Corporation, Qatar

Ruth Capewell
(*Chapter 28*)
MacMillan Gynaecology Clinical
Nurse Specialist (Oncology)
University Hospitals Coventry
and Warwickshire NHS Trust, UK

Anna Casey
(*Chapter 14*)
Clinical Research Scientist
University Hospitals Birmingham
NHS Foundation Trust, UK

Kirsty Cotterill
(*Chapter 28*)
Gynaecology Clinical
Nurse Specialist
University Hospitals Coventry
and Warwickshire NHS Trust, UK

Kevin Crimmons
(*Chapter 25*)
Head of Adult Nursing
Birmingham City University, UK

Patricia Davies
(*Chapter 12, Chapter 13*)
Senior Lecturer
Birmingham City University, UK

Suzanne Davies
(*Chapter 21*)
Vascular Nurse Specialist
University Hospitals Coventry
and Warwickshire NHS Trust, UK

Helen Gibbons
(*Chapter 17*)
Senior Lecturer
City University, London, UK

Suzanne Hammond
(*Chapter 28*)
Urogynaecology Clinical
Nurse Specialist
University Hospitals Coventry
and Warwickshire NHS Trust, UK

Kim Harley
(*Chapter 20, Chapter 23*)
Formerly Senior Lecturer
Birmingham City University, UK

Susan Harrington
(*Chapter 28*)
Modern Matron—Gynaecology
University Hospitals Coventry
and Warwickshire NHS Trust, UK

Helen Holder
(*Chapter 10*)
Senior Lecturer
Birmingham City University, UK

Louise Jennings
(*Chapter 28*)
Clinical Nurse Specialist
Gynaecology Outpatient
Department, University
Hospitals Coventry and
Warwickshire
NHS Trust, UK

Sue Jones
(*Chapter 23*)
Formerly Senior Lecturer
Birmingham City University, UK

Amanda Kirkman
Clinical Nurse Specialist for Early
Pregnancy and Miscarriage
University Hospitals Coventry and
Warwickshire NHS Trust, UK

Aaron Kisiel
(*Chapter 1*)
CT1 General Surgery
University Hospitals Birmingham
NHS Foundation Trust, UK

Maria Kisiel
(*Chapter 1, Chapter 26*)
Formerly Head of Department of
Adult and Critical Care Nursing
Birmingham City University, UK

Alison Kite
(*Chapter 21*)
Clinical Nurse Specialist—
Vascular Surgery
University Hospitals Coventry and
Warwickshire NHS Trust, UK

Jane Leaver
(*Chapter 24*)
Senior Lecturer
Birmingham City University, UK

Lorraine Marsons
(*Chapter 25*)
Senior Lecturer
Birmingham City University, UK

Ross Palmer
(*Chapter 8*)
Modern Matron—Trauma and
Orthopaedics
University Hospitals Coventry
and Warwickshire NHS Trust, UK

Claire Perkins
(*Chapter 15, Chapter 16*)
Senior Lecturer
Birmingham City University, UK

Mike Phillips
(*Chapter 5*)
Lead Anaesthesia Practitioner
Heart of England NHS
Foundation Trust, UK

Mark Radford
(*Chapter 3, Chapter 4, Chapter 7*)
Chief Nursing Officer
University Hospitals Coventry
and Warwickshire NHS Trust,
and Professor Birmingham City
University, UK

Anna Rudkin
(*Chapter 28*)
Gynaecology Clinical Nurse Specialist
University Hospitals Coventry
and Warwickshire NHS Trust, UK

Debbie Shreeve
(*Chapter 22*)
Urology Nurse Specialist
University Hospitals Coventry
and Warwickshire NHS Trust, UK

Alison Smith
(*Chapter 1, Chapter 6, Chapter 8,
Chapter 11, Chapter 18, Chapter 26*)
Lecturer
University of Birmingham, UK

Dion Smyth
(*Chapter 27*)
Senior Lecturer
Birmingham City University, UK

Richard Stock
(*Chapter 20*)
Senior Lecturer
Birmingham City University, UK

Meriel Swann
(*Chapter 9*)
Senior Lecturer
Birmingham City University, UK

Iain Wharton
(*Chapter 22*)
Consultant Urologist
University Hospitals Coventry
and Warwickshire NHS Trust, UK

Maddie White
(*Chapter 19*)
Colorectal Nursing Team Leader
University Hospitals Birmingham
NHS Foundation Trust, UK

Annette Wye
(*Chapter 21*)
Vascular Nurse Specialist
University Hospitals Coventry
and Warwickshire NHS Trust, UK

Symbols and abbreviations

▶	important
▶▶	act quickly
⊖	cross-reference
℘	website
AAA	abdominal aortic aneurysm
ABPI	Ankle Brachial Pressure Index
ACE	angiotensin-converting enzyme
ACS	acute coronary syndrome
ADH	antidiuretic hormone
AED	automated external defibrillator
AF	atrial fibrillation
AFP	alpha-fetoprotein
AIDS	acquired immunodeficiency syndrome
AKI	acute kidney injury
ALI	acute lung injury
ALT	alanine transaminase
ANTT	aseptic non-touch technique
AP	anteroposterior
APC	activated protein C
APTT	activated partial thromboplastin time
ARDS	acute respiratory distress syndrome
ASA	American Society of Anesthesiologists
ASI	acute spinal injury
AST	aspartate transaminase
ATP	adenosine triphosphate
AUR	acute urinary retention
AV	atrioventricular
AVPU	Alert, Voice, Pain, Unresponsive
BAPEN	British Association for Parenteral and Enteral Nutrition
BCC	basal-cell carcinoma
BMI	body mass index

BMT	best medical therapy
BPH	benign prostatic hyperplasia
BSE	bovine spongiform encephalopathy
CABG	coronary artery bypass graft
CAPD	continuous ambulatory peritoneal dialysis
CBT	cognitive behavioural therapy
CD	controlled drug
CJD	Creutzfeldt–Jakob disease
CK	creatinine kinase
CMV	cytomegalovirus
CNS	central nervous system
COPD	chronic obstructive pulmonary disease
CPAP	continuous positive airway pressure
CPE	carbapenemase-producing Enterobacteriaceae
CPET	cardiopulmonary exercise testing
CPR	cardiopulmonary resuscitation
CQC	Care Quality Commission
CRP	C-reactive protein
CSF	cerebrospinal fluid
CT	computed tomography
CUR	chronic urinary retention
CVA	cerebrovascular accident
CVP	central venous pressure
DAI	diffuse axonal injury
DBS	deep brain stimulation
DCIS	ductal carcinoma *in situ*
DIC	disseminated intravascular coagulopathy
DKA	diabetic ketoacidosis
DVT	deep vein thrombosis
DXA	dual-energy X-ray absorptiometry
ECF	extracellular fluid
ECG	electrocardiogram
ED	erectile dysfunction
EDTA	ethylene diamine tetra-acetic acid
EEG	electroencephalography

EMDR	eye movement desensitization and reprocessing
ERAS	enhanced recovery after surgery
ERCP	endoscopic retrograde cholangiopancreatography
ERP	Enhanced Recovery Programme
ERPOC	evacuation of retained products of conception
ERV	expiratory reserve volume
ESBL	extended-spectrum β-lactamase
ESR	erythrocyte sedimentation rate
ETF	enteral tube feeding
FAP	familial adenomatous polyposis
FAST	focused assessment with sonography for trauma
FBC	full blood count
FDP	fibrin degradation product
FES	fat embolism syndrome
FEV1	forced expiratory volume in 1 s
FFP	fresh frozen plasma
FRC	functional residual capacity
FRCA	Fellow of the Royal College of Anaesthetists
FRCS	Fellow of the Royal College of Surgeons
FVC	forced vital capacity
FVD	fluid volume deficit
GALS	gait, arms, legs, and spine
GCS	Glasgow Coma Scale
GI	gastrointestinal
GMC	General Medical Council
GORD	gastro-oesophageal reflux disease
GTN	glyceryl trinitrate
HAART	highly active antiretroviral therapy
Hb	haemoglobin
HbA1c	glycated haemoglobin
HCAI	healthcare-associated infection
HER2	human epidermal growth factor receptor-2
HHS	hyperosmolar hyperglycaemic state
HIV	human immunodeficiency virus
HPV	human papilloma virus

HRT	hormone replacement therapy
HSDU	Hospital Sterilization and Disinfection Unit
HSV	herpes simplex virus
IABP	intra-aortic balloon pump
IBD	inflammatory bowel disease
IC	inspiratory capacity
ICF	intracellular fluid
ICP	intracranial pressure
IHD	ischaemic heart disease
IM	intramuscular
INR	international normalized ratio
IOL	intra-ocular lens
IOP	intra-ocular pressure
IPC	infection prevention and control
IPH	inadvertent peri-operative hypothermia
IPPV	intermittent positive pressure ventilation
IRV	inspiratory reserve volume
IV	intravenous
JVP	jugular venous pressure
LBO	large bowel obstruction
LDH	lactate dehydrogenase
LFT	liver function test
LMA	laryngeal mask airway
LV	left ventricle
MAP	mean arterial pressure
MDT	multidisciplinary team
MET	metabolic equivalent
MHRA	Medicines and Healthcare products Regulatory Agency
MI	myocardial infarction
MODS	multiple organ dysfunction syndrome
MRI	magnetic resonance imaging
MRSA	meticillin-resistant *Staphylococcus aureus*
MSSA	meticillin-sensitive *Staphylococcus aureus*
MUST	Malnutrition Universal Screening Tool

NAI	non-accidental injury
NBM	nil by mouth
NCEPOD	National Confidential Enquiry into Patient Outcome and Death
NEWS	National Early Warning Score
NICE	National Institute for Health and Care Excellence
NIPPV	non-invasive positive pressure ventilation
NMC	Nursing and Midwifery Council
NPA	nasopharyngeal airway
NPSA	National Patient Safety Agency
NRS	numerical rating scale
NSAID	non-steroidal anti-inflammatory drug
NSTEMI	non-ST-segment-elevation myocardial infarction
NYHA	New York Heart Association
ODP	operating department practitioner
OGTT	oral glucose tolerance test
ONS	oral nutrition supplements
OPA	oropharyngeal airway
ORIF	open reduction and internal fixation
PA	posteroanterior
$PaCO_2$	partial pressure of carbon dioxide
PAD	peripheral artery disease
PaO_2	partial pressure of oxygen
PCA	patient-controlled analgesia
PCI	percutaneous coronary intervention
PEEP	positive end-expiratory pressure
PEG	percutaneous endoscopic gastrostomy
PEJ	percutaneous endoscopic jejunostomy
PET	positron emission tomography
PET-CT	positron emission tomography with computed tomography
PGD	patient group direction
PICC	peripherally inserted central catheter
PID	pelvic inflammatory disease
PII	period of increased incidence
PMC	pseudomembranous colitis

PMPS	post-mastectomy pain syndrome
PN	parenteral nutrition
PONV	post-operative nausea and vomiting
PPE	personal protective equipment
PPV	positive pressure ventilation
PSA	prostate-specific antigen
PSC	primary sclerosing cholangitis
PT	prothrombin time
PTSD	post-traumatic stress disorder
PTT	partial thromboplastin time
PVL	Panton–Valentine leucocidin
RAS	renal artery stenosis
RCA	root cause analysis
RCC	renal-cell carcinoma
REMS	regional examination of the musculoskeletal system
RICP	raised intracranial pressure
RIG	radiologically inserted gastrostomy
RN	registered nurse
RRT	renal replacement therapy
RSI	rapid sequence induction
RTT	referral to treatment time
RV	residual volume
SA	sinoatrial
SAH	subarachnoid haemorrhage
SALT	speech and language therapy
SBAR	Situation–Background–Assessment–Recommendation
SBC	standard bicarbonate concentration
SBO	small bowel obstruction
SCC	squamous-cell carcinoma
SGOT	serum glutamic oxaloacetic transaminase
SHOT	Serious Hazards of Transfusion
SICP	Standard Infection Control Precautions
SIGN	Scottish Intercollegiate Guidelines Network
SIRS	systemic inflammatory response syndrome
SSI	surgical site infection

STEMI	ST-segment-elevation myocardial infarction
STI	sexually transmitted infection
SUFE	slipped upper femoral epiphysis
TBI	traumatic brain injury
TBP	Transmission-Based Precautions
TBSA	total body surface area
TBW	total body water
TCI	target-controlled infusion
TENS	transcutaneous electrical nerve stimulation
TIPS	transjugular intrahepatic portosystemic shunt
TIVA	total intravenous anaesthesia
TLC	total lung capacity
TNF	tumour necrosis factor
TNP	topical negative pressure
TPN	total parenteral nutrition
TRALI	transfusion-related acute lung injury
TSH	thyroid-stimulating hormone
tTGA	tissue transglutaminase
TV	tidal volume
U&E	urea and electrolytes
UTI	urinary tract infection
VAD	venous access device; ventricular assist device
VAS	visual analogue scale
VATS	video-assisted thoracic surgery
VC	vital capacity
V/Q	ventilation/perfusion
VRE	vancomycin-resistant enterococci
VTE	venous thromboembolism
WCC	white cell count
WFNS	World Federation of Neurological Surgeons
WHO	World Health Organization

Chapter 1

Introduction to the surgical patient

The surgical patient

Surgical patients receive physical treatment in the form of operative procedures to remove or replace diseased organs and/or tissues. This means that specific aspects of the care of these patients may differ from those of medical patients. In addition, surgical patients are at risk of complications following a surgical procedure.

Psychological support

Psychological support is required throughout the peri-operative period, in order to ensure that the patient:
- is able to express any fears and anxieties
- has a clear understanding of the processes involved in the pre-operative assessment and preparation for surgery
- understands the surgical procedure that is being undertaken and the potential risks and complications
- is aware of the interventions and monitoring required in the post-operative period
- has access to specialist nursing teams in order to discuss any concerns and anxieties they may have relating to altered body image (e.g. scarring, prosthesis)
- knows who to contact if they have a query or concern after discharge from hospital.

Pain management

Surgical patients require good-quality pain management interventions both following surgical procedures and prior to surgery. If a patient's pain is poorly controlled, the following complications may occur:
- emotional and physical suffering, which can result in the breakdown of the nurse–patient relationship
- cardiovascular effects, tachycardia, and hypertension
- increased oxygen demand
- reduced respiratory function, and consolidation or collapse of the alveoli
- reduced mobility, which increases the risk of developing a venous thromboembolism
- sleep disturbance
- delayed discharge.

Wound care and infection control

Surgical site infections represent 16% of all healthcare-associated infections, and can have both physical and psychological effects on the patient.[1] Most surgical site infections are preventable, and it is the responsibility of all members of the multidisciplinary team (MDT) to ensure that measures are taken to reduce the risk of infection. Best practice should be adhered to at all times, while also taking into consideration the patient's individual needs and preferences.

Nutrition

Following surgery the patient may have a reduced appetite due to nausea and vomiting, which are side effects of analgesic and anaesthetic drugs. It is important that the surgical patient has a diet rich in protein and vitamins, to promote wound healing. The body has an increased metabolic demand for protein following surgery, due to the stress response releasing catecholamines such as cortisol. A diet rich in fibre is also required to prevent constipation, which can occur as a result of reduced mobility or after the administration of opioid analgesia.

Reference

1 National Institute for Health and Care Excellence (NICE). *Surgical Site Infection*. QS49. NICE: London, 2013. ℘ www.nice.org.uk/guidance/qs49

The surgical team

The surgical team consists of a range of healthcare professionals who are involved in the patient's care throughout the peri-operative period. Patient safety is at the centre of care provision, and requires effective leadership and teamworking by all clinical staff. The surgical team and wider members of the MDT have an obligation to support each other while delivering patient care in wards, theatre, clinics, and community settings following discharge. It is imperative that there is effective communication between all team members with regard to the patient's care, in order to maintain high standards of patient care and reduce the risk of errors.

Key members of the general intra-operative team include the following:

- surgeon
- surgical care practitioner
- anaesthetist
- anaesthetic practitioner
- advanced scrub practitioner
- circulating practitioner
- recovery practitioner.

Surgeon

In the operating department, the surgeon is the lead member of the MDT. He or she is responsible for performing the surgery safely and effectively, while at the same time maintaining a good level of communication with the scrub practitioner and the anaesthetist. The consultant surgeon is responsible for the patient's care throughout the peri-operative period.

Surgical care practitioner

The surgical care practitioner was defined by the Royal College of Surgeons of England[2] as 'a registered non-medical practitioner who has completed a Royal College of Surgeons accredited programme (or other previously recognized course) working in clinical practice as a member of the extended surgical team, who performs surgical intervention, pre-operative and post-operative care under the direction and supervision of a consultant surgeon.'

The role includes the provision of care and appropriate interventions within the peri-operative, ward, and clinic settings.

Anaesthetist

The anaesthetist administers the anaesthetic, maintains the patient's airway, and monitors and acts upon the patient's vital signs throughout the intra-operative period. He or she is responsible for assessing the patient prior to surgery and putting in place a plan of pain management interventions for the initial post-operative period.

Anaesthetic practitioner

The anaesthetic practitioner provides skilled assistance to the anaesthetist. He or she may be an operating department practitioner (ODP) or a nurse who has undertaken further training. Such nurse training may be an in-house competency-based programme or a university degree-level anaesthetics course.

Advanced scrub practitioner

A nurse or ODP undertakes post-registration training to enable them to take on the role of advanced scrub practitioner, which is defined by the Perioperative Care Collaboration[3] as 'the role undertaken by a registered peri-operative practitioner providing competent and skilled assistance under the direct supervision of the operating surgeon while not performing any form of surgical intervention.' They are responsible for draping the patient and handling sterile instruments and supplies. The scrub practitioner is also responsible for ensuring that all swabs, needles, and instruments are accounted for at the end of the procedure.

Circulating practitioner

The circulating practitioner acts as a 'runner', ensuring that adequate supplies are available and providing the scrub practitioner with any equipment that is not available on the scrub trolley. They need to have a good knowledge of where equipment is stored, in order to minimize delays in treatment during surgery. Circulating practitioners also assist with positioning of the patient and repositioning of equipment (e.g. lighting, cameras) for the surgical team.

Recovery practitioner

The recovery practitioner works in the recovery area of the operating theatre, and may be an ODP or a nurse who has undertaken further training. They ensure that the post-operative patient is able to maintain his or her airway and is receiving adequate analgesia. They also monitor the patient's vital signs, wound site, and wound drain, and complete all documentation according to trust policy. They will hand over to the ward nurse, providing details of the patient's intra-operative care and specific instructions from the surgeon and anaesthetist for patient care during the post-operative period.

References

2 Royal College of Surgeons of England. *The Curriculum Framework for the Surgical Care Practitioner*, 2nd edn. Royal College of Surgeons of England: London, 2014.
3 Perioperative Care Collaborative. *The Role and Responsibilities of the Advanced Scrub Practitioner*. Perioperative Care Collaborative: London, 2007.

The role of the surgical nurse

Surgical nurses are skilled in preparing patients for surgical procedures and caring for them after surgery. They need to have a good theoretical knowledge of the following:

- anatomy and physiology
- complications associated with surgical procedures
- asepsis
- infection control
- pharmacology, including pain management
- anxiety and coping mechanisms
- patient education
- discharge planning.

All surgical nurses should be competent to provide care for patients in the pre-operative and post-operative period. Nursing care should be evidence-based and comply with local or national policy, to ensure that the patient receives optimum care in order to reduce the risks associated with surgery.

When further developing their skills, the surgical nurse should consider whether:

- the skill will benefit the quality of patient care that they deliver
- they are the best person to develop this skill
- when they have acquired the skill they will use it often enough in clinical practice to remain competent.

A good knowledge of ethical, legal, and professional issues is essential within surgical nursing. The Nursing and Midwifery Council (NMC) Code of Conduct[4] is a professional document that is based on ethical principles within the laws of the UK. The four key ethical principles within healthcare are:

- beneficence—balancing the benefits of treatment against the risks and costs that it incurs
- non-maleficence— avoiding harm; all treatment incurs a small amount of harm, but the harm should not be disproportionate to the benefits of treatment
- autonomy—enabling an individual to make reasoned and informed decisions about their care
- justice—the act of being just and fair.

A good working knowledge of consent is imperative for surgical nurses, particularly in special circumstances (e.g. when the patient is unconscious).

Reference

4 Nursing and Midwifery Council (NMC). *The Code: professional standards of practice and behaviour for nurses and midwives.* NMC: London, 2015.

Classification of surgery

In December 2004, the National Confidential Enquiry into Patient Outcome and Death (NCEPOD)[5] issued new classifications of interventions. These are as follows:
- immediate
- urgent
- expedited
- elective.

They replace the old categories of surgery, which were as follows:
- emergency
- urgent
- scheduled
- elective.

These classifications exist to ensure that patients receive surgery within the time frame necessary for their condition, and also to ensure that medical staff only perform surgery out of hours when it is appropriate to do so. The classification should be assigned by the consultant caring for the patient, at the time when the decision to operate is taken. Specific conditions or types of surgery cannot be pre-assigned to these categories, as individual patient need will vary on a case-by-case basis.

Immediate surgery

Surgery takes place within minutes of the decision to operate, in order to save life, an organ, or a limb. It should take place in the next available operating theatre, and can necessitate interrupting existing theatre lists. Examples of this category include:
- a ruptured aortic aneurysm that requires repair
- a myocardial infarction that requires a coronary angioplasty to restore the blood supply to the myocardium.

Urgent surgery

The surgical intervention normally takes place within hours of the decision to operate, in order to treat the acute onset or the clinical deterioration of a potentially life-threatening condition. It also includes the fixation of fractures, and the relief of pain or other distressing symptoms. Patients who are to undergo this category of surgery should be added to the emergency theatre list. Examples include:
- a laparotomy for a perforated large bowel
- the debridement and fixation of a compound fracture.

Expedited surgery

The surgical intervention takes place within days of the decision to operate for a condition that requires early intervention but which does not pose an immediate threat to life, a limb, or an organ. The patient should either be added to an elective theatre list which has spare capacity, or be included on a daytime emergency list. Examples include:
- a developing large bowel obstruction that requires excision of a tumour
- surgery to correct a retinal detachment that could lead to loss of vision in the affected eye.

Elective surgery

This type of surgery is planned in advance of a routine admission, at a time to suit the patient and the hospital. It takes place on an elective theatre list, having been booked in advance. Examples include:

- a knee replacement for a patient with degenerative knee joint disease
- varicose vein surgery.

Reference

5 National Confidential Enquiry into Patient Outcome and Death. *The NCEPOD Classification of Intervention*. NCEPOD: London, 2004.

Terminology in surgery

Many different terms are used within surgery, and some of the main terms are defined here. Other surgical terminology will be discussed in subsequent chapters.

Abscess
An accumulation of pus that forms within a tissue when the body tries to fight an infection.

Adhesion
A band of scar tissue that joins together organs or tissues that would normally be separate.

Amputation
The removal of all or part of a limb or body extremity (e.g. a finger), either by surgery or as a result of trauma.

Anastomosis
The joining of two structures that would not normally be connected.

Biopsy
The process of taking a sample of living tissue to be examined under the microscope.

Debridement
The removal of dead, damaged, contaminated, or infected tissue from a wound.

Diathermy
A surgical technique in which heat produced by electric currents is used to cut body tissue or seal bleeding vessels.

-ectomy
The surgical removal of an anatomical structure (e.g. appendectomy is the surgical removal of the appendix).

Excision
The surgical removal of all or part of an anatomical structure by cutting it out.

Fistula
An abnormal connection consisting of a passage or duct between an organ, vessel, or tissue and another anatomical structure.

Hernia
The abnormal bulging or protrusion of a tissue or organ through a weakened area in the muscle or other tissue that normally surrounds it.

Incision
A cut made through skin or other tissue in order to expose the underlying tissue, organ, or bone.

Laparoscopy
A surgical procedure in which a viewing instrument (laparoscope) is used to visualize the organs and tissues in the abdomen without the need to make a large incision.

Laparotomy
A surgical procedure in which a large incision is made through the abdominal wall to provide access to the abdominal cavity.

Microsurgery
The use of a microscope and specialized instruments to allow very small structures to be visualized and operated on.

Minimally invasive
A surgical technique that is considered to be less traumatic than the traditional technique. Keyhole surgery is a widely used minimally invasive technique.

Necrosis
The death of cells within a tissue. Necrotic tissue cannot be treated and must be excised.

-oscopy
The use of a viewing instrument to examine an organ or tissue (e.g. bronchoscopy of the lungs).

-ostomy
A surgically created opening in the body to allow the discharge of body waste (e.g. colostomy).

Paralytic ileus
Obstruction of the intestine caused by paralysis of the intestinal muscles.

Peri-operative
Relating to a procedure or treatment that occurs at or around the time of a surgical operation.

-plasty
The surgical repair, restoration, or reshaping of a tissue, organ, or anatomical structure (e.g. rhinoplasty following nasal surgery).

Resection
The surgical removal of part or all of an organ or anatomical structure.

Sigmoidoscopy
A minimally invasive procedure that is used to examine the large intestine from the rectum to the colon.

Stricture
An abnormal narrowing of a tubular structure in the body (e.g. urethral stricture).

Basic anatomy of the chest

The anatomy of the chest (thorax) can be subdivided into two distinct regions:
- the thoracic wall
- the thoracic viscera.

The thoracic wall

The thoracic wall is composed of a large number of structures, which are summarized briefly here.

Bones
- Twelve pairs of ribs:
  - seven true pairs of ribs (ribs that have their own costal cartilage to directly attach to the sternum)
  - three false pairs of ribs (ribs that share a costal cartilage to indirectly attach to the sternum)
  - two floating pairs of ribs (ribs that are not attached to the sternum).
- Twelve thoracic vertebrae.
- The sternum.

Muscles
- Intercostal muscles, which are involved in elevating and depressing the ribs during respiration.
- Pectoralis major and minor muscles, which are mainly involved in upper limb movements.

The thoracic viscera

The thoracic cavity contains the two lungs in the pulmonary cavities, and the heart, great vessels, and other structures in the mediastinum.

The lungs

The lungs are situated on either side of the mediastinum, and are covered by a serous membrane known as the pleura.
- The right lung consists of three lobes—the upper, middle, and lower lobe.
- The left lung has only two lobes—the upper and lower lobe.

The lungs contain the small airways and alveoli that are responsible for gaseous exchange. Inspired air reaches these structures through the large airways situated in the mediastinum.

The mediastinum

The mediastinum is the volume within the thoracic cavity that is not occupied by the lungs. It consists of loose connective tissue surrounding a number of organs and structures, which include the heart, the great vessels, the proximal oesophagus, the trachea, and the main bronchi.

The heart consists of four chambers. Blood from the superior vena cava and the inferior vena cava drains into the first chamber of the heart, which is called the right atrium. The blood then passes through the tricuspid valve into the right ventricle before being pumped to the lungs for oxygenation. To reach the lungs, blood is pumped through the pulmonary valve and into the pulmonary artery, which then transports the blood to the lungs. Blood is drained from the lungs via the pulmonary vein into the left atrium. It then flows through the mitral valve into the left ventricle, which is responsible for pumping blood through the aortic valve into the aorta, around the aortic arch and to the rest of the body in order to supply all of the tissues with oxygen and other necessary nutrients.

The heart is continually beating, and consequently it has a high metabolic demand. In order to meet this demand, the heart has an excellent blood supply. Two coronary arteries—the right and left coronary arteries—branch off the aorta in order to supply the muscular layer of the heart (the myocardium).

Basic anatomy of the abdomen

The abdominal cavity is located in the space between the diaphragm, the pelvic inlet, and the anterior, lateral, and posterior abdominal walls.

The anterior and lateral abdominal walls are formed entirely from muscles and their tendons, and normally hold the abdominal organs within the abdominal cavity. The posterior abdominal wall also contains the components of the lumbar spine, consisting of the lumbar vertebrae, the intervertebral discs, the spinal cord, and the meninges that cover the spinal cord.

The abdominal cavity is lined by a special membrane known as the peritoneum which lies beneath the abdominal walls. The numerous important organs that are located within the abdominal cavity will be briefly outlined here.

The digestive system consists of the following organs:
- distal oesophagus
- liver and biliary tree
- stomach
- small intestine
- large intestine/colon, including the appendix but excluding the rectum.

The haematological system consists of the spleen.

Some organs and systems are located behind the peritoneum lining of the posterior abdominal wall, in a space called the retroperitoneal space. These consist of the following:
- genito-urinary system
- kidneys
- proximal ureters
- digestive system
- pancreas
- endocrine system
- suprarenal glands and adrenal glands.

Divisions of the abdomen

In order to help to establish the site of injury or pain, the abdomen can be divided into either four quadrants (see Figure 1.1) or nine regions (see Figure 1.2).

If it is divided into four quadrants, these are named as follows:
- right upper quadrant
- left upper quadrant
- left lower quadrant
- right lower quadrant.

Alternatively, if the abdomen in divided into nine regions, these are named as follows:
- right hypochondrium
- epigastrium
- left hypochondrium
- right lumbar region

- umbilical region
- left lumbar region
- right inguinal region
- suprapubic region
- left inguinal region.

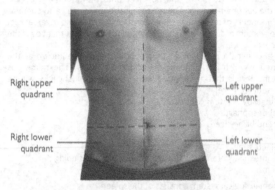

Figure 1.1 The four quadrants of the anterior abdominal wall. Reproduced from James Thomas and Tanya Monaghan, *Oxford Handbook of Clinical Examination and Practical Skills*, 2007, with permission from Oxford University Press.

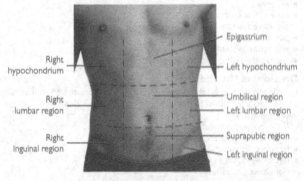

Figure 1.2 The nine regions of the anterior abdominal wall. Reproduced from James Thomas and Tanya Monaghan, *Oxford Handbook of Clinical Examination and Practical Skills*, 2007, with permission from Oxford University Press.

Basic anatomy of the upper limb

The upper limb consists of the arm, forearm, and hand (see Figure 1.3). Each of these parts is separated from the next by a joint.

The upper limb contains 32 bones in total (including those that form the pectoral girdle):

- clavicle
- scapula
- humerus
- radius
- ulna
- 8 carpal bones
- 5 metacarpals
- 14 phalanges.

The upper limb contains a number of joints, which all allow movement. The most important of these are:

- the shoulder joint, which attaches the arm to the thorax
- the elbow joint, which attaches the arm to the forearm
- the wrist joint, which attaches the forearm to the hand.

The shoulder joint

The shoulder joint is between the pectoral girdle and the arm and it allows an extremely wide range of movement, including flexion,

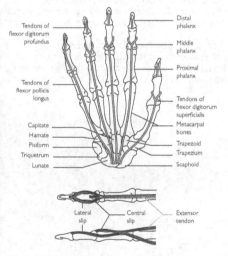

Figure 1.3 The hand. Reproduced from Rebecca Jester, Julie Santy, and Jean Rogers MSC, *Oxford Handbook of Orthopaedic and Trauma Nursing*, 2011, with permission from Oxford University Press.

extension, internal and external rotation, and adduction and abduction of the arm.

The pectoral girdle is formed by the scapula and the clavicle, and it is part of the scapula, known as the glenoid cavity, that articulates with the head of the humerus to form the shoulder joint (the glenohumeral joint).

The elbow joint

The elbow joint allows only flexion and extension of the forearm. It joins the arm, which contains the humerus, to the forearm, which contains the radius and ulna bones. The head of the radius and the trochlear notch of the ulna articulate with the capitulum and trochlea of the humerus, respectively.

The wrist joint

The wrist joint is also known as the radiocarpal joint, and is formed between the four most proximal carpal bones and the radius. Movement at the wrist is limited to flexion, extension, adduction, and abduction.

Blood supply and venous drainage

The blood supply to the upper limb is provided by a number of branches of the subclavian artery. As the subclavian artery passes under the clavicle it changes its name to the axillary artery, and then as the axillary artery leaves the axilla (the armpit) it becomes the brachial artery.

The brachial artery then bifurcates just distal to the elbow joint, to form the radial and ulnar arteries. These arteries rejoin in the hand as they form the deep and superficial palmar arches, respectively.

The axillary, brachial, ulnar, and radial arteries each give off many small branches to ensure that every structure in the upper limb is supplied with blood.

The upper limb is drained by both superficial and deep veins. The deep veins run with the arteries of the upper limb and have the same names as the arteries. The superficial veins—the cephalic (lateral) and basilic (medial) veins—eventually drain into the axillary and brachial veins, respectively.

Basic anatomy of the lower limb

The lower limb consists of the thigh, leg, and foot (see Figure 1.4). Each of these parts is separated from the next by a joint.

The lower limb contains 32 bones in total (including those that form the pelvic girdle):

• ischium
• ilium
• pubis
• femur
• tibia
• fibula
• talus
• calcaneus
• cuboid
• navicular
• 3 cuneiform bones
• 5 metatarsals
• 14 phalanges.

The lower limb contains a number of joints, which all allow movement. The most important of these are:

• the hip joint, which attaches the thigh to the pelvis
• the knee joint, which attaches the thigh to the leg
• the ankle joint, which attaches the leg to the foot.

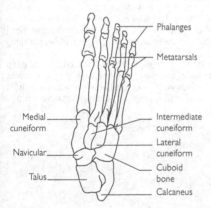

Figure 1.4 The foot. Reproduced from Rebecca Jester, Julie Santy, and Jean Rogers MSC, *Oxford Handbook of Orthopaedic and Trauma Nursing*, 2011, with permission from Oxford University Press.

The hip joint

The hip joint is between the pelvic girdle and the thigh, and it allows an extremely wide range of movement, including flexion, extension, internal and external rotation, and adduction and abduction of the thigh.

The pelvic girdle is formed by the ischium, the pubis, and the ilium. In adults these are fused to form the innominate bone. The three bones fuse at the acetabulum, and this is the part of the pelvis that articulates with the head of the femur to form the hip joint.

The knee joint

The knee joint allows flexion and extension of the leg, together with extremely small amounts of rotation. The lateral and medial condyles of the tibia articulate with the lateral and medial condyles, respectively, of the femur, to form the knee joint. The knee joint also contains another important articular surface, between the patella and the femur.

The ankle joint

The ankle joint is also known as the talocrural joint, and is formed between the talus of the foot and the distal ends of both the tibia and the fibula. Movement at the ankle is mainly limited to dorsiflexion and plantar flexion. However, some rotation, adduction, and abduction are available when the foot is plantar flexed.

Blood supply and venous drainage

The blood supply to the lower limb is provided by a number of branches of the external iliac artery. As the internal iliac artery passes under the inguinal ligament, it changes its name to the femoral artery.

The femoral artery then continues down to the knee, where it becomes the popliteal artery. The popliteal artery then bifurcates to form the anterior tibial and posterior tibial arteries. The posterior tibial artery branches again to form the fibular artery. These arteries all supply different areas of the leg and foot.

The lower limb is drained by both superficial and deep veins. The deep veins run with the arteries of the lower limb and have the same names as the arteries. The superficial veins—the long (anteriomedial) and short (posteriolateral) saphenous veins—eventually drain into the femoral and popliteal veins, respectively.

Basic anatomy of the head and neck

The head consists of a vast number of highly detailed and intricate structures, including the following:
- cranium (skull)
- scalp
- face
- brain, meninges (the membranes that enclose the brain), and cerebrospinal fluid
- special sense organs for sight, smell, hearing, and taste.

The cranium (skull)

This is the framework of the head and face. It consists of 22 bones and can be divided into two parts:
- the neurocranium, which houses the brain
- the viscerocranium, which forms the facial skeleton.

The brain

The brain is enclosed by three membranes (the meninges), and can be divided into three main structures—the cerebrum, the cerebellum, and the brainstem.

The cerebrum forms the largest part of the brain, and consists of two cerebral hemispheres, each of which contains four lobes:
- frontal lobe
- parietal lobe
- temporal lobe
- occipital lobe.

The cerebellum sits beneath the occipital lobe of the cerebrum at the posterior aspect of the brain and, like the cerebrum, it consists of two hemispheres.

The brainstem joins the cerebrum to the spinal cord, and consists of three parts:
- midbrain
- pons
- medulla oblongata.

All of these structures lie in the cranium and are surrounded by cerebrospinal fluid (CSF), which cushions the brain tissue from the rigid walls of the cranial vault.

The neck

The neck contains many important structures that connect the head to the rest of the body. The superficial layers of the neck can be divided into two triangles—the anterior and posterior triangles.

The anterior triangle is the area below the mandible, lateral to the midline and medial to the anterior border of the sternocleidomastoid muscle. It contains:
- blood vessels that supply blood to and drain it from the brain
- nerves
- salivary and endocrine glands, including the thyroid and parathyroid glands.

The posterior triangle is the area in front of the anterior border of the trapezius muscle, behind the posterior border of the sternocleidomastoid muscle and above the clavicle. It contains:
• veins that drain blood from the face
• nerves
• blood vessels that supply blood to and drain it from the upper limbs
• nerves that innervate the upper limbs.

Deeper structures

The neck is also the site at which the lower respiratory tract starts. The larynx (the voice box) sits in the neck on top of the trachea (the windpipe). The larynx is an extremely complex organ that consists of a number of cartilages and muscles. It allows humans to talk and communicate, and also provides some protection to the airway.

The spinal cord also extends down from the neck. It is protected by seven cervical vertebrae before it enters the thorax. The cervical spinal cord is extremely important, as it gives off the phrenic nerve, which innervates the diaphragm, allowing ventilation.

Basic anatomy of the gastrointestinal tract

The gastrointestinal tract extends from the oral cavity to the anus, and has many different components, all of which have distinct functions (see Figure 1.5).

The oral cavity

The mouth forms the opening to the oral cavity. Saliva, which is formed by the sublingual, submandibular, and parotid glands, drains into the oral cavity and aids the digestive process after ingested food has been masticated (chewed).

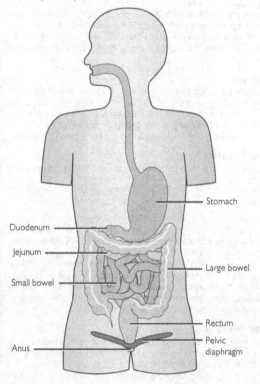

Figure 1.5 The gastrointestinal tract. Reproduced from Norton C et al. (eds) (2008) *Oxford Handbook of Gastrointestinal Nursing*, Figure 1.1, p. 3. Oxford University Press, Oxford, with permission from the Burdett Institute of Gastrointestinal Nursing, King's College, London.

The pharynx

The next part of the gastrointestinal tract is the pharynx, which consists of three parts:
- the nasopharynx
- the oropharynx
- the laryngopharynx.

The oropharynx lies directly posterior to the oval cavity, and inferior to this is the laryngopharynx. Both of these structures have the function of transporting ingested food from the oral cavity to the oesophagus during swallowing.

The oesophagus

The oesophagus is a muscular structure that starts in the neck, inferior to the larygnopharynx, passes through the thorax and the diaphragm, and finally terminates as it joins the stomach in the abdominal cavity. It allows food to pass from the pharynx to the stomach, and is aided by a series of wave-like muscular contractions along its length (a process known as peristalsis).

The stomach

The stomach is the organ that receives food from the oesophagus. The muscular layers of the stomach help to churn the stored food so that it becomes coated by the digestive enzymes that are secreted by the lining of the stomach. The churned partially digested food leaves the stomach via the pyloric sphincter, and enters the first part of the small intestine.

The small intestine

The small intestine is the main site of digestion, and consists of three parts:
- the duodenum
- the jejunum
- the ileum.

The duodenum is the shortest part of the small intestine, and it accepts the biliary and pancreatic secretions from the common bile duct and pancreatic duct, respectively. These secretions aid the digestive process.

The majority of the small intestine is comprised of the jejunum and ileum, which are attached to the posterior abdominal wall by a fold of membrane known as a mesentery. This mesentery, in addition to securing the small intestine within the abdominal cavity, carries within it the major arteries, veins, and lymphatics that supply and drain the small intestine, and also the nerves that innervate the latter.

The large intestine

The large intestine can be differentiated from the small intestine by its visible pouch-like structures known as haustra, and small projecting sacs (containing fatty tissue) called omental appendices, along its length. The large intestine contains the following (starting from the point at which the ileum joins the large intestine):
- the caecum and appendix
- the ascending colon

- the transverse colon
- the descending colon
- the sigmoid colon
- the rectum
- the anal canal and anus.

Like many other parts of the digestive system, including the small intestine and the oesophagus, the large intestine has a muscular wall that helps to move digested food along by peristalsis.

Basic anatomy of the vascular system

The human body relies on a continuous supply of oxygen and glucose in order to function. Blood is a specialized substance that meets this demand by transporting glucose and oxygen to tissues and then removing waste metabolites from the tissues.

Tissues are supplied with blood by arteries and drained by veins. These two components of the vascular system are joined by a microcirculation that consists of arterioles, capillaries, and venules. Arterioles carry blood from the arteries to the capillaries, and venules drain the capillary beds.

The arterial tree

The whole arterial tree arises from the aorta, the main artery in the body, which in turn arises from the outflow tract of the left ventricle. All of the blood that is pumped out of the heart travels into the aorta and then through its various branches to the rest of the body.

The very first vessels that branch off the aorta—the right and left coronary arteries—have the important role of supplying the heart with the nutrients that it requires in order to keep beating.

The aorta then extends up towards the head as the ascending aorta, arches over to form the arch of the aorta, and then extends back down the body on the posterior thoracic and abdominal walls as the descending aorta.

The arch of the aorta is the point at which a number of important arteries originate, including the right and left common carotid arteries and the right and left subclavian arteries. These vessels branch further to form all the vessels that supply the head, neck, and upper limbs.

The descending aorta is responsible for supplying the abdominal organs via the coeliac trunk, the superior mesenteric artery, the inferior mesenteric artery, and the renal arteries. At the end of its course, the aorta bifurcates to form the right and left common iliac arteries, and these branch to form the external and internal iliac arteries.

The internal iliac arteries supply the majority of the pelvic organs, whereas the external iliac arteries supply the lower limbs.

The venous tree

The venous tree does not have a single starting point. However, all of the veins eventually drain blood back to the right atrium. Two major veins—the superior vena cava and the inferior vena cava—drain into the right atrium. Blood from the head, neck, and upper limbs drains into the superior vena cava via the internal and external jugular veins and the subclavian veins. Blood from the abdominal organs, pelvic organs, and lower limbs drains into the inferior vena cava via the renal veins, the hepatic veins, and the right and left common iliac veins.

In addition to these systemic veins, there is a network of veins known as the portal venous system which drains blood from the gastrointestinal tract and the spleen to the liver. This means that absorbed nutrients can be processed by the liver before they enter the systemic circulation. Blood from the liver is then drained into the systemic circulation via the hepatic veins.

Basic anatomy of the genito-urinary system

The genito-urinary system consists of the urinary and reproductive systems (see Figure 1.6).

The urinary system

The urinary system consists of the two kidneys, the bladder, the two ureters, and the urethra.

Blood from the renal arteries is filtered by the kidneys. The tubules in the kidneys are responsible for excreting any nitrogenous waste products and excess water and electrolytes. These three substances are the main components of the urine that leaves the kidney via the renal pelvis (the top part of the ureter).

The right and left ureters are muscular tubes that connect the right and left kidneys to the bladder. Their muscular walls allow peristalsis to occur to move urine through the urinary system.

The bladder is a muscular organ that acts as a reservoir for storing urine. Its muscular wall allows the bladder to stretch and increase in size as it fills with urine. At the base of the bladder is the top part of the urethra. At this point there is a sphincter, known as the internal urethral sphincter, which controls the flow of urine from the bladder into the urethra.

The urethra is much longer in males than in females. In males it also passes through the prostate as it leaves the bladder. At the end of the urethra, in both males and females, there is a second sphincter, known as the external urethral sphincter. This is the sphincter that we consciously control to allow or prevent the act of urination.

The reproductive system

The male and female reproductive systems both consist of external genitalia and internal reproductive organs.

Male reproductive system

Sperm (the male reproductive cells) are produced in the testes, which are located in the scrotum. The sperm then pass into a structure called the epididymis, where they undergo a process of maturation and are stored.

During ejaculation, stored sperm enter a thin tube called the vas deferens. They travel through the vas deferens out of the scrotum into the pelvic cavity and then join the urethra as it passes through the prostate gland.

The sperm cells are supplied with nutrients by secretions from the prostate gland and the seminal vesicles. These secretions, together with the sperm cells, form semen. Semen travels through the urethra and leaves the body via the external urethral sphincter at the end of the penis.

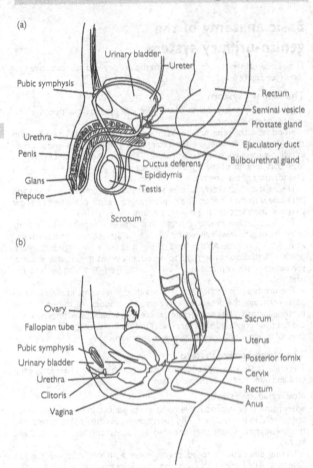

Figure 1.6 (a) Male reproductive system. (b) Female reproductive system. Reproduced from Edward Alan Glasper, Gillian McEwing and Jim Richardson, *Oxford Handbook of Children's and Young People's Nursing*, 2007, with permission from Oxford University Press.

Female reproductive system

The external female genitalia consist of the labia majora, the labia minora, the clitoris, and the mons pubis. Collectively they are often referred to as the vulva, and are situated in the perineum anterior to the anus. Between the labia minora is the vestibule, which contains the opening of the vagina, the external urethral orifice, and the ducts of the vestibular glands.

The internal reproductive organs consist of the ovaries, oviducts, uterus, cervix, and vagina. The ova are formed in the ovaries, where they are stored until they are released during ovulation. The uterus is the site of implantation of fertilized ova, and of growth and development of the embryo.

Further reading

Moore KL, Agur AMR and Dalley AF. *Essential Clinical Anatomy*, 5th edn. Lippincott Williams & Wilkins: Philadelphia, PA, 2015.

Managing
the surgical ward

The ward structure

In most hospitals, patients with similar types of illness or surgical problems are nursed together in the same ward (e.g. colorectal or urology patients). Depending on the size and layout, wards have different numbers of patients for the ward nursing team to look after, and a number of different nursing roles, which are listed in Table 2.1.

The severity of illness of patients on a ward will influence the staffing of the ward and the ward hierarchy. It may also influence where the patients are cared for (e.g. closer to the nurses' station).

There are a variety of medical roles that are part of the surgical multidisciplinary team (MDT), and with whom surgical ward nurses will be expected to work to ensure that the patients' health needs are met. These medical roles are listed in Table 2.2.

Table 2.1 Members of the surgical ward nursing team

Team role	Qualification and experience
Healthcare assistant	Unregistered but trained staff responsible for providing direct patient care under the supervision of qualified nurses
Staff nurse	The basic grade of qualified nursing staff. These nurses are responsible for caring for a group of patients (e.g. one bay of a ward). The staff nurse will also undertake specific tasks (e.g. administering medications)
Senior staff nurse	These nurses carry out many of the same roles as staff nurses, but are more experienced and senior. They are often in charge of the ward or department area during a shift
Junior/deputy sister, charge nurse, ward manager	These nurses are responsible for the day-to-day running of the ward, and they may also have specific responsibilities for the overall running of the ward (e.g. organizing mandatory training in accordance with the wishes of the ward manager)
Sister/charge nurse, ward manager	These nurses are responsible for running a ward or unit, and usually have budgetary control. They will employ staff, and be responsible for all the local management (e.g. rostering, approving pay claims, purchasing equipment, delegation of duties or tasks)
Senior sister/charge nurse, senior ward manager	In some large wards or complex areas (e.g. Accident and Emergency, critical care areas) there may be a need to employ several nurses at ward manager level. In this situation usually one nurse is the senior manager in the area
Modern matron	This role was developed to ensure that nursing standards were raised. The modern matron is responsible for overseeing all nursing standards within a department or directorate

For most wards there is also an individual who provides administrative support, such as processing the patients' paperwork and organizing appointments for the patients (e.g. diagnostics) and discharge. This role is vital for the ward to run smoothly.

Another important role on the ward is that of ward domestics or cleaners. This role is an integral part of providing a safe clean environment and reducing the risk of infection, thereby enhancing patient safety.

Table 2.2 Medical staff roles

Team role	Qualification and experience
Consultant anaesthetist	A qualified doctor who has completed post-basic training in anaesthesia and intensive care
Anaesthetic trainee	A qualified doctor on a training programme to become a consultant. Training is dependent upon FRCA qualification, assessment and over 8 years' clinical experience
F1 and F2 doctors	Junior doctors who will be on placement as part of their training rotations
Consultant surgeon	A qualified doctor who has completed a post-basic training programme as a trainee in surgery. Consultant surgeons will subspecialize during their training in the chosen field, including general surgery, trauma, orthopaedics, colorectal, breast, vascular, urological, transplant, cardiothoracic, and gynaecological surgery

FRCA, Fellowship of the Royal College of Anaesthetists; F1, foundation year 1; F2, foundation year 2.

Surgical ward leadership

The role of the surgical ward manager is key to ensuring that patients receive high-quality care. This individual is responsible for the care that patients receive and for managing the staff who are providing front-line care, as well as being the interface between clinical care delivery and healthcare management.

Patient care

The ward manager role is pivotal in the hospital system, as it is at the centre of the patient experience and can oversee and coordinate the different dimensions of service provision for patients.

There is extensive research evidence that links the impact of the ward manager's leadership role to the standards of care that patients receive on a ward.[1] Research shows that there are identifiable characteristics of a good ward leader.[2,3] These include:

• being passionate
• being motivational
• having problem-solving skills
• having a desire to develop others.

There is a correlation between effective ward manager leadership, patient outcomes, and staff performance and satisfaction.

Staff leadership

The ward manager has a responsibility to develop the skills of all the nurses on their ward. This includes promoting professional development and undertaking appraisals. In a nursing team with good leadership, people often feel more valued, which can help to lower staff absence and sickness rates. Staff who feel that they belong to a good team will often work more closely together to provide excellent patient care.

References
1 Hay Group. *Nurse Leadership: being nice is not enough.* Hay Group: London, 2006.
2 Mahoney J. Leadership skills for the 21st century. *Journal of Nursing Management* 2001; 9: 269–71.
3 Bondas T. Paths to nursing leadership. *Journal of Nursing Management* 2006; 14: 332–9.

Understanding nursing establishments

Having a mechanism for ensuring that there are the correct numbers of nurses on a ward to care for patients is one of the most important factors for any nurse manager. With studies indicating that there is a relationship between staffing levels and patient outcomes, safe staffing is paramount.[4,5] In 2014, the National Institute for Health and Care Excellence (NICE) produced guidance on safe nurse staffing for acute adult inpatient wards.[6] Recommendation 1 stated that ward nursing staff establishments should be at sufficient levels to be able to provide safe nursing care to each patient at any time.

There is no one widely accepted model across different healthcare systems. Hospitals benchmark their staffing levels with peers or via bodies to gauge how their staffing levels compare. In some areas of nursing (e.g. paediatrics) there may be professional guidance to assist in this process.[7]

There are five approaches that can be used to calculate nurse staffing.[8]

- The *professional judgement approach* is used by experienced and senior practitioners, who review the nurses' workload and decide the numbers of nurses required.
- The *ratio of nurses to occupied beds* is a top-down approach that reviews the number of patients, bed occupancy, and the hours/ratio of nurses to patients (i.e. hours of care per patient day and nurse ratios). Non-direct patient care hours are added into some models.
- The *acuity-dependency method* uses a categorization of patients to understand the amount of care that the patients require.
- The *time/task activity model*, in which the time and frequency of nurse interventions become a template for staffing levels, has been incorporated into computer programs (e.g. Grasp and Trend Care).
- *Regression analysis* is a statistical method for reviewing how many nurses are needed for a given activity.

Each approach has advantages and disadvantages. The models have different components, different weights of time for tasks, or slightly different patient categories, and some models do not incorporate dependency and acuity elements. Typically the number of patients, the bed occupancy, and the number of hours per day that the area or ward is open are standard in the methods of calculation. The throughput or bed utilization is accounted for in some models, but not all of them. In 2013, the National Quality Board produced a guide on nursing staff capacity and capability.[9] Expectation 3 states that 'Evidence based tools are used to inform nursing, midwifery and care staffing capacity and capability.'

The surgical nurse manager should understand the method that is being used to calculate the nursing establishment, sometimes referred to as whole-time equivalents (WTE) or full-time equivalents (FTE), and in each care environment nurses should be able to discuss the rationale for calculation of the nursing numbers, and participate in this process. It is important that nursing establishments are reported at every level of the organization. This provides clarity on how the nursing workforce is created.

References

4 Royal College of Nursing (RCN). *Guidance on Safe Nurse Staffing Levels in the UK*. Policy Unit, RCN: London, 2010.
5 Ford S. Dr Foster reveals link between nursing levels and patient care. *Nursing Times* 31 March 2009.
6 National Institute for Health and Care Excellence (NICE). *Safe Staffing for Nursing in Adult Inpatient Wards in Acute Hospitals*. SG1, NICE: London, 2014. ♪℗ www.nice.org.uk/guidance/sg1
7 Royal College of Nursing (RCN). *Defining Staffing Levels for Children and Young People's Services: RCN standards for clinical professionals and service managers*. RCN: London, 2013.
8 Hurst K. *Selecting and Applying Methods for Estimating the Size and Mix of Nursing Teams*. Nuffield Institute for Health: Leeds, 2003.
9 National Quality Board. *How to Ensure the Right People, with the Right Skills, are in the Right Place at the Right Time: a guide to nursing, midwifery and care staffing capacity and capability*. NHS England: Redditch, 2013.

Staffing rotas

Nurse staffing rotas are vital to ensure that the right number and skill mix of nurses are on duty across the 24-h period. The demand for better alignment of nurse hours with patient care has continued to be a challenging issue for the profession and organizations to resolve.

The nursing rota combines the need for efficiency, cost-effectiveness, and patient safety. Understanding the finance, patient acuity/dependency, and the nursing hours per patient day will influence how the resources required to care for patients are used. To assist in bringing these components together, good nurse scheduling/rostering practices are essential. The importance of efficiency and productivity alongside the quality of care is something that nurse managers constantly have to balance when reviewing how they allocate nurses to shifts.

The NHS has seen a recent re-examination of rotas in the light of European working time legislation.[10] This highlights the rest periods and the times between shifts that nurses should expect.

Examples of these rules include:
- a daily rest period of 11 h per 24-h period
- an average working time that does not exceed 48 h for each 7-day period
- annual leave of at least 4 weeks (i.e. 20 days on a full-time basis).

The lack of clarity of rotas in large organizations has led to the need for robust information systems, in order to determine whether the establishment agreements are being followed by managers. By using electronic systems, nurses with specific skills or experience can be more easily identified and can be allocated to the right location at the right time, thus matching skills more accurately. This is particularly important on night shifts and at weekends when there may be less staff available. This has led to the development of software solutions, which can provide a better assessment of the number and skills of available staff, thus having the potential to promote better patient care and quality outcomes.

Not only can effective electronic rosters assist in ensuring that the correct number of staff are on duty to promote good patient care, but also they can help to reduce hospitals' costs. In the UK, implementation of an electronic rostering system can also yield annual savings.

Matching staffing levels to patient demand can be challenging, as variations occur as a result of constant fluctuations in patient volume and disease demographics. Having an efficient system that is able to show the skills of nurses on a particular shift across a hospital enhances the ability to provide optimal staffing of a patient area. Consistency and accuracy with regard to placing skilled personnel in a scheduled roster alleviates concerns about inexperienced staff or an under-supply of staff. Rostering rules are also essential to ensure equity in the nursing team and a shared understanding of an appropriate skill mix and how and when to ask for additional support.

Applying rules to systems provides transparency and demonstrates how the allocation of rosters is constructed, rather than the flexibility being awarded to some staff and resulting in inflexibility for others. This creates greater staff contentment, current staff are more likely to be retained, and recruitment is more successful.

Accurate rosters also provide information on the number of hours that nurses are working, as this is linked to adverse events such as needlestick injuries and medication errors.

Reference

10 The European Parliament and the Council of the European Union. *Directive 2003/88/EC of the European Parliament and of the Council of 4 November 2003 Concerning Certain Aspects of the Organization of Working Time.* The European Parliament and the Council of the European Union: Brussels, 2003.

Clinical governance

The main aim of clinical governance is to achieve continuous quality improvement. When put into practice, clinical governance should provide a framework for health organizations to work towards improvement and provide assurance of the quality of clinical services for patients.

During the 1990s, the concept of governance evolved to provide assurance that the care which patients were receiving was effective, safe, and also paid attention to the individual as a person.

Nursing governance is defined as 'the elements related to nursing that are required in an organization to ensure that the nursing care is safe and effective.'

Nursing governance should work as an integrated system across an organization from ward to board. This involves checking and demonstrating that quality assessment, improvement, and patient safety are part of the everyday routine and practice of everyone. A primary function of clinical governance includes early detection of and intervention with regard to any poor performance, with subsequent provision of support and feedback as necessary, to ensure that a safe system of care is being provided to patients.

Nurses who are leading a team, a ward, a department, or even a hospital often need practical advice on how to deliver a comprehensive nursing governance approach. For a nurse, the following fundamental questions need to be considered:

- How do I know that the care in my area is safe?
- How would I prove this to my patients?
- What does my executive nurse need to understand in terms of risks?
- What do my patients think about the care that they received today?

When answering the above questions, nursing governance across a hospital can be subdivided into three main categories—people, systems, and tools (see Table 2.3).

It is important at a ward level that information from each of these categories is discussed by the ward manager and displayed, to enable nurses to understand the patient outcomes and how nursing influences patient care and outcomes on the ward in which they are working.

Table 2.3 Nursing governance across a hospital

People	Nursing structure—operational and professional
	Models of nursing care
	Nurse staffing levels and establishments to deliver the model of care
	Developing the nursing workforce
	The nursing voice and culture
Systems	Nursing meetings
	Key performance indicators
	Nursing research
	Nurse education
	Patient safety and quality
Tools	Nursing audits/reviews of practice
	Nursing metrics
	Patient experience and feedback

Medicine management

The improvement of medicine management services in hospitals is central to improving the care provided for patients. Medicines management is a term that encapsulates all of the steps involved in administering a drug,[11] including:

• selection
• procurement
• delivery
• prescription
• administration
• review.

Nursing is central to the way that medicines are stored, prescribed, and administered, and these steps are vital both for safety and for medicines to have the desired outcomes for patients. Medicines management is central to the quality of healthcare. Nearly all patients are given medication as a result of a visit to hospital, and nearly 7000 doses are administered daily in a typical hospital.

A key focus in effective medicines management is teamwork within organizations. Nurses will need to work effectively with the pharmacy service to ensure that drugs are stored and administered correctly.

All nurses, when commencing work with an organization, must read the medicines management guidance to ensure that they fully understand the hospital policy. One important aspect of medicines that nurses should learn about is the storage and administration of controlled drugs (CDs). These medicines are classified by law, based on their benefit when used in medical treatment and their harm if misused. There are many rules that nurses need to comply with. For example, within a hospital all wards must keep their own CD register and all healthcare professionals are personally responsible, when checking and administering CDs, for keeping the relevant CD registers up to date.

These practices should be audited regularly to ensure that improvements are continuous. The aim is for staff who are directly caring for patients to have ownership of priorities for improvement and to progress work in their own clinical environments, thus promoting a 'bottom-up' approach.

On all wards it is vital that the nurses participate in raising the profile and understanding of medicines management among staff, patients, and carers. There should be strict routines to ensure that medicines administration is as interruption free as possible, and safety checks to ensure that medicines storage is appropriate. Nurses should work with pharmacists and portering staff to ensure the drugs are delivered to the wards in a timely way and that there is minimal drug wastage on wards.

Nurses are also central to the patient admission and discharge process. During this time the nurse can help the patient to gain an understanding of the importance of medications, compliance, and side effects or drug reactions. Patient information leaflets are also valuable as an aid to understanding drugs and their side effects.

Nurses should understand how the pharmacy department works, as this knowledge has major benefits in allowing them to appreciate some of the steps involved in medicines management that nurses do not usually see, such as procurement and dispensing.

Reference

11 Audit Commission. *A Spoonful of Medicine: medicines management in NHS hospitals*, Audit Commission: London, 2001.

Ward and local risk registers

Risk registers

A risk register is a management tool that enables an organization to understand its risk profile. Each ward and department should also have a risk register for its area. Ward managers will be responsible for the management of risk relating to the staff whom they supervise, the workplace that they control, and the patients for whom they provide care within their level of competency.

Risk identification

It is the surgical ward manager's responsibility to minimize the likelihood and severity of risk events by recording all incidents or near misses through the incident recording system. Hospitals have different systems, but incidents are either recorded on a paper form or via an electronic system. All staff should be encouraged to report incidents that do or could pose a hazard.

The surgical ward manager will also be expected to undertake a regular 'horizon scan' to proactively identify potential risks as part of the risk register. They can then raise awareness across the ward and plan and record actions to reduce or eliminate the risk.

If there is an immediate risk that is causing nurses concern, it should be escalated immediately to a senior member of the ward staff or to the appropriate hospital bleep holder or manager to ensure that action can be taken. It is important to emphasize that if there is a concern, this should be escalated immediately to ensure that advice and help are sought and patient safety is maintained.

Within an organization, all risks should use a standard classification matrix or system, which will involve the risk being described in terms of its consequences and likelihood of occurrence, which will often produce a score to help others to understand the severity of the risk.

When nurses look at a risk register there should be a number of components. These include:
• dates—the register is a live document and it is important to record the dates when the risks are identified and the target or completion dates
• a description of the risk—this will include the likelihood of the occurrence (e.g. whether the risk is low, medium, or high) plus the severity of the risk, which provides an assessment of the impact that the occurrence would have on the ward
• countermeasures or actions—these are the actions that are being taken to reduce, prevent, or mitigate the risk
• the risk owner—a named individual should be responsible for ensuring that the risks are communicated and understood, and that countermeasures are being implemented. The risk manager will have a plan of action to mitigate the risk (e.g. removal of certain equipment). This action will be reviewed to ensure completion at the appropriate hospital committee or meeting.

Corporate risks

A corporate risk is one that can affect the objectives of a whole business or hospital. This could be a clinical safety, financial, or environmental issue. Therefore identification and management of the risks is vital for the business and hospital objectives. The risks that are received from the organization and the trust board will be reviewed and graded as a corporate risk at the appropriate hospital forum.

Serious untoward incidents

Serious incidents in hospitals can be reported in a variety of ways, including the hospital's incident reporting system, complaints, or coroners' cases.

Serious incidents include the following:

- a serious event in which a patient or patients were harmed or could have been harmed
- an event that was unexpected
- an event that would be likely to give rise to serious public concern or criticism of the service involved.

Hospitals have policies that describe their systems for dealing with serious incidents, including the action to be taken by staff in the event of an incident. The policy will include information about who is responsible for initiating further communication or enquiries and ensuring that appropriate action is taken.

'Never events'

These are events that should never happen in NHS hospitals, as they are mainly preventable and are of serious concern because they cause patients harm. There is a list of 'never events' that hospitals are required to report if they should occur. These range from entrapment in bed rails to wrong site surgery.

There are 25 'never events' on the expanded list:

- wrong site surgery
- wrong implant or prosthesis
- retained foreign object post-operation
- wrongly prepared high-risk injectable medication
- maladministration of potassium-containing solutions
- wrong route of administration of chemotherapy
- wrong route of administration of oral or enteral treatment
- intravenous administration of epidural medication
- maladministration of insulin
- overdose of midazolam during conscious sedation
- opioid overdose in an opioid-naive patient
- inappropriate administration of daily oral methotrexate
- suicide using non-collapsible rails
- escape of a transferred prisoner
- falls from unrestricted windows
- entrapment in bed rails
- transfusion of ABO-incompatible blood components
- transplantation of ABO- or HLA-incompatible organs
- misplaced nasogastric or orogastric tubes
- administration of the wrong gas
- failure to monitor and respond to oxygen saturation
- air embolism
- misidentification of patients
- severe scalding of patients
- maternal death due to postpartum haemorrhage after elective Caesarean section.

Complaints

There are times when a person's healthcare experience is not as he or she expected, and occasions when processes or procedures go wrong. In 1996 a single NHS complaints system was introduced for healthcare providers, and although this has been amended slightly, it remains a framework in which people should expect a response to their concerns.

Informal complaint and resolution

The first line of response is from the local service or ward, with the aim of resolving the issue either formally or informally as quickly as possible. Nurses who listen and who are open to discussing the complaint with the patient and their family or carer may find that resolution and an agreed way forward are possible. If this is not the case, a formal written complaint may be made to the organization. If this complaint concerns the care on a ward, the ward manager or the modern matron will often be asked to ascertain the facts of the incident. The ward manager will ask the staff involved in the incident to make a statement of what they can recall, so that he or she can respond accurately to the person.

Formal complaint

If after discussion and a written response the individual feels that the complaint is still unresolved or there has been poor practice, they can refer the complaint to the Health Service Ombudsman for further review. Here it will be decided whether further review of the complaint is required. For those cases that are reviewed, reports may make comments and recommendations about the circumstances of the complaint and the need for service improvements.

It is vital that nursing staff listen to the feedback they receive from patients so that they can learn from mistakes and improve the care that they provide. A common theme in complaints is poor communication, when patients feel that they were not given the information they required. It is important at ward meetings to discuss complaints so that there can be agreement on the best way to improve the service across the team. Actions to address the cause of the complaints may be given to the team so that the solution is a shared response.

Patient feedback

The views of patients receiving care in some hospitals have led to a refocusing on quality and safety systems across healthcare, and have highlighted the importance of listening to patients and putting them at the centre of decision-making processes. Patient feedback is important, and both complaints and suggestions need to be routinely reviewed by nurses at all levels throughout the organization. It is important not only to review the number of complaints being received, but also to define themes or trends where the patient experience is suboptimal.

Patient surveys

Patient surveys provide important and standardized information across a healthcare system. Often at an organizational level the sample selected is small and much of the data is high level, and may not relate directly back to a ward or department for them to undertake a review or an improvement cycle. Therefore more regular feedback, such as an online system whereby patients can not only score their experience but also input free text comments, is important to ensure that all wards or areas are receiving timely feedback on which they can act.

Patients' stories

Another powerful means of understanding the care experience from the patients' perspective is to invite them to tell their stories. This approach is extremely useful for staff education sessions, to enable them not only to understand the patient's perspective but also to learn how to receive feedback and use it constructively. Often junior nurses are not exposed to this experience and may find criticism difficult if they are not aware of the importance of receiving feedback.

Service design

Including patients at the beginning of a new service or plan is essential, and a 'fresh pair of eyes' can bring a new perspective. The use of local improvement networks to represent the views of patients and voluntary bodies provides another opportunity to develop improvements in care.

Financial management

The ward manager is responsible for ensuring that care is delivered effectively and safely. Each ward area has a budget for paying the staff who are working on the ward and a budget for stock items. The latter is often described as the non-pay budget.

Agreeing a budget

At the beginning of the financial year the ward manager should have the opportunity to discuss the ward budget with the appropriate manager to review whether anything is likely to affect the budget in the coming year.

Influences on the budget

Influences on the pay budget include:
- vacancies—if these are not filled in a timely manner, temporary staffing solutions may have to be found, which may cost more than substantive staff
- rotas—if these are not managed well, this may lead to an overspend on pay.

Influences on the non-pay budget include:
- holding too much stock on the ward
- the introduction of a new procedure that requires an expensive non-pay item
- staff not being educated about the cost of non-stock items.

Ongoing budgetary management

Ward managers will often have to meet monthly with accounts and managers, to ensure that budgets are not overspent. At ward meetings this should be discussed, to ensure that all staff are aware of the cost of items. To facilitate this, the costs are often displayed on shelving next to the item, to remind staff of the cost of the product.

Care audit and evaluation

Understanding nursing-sensitive indicators

Nurses need to understand the outcomes for the patients for whom they provide care. It is essential to measure the care that healthcare professionals deliver, in order to provide evidence of the impact on patient outcomes. The decision as to what to measure may be influenced by a variety of factors, including national and political priorities or the immediate healthcare setting of a hospital or a ward. Depending on the country of work, there may be national nursing data sets that need to be submitted.

The measurement of care has been discussed by nurses for over 150 years.[12] Methods of measuring care include mortality statistics, access times, and patient views. The evidence base is important to ensure that professionals not only know what they are doing well, but also understand where improvements are needed. To ensure that the quality of nursing care is understood across a ward, hospital, or geographical area (e.g. country) it is important that the nursing information is consistently collected. Nursing performance can then be discussed across the nursing community and provide evidence that enables non-nurses to understand the quality of nursing care.

Providing a range of nursing key performance indicators or a nursing dashboard can allow information about nursing safety and outcomes to be simply and quickly understood. For example, it could be made electronically available at ward level or displayed in wards, so that nurses and patients can see this information. There should be a variety of indicators that include structure, process, and outcome measures. Irvine and colleagues[13] based their work on Donabedian's structure–process–outcome quality of care model[14] (see Table 2.4).

The exact indicators that are used will depend upon priorities or areas where nurses feel that practice requires improvement. Nursing key performance indicators should be a selection of measures to reflect the quality of nursing care in the organization. Nurses should be able to articulate why a particular set of measures were chosen. These need to be challenging and drive performance, and are likely to change over time. Nursing indicators should be shared with all levels of the organization, from the ward nurse to the executive nurse.

There is a range of evidence-based indicators or outcomes which can be linked to the quality of nursing care. These include failure to rescue, falls, and healthcare-associated infections.[15] Some studies show an association between registered nurse (RN) numbers and patient outcomes, including mortality, adverse events, and failure to rescue.[16,17]

The practicalities of collecting nursing key performance indicators across an organization need to be considered. Much of the information or data source is likely to have already been collected within an organization. It may just need to be drawn together into a matrix or dashboard.

The validation of the data is important, so that measurements are reliable and there is clinical agreement on the data.[18] As the organization checks and replicates the information, this process becomes easier.

Table 2.4 Structure–process–outcome quality of care model

Donabedian category	Translation of Donabedian's model for nursing
Structure	Patients' acuity and dependency
	Nurse and education
	Nursing numbers/skill mix
	Environment
Process	Nursing interventions
	Organization of care
	Interdependent care roles with other professional teams
Outcome	Patient outcomes, including:
	Functional status
	Adverse events
	Patient satisfaction
	Symptom control

References

12 Nightingale F. *Notes on Hospitals*, 3rd edn. Longman, Green, Longman, Roberts and Green: London, 1863.

13 Irvine D, Sidani S and Hall L. Linking outcomes to nurses' roles in health care. *Nursing Economics* 1998; 16: 58–64, 87.

14 Donabedian A. *The Definition of Quality and Approaches to Its Assessment*. Health Administration Press: Ann Arbor, MI, 1980.

15 Griffiths P. RN + RN = better care? What do we know about the association between the number of nurses and patient outcomes? *International Journal of Nursing Studies* 2009; 46: 1289–90.

16 Kane RL et al. The association of registered nurse staffing levels and patient outcomes: systematic review and meta-analysis. *Medical Care* 2007; 45: 1195–204.

17 Lang TA, Hodge M and Olsen V. Nurse patient ratios: a systematic review on the effects of nurse staffing on patient, nurse employee, and hospital outcomes. *Journal of Nursing Administration* 2004; 34: 326–37.

18 Doran D and Almost J. *Nursing-Sensitive Outcomes: state of the science*. Jones & Bartlett Learning: Toronto, 2003.

Recruitment and selection

A ward is only as good as the nurses who work on it. All surgical wards will have a number of different nursing roles and grades to ensure that patients receive the best possible care. The recruitment and selection process is crucial to the functioning of the surgical ward team. It is vital that the team as a whole has the skills and capabilities required to care for patients on a surgical ward.

The recruitment process

Each nursing role will have a job description and a person specification. The ward manager will advertise vacant posts once they have been agreed internally according to the hospital process. The post will be advertised for a period of time and the candidates will have to complete a specific form or alternatively send their CV (curriculum vitae) when applying. Once the advert is closed there will be a short-listing process to ascertain which of the candidates meet the role criteria.

During the interview, each candidate will be asked the same questions against the person specification and the criteria for the role. Each member of the interview panel will use a scoring matrix to provide consistency and choose the candidate who is most suitable for the role. After the interview the successful candidate's references will be checked to ensure that they are satisfactory.

Occupational health

For nursing roles, candidates will be asked to complete an occupational health form, which will give the candidate's health history. This will include questions about obligatory communicable disease, immunization, and vaccination history. Some candidates may be asked to discuss their health with the occupational health nurse or doctor.

Disclosure and Barring Service (DBS) check

All successful candidates will be required to undergo a Disclosure and Barring Service (DBS) check—previously known as a Criminal Records Bureau (CRB) check—and will be given a form to complete. Nursing is a regulated activity, which means that the employing hospital must check that the candidate is not barred from working with children and/or vulnerable adults.

Qualifications and professional registration

When applying for a nursing role, candidates must prove to the employer that their registration is valid and up to date. If registration is not confirmed, employment cannot commence.

Ward routines and ward rounds

Each ward has its own routines, which will be dependent on the following factors, among others.

The type of patients on the ward

Each ward has different types of patients, and their care needs will alter the daily routine. This will affect the nursing workload at different times of the day. A simple example would be the frequency of observations or dressing changes.

Shift patterns

Shift patterns across wards may be different, or they may be standardized across a hospital. Often nursing shifts are 7.5, 10, or 12 h in duration, although some nurses may work part-time hours. Surgical wards that use a two-shift system will have different handover and nursing break (drink and mealtime) routines to those that use a three-shift system.

The organization of nursing care

Nursing care is organized differently on each ward. Often the ward manager in each area decides this, or alternatively it may have been a corporate nursing decision. Some areas will nurse patients in teams, whereas other wards may assign different levels of experienced nurses to carry out different tasks, so the organization of care is task based. In some wards where patients have a high acuity and dependency, a nurse may care for all the needs of one or two patients. Each care model will affect the ward routine.

Consultant ward rounds

Consultant ward rounds occur on a regular basis on surgical wards, with most consultants seeing their patients on a daily basis. Some of these ward rounds may be teaching rounds, and others may be much shorter. It is vital that nurses participate in these activities to ensure that they can adequately report and plan the care of patients with the medical staff. If there is a regular teaching round this should be agreed with the ward manager to ensure that the nursing off-duty can reflect the need for this time commitment. If the ward cares for the patients of a variety of consultants, a discussion is required to ensure that the ward rounds do not all occur at the same time. If nurses do not discuss the care of their patients with the consultants, patient care may become disjointed and the patients' length of stay and the quality of care that they receive are likely to be affected.

Hospital policies and procedures

A hospital's policies and procedures may affect the ward's routines, so these should be considered when providing care. Examples of this are numerous, and may range from the theatre start time to the availability of medical staff on an audit day. Mealtimes for patients on surgical wards or the routine times at which drugs are delivered to wards will affect when patients have procedures or the best time for relatives to collect the patient from the ward.

Advanced skills of the team

The skills of the nursing team on the ward will affect the ward routines. Many nurses today have gained additional skills and competencies to carry out roles that would have traditionally been the domain of the medical staff. Nurses are competent in some wards to admit and discharge patients and prescribe medication. This enables patients to be effectively cared for, but alters the ward routine by often reducing the waiting times for patients to receive care and to be discharged.

Communication with other healthcare professionals

A patient on a surgical ward will need expert help and advice from a variety of professionals, including physiotherapists, social workers, occupational therapists, dietitians, and speech and language therapists. It is vital that the surgical nurse assesses and evaluates the needs of patients in their care and refers them to the appropriate professional in a timely way. Depending on the ward, there may be daily meetings with all of the professional groups to ensure that care is appropriately coordinated. It is important that the nurse explains to the patient the roles of the different members of the healthcare team, so that the patient has an understanding of how these individuals can help their rehabilitation and their journey home.

Chapter 3

Surgical care models

Surgical care models

The increasing specialization of surgery has seen a radical shift in the organization of surgical care. This has resulted in fewer surgeons maintaining general skills, and an increasing number having a more organ-specific focus (e.g. breast, pancreatic, trauma, orthopaedic, or colorectal surgery). This shift has occurred during a period when perioperative pathways have changed due to increasing use of technology, pharmacology, and refined techniques that result in reduced pre-operative and overall length of stay. Soreide[1] has highlighted how day-case, short-stay, inpatient, emergency, and trauma surgery have all developed significantly in recent years with an integrated model of surgery as outlined in Figure 3.1.

Significantly, the intensity of care is higher, with greater throughput of patients in fewer hospital beds. The combined effect has resulted in the development of surgical models that require healthcare professionals to deliver care to patients in different environments and modalities. The traditional role of the ward-based surgical nurse has evolved in response to these changes to the clinical pathway, where a range of healthcare professionals now provide surgical expertise in the pre-operative phase. This chapter will focus on the key defining aspects of the following care models:
- day-case surgery
- day-of-surgery admission
- short-stay surgery
- inpatient (elective and emergency) surgery.

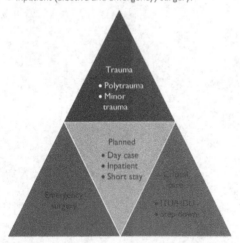

Figure 3.1 Models of surgical care.

Reference
1 Soreide K. Trauma and the acute care surgery model—should it embrace or replace general surgery? *Scandinavian Journal of Trauma, Resuscitation and Emergency Medicine* 2009: **17**: 4.

Day-case surgery

Day-case surgery evolved in the early 1900s, but underwent rapid expansion during the 1980s. The development of minimally invasive techniques and analgesia supported its practice. Day-case surgery is defined as hospital treatment that requires some form of preparation or period of recovery, or both, involving the provision of accommodation and other services but not involving an overnight stay, and where the patient is admitted to the care of the hospital.

Day-case procedures normally:
• are of short duration
• have a low incidence of complications
• have a low risk of transfusion
• do not require significant post-operative analgesia.

Day-case surgery procedures are often performed on a preselected group of patients who have undergone a thorough pre-operative assessment (see ➜ p. 62) and have had identified comorbidity evaluated and treated or controlled. This includes investigating potential threats to the patient's health and well-being. Patient selection criteria vary from one unit to another, but the key criteria are as follows:
• suitable as a day-case procedure
• American Society of Anesthesiologists (ASA) grade 1–2 (although grade 3 is possible)
• body mass index (BMI) < 40 kg/m^2
• social criteria (e.g. carers available for 24 h post discharge)
• access to a telephone during the post-operative period
• living within an hour's travel time to the hospital.

Age is not a contraindication to day-case surgery, unless the patient does not meet any of the selection criteria listed.

Day-case emergency surgery

Development of surgical and anaesthetic techniques has allowed the development of day-case emergency surgery. Similar principles are applied to patient selection as for day-case surgery, but may also include the following.

It should be clinically appropriate to undertake the proposed surgery as a day procedure. Examples include:
• trauma and orthopaedics—simple manipulation under anaesthesia, minimal debridement, and removal of foreign bodies
• plastic surgery
• gynaecology—evacuation of retained products of conception (ERPOC) and Bartholin's abscess
• general surgery—pilonidal, (some) perianal, and other non-septic localized abscesses.

To improve efficiency and patient experience, patients are assessed on one day, discharged, and readmitted as a planned emergency the following day. Patients in these cases require:
• appropriate clinical review prior to discharge
• analgesia and other medications (e.g. antibiotics)
• appropriate fasting advice (see ➔ p. 113)
• an advice sheet and the contact details of a healthcare professional.

Day-of-surgery admission

Inpatient surgery has also seen a change whereby patients are pre-assessed prior to admission (see ➔ p. 62), so that the requirement for admission the day before surgery is often limited to a few clinical cases.

Now the majority of inpatients will arrive in hospital on the day of surgery. Day-of-surgery admission areas have developed to provide an environment away from busy wards, where pre-procedure checks can be undertaken and the patient and their relatives can wait, thus reducing anxiety and stress.

Same-day admission units also:
- improve patient scheduling for surgery through staggered start times for theatre sessions
- provide a central area where clinicians can see patients on the day of surgery
- allow improved communication with patients and their relatives.

Once they have been prepared for surgery, patients often walk from the same-day admissions unit to the operating theatre (this has been shown to reduce anxiety).

Further reading

Kulasegarah J et al. Day of surgery admission—is this safe practice? *Irish Medical Journal* 2008; 101: 218–19.

Ortiga B et al. Effectiveness of a Surgery Admission Unit for patients undergoing major elective surgery in a tertiary university hospital. *BMC Health Services Research* 2010; 10: 23.

Short-stay surgery

Short-stay surgery is defined as a procedure that requires the patient to remain in hospital for more than 12 h and less than 48 h. Pre-operatively they require the same preparation before their procedure as a day case.

As an extension to day-surgery procedures, more complex operations on patients with greater comorbidity can be conducted within this time frame.

This also allows increased shorter-duration opiate analgesia to be given to the patient during this period.

Further reading
Verma R et al. Day case and short stay surgery: 2. *Anaesthesia* 2011; 66: 417–34.

Inpatient (elective and emergency) surgery

Inpatient surgery is focused on more complex surgery and on those patients with significant comorbidity (> ASA grade 3) in both the planned and emergency pathways.

The National Confidential Enquiry into Patient Outcome and Death (NCEPOD) classification of surgical urgency[2] will determine the speed with which the surgery is to take place (see ➔ p. 7). This in turn will determine the required preparation prior to the procedure.

Planned surgery

Also commonly referred to as elective surgery, a planned surgical procedure is booked in advance of routine admission to hospital. Patients are often referred by their GP to a hospital specialist for assessment, investigation, diagnosis, and a definitive treatment plan. Following this, they will require pre-operative assessment (see ➔ p. 62), consenting (see ➔ p. 68), and admission to hospital.

In England, NHS patients with a potential cancer diagnosis are referred quickly to a specialist via the '2-week wait' system.[3] This ensures that they receive a prompt diagnosis. Further treatment is mandated as early as possible, but may include adjunct therapy such as radiotherapy prior to the procedure. Definitive treatment (surgery or adjunct therapy) must begin within 62 days of referral.

An 18-week referral to treatment time (RTT) is the NHS standard applied to patients having their surgery following outpatient assessment.[4]

Emergency surgery

The NCEPOD classification[2] subdivides emergency surgery as follows:

• *Immediate* surgery may include ruptured aortic aneurysm, major trauma to the abdomen or thorax, fracture with major neurovascular deficit or a compartment syndrome, and requires surgery within minutes of the decision to operate. Resuscitation and surgery occur simultaneously.

• *Urgent* surgery may include compound fractures, perforated bowel with peritonitis, critical organ or limb ischaemia, and perforating eye injuries. Surgery in these patients can be delayed for a few hours until resuscitation is completed.

References

2 National Confidential Enquiry into Patient Outcome and Death (NCEPOD). *Knowing the Risk: a review of the peri-operative care of surgical patients.* NCEPOD: London, 2011.

3 Department of Health. *Review of Cancer Waiting Times Standards: improving outcomes: a strategy for cancer.* Department of Health: London, 2011.

4 Department of Health. *Referral to Treatment Consultant-Led Waiting Times.* Department of Health: London, 2012.

Pre-operative assessments and preparation

Elective pre-operative assessment

Pre-operative assessment is an integral part of preparation for patients prior to surgery. If performed well, it decreases cancellations on the day of surgery, improves the patient's experience of their hospital admission, and reduces complication rates and mortality.[1]

Pre-operative services should:[2]

- ensure that every patient is fully informed about their proposed procedure and the interventions that will need to be undertaken
- estimate the level of risk for every patient
- ensure that every patient understands their own individual risk so they can make an informed decision about whether to proceed to surgery
- identify coexisting medical illnesses and optimally prepare every patient while taking into account the urgency of the operation
- identify patients at high risk of complications in the peri-operative period, and define the appropriate post-operative level of care (i.e. day stay, inpatient, ward, or critical care).
- plan discharge.

The pre-operative process of assessment and optimization is guided by the urgency of surgery and the relative comorbidity of the patient. Elective operations can be performed on patients who are ASA grade 1–4. The optimization process will focus on acute and chronic conditions as outlined in Table 4.1, ensuring that the time is taken to improve the patient's condition and outcomes.

Table 4.1. The pre-operative process of assessment and optimization for elective surgery

Surgical urgency	Acute pre-operative optimization considerations	Chronic disease pre-operative optimization considerations	
		New onset/ exacerbation	Long-term conditions
Elective	Pain control, hydration, nutritional and gastrointestinal considerations, including bowel preparation and gastro-oesophageal reflux disease (GORD)	Consideration is given to delaying surgery (if appropriate) until condition has stabilized	Conditions such as asthma, hypertension, and diabetes are often optimized by pre-operative assessment services prior to surgery. Maintain normal treatment regime unless contraindicated by surgery or acute optimization

However, some procedures, such as cancer surgery, require an operation in an expedited time frame. The pre-operative assessment and optimization strategy are altered accordingly as outlined in Table 4.2.

Table 4.2. The pre-operative process of assessment and optimization for expedited surgery

Surgical urgency	Acute pre-operative optimization considerations	Chronic disease pre-operative optimization considerations	
		New onset/ exacerbation	Long-term conditions
Expedited	Pain control, hydration, haematological and biochemical conditions, and gastrointestinal considerations (bowel preparation and GORD)	Condition is actively treated and improved prior to surgery. Delay can be required if an improvement that reduces risk can be achieved (e.g. chest infection, atrial fibrillation, urinary tract infection)	Maintain normal treatment regime unless contraindicated by surgery or acute optimization

References

1 Radford M, Williamson A and Evans C. *Preoperative Assessment and Perioperative Management.* M&K Publishing: Keswick, 2012.
2 Association of Anaesthetists of Great Britain and Ireland (AAGBI). *Pre-Operative Assessment and Patient Preparation.* AAGBI: London, 2010.

Emergency inpatient assessment

Patients who require surgery after an unplanned admission, such as an emergency or trauma admission, are at higher risk of peri-operative complications. The standards and principles of care for elective patients apply equally to those admitted in an emergency, even though it is often more difficult to achieve them due to time constraints prior to their operation.

The NCEPOD classification (see ➔ p. 7) highlights immediate and urgent surgery groups. Each requires different assessment and optimization strategies to manage their care. It is critical that clear pathways of care for unplanned admissions include surgeons, emergency departments, and theatre departments. The purpose of these pathways should be to enable a high standard of care, avoid omissions, and improve optimization, particularly in vulnerable groups such as the elderly.

An assessment plan for immediate surgery (e.g. ruptured aortic aneurysm, laparotomy for bleeding) is outlined in Table 4.3.

For urgent surgery (e.g. debridement plus fixation of fracture, laparotomy for perforation) the clinical team has a limited window of opportunity in which to assess and optimize the patient (see Table 4.4).

Table 4.3. The pre-operative process of assessment and optimization for immediate surgery

Surgical urgency	Acute pre-operative optimization considerations	Chronic disease pre-operative optimization considerations	
		New onset/ exacerbation	Long-term conditions
Immediate	Optimization in the immediate surgical category is primarily aimed at treating the surgical condition simultaneously with resuscitation (e.g. fluid resuscitation for massive haemorrhage, severe sepsis, and pain control)	Long-term conditions may require active treatment as a result of their deterioration as part of surgical/ trauma insult (e.g. cardiac ischaemia, diabetes, chronic renal insufficiency)	

Table 4.4. The pre-operative process of assessment and optimization for urgent surgery

Surgical urgency	Acute pre-operative optimization considerations	Chronic disease pre-operative optimization considerations	
		New onset/ exacerbation	Long-term conditions
Urgent	Optimization in the urgent surgical category is aimed at stabilizing the surgical condition prior to surgery taking place (e.g. fluid resuscitation for haemorrhage, shock, sepsis, and pain control)	The condition is actively treated and improved prior to surgery. A delay of only hours may be required if an improvement that reduces risk can be achieved	Maintain normal treatment regime unless contraindicated by surgery or acute optimization

Surgical nursing process

The modern surgical facility has evolved to segregate patients by pathway and acuity. This has resulted in the development of independent day units and short-stay facilities that are separate from the main hospital wards. Patients are routinely pre-assessed prior to admission. Nursing care may be required over a 24 hour period for the few patients who are admitted before surgery, and can include drug therapy, bowel preparation, and management of coagulation disorders.

The majority of inpatients will arrive in the hospital on the day of surgery. Day-of-surgery admission areas have developed to provide an environment away from busy wards, where pre-procedure checks can be undertaken, and the patient and their relatives can wait, reducing anxiety and stress.[3,4]

The surgical nursing admissions process must be focused and thorough so that the patient is prepared safely. A structured approach to admissions must incorporate surgical needs as well as holistic needs.

The first step should be to familiarize the patient and their carers with the ward environment, including:
- orientating the patient to the ward area, including reception, toilets, day room, and exits
- introducing staff, their roles, and their uniforms to ensure recognition
- explaining the ward timetable, including ward rounds, mealtimes, visiting times, and other likely events
- explaining the expected processes in the admission process
- explaining how equipment works (e.g. nurse call-bells, the bed, and communication equipment).

Pre-operative care assessment

The care and admission assessment is often completed when the patient first arrives. This assessment includes evaluation of the patient's current health status, the impact of the surgical procedure, and the health benefits that the procedure is expected to achieve.

This baseline information draws upon risk assessments so that care plans can be drawn up. Examples of common care assessments include:
- tissue viability—measures the risk of developing pressure damage
- venous thromboembolism (VTE)—measures the risk of developing thromboemboli and the associated risk of pulmonary emboli
- nutrition—measures the risk of developing malnutrition while in hospital
- falls—measures the risk of a patient suffering a fall.

The nursing assessment that is completed on admission should consider all aspects of the patient, their health needs, personal preferences, lifestyle choices, and social circumstances. The structure around which this assessment is completed may vary (e.g. with the use of care and nursing models). However, the aim is always to assess each aspect of the person as a whole.

Consideration needs to be given to areas such as the patient's surgical history and medical conditions, as these may have a direct impact on the care that the patient receives. Equal importance must be given to other aspects of the patient's lifestyle, as the impact of these may not be so readily apparent or influence the patient's surgery, but may affect their recovery and/or discharge.

References

3 Kulasegarah J et al. Day of surgery admission—is this safe practice? *Irish Medical Journal* 2008; 101: 218–19.

4 Ortiga B et al. Effectiveness of a Surgery Admission Unit for patients undergoing major elective surgery in a tertiary university hospital. *BMC Health Services Research* 2010; 10: 23.

Consent for surgery

Consent for surgery must be obtained by a trained and qualified practitioner prior to the procedure taking place. Consent in its basic form refers to the provision of approval or agreement *after thoughtful consideration*. For this to be achieved, the patient needs access to as much information as possible, so that they can fully evaluate and formalize a decision.

Consent is required for any procedure that is performed on or on behalf of the patient. It needs to cover:

- the exact nature of the planned procedure, including the intended benefits and serious or frequently occurring risks
- any extra procedures that may become necessary during the procedure (e.g. blood transfusion)
- alternative treatments and their outcomes that could be considered
- the anaesthesia to be used, the reason for this choice, and the complications that may occur
- ongoing peri-operative and post-operative care, where this will be delivered, and what is to be expected.

The General Medical Council (GMC)[5] guidelines on consent include the following useful principles:

- Listen to the patient and respect their views about their health.
- Discuss with the patient what their diagnosis, prognosis, treatment, and care involve.
- Share with the patient the information that they want or need in order to make their decisions.
- Maximize the patient's opportunities and ability to make decisions for him- or herself.
- Respect the patient's decisions.

The formal consenting process will involve a written document which confirms that the above procedure has taken place and the patient is fully informed.

Emergency treatment

If a person requires emergency treatment to save their life, and they are unable to give consent as a result of being physically or mentally incapacitated (e.g. they are unconscious), treatment will be carried out. It is important that, once the patient has recovered, they are given a full explanation.

Additional procedures

There may be some circumstances in which, during a procedure, the patient requires an additional procedure that was not included or discussed in their original consent. For example, during abdominal surgery the surgeon may notice that the patient's appendix is infected, and therefore needs to be removed because there is a risk that it may rupture. If the surgeon believes that a delay would cause further harm, the additional procedure can go ahead if it is considered to be in the patient's best interest.

Consent for children

Consent for children will involve their parents or legal guardians, although in the UK it is required that children are central to the discussions prior to surgery. Children under 16 years of age are able to consent for themselves if they are deemed to be 'Gillick competent'[6] (i.e. if they fully understand the nature of their condition and the proposed treatment). Consent can be formally accepted by children aged 16–18 years, although refusal of surgery can be overturned by the parent or guardian.

Consent and patients with mental health conditions

Patients with long-term mental health conditions can be consented against their will under the Mental Health Act.[7] Where a procedure is deemed to be the right course of action and in the patient's best interests, healthcare professionals undertake this procedure. This requires a full psychiatric and medical assessment. Individuals covered under the Mental Health Act will have an Independent Mental Capacity Advocate as per the Mental Capacity Act (2005).[8] Where acute confusion or lack of capacity exists, extra care needs to be taken in involving patient advocates, who may be family members or alternative professionals, and ensuring that the patient's best interests are maintained throughout.

Lasting Power of Attorney

A Lasting Power of Attorney[8] (LPA) allows the individual (the donor) to give authority to someone else (the attorney) to make decisions on the donor's behalf. There are two types of LPA—the property and affairs LPA and the personal welfare LPA. The personal welfare LPA covers personal, welfare, and healthcare decisions, including decisions relating to medical treatment.

References

5 General Medical Council. *Good Medical Practice: explanatory guidance.* ℛ www.gmc-uk.org/guidance/ethical_guidance.asp
6 Gillick v West Norfolk and Wisbech AHA (1986) AC 112 (HL).
7 Department for Constitutional Affairs. *Mental Health Act 2007.* The Stationery Office: London, 2007.
8 Department for Constitutional Affairs. *Mental Capacity Act 2005: code of practice.* The Stationery Office: London, 2007.

Taking a clinical history

It is critically important to obtain an accurate and comprehensive patient history during the pre-operative assessment. The aim should be to assess the patient's pre-operative condition, and diagnose and correct any disease or abnormality, or at least optimize a condition that is relevant to the ensuing surgery and anaesthetic.

When evaluating the health status of the patient, the following aspects of the history should be covered in detail:

• the presenting complaint and its symptoms
• the diagnosis (if relevant)
• the past medical history
• the previous surgical history
• the anaesthetic history, including any problems experienced and the family history of anaesthetic problems
• medications
• allergies
• family history
• social and psychological history
• activities of daily living
• systems enquiry, with a particular focus on:
  • cardiovascular function (metabolic equivalents and functional capacity and symptomatology)
  • respiratory function.

In addition, there may be a number of special considerations relating to the individual patient, such as:

• children
• older adults
• mental illness
• learning disability
• cultural considerations.

Once the history has been obtained, it can act as a guide to appropriate physical examination, as well as to relevant investigations and observations. The main purpose of observations and diagnostic tests is to provide additional information to the clinical history of a patient, with the aim of:

• providing information that may confirm or question the correctness of the current course of clinical management
• using this information to reduce the possible harm or increase the benefit to the patient, by altering their clinical management if necessary
• using this information to help to assess the risk to the patient and provide an opportunity to discuss potentially increased risks with the patient
• predicting post-operative complications
• establishing a baseline measurement for later reference in the surgical care period
• allowing opportunistic screening that is unrelated to the surgery.

Broadly speaking a range of investigations would be required as outlined in Table 4.5. Following reviews of the available evidence of the value of routine pre-operative testing in healthy or asymptomatic adults, the National Institute for Health and Care Excellence (NICE) has produced guidelines on the subject.[9]

Table 4.5 Investigations required prior to surgery

Test	Age 16–40	Age 40–60	Age 60–80	Age > 80
Chest X-ray	No	No	Consider	Consider
ECG	No	Consider		
Full blood count				
Haemostasis	Consider	Consider	Consider	Consider
Renal function				
Random glucose	Consider	Consider	Consider	Consider
Urinalysis	Consider	Consider	Consider	Consider

Reference

9 National Institute for Health and Care Excellence (NICE). *Preoperative Tests: the use of routine preoperative tests for elective surgery*. CG3. NICE: London, 2003. ℬ www.nice.org.uk/guidance/cg3

Clinical examination

Approximately 70% of the information that is needed to make a diagnosis is obtained during the history taking process. The subsequent clinical examination is designed to confirm the diagnosis suggested by the history, and determine the plan of care.

Adopting a systematic approach is the key to effective clinical examination. The following is a suggested methodology.

1. Greeting and introduction:
   - If the patient is able to walk, examine their gait.
   - Note their posture, stature, height, and weight.
   - Note any limb amputations or obvious deformities.
   - Is the patient's physique appropriate for their age?
2. Note the patient's general appearance:
   - Neurological condition and alertness, using the AVPU classification, National Early Warning Score (NEWS), or Glasgow Coma Scale (GCS) as appropriate.
   - Hands and nails.
   - Jugular venous pressure (JVP).
   - Face and eyes.
   - Mouth and dental condition.
3. Anterior chest:
   - Lungs.
   - Heart.
4. Posterior chest and back.
5. Lungs.
6. Respiratory system—abnormal breath sounds.
7. Spine and sacral area.
8. Abdomen.
9. Gastrointestinal system:
   - Abdominal masses.
   - Previous scars.
10. Lower limbs:
    - Oedema.
    - Circulation and pulses.
    - Movement.
    - Neurology.
11. Upper limbs:
    - Circulation and pulses.
    - Movement.

Airway assessment

The induction of anaesthesia results in the loss of reflexes and respiratory function, due to the effect of the anaesthetic agents. This requires rapid control of the airway to ensure continued oxygenation and prevention of complications. Prior to anaesthesia it is important that the airway is assessed for any potential problems. This assessment should consider the following factors.

Patient history

- Previous history of difficult intubation.
- Tumours of the head and neck.
- Arthritis.
- Pregnancy.
- Trauma—cervical spine, full stomach.

Physical examination

- Tongue versus pharyngeal size.
- Atlanto-occipital joint extension.
- Cervical spine mobility (normally 35°).
- Anterior mandibular space and mobility:
  - thyromental distance (normal value is > 6 cm)
  - ability to sublux the jaw.
- Dental examination—loose teeth, prostheses.
- Mallampati score.

The Mallampati score (see Figure 4.1) is extensively used and involves the patient opening their mouth wide while sitting in front of the anaesthetist. The patient is then assigned a grade according to the best view obtained. Grade 1 usually predicts an easy intubation, whereas grades 3 or 4 suggest a significant likelihood that the patient will prove difficult to intubate. The results of this test are influenced by the ability to open the mouth, and by the size and mobility of the tongue and other intra-oral structures.

The type of airway that is utilized will depend on a number of factors, including the type of surgery, its duration, and the potential for complications.

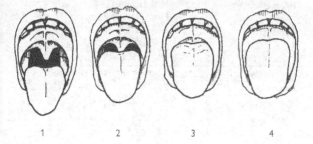

1   2   3   4

Figure 4.1 Mallampati grade 1, 2, 3, and 4. Reproduced from Keith Allman and Iain Wilson, *Oxford Handbook of Anaesthesia*, 3rd edition, 2011, with permission from Oxford University Press.

Haematology tests

Haematology tests are critically important for assessing the presence of a variety of clinical conditions prior to surgery. A number of haematological tests can be performed, including the full blood count (FBC) and sickle-cell assay.

Full blood count (FBC)

This assesses several different parameters and can provide a large amount of information prior to surgery. The blood sample is taken from the patient and stored in a blood EDTA tube. The sample should be analysed in the laboratory within 4 h.

The main parameters that are measured by an FBC are listed in Table 4.6.

An FBC is recommended for the following patients prior to surgery:
- all patients over 60 years of age
- all adult women
- all patients undergoing intermediate or major surgery
- all patients undergoing major surgery or with suspected or known low Hb (< 12 g/dL)—these individuals should also have ferritin and C-reactive protein (CRP) levels measured.

In addition, an FBC is required for patients with:
- known or suspected anaemia
- chronic blood loss
- a known history of heart disease, including hypertension
- a known history of chest disease
- known renal impairment
- chronic disease (e.g. rheumatoid arthritis)

An FBC is also needed for patients known to the haematologist.

Table 4.6. Parameters measured with a full blood count (FBC) assay

Parameter	Reference range
Haemoglobin (Hb)	Male: 13.5–18.0 g/dL Female: 11.5–16.0 g/dL
Red cell count	Male: $4.5-6.5 \times 10^{12}$/L Female: $3.9-5.6 \times 10^{12}$/L
White cell count (WCC)	$4.0-11.0 \times 10^9$/L
Lymphocytes	$1.3-3.5 \times 10^9$/L; 20–45% WCC
Neutrophils	$2.0-7.5 \times 10^9$/L; 40–75% WCC
Eosinophils	$0.04-0.44 \times 10^9$/L; 1–6% WCC
Basophils	$0.0-0.10 \times 10^9$/L; 0–1% WCC
Monocytes	$0.2-0.8 \times 10^9$/L; 2–10% WCC
Platelet count	$150-400 \times 10^9$/L

C-reactive protein (CRP)

CRP is a protein that is produced by the liver and which is found in blood plasma. Its levels rise in response to inflammation. Conditions that can cause elevated CRP levels include:

- bacterial infections
- autoimmune conditions (e.g. arthritis)
- tissue injury (e.g. wound)
- cancer
- myocardial infarction.

Sickle-cell assay

It is important to offer sickle-cell testing pre-operatively in order to iden-tify this risk before the anaesthetic is administered. This is essential for ethnic groups who have a family history of homozygous sickle-cell anae-mia or sickle-cell trait, particularly if there is no previous surgical history. The following ethnic groups are at risk:

- African
- Caribbean
- Eastern Mediterranean
- Middle Eastern
- Asian.

Sickle cell has also been identified in patients of Cypriot origin.

Appropriate counselling is essential, so that the patient realizes the implications of both positive and negative results and is able to give their informed consent.

Clotting tests

Coagulation studies or clotting tests are required in patients who:
- have known or suspected liver disease
- have a history of abnormal bleeding
- have chronic renal impairment
- have advanced malignancy
- are scheduled for major surgery (grade 3 severity or higher)
- have inherited clotting factor deficiencies.

All patients on long-term warfarin therapy must have their international normalized ratio (INR) checked in the clinic.

Clotting tests

Clotting tests consist of the following:
- plasma protein (fibrinogen)
- clotting times—prothrombin time (PT) and activated partial thromboplastin time (APTT)
- INR and partial thromboplastin time (PTT).

Fibrinogen is one of the more important blood proteins involved in clotting. It is produced in the liver, and is converted into fibrin by an enzyme called thrombin which is derived from prothrombin, and is also produced by the liver and has a crucial role in clot formation.

PT and PTT are measures of the ability of blood plasma to form an artificial clot in the laboratory. (Some laboratories place an 'A' for 'activated' in front of the PTT, and it is referred to as APTT.)

PT and PTT measure different parts of the clotting pathway, and they are used to investigate bleeding disorders and monitor the effects of different drugs that interfere with different parts of the coagulation system. The effectiveness of unfractionated heparin is monitored by its effect on prolonging the PTT.

The PT is commonly used to assess the efficacy of the oral anticoagulant warfarin. The INR is the ratio between the normal PT and the patient's PT while on warfarin therapy. Its value varies depending on the condition (see Table 4.7).

Table 4.7 INR reference ranges for different conditions

Indication	Reference range
Treatment of venous thrombosis	2.0–3.0
Treatment of pulmonary embolism	2.0–3.0
Prophylaxis of venous thrombosis (high-risk surgery)	2.0–3.0
Prevention of systemic embolism	2.0–3.0
Tissue heart valves	2.0–3.0
Acute myocardial infarction (to prevent systemic embolism)	2.0–3.0
Valvular heart disease	2.0–3.0
Atrial fibrillation	2.0–3.0
Bileaflet mechanical valve in aortic position	2.0–3.0
Mechanical prosthetic valves (high risk)	2.5–3.5
Systemic recurrent emboli	2.5–3.5

Biochemistry tests

Urea and electrolytes (U&E) are a routine blood test conducted on pre-operative patients:
- over 60 years of age
- undergoing intermediate and major surgery
- with known or suspected renal disease
- with hepatic failure
- with cardiovascular disease
- with hypertension
- with diabetes
- with liver disease
- with advanced malignancy
- with a cardiac pacemaker
- with disturbed fluid balance, dehydration, vomiting, or diarrhoea
- taking any of the following medications:
  - digoxin or other anti-dysrhythmic agents
  - diuretics
  - ACE inhibitors or other anti-hypertensive agents
  - lithium
  - systemic steroids.

Reference ranges for U&E and liver function tests (LFTs) are listed in Tables 4.8 and 4.9, respectively. It is important to check local laboratory ranges, as variations in reference values can occur.

Table 4.8 Urea and electrolyte (U&E) tests

Parameter	Reference range
Sodium	135–145 mmol/L
Potassium	3.5–5 mmol/L
Creatinine	70–150 µmol/L
Urea	2.5–6.7 mmol/L
Calcium	2.12–2.65 mmol/L
Albumin	35–50 g/L
Protein	60–80 g/L

Table 4.9 Liver function tests (LFTs)

Parameter	Reference range
Bilirubin	3–17 µmol/L
Alanine transaminase (ALT)	3–35 U/L
Aspartate transaminase (AST)	3–35 U/L
Alkaline phosphatase	30–35 U/L (adults)
Creatine kinase	25–195 U/L
Lactate dehydrogenase (LDH)	70–250 U/L

Endocrine tests

Patients with endocrine disease who present for anaesthesia and surgery can pose significant clinical challenges. A detailed clinical history can help to detect endocrine disease in patients with undiagnosed conditions, as well as aiding the management of those with established disease. Endocrine tests are performed pre-operatively for patients:

- who have a history of diabetes, polydipsia (excessive thirst), and polyuria, and these conditions have not been checked recently
- on medication, including steroids, if a random blood glucose measurement is > 7 mmol/L
- with a BMI of > 35 kg/m^2 and random blood glucose > 7 mmol/L
- with a history of hypothyroidism or hyperthyroidism
- with a history of thyroidectomy.

It is important to undertake condition-specific testing for known endocrine conditions prior to surgery.

Diabetes

- A random plasma glucose measurement of ≥ 8 mmol/L followed up with fasting blood glucose.
- An oral glucose tolerance test (OGTT) may be appropriate alongside previous abnormal or equivocal blood glucose results.
- A random blood glucose level of ≥ 11.1 mmol/L or fasting blood glucose level of ≥ 7.0 mmol/L is diagnostic for diabetes in a symptomatic patient. In an asymptomatic patient, a further test is required.
- An HbA1c measurement can be useful for patients with previously undiagnosed diabetes, as it enables identification of those who require intervention to improve diabetes control prior to surgery.

Hypothyroidism

For pre-operative assessment, measurement of thyroid-stimulating hormone (TSH) alone is recommended. If the TSH level is above or below the reference range, a free T$_4$ measurement may be required. Uncontrolled hypothyroidism and hyperthyroidism both represent significant risks for anaesthesia and surgery.

Cushing's syndrome

Non-iatrogenic Cushing's syndrome (i.e. occurring in patients who are not on steroids) is rare, and requires specialized endocrine input prior to operation. However, U&E and plasma glucose levels should be checked in patients with suspected Cushing's syndrome, in order to exclude hypokalaemia and diabetes (see Table 4.10).

Table 4.10 Endocrine blood tests

Parameter	Reference range
Cholesterol	< 6 mmol/L
Triglycerides	0.5–1.9 mmol/L
Amylase	0–180 Somogyi U/dL
C-reactive protein (CRP)	< 10 mg/L
Fasting glucose	3.5–5.5 mmol/L
Prostate-specific antigen (PSA)	0–4 ng/mL
T₄ (total thyroxine)	70–140 mmol/L
TSH	0.5–5 mU/L

Pre-operative electrocardiogram (ECG)

A 12-lead ECG is a common pre-operative investigation, and is conducted on patients:
- over the age of 60 years
- undergoing major surgery
- with any cardiac history.

More specifically, an ECG is indicated for patients:
- with hypertension (treated or not)
- on any anti-hypertensive medication
- with a history of previous myocardial infarction
- with a history of angina or breathlessness on exertion
- with a history of a dysrhythmia or palpitations
- with other known or suspected cardiac disease
- with diabetes or hyperlipidaemia and aged ≥ 40 years
- with renal disease.

ECG morphology

The P wave is the result of the atrial depolarization which starts in the sinoatrial (SA) node. The signal produced by pacemaker cells in the SA node is conducted to the right and left atria. The QRS complex represents ventricular depolarization, and the T wave represents the repolarization of the ventricles. There is no cardiac muscle activity during the T wave. Figure 4.2 shows the normal ECG waveform.

Positioning of 12-lead ECG

A 12-lead ECG is designed to take a range of readings from the heart, and each of the 10 leads is mapped to a specific segment of the heart in order to produce a 12-lead picture in the horizontal and vertical planes. This enables a trained clinician to interpret a variety of conditions, depending upon the position and ECG morphology.

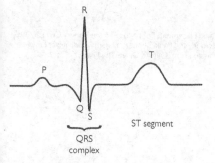

Figure 4.2 A normal ECG waveform. Reproduced from James Thomas and Tanya Monaghan, *Oxford Handbook of Clinical Examination and Practical Skills*, 2007, with permission from Oxford University Press.

There are six chest leads, which are labelled V1–V6 (see Figure 4.3):
- V1: fourth intercostal space on right sternal border
- V2: fourth intercostal space on left sternal border
- V3: midway between V2 and V4
- V4: fifth intercostal space at the left mid-clavicular line
- V5: left anterior axillary line at the same horizontal level as V4
- V6: left mid-axillary line at the same horizontal level as V4 and V5.

There are four limb leads (see Figure 4.4), which are either colour coded or labelled as follows:
- red lead: right arm (RA)
- yellow lead: left arm (LA)
- green lead: left leg (LL)
- black lead: right leg (RL).

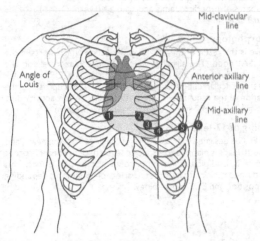

Figure 4.3 ECG chest lead placement. Reproduced from Robert Crouch OBE, Alan Charters, Mary Dawood, and Paula Bennett, *Oxford Handbook of Emergency Nursing*, 2009, with permission from Oxford University Press.

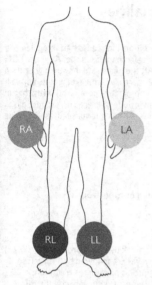

Figure 4.4 ECG limb lead placement. RA, right arm; LA, left arm; RL, right leg; LL, left leg. Reproduced from Robert Crouch OBE, Alan Charters, Mary Dawood, and Paula Bennett, *Oxford Handbook of Emergency Nursing*, 2009, with permission from Oxford University Press.

Common ECG abnormalities

Tachyarrhythmia

Atrial fibrillation (AF) is a heart condition that causes an irregular and often abnormally fast heart rate, arising from the SA node. A typical ECG waveform is shown in Figure 4.5. In AF, the heart rate may be higher than 140 beats/min. The prevalence of AF increases with age, and its appearance is associated with a doubling of mortality compared with that in individuals without AF. Symptoms can include palpitations, fatigue, dyspnoea, dizziness, and decreased stamina. AF has multiple causes, including the following conditions:

* valvular heart disease
* hypertension
* coronary artery disease
* hyperthyroidism
* pericarditis
* myocarditis, cardiomyopathy (dilated or hypertrophic)
* excessive alcohol consumption
* post-coronary bypass surgery.

Bradyarrhythmia

* In first-degree atrioventricular (AV) block there is a prolonged (> 0.2 s) but constant PR interval, and all P waves are followed by a QRS (see Figure 4.6). It rarely causes any symptoms or requires treatment.
* In second-degree AV block Mobitz type 1 (Wenckebach), the PR interval becomes progressively longer after each beat until a QRS is dropped and the pattern starts again (see Figure 4.7). The need for treatment is dictated by the effect on the patient and the risk of developing more severe AV block or asystole.

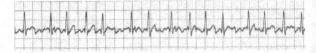

Figure 4.5 Atrial fibrillation. Reproduced from Kate Olson, *Oxford Handbook of Cardiac Nursing*, 2014, with permission from Oxford University Press.

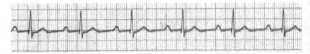

Figure 4.6 First-degree AV heart block. Reproduced from Kate Olson, *Oxford Handbook of Cardiac Nursing*, 2014, with permission from Oxford University Press.

- In second-degree AV block Mobitz type 2, the PR interval is prolonged but at regular intervals, such as every third or fourth P wave, and the P wave is not followed by a QRS (see Figure 4.8). There is an increased risk of developing third-degree AV block and asystole.
- In third-degree AV block there is complete AV dissociation, with no relationship between the P waves and the QRS complexes (see Figure 4.9). They are fired from different pacemakers within the heart in an uncoordinated manner, and there is a high risk of developing asystole.

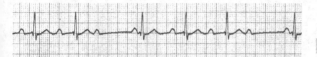

Figure 4.7 Second-degree AV block, Mobitz type 1(Wenckebach). Reproduced from Kate Olson, *Oxford Handbook of Cardiac Nursing*, 2014, with permission from Oxford University Press.

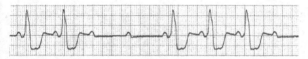

Figure 4.8 Second-degree AV block, Mobitz type 2. Reproduced from Kate Olson, *Oxford Handbook of Cardiac Nursing*, 2014, with permission from Oxford University Press.

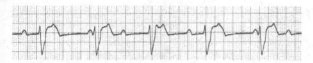

Figure 4.9 Third-degree AV block. Reproduced from Kate Olson, *Oxford Handbook of Cardiac Nursing*, 2014, with permission from Oxford University Press.

ST depression
- Acute ST depression can be associated with ischaemia, non-Q-wave infarction, electrolyte abnormalities, osmolality changes, hyperventilation, standing, and certain drugs. An ECG should be obtained in any patient with chest pain of uncertain aetiology, because an acute ST shift can confirm that it is due to ischaemia. The amount of ST depression is measured from the PR segment (the isoelectric line).
- Chronic ST depression is a non-specific marker for cardiac disease, but is associated with a poor outcome. It can be due to electrolyte abnormalities and drugs, particularly digoxin.

Other cardiology investigations

Echocardiography

An 'echo' can be either percutaneous or transoesophageal, producing a visual picture of the heart. Two-dimensional echocardiography allows assessment of:

• the muscle mass of the heart
• ventricular function/ejection fraction
• end-diastolic and end-systolic volumes
• valvular function
• segmental defects.

Doppler ultrasound allows assessment of valvular flow and pressure gradients.

The echo will give some indication of ventricular function, but this does not always correlate well with capacity or outcome. An ejection fraction of less than 50% is abnormal, and is compatible with a diagnosis of systolic heart failure. However, two-thirds of patients over the age of 80 years with heart failure will have diastolic dysfunction and a normal left ventricle (LV) ejection fraction.

Heart failure (either systolic or diastolic dysfunction) is a major perioperative risk factor. The presence of heart failure doubles the risk of death after major surgery.

An echo should also be performed if the clinical examination identifies a new murmur, especially if the patient presents with any of the following:

• poor functional capacity
• syncope or dizzy spells
• angina
• left ventricular hypertrophy or ST changes on an ECG
• a history of major surgery
• known aortic stenosis or mitral stenosis with no recent imaging (i.e. within the last 12 months), or with deterioration in symptoms
• suspected heart failure, and shortness of breath on climbing a flight of stairs (< 4 METs)
• known heart failure with no recent echo and/or a change in symptoms
• known ischaemic heart disease, and without a formal assessment of left ventricular function.

Reviewing a chest X-ray

A routine pre-operative chest X-ray is not recommended. It is only indicated in the presence of the following cardiorespiratory symptoms or signs elicited during history taking:
• chest pain
• increasing dyspnoea
• paroxysmal nocturnal dyspnoea
• a known respiratory condition (e.g. asthma).

The following types of surgery do require a chest X-ray, if it has not already been performed as part of the pre-operative asssessment:
• abdominal, cardiac, thoracic, and some oesophageal surgery
• thyroidectomy or head and neck surgery
• neurosurgery (due to the prolonged nature of anaesthesia and the need for post-operative critical care)
• lymph node surgery.

Review of a chest X-ray requires a systematic approach, which will now be summarized.

Housekeeping
• Patient's name.
• Date on which the examination was performed—this is important if comparing with previous examinations.
• Check for position markers—right vs. left, upright.
• Projection—posteroanterior (PA), anteroposterior (AP).

Image
• Type of film—plain, computed tomography (CT), angiography, magnetic resonance imaging (MRI).
• Patient's position—supine, upright, lateral, decubitus.
• Inspiration vs. expiration.
• Technical quality of examination—a subtle pneumothorax can be missed if the patient moves or the film is overexposed.

Primary survey
• General body size, shape, and symmetry.
• Male vs. female.
• Patient age—infant, child, young adult, or older adult.
• Survey for foreign objects—for example, chest drain, intravenous lines, nasogastric tube, ECG leads, surgical drains, prosthesis, as well as non-medical objects, bullets, shrapnel, glass, etc.

Secondary survey
• Bones and soft tissue:
  • fractures or dislocations
  • surgical emphysema
  • bone density
  • thoracic spine
  • position and shape of diaphragm
  • cardiac anatomy.
• Lung anatomy.

Respiratory tests and investigations

Respiratory function

Lung function tests should be able to predict the type and severity of lung disease. They can predict the risk of complications and post-operative mortality. These tests fall into three categories:
- lung mechanics
- gas exchange
- control of breathing.

Useful radiological investigations include:
- chest X-ray
- high-resolution thoracic CT.

Arterial blood gas analysis may be invaluable. Lung function tests allow assessment of:
- lung volumes
- airway calibre
- gas transfer.

Lung volumes

Lung volumes are assessed by spirometry. Volumes measured include:
- inspiratory capacity (IC)
- inspiratory reserve volume (IRV)
- tidal volume (TV)
- vital capacity (VC)
- functional residual capacity (FRC)
- residual volume (RV)
- expiratory reserve volume (ERV)
- total lung capacity (TLC).

Airway calibre

Airway calibre can be assessed by peak flow measurements (absolute values depend on height, weight, age, gender, and ethnic origin), which require cooperation and maximum voluntary effort by the patient.

Flow rates that are measured include:
- forced vital capacity (FVC)
- forced expiratory volume in 1 s (FEV1)
- the FEV1/FVC ratio is important.

Lung function can be classified as normal, restrictive, or obstructive.
- In restrictive lung disease, FVC is reduced but FEV1/FVC is normal.
- In obstructive lung disease, FVC is normal or reduced, and FEV1/FVC is reduced.

Gas transfer

Arterial blood gases are the best available measure of gas transfer, and they also allow assessment of ventilation/perfusion mismatch.

Important parameters to measure include:

- pH
- partial pressure of oxygen
- partial pressure of carbon dioxide.

Pulse oximetry provides an indirect estimate of gas transfer. However, the technique is unreliable in the presence of other medical problems (e.g. anaemia).

Cardiovascular testing

A number of cardiovascular assessment tools are available for risk stratification of a patient's cardiac disease. The Canadian Cardiovascular Society's angina classification system (see Table 4.11) is used to determine the symptoms in line with functional capacity.

The New York Heart Association (NYHA) scoring system (see Table 4.12) is widely used in pre-operative assessment and cardiology to determine symptomology (e.g. angina, dyspnoea) linked to functional capacity and known metabolic equivalent (MET) values.

Table 4.11 Canadian Cardiovascular Society's angina classification system. © Canadian Cardiovascular Society

Grading of angina pectoris by the Canadian Cardiovascular Society classification system	
Class I	Ordinary physical activity, such as walking and climbing stairs, does not cause angina. Angina occurs with strenuous, rapid, or prolonged exertion at work or during recreation
Class II	Slight limitation of ordinary activity. Angina occurs on walking or climbing stairs rapidly, walking uphill, walking or stair climbing after meals, and in cold, or in the wind, or under emotional stress, or only during the few hours after awakening. Angina occurs on walking more than two blocks on the level and climbing more than one flight of ordinary stairs at a normal pace and in normal conditions
Class III	Marked limitation of ordinary physical activity. Angina occurs on walking one to two blocks on the level and climbing more than one flight of ordinary stairs in normal conditions and at a normal pace
Class IV	Inability to carry out any physical activity without discomfort—anginal symptoms may be present at rest

Table 4.12 New York Heart Association classification of heart failure

Class I	Can perform activities that require > 7 METs	Cardiac disease but without resulting limitation of physical activity. Ordinary physical activity does not cause undue fatigue, palpitations, dyspnoea, or anginal pain
Class II	Can perform activities that require > 5 METs but < 7 METs	Cardiac disease resulting in slight limitation of physical activity. Comfortable at rest. Ordinary physical activity results in fatigue, palpitations, dyspnoea, or anginal pain
Class III	Can perform activities that require > 2 METs but < 5 METs	Cardiac disease resulting in marked limitation of physical activity. Comfortable at rest. Less than ordinary physical activity results in fatigue, palpitations, dyspnoea, or anginal pain
Class IV	Patient cannot perform activities that require > 2 METs	Cardiac disease resulting in inability to carry out any physical activity without discomfort. Symptoms of cardiac insufficiency or of anginal syndrome may be present even at rest. If any physical activity is undertaken, discomfort is increased

Cardiopulmonary exercise testing

Cardiopulmonary exercise testing (CPET, or CPEx) has been demonstrated to improve outcomes of surgery in terms of morbidity and mortality.[10] CPET directly measures the aerobic capacity of an individual while they exercise, usually on either a treadmill or a bicycle.

The CPET test measures breath volume, oxygen consumption, and carbon dioxide production during exercise. An ECG with ST-segment analysis and pulse oximetry is recorded throughout, along with intermittent non-invasive blood pressure measurements. Rarely, arterial blood gases are sampled. Power increases throughout the CPET test by increased braking on the bicycle and by increased speed and gradient on the treadmill, until the person stops. Incremental exercise should last at least 5 min, and preferably 10 min, in order to accurately gauge the prognosis.

The more complete prognostic information provided by CPET tests is probably of use if it:
- helps clinicians to determine whether surgery is more likely to harm or benefit a patient
- helps the patient to decide whether to have surgery
- helps to determine the efficient use of scarce resources (e.g. critical care, transplants)
- helps to determine the likelihood that interventions could improve outcomes.

Reference

10 Goodyear SJ et al. Risk stratification by pre-operative cardiopulmonary exercise testing improves outcomes following elective abdominal aortic aneurysm surgery: a cohort study. Perioperative Medicine 2013; 2: 10.

American Society of Anesthesiologists (ASA) grading

The American Society of Anesthesiologists (ASA) has developed a risk scoring system that is commonly used to determine patient risk in relation to existing conditions, which can be used as a guide for the patient undergoing anaesthesia.

This simple tool is widely used within pre-operative assessment. The classification system subjectively categorizes patients into six groups according to their pre-operative level of physical fitness:

- ASA Physical Status 1: normal healthy patient
- ASA Physical Status 2: patient with mild systemic disease
- ASA Physical Status 3: patient with severe systemic disease
- ASA Physical Status 4: patient with severe systemic disease that is a constant threat to life
- ASA Physical Status 5: moribund patient who is not expected to survive without the operation
- ASA Physical Status 6: patient who is declared brain-dead and whose organs are being removed for donor purposes.

Venous thromboembolism (VTE) assessment

It is critically important to conduct a VTE assessment prior to surgery. The current national guidelines from the Department of Health, NICE, the Royal College of Obstetricians and Gynaecologists, and NHS England[11-17] are as follows:

- Routinely assess all patients for their level of mobility on admission to hospital.
- All surgical patients, and all medical patients with significantly reduced mobility, should be considered to be potentially at risk of developing VTE, and should be regularly monitored and further risk assessed.
- Consider the factors which may indicate that a patient is likely to develop a deep vein thrombosis (DVT). For example:
  - Do they have a previous history of blood clots?
  - Are they obese?
  - Have they undergone surgery?
  - Are they pregnant?
  - Are they taking an oral contraceptive?

If at least one of these factors is present, the patient may require an anticoagulant medicine such as heparin in accordance with NICE guidelines, but only if they are not at risk of bleeding.

- Provide the patient and their carer with verbal and written information about the symptoms, risks, and possible consequences of VTE, including information on the various forms of prophylaxis.

References

11 National Institute for Health and Care Excellence (NICE). *Venous Thromboembolism in Adults Admitted to Hospital: reducing the risk*. CG92. NICE: London, 2010.

12 Department of Health. *Venous Thromboembolism Prevention: a patient safety priority*. Department of Health: London, 2009. ℘ http://webarchive.nationalarchives.gov.uk/20130107105354/   http://www.dh.gov.uk/en/Publicationsandstatistics/Publications/PublicationsPolicyAndGuidance/DH_101398

13 House of Commons Health Committee. *The Prevention of Venous Thromboembolism in Hospitalised Patients*. The Stationery Office: London, 2005. ℘ www.publications.parliament.uk/pa/cm200405/cmselect/cmhealth/99/99.pdf

14 National Institute for Health and Care Excellence (NICE). *Venous Thromboembolism Prevention Quality Standard*. QS3. NICE: London, 2010. ℘ www.nice.org.uk/guidance/qs3

15 Royal College of Obstetricians and Gynaecologists (RCOG). *Reducing the Risk of Venous Thromboembolism during Pregnancy and the Puerperium*. Green-top Guideline No. 37a. RCOG: London, 2015. ℘ www.rcog.org.uk/globalassets/documents/guidelines/gtg-37a.pdf

16 Department of Health. *Using the Commissioning for Quality and Innovation (CQUIN) Payment Framework: an addendum to the 2008 policy guidance for 2010/11*. Department of Health: London, 2010. ℘ www.londonsexualhealth.org/uploads/CQUIN%20addendum%20201011.pdf

17 NHS England. *Venous Thromboembolism (VTE) Risk Assessment*. NHS England: Redditch, 2015. ℘ www.england.nhs.uk/statistics/statistical-work-areas/vte/

Falls assessment

Falls are an increasing challenge for healthcare providers. The increasing size of the older population, with more complex comorbidities, who are being admitted to hospital for surgery or medical problems necessitates a thorough assessment of the patient to identify any risk of falls. A report from the National Patient Safety Agency (NPSA) in 2011 stated that each year around 280 000 patient falls are reported to NHS England's Patient Safety division by hospitals and mental health units.[18] In 2015, NICE produced a quality standard[19] relating to falls in older adults, as people over the age of 65 years are at highest risk of falling. Among adults aged over 80 years, around 50% will suffer at least one fall a year either at home or in residential care.

The causes of falls are multifactorial, but require comprehensive assessment, including both common and uncommon reasons for falls.

Common causes of falls

- Visual impairment.
- Peripheral sensory neuropathy.
- Cerebrovascular accident.
- Transient ischaemic attack.
- Joint buckling or instability.
- Deconditioning.
- Effects of medicine or polypharmacy.
- Environmental or home hazards.

Uncommon causes of falls

- Vestibular dysfunction.
- Gait disorders.
- Dementia.
- Delirium.
- Depression.
- Seizure.
- Subdural haematoma.
- Syncope.
- Orthostatic hypotension.
- Mechanical mobility or gait disorder.
- Substance abuse.
- Carotid sinus sensitivity.
- Postprandial hypotension.

Assessment questions

1. Is there any history of falls in the previous year?
2. Is the patient taking four or more medications per day?
3. Does the patient have a diagnosis of stroke or Parkinson's disease?
4. Does the patient report any problems with their balance?
5. Is the patient unable to rise from a chair of knee height?

References

18 National Patient Safety Agency (NPSA). *Essential Care after an Inpatient Fall*. NPSA: London, 2011.
19 National Institute for Health and Care Excellence (NICE). *Falls in Older People: assessment after a fall and preventing further falls*. QS86. NICE: London, 2015. ℗ www.nice.org.uk/guidance/qs86

Post-operative delirium assessment

Post-operative delirium is the inability to maintain a coherent sequence of thoughts, usually accompanied by inattention and disorientation, associated with surgery and/or treatment regimes. It is one of the most common post-operative complications, with an incidence of 37%, and 20% of cases of post-operative delirium occur in the elderly. Delirium increases morbidity and mortality following surgery, and results in:

- higher post-operative complication rates
- delayed functional recovery
- increased length of stay.

Causes of post-operative delirium

- Infections.
- Withdrawal (e.g. from ethanol, sedative hypnotics, barbiturates).
- Acute metabolic causes (e.g. dehydration).
- Acid–base disorders.
- Electrolyte disturbance.
- Elevated or lowered levels of sodium, calcium, phosphate, or glucose.
- Hepatic or renal disease.
- Trauma (e.g. burns, head injury).
- CNS disease.
- Cerebrovascular accident (CVA), ischaemic or haemorrhagic stroke.
- Seizures
- Tumour.
- Vasculitis.
- Hypoxia—due to myocardial infarction, congestive heart failure, pulmonary embolus, pneumonia, or chronic obstructive pulmonary disease (COPD).
- Deficiencies (e.g. vitamin B_{12}, niacin, thiamine, or folate deficiency due to malnourishment).
- Environmental (e.g. raised or lowered body temperature).
- Endocrinopathies (e.g. thyroid disorders, diabetes, adrenal disorders).
- Acute vascular causes (e.g. hypertensive emergency, subarachnoid haemorrhage).
- Toxins and/or drugs (e.g. substance abuse, medications, carbon monoxide poisoning).
- Heavy metals (e.g. lead, mercury).

Predisposing factors

- Elderly age group—pre-existing dementia or decreased cognitive ability.
- Polypharmacy and reduced ability to metabolize drugs.
- Visual and/or hearing impairment.
- Higher incidence with COPD, coronary artery disease, and cerebrovascular disease.
- Underlying brain disease (e.g. CVA, seizures, dementia).
- Psychiatric illness, especially depression.

- Comorbid illness (e.g. congestive heart failure, coronary heart disease, chronic renal failure, liver disease, COPD, diabetes mellitus).
- Medications:
  - anticholinergics (e.g. tricyclic antidepressants, neuroleptics, antihistamines, benzatropine)
  - opioids (e.g. morphine, codeine)
  - benzodiazepines (e.g. diazepam, lorazepam)
  - antiparkinsonian agents (e.g. levodopa, amantadine, bromocriptine)
  - H_2-receptor blockers (e.g. ranitidine, famotidine)
  - cardiovascular drugs (e.g. beta blockers, digoxin, diuretics, calcium-channel blockers)
  - antibiotics (e.g. penicillin, cephalosporins, gentamicin)
  - anticonvulsants (e.g. phenytoin, carbamazepine)
  - anti-inflammatory agents (e.g. steroids, NSAIDs)
  - oral hypoglycaemic agents (e.g. glibenclamide, glipizide).

Other factors
- Length and complexity of surgery.
- Type and possible complications of surgery:
  - cardiac surgery—hypoperfusion, emboli, ischaemia
  - orthopaedic surgery—fat emboli
  - ophthalmic surgery—vision loss, anticholinergics.
- Unfamiliar surroundings in recovery and in the ward.
- Sensory overload.

Management
- Prevention:
  - pre-operative optimization of comorbidities
  - elimination of treatment that can predispose to delirium
  - optimization of fluid status
  - aggressive treatment of pain
  - promotion of early ambulation
  - provision of familiar, tranquil post-operative care settings.
- Identification and treatment of underlying disorders:
  - may be multifactorial
  - identification of risk factors and potential post-operative complications
  - vital signs, fluid status, signs and symptoms of infection and focal neurological deficits.
- Supportive care:
  - frequent reorientation and reassurance (verbal and visual)
  - staff and family, clocks, calendars
  - glasses, hearing aids
  - room lighting—mimic the day–night cycle
  - early ambulation.

Further reading
National Institute for Health and Care Excellence (NICE). *Delirium; diagnosis, prevention and management.* CG103. NICE: London, 2010.

Inadvertent peri-operative hypothermia (IPH) assessment

IPH is a common but preventable complication of peri-operative procedures, and is associated with poor outcomes for patients. During the first 30–40 min of anaesthesia the patient's temperature can drop to below 35.0°C. The reasons for this include loss of the behavioural response to the cold, and impairment of thermoregulatory heat-preserving mechanisms under general or regional anaesthesia, anaesthesia-induced peripheral vasodilation (with associated heat loss), and the patient becoming cold while waiting for surgery on the ward or in the emergency department.

Pre-operative assessment

Each patient should be assessed for their risk of inadvertent peri-operative hypothermia and potential adverse consequences before they are transferred to the theatre suite. The patient should be managed as higher risk if any two of the following apply:

- ASA grade 2–5 (the higher the grade, the greater the risk)
- the patient's pre-operative temperature is below 36.0°C, and pre-operative warming is not possible because of clinical urgency
- the patient is undergoing combined general and regional anaesthesia
- the patient is undergoing major or intermediate surgery
- the patient is at risk of cardiovascular complications.

Forced air warming should be started pre-operatively on the ward or in the emergency department, unless there is a need to expedite surgery because of clinical urgency (e.g. due to bleeding or critical limb ischaemia). Forced air warming should be maintained throughout the procedure.

In 2013, NICE produced a quality standard on surgical site infection, which states that 'people having surgery under general or regional anaesthesia have normothermia maintained before, during (unless active cooling is part of the procedure) and after surgery.'[20]

Reference

20 National Institute for Health and Care Excellence (NICE). *Surgical Site Infection*. QS49. NICE: London, 2013. ℘ www.nice.org.uk/guidance/qs49

Further reading

National Institute for Health and Care Excellence (NICE). *Inadvertent Perioperative Hypothermia: the management of inadvertent perioperative hypothermia in adults*. CG65. NICE: London, 2008. ℘ www.nice.org.uk/guidance/cg65

Discharge assessment

Preparing for discharge

Admission on the day of surgery is now a key element of the delivery of timely and cost-efficient care. Linked to this is the obvious need to discuss discharge at the earliest opportunity, namely on admission. As well as discussing this and advising the patient about the events that are expected to occur during the peri-operative period, assessment of the patient's discharge needs should be undertaken. This should include all aspects of the discharge, from medication needs to referral to external agencies for home care. This highlights the need for a multidisciplinary approach to the admission process, both in its design and in its execution.

The admission process is not just a time for assessment, and all discussions should be two-way (i.e. it is important to listen to the patient's concerns, worries, and fears, and to address these as thoroughly as possible in order to reduce anxiety and stress).

Uncomplicated discharge: day-case and short-stay surgery

- Suitable transport home (not public transport) should be arranged.
- The home environment should be suitable for the patient following the procedure or surgery that has been undertaken (e.g. access to a telephone or lift if the patient is living in a flat). If the patient is a child, check their sleeping arrangements (e.g. whether they will be sharing with a sibling).
- Parents and carers should make arrangements for taking time off work or arranging care of other children.
- Suitable arrangements should be made with the general practitioner, community or children's community nurse, health visitor, or school nurse.[21]

Complex discharge

This is a discharge process that deviates from the simple discharge pathway and requires complex coordination of services to enable a safe discharge. Staff with the necessary skills and responsibilities must be involved in the patient's care and/or discharge.

The team includes:
- specialist nursing staff
- consultants and their teams
- physiotherapists
- occupational therapists
- dietitians
- speech and language therapists
- transfer team service
- social services
- intermediate care services.

Reference

21 Royal College of Nursing (RCN). *Day Case Discharge Guide*. RCN: London, 2009.

Spiritual assessment

Spiritual care[22] is defined as that which recognizes and responds to the needs of the human spirit when faced with trauma, ill health, or sadness. It can include the need for meaning, for self-worth, to express oneself, for faith support, perhaps for rites or prayer or sacrament, or simply for a sensitive listener. Spiritual care begins with encouraging human contact in compassionate relationships, and moves in whatever direction is dictated by need.

Spirituality is concerned with:[23]
- hope and strength
- trust
- meaning and purpose
- forgiveness
- belief and faith in self and others—for some this includes belief in a deity or higher power
- people's values
- love and relationships
- morality
- creativity and self-expression.

Meeting the patient's spiritual needs is part of daily nursing care, yet many nurses feel uncomfortable performing a spiritual assessment. This is especially difficult when the patient presents no clues to their spiritual or religious preference, or has a spiritual belief that is unfamiliar to the nurse. However, there are simple, easy-to-use assessment tools that can help the nurse to quickly assess and plan for spiritual need.

One popular tool uses the FICA model.[24] The areas of assessment and possible questions that can be asked are listed in Box 4.1.

> **Box 4.1 Spiritual assessment using the FICA model**
>
> Faith or beliefs: What are your spiritual beliefs? Do you consider yourself spiritual? What things do you believe in that give meaning to life?
>
> Importance and influence: Is faith/spirituality important to you? How has your illness and/or hospitalization affected your personal practices and/or beliefs?
>
> Community: Are you connected with a faith centre in the community? Does it provide support and comfort for you during times of stress? Is there a person, group, or leader who supports and assists you in your spirituality?
>
> Address: What can I do for you? What support and guidance can healthcare provide to support your spiritual beliefs and/or practices?

References
22 NHS Education for Scotland. *Spiritual Care Matters: an introductory resource for all NHS Scotland staff.* NHS Education for Scotland: Edinburgh, 2009.
23 Royal College of Nursing (RCN). *RCN Spirituality Survey 2010.* RCN: London, 2011.
24 Mauk K and Schmidt N. *Spiritual Care in Nursing Practice.* Lippincott Williams & Wilkins: New York, 2004.

Pre-operative teaching

Pre-operative teaching is the physical and psychological preparation of a patient prior to surgery. It includes instruction about the pre-operative period, the surgery itself, and post-operative care.

Patients who are physically and psychologically prepared for surgery tend to have better surgical outcomes. Pre-operative teaching can alleviate most patient fears. Patients who know more about what to expect after surgery often cope better with pain and post-surgery lifestyle changes.

The 'Making Every Contact Count' initiative was launched by NHS Midlands and East,[25] and involves utilizing every opportunity to encourage people to make healthier lifestyle choices. Such counselling most commonly involves encouraging people to:

• stop smoking
• adopt a healthy diet
• maintain a healthy weight
• limit alcohol consumption to within the recommended daily limits
• undertake the recommended weekly amount of physical activity.

The pre-operative phase is an ideal opportunity for counselling the patient about a number of other lifestyle issues relating to surgery, including:

• complications of surgery
• body image following surgery
• weight loss or gain
• stoma formation
• end-of-life care.

Reference

25 Varley E and Murfin M. *An Implementation Guide and Toolkit for Making Every Contact Count: using every opportunity to achieve health and wellbeing.* NHS Derbyshire County: Derby, 2012.

Smoking cessation

Compared with non-smoking patients, patients who smoke pre-operatively have been shown to experience more problems. Smoking has been associated with local wound complications, pulmonary and cardiac complications, an increased need for post-operative critical care, and longer periods of hospitalization.[26]

Smoking cessation interventions have been proved to be effective for hospitalized patients in general,[27] and specifically for surgical patients.[28,29] In order to gain maximum benefit, any attempt to give up smoking must begin at least 8 weeks before surgery, and lead to permanent abstinence. However, temporary abstinence beginning immediately around the time of surgery and lasting until the patient has recovered may still have significant benefits.

Smoking cessation interventions increase the rate of long-term abstinence from smoking if they include regular behavioural support and pharmacotherapy which is continued at least 1 month after discharge.

NICE[30] has recommended that smoking cessation interventions should be offered to surgical patients, and healthcare professionals are encouraged to access training, deliver brief advice, offer pharmacological support, and refer patients to local specialist services.

References

26 Lindstrom D. *The Impact of Tobacco Use on Postoperative Complications.* Karolinska Institute: Stockholm, 2008.

27 Rigotti N, Clair C, Munafo MR and Stead LF, Interventions for smoking cessation in hospitalised patients. *Cochrane Database of Systematic Reviews* 2012; 5: CD001837.

28 Thomsen T, Villebro N and Moller A, Interventions for preoperative smoking cessation. *Cochrane Database of Systematic Reviews* 2010; 7: CD002294.

29 Cropley MT. The effectiveness of smoking cessation interventions prior to surgery: a systematic review. *Nicotine and Tobacco Research* 2008; 10: 407–12.

30 National Institute for Health and Care Excellence (NICE). *Smoking Cessation in Secondary Care: acute, maternity and mental health services.* PH48. NICE: London, 2013. www.nice.org.uk/guidance/ph48

Pre-operative optimization

Assessing the high-risk surgical patient

One of the many purposes of assessing the high-risk surgical patient is to ascertain the likelihood of the patient experiencing morbidity as a result of their intervention. In patients with significant pre-existing comorbidities, or in those undergoing certain types of major surgery, this would be considered alongside an assessment of the likelihood of mortality. The key factors that affect the risk of such occurrences in the surgical patient are:

• age
• socio-economic background
• pre-operative fitness
• pre-existing disease (e.g. cardiovascular disease, respiratory disease, diabetes)
• classification or type of surgery
• lifestyle factors (e.g. smoking, alcohol intake, sedentary lifestyle).

The presence of acute illness in a patient who requires surgery can significantly increase the risk of both morbidity and mortality. Recognition and stabilization of the acute signs and symptoms should be attempted prior to surgery in all but the most urgent of cases, or where the only significant benefit to be achieved is through surgical intervention.

The most useful clinical method of assessing the high-risk surgical patient is to gain an understanding of the patient's premorbid functional capacity, or their ability to perform physical exercise. A patient's functional capacity is indicative of how well their heart and lungs are likely to perform under the physical stress of anaesthesia and surgery. This can be assessed in a number of ways:

• assessment of the patient's ability to perform everyday tasks
  (e.g. walking, climbing stairs, housework, shopping, sports)
• exercise/stress tolerance tests, often branded as CPEx/CPET
  (cardiopulmonary exercise tests)
• specific tests of the heart and lungs, such as coronary angiography, trans-thoracic or trans-oesophageal echocardiography, and pulmonary function tests.

Once an assessment of the patient has been made, the results can be used to determine and evaluate risk, so that peri-operative teams can then examine how elevated levels of risk can be reduced through pre-operative optimization.

Cardiovascular monitoring

Advances in technology in recent years have facilitated more accurate cardiovascular monitoring in a variety of forms, ranging from the traditionally invasive to some of the safer non-invasive devices now available.

Monitoring of the cardiovascular system pre-operatively can provide an opportunity to undertake interventions that serve to enhance the heart and vascular system, in order to enable it to cope with the intense stress placed upon it through anaesthesia and surgery.

- A 12-lead electrocardiogram (ECG) is the most common form of pre-operative testing, and it serves to identify patients who have a degree of dysfunction of the heart caused by ischaemia or infarct, such as a myocardial infarction (MI), or dysfunction due to inadequate passage of electricity through the heart's conduction system, such as occurs in atrial fibrillation (AF).
- An echocardiogram using either trans-thoracic or trans-oesophageal scanning assesses global function of the heart muscle. In addition, assessment can be made of the function of the heart valves and of the blood flow through the heart.
- An arterial line is most commonly inserted in the radial artery if continuous arterial blood pressure monitoring is required. This is used in an acutely ill patient who has cardiovascular instability and/or is receiving inotropic drugs to support cardiac function.
- A central line inserted into a large central vein, such as the subclavian vein, enables monitoring of the patient's central venous pressure. (CVP). The tip of the central line sits in the right atrium and can be transduced via a cardiac monitor in order to monitor the CVP, which measures the pressure in the right side of the heart. The pressure in the right side of the heart is determined by the volume of blood returning to the heart and the ability of the heart to pump the blood. A low CVP may indicate hypovolaemia and the need for fluid replacement, whereas a high CVP may indicate fluid overload or right-sided heart failure.
- Cardiac output flow monitoring is used to assess the function of the cardiovascular system. It provides accurate measurements of a variety of cardiac parameters, including stroke volume, cardiac output, and systemic vascular resistance. Cardiac output studies can be used to guide treatment, including fluid resuscitation, the use of an intra-aortic balloon pump in cardiogenic shock, and inotropic therapy in the patient with septic shock. Techniques such as oesophageal doppler monitoring and lithium dilution cardiac output monitoring are also available.

Fluid and electrolyte optimization

The body of an average adult patient weighing 70 kg contains 42 L of body fluid. This is composed of:
• 28 L of intracellular body fluid
• 14 L of extracellular body fluid (of which 3 L are within the vascular system).

The necessary daily maintenance fluid requirement is:
• 2.5–3 L of water
• 120–140 mmol/L of sodium
• 70 mmol/L of potassium.

The surgical patient's fluid and electrolyte status should be assessed pre-operatively to ensure that an optimum hydration status is achieved. In this way the following complications can be minimized:
• pre-operative dehydration from fasting
• intra-operative blood loss
• post-operative vomiting
• losses from surgical drains, stomas, etc.
• insensible losses (e.g. evaporation from an open abdomen).

If pre-operative correction or intra-operative replacement is required, the appropriate intravenous fluid should be administered. The most common crystalloid intravenous fluids, together with their electrolyte content, are listed in Table 5.1.

It is not uncommon to see disruption to the plasma concentrations of both sodium and potassium in the surgical patient. Therefore electrolyte levels need to be closely monitored and any abnormalities corrected.

Hyponatraemia
The treatment of hyponatraemia will depend on the cause, but only rarely are reduced serum sodium levels the true cause of hyponatraemia. More commonly the cause is a dilutional effect due to fluid retention. Treatment of hypervolaemic hyponatraemia will include fluid and salt restriction and the use of diuretics.

Table 5.1 Electrolyte content of common crystalloid intravenous fluids

	Hartmann's solution	Normal saline 0.9%	Glucose
Sodium (mmol/L)	131	150	30
Chloride (mmol/L)	111	150	30
Potassium (mmol/L)	5	—	—
Bicarbonate (mmol/L)	29	—	—
Calcium (mmol/L)	2	—	—

Correction of the low sodium concentration should be done slowly (an increase of less than 8 mmol/L within a 24 hour period) in order to avoid the development of a potentially catastrophic neurological condition known as central pontine myelinolysis.

Hypernatraemia

Hypernatraemia is most commonly associated with dehydration, and will often manifest in the surgical patient as a strong thirst, with lethargy and weakness. Acute hypernatraemia should be treated rapidly (within < 24 h) with fluid replacement, but chronic hypernatraemia should be treated more slowly (over a period of > 48 h), due to the risk of development of cerebral oedema.

Hypokalaemia

Hypokalaemia occurs if the body loses too much serum potassium, and may be caused by:
- diarrhoea and/or vomiting
- a high-output stoma (e.g. ileostomy)
- diuretic therapy (e.g. furosemide)
- diabetic ketoacidosis
- poor dietary intake of potassium.

Potassium is essential for many body functions, including muscle and nerve activity. Hypokalaemia can cause muscle weakness, muscle cramps, cardiac arrhythmias, and ultimately cardiac arrest.

Treatment will initially be aimed at addressing the cause of the imbalance, followed by replacement of the lost serum potassium. Treatment will be with either oral or intravenous potassium chloride supplements. The route of administration will be dependent on the severity of the potassium deficit and the patient's condition.

Hyperkalaemia

Hyperkalaemia occurs if the body does not excrete excess potassium, and may be caused by:
- renal insufficiency—acute kidney injury or chronic renal failure
- medications that interfere with renal excretion of potassium, such as angiotensin-converting enzyme (ACE) inhibitors, potassium-sparing diuretics, and non-steroidal anti-inflammatory drugs (NSAIDs)
- Addison's disease
- aldosterone deficiency
- massive blood transfusion
- rhabdomyolysis secondary to burns or rapid tissue necrosis.

Treatment of this potentially fatal condition can be through increasing elimination via dialysis or haemofiltration, or by pharmacological methods to temporarily lower the potassium concentration while elimination can be facilitated.

Pharmacological optimization

Surgical patients may be prescribed complex medications for management of their pre-operative comorbidities. The importance of continuing, or in some cases substituting, the regular medications of patients who present for surgery cannot be over-emphasized, and should be considered within the clinical context.

Any changes to a patient's regular medications should be based on local hospital policies. The following drug groups most commonly require manipulation:

- drugs used to treat cardiovascular disorders:
  - ACE inhibitors (e.g. ramipril, perindopril, lisinopril)
  - angiotensinogen II drugs (e.g. losartan, irbesartan)
  - beta blockers (e.g. atenolol, sotalol, propranolol)
- drugs used to treat respiratory disorders:
  - inhalers/nebulizers (e.g. salbutamol, ipratropium bromide, beclometasone dipropionate)
  - steroids (e.g. oral prednisolone)
- drugs used to treat endocrine disorders:
  - oral hyperglycaemic agents
  - insulin therapy
  - levothyroxine
- hormone therapy:
  - oral contraceptive pill
  - hormone replacement therapy (HRT).

In the extremely unwell surgical patient, pharmacological optimization may need to be undertaken with drugs to stabilize the cardiovascular system. Inotropes are prescribed in order to restore, maintain, or improve perfusion to the vital organs prior to the insult of anaesthesia and surgery.

Respiratory optimization

Patients who present with a chronic respiratory condition have an increased risk of post-operative pulmonary complications. Factors that may exacerbate their inherent risk include:

- the use of anaesthetic gases which can cause irritation to the mucosal lining of the airways and the lungs
- reduced post-operative respiratory effort, which is common especially after thoracic or abdominal surgery, due to post-operative pain-limiting chest expansion
- pulmonary infection
- smoking, which increases the risk of peri-operative and post-operative complications.

In order to reduce the risk of post-operative pulmonary complications, the following should be considered:

- Acute respiratory conditions should be treated and all but the most urgent surgery postponed until the symptoms have been eradicated and a period of 2–4 weeks has elapsed, in order to allow airway irritability to settle.
- In patients with chronic respiratory conditions, such as asthma, chronic obstructive pulmonary disease (COPD), emphysema, or bronchiectasis, supplementation of the normal pharmacological regime may be considered in order to achieve optimal peak flow. This may include increasing the dose of orally inhaled steroids for a week prior to surgery. In patients with severe respiratory disease, pre-operative supplementation of oral steroids and antibiotic therapy may be considered beneficial.
- Smoking cessation can reduce the peri-operative risk. However, for a smoker to return to the level of risk equivalent to a non-smoker, a minimum cessation period of 6 months is required. There are benefits to be gained from a shorter period of cessation, such as a decrease in the blood concentration of carbon monoxide and a reduction in upper and middle airway secretions.

Haematological optimization

A patient's haematological function requires assessment pre-operatively in order to identify and correct anaemia, coagulation problems, and platelet dysfunction. Anaemia will reduce the oxygen-carrying capacity of the blood, and coagulation problems and platelet dysfunction will increase the risk of peri-operative or post-operative haemorrhage and/or venous thromboembolism formation.

Anaemia

Anaemia can be due to:
- iron deficiency caused by poor dietary input or poor absorption of iron in the gut (e.g. coeliac disease, Crohn's disease)
- pregnancy
- haemorrhage
- sickle-cell disease
- leukaemia
- chronic kidney disease
- trauma (fractures)
- pernicious anaemia.

Treatment will be based on the severity of the anaemia and will also involve treating the underlying cause as follows:
- iron supplements in the form of ferrous sulfate
- iron-rich diet
- vitamin B_{12} injections for pernicious anaemia
- erythropoietin injections for chronic kidney disease
- blood transfusion if the Hb concentration is < 8 g/dL or active bleeding is causing cardiovascular compromise.

Clotting disorders

Clotting disorders can result in either an increased risk of bleeding or an increased risk of thrombus formation. These disorders can be due to underlying medical conditions or result from taking specific medication.

Causes of an elevated clotting time leading to an increased risk of haemorrhage, and the possible treatments of these causes, include:
- haemophilia A—injection of Factor VIII
- acute or chronic liver disease—consider giving FFP
- heparin therapy—consider giving protamine as reversal agent
- warfarin therapy—consider giving vitamin K/FFP as reversal agent
- vitamin K deficiency—consider giving vitamin K orally or intravenously.

Where suspension or reversal of anticoagulant drugs is indicated, consideration has to be given to the reason for this medication having been commenced (e.g. atrial fibrillation, CVA, prosthetic heart valve) and the need for a safe level of prophylactic anticoagulant therapy.

Potential risk factors for venous thromboembolism include:
- oral contraceptive pill/HRT—depending upon the type of surgery and other risk factors, hormone therapy may be stopped 1 month before surgery in order to reduce the risk
- obesity—weight loss and early mobilization post-operatively are imperative
- dehydration—optimize hydration with oral or intravenous fluids
- malignancy
- atheroma.

Platelet dysfunction

Platelet dysfunction can lead to problems with clot formation and wound healing following surgery. The main causes of platelet dysfunction are thrombocytopenia (low platelet count) and antiplatelet aggregation therapy, which is used to inhibit clot formation in cardiovascular disease. Treatment for platelet dysfunction in the surgical patient mainly involves the use of platelet transfusion.

Causes of thrombocytopenia include:
- aplastic anaemia
- chemotherapy
- radiotherapy
- vitamin deficiency (e.g. folate, vitamin B_{12})
- heparin-induced thrombocytopenia
- disseminated intravascular coagulopathy (DIC).

Antiplatelet aggregation therapy includes:
- aspirin
- clopidogrel.

Premedication prior to surgery

Premedication prior to surgery aims to prepare the patient for anaesthesia and provide optimization for surgery. The choice of drugs used for premedication will depend on the surgical procedure, the patient, and the anaesthetic technique.

The main aims of premedication are:
- to reduce anxiety prior to anaesthesia
- to promote amnesia in young patients and in those receiving repeated general anaesthetics
- to reduce pain in the immediate post-operative period
- to reduce the volume and pH of the gastric contents
- to reduce post-operative nausea and vomiting

The following main groups of drugs are given as premedication:
- Anxiolysis is given in the form of benzodiazepines (e.g. diazepam, temazepam). These agents are given 1–2 h prior to induction of anaesthesia.
- Amnesia is induced using lorazepam or midazolam.
- Analgesic drugs that are used include opioids, paracetamol, and NSAIDs (e.g. ibuprofen, diclofenac).
- Anti-emetics (e.g. domperidone, cyclizine, granisetron, chlorpromazine) reduce the emetic effects of anaesthetic agents. Metoclopramide acts by enhancing gastric emptying.
- Proton pump inhibitors (e.g. lansoprazole, pantoprazole) reduce gastric acidity. They are beneficial if there is a risk of regurgitation of gastric contents, or in procedures associated with a high incidence of nausea and vomiting (e.g. laparoscopy).

Useful website
www.medicinescomplete.com

Surgical fasting: elective and emergency

The purpose of pre-operative fasting is to minimize the risk of regurgita-tion of the stomach contents, which could lead to pulmonary aspiration. The complications of pulmonary aspiration of the acid contents of the stomach can be severe, and indeed fatal in some circumstances.

The Association of Anaesthetists of Great Britain and Ireland and the Royal College of Anaesthetists have provided clear, evidence-based guidelines[1] on pre-operative fasting:
- 6 h before surgery for food
- 2 h before surgery for clear fluids.

In patients who have a surgical pathology that requires intervention sooner than these pre-operative fasting guidelines would permit, it is clearly in the patient's best interests to proceed with surgery. A nasogastric tube can be passed in order to aspirate the stomach contents and reduce the risk of pulmonary aspiration.

Over-fasting of some patient groups can be detrimental to outcomes, due to increasing the risk of post-operative nausea and vomiting and pre-cipitating complications in diabetic patients.

The Royal College of Anaesthetists has produced surgical guidelines on the management of adults with diabetes.[2] The main points in these guidelines which relate to pre-operative fasting are as follows:
- Minimize starving times by prioritizing diabetic patients on the operating list.
- Patients with a planned short starvation time should be managed with a modification of their usual diabetic medication.
- If a patient is expected to miss more than one meal, they should have a variable-rate intravenous insulin infusion.
- The first choice of intravenous fluid to be administered alongside the insulin infusion is 0.45% sodium chloride with 5% glucose and 20 mmol potassium chloride.
- Maintain blood glucose levels in the range 6–10 mmol/L.

During the pre-operative fasting period the patient may require their regular medications. Follow local policies on administering regular medi-cations to the pre-operative fasting patient.

References
1 Association of Anaesthetists of Great Britain and Ireland and the Royal College of Anaesthetists (AAGBI). *AAGBI Safety Guideline. Pre-operative assessment and patient prepara-tion: the role of the anaesthetist. 2.* AAGBI: London, 2010.
2 Royal College of Anaesthetists (RCOA). *Management of Adults with Diabetes Undergoing Surgery and Elective Procedures: improving standards.* RCOA: London, 2011.

Nutritional optimization

Optimization of nutritional status and metabolic function is now under-stood to have a positive impact on surgical outcomes. Recognition of patients who are malnourished, or who are at risk of pre-operative mal-nourishment, is generally poor. In the UK, initiatives such as Enhanced Recovery Programmes[3] have served to encourage screening of patients to identify this cohort. These patients are targeted pre-operatively for optimization of their nutritional state, in order to reduce post-operative complications associated with malnutrition.

Patients who may be at particular risk and who should be considered for nutritional optimization include:
- the elderly
- patients with inflammatory bowel disease
- patients who require bowel preparation with laxatives
- oncology patients
- neonates.

Good practice with regard to improving peri-operative nutritional state includes:
- use of screening tools pre-operatively—for example, the Malnutrition Universal Screening Tool (MUST) should be used to identify those who are malnourished prior to entering the peri-operative journey
- adherence to local and national guidelines on pre-operative fasting
- avoidance of bowel preparation with laxatives where possible.

For all patients who are identified as malnourished in the pre-operative setting:
- arrange referral to a dietitian for nutritional assessment and ongoing dietary advice
- maintain an accurate food diary
- give oral nutritional supplements as prescribed
- ensure that the patient receives any special diets prescribed by the dietitian (e.g. high protein, high carbohydrate).

For some patients the oral feeding route may not be the optimal route for establishing an improved nutritional state prior to or during the operative phase. Enteral feeding offers an alternative whereby a mixture of nutrients is delivered directly into the gut via a tube placed either in the stomach (nasogastric tube) or in the jejunum (naso-jejunal tube). The nutrients are then absorbed through the distal gut wall, thus avoiding reliance on the upper gastrointestinal tract, which may be performing suboptimally.

In slightly more severe cases of malnourishment where the gastro-intestinal tract is not functioning, total parenteral feeding may be required in order to optimize the surgical patient. Total parenteral nutri-tion (TPN) involves the administration of a patient-specific mixture of nutrients directly into a large vein via an indwelling cannula. Systemic absorption of these nutrients can facilitate an improved outcome when used in either the short or long term.

Reference

3 Royal College of Anaesthetists (RCOA). *Guidelines for Patients Undergoing Surgery as Part of an Enhanced Recovery Programme (ERP): helping you to get better sooner after surgery.* RCOA: London, 2012.

Transfer to other departments or theatre

Pre-transfer assessment

Before transferring a patient to another department or theatre, it is essential that their clinical condition is assessed. This is to ensure both that the benefits of transfer outweigh the risks involved, and that there are minimal interruptions to planned care. Patients who are acutely ill often require a higher level of planning prior to transfer. It is important that advice is sought from relevant clinical teams (surgeons, acute pain team, and critical care) to ensure the patient's safety and optimal standard of care throughout. The following factors should also be considered:

• Critical care stabilization on the ward prior to transfer is essential.
• Infection risks (e.g. *Clostridium difficile*, MRSA) to the receiving department should be reviewed with the infection control team.
• Ensure adherence to local policy on patient transfer.
• Be aware of the difference between 'in-hours' and 'out-of-hours' transfers. The latter carry greater risks due to lower staffing levels in all wards and departments of the hospital at night and at weekends.

Patient assessment

• Use the ABCDE assessment process[1] to check the patient's condition and suitability for transfer.
• Within the ABCDE assessment, perform a full set of observations and document them, including at the very minimum:
  • blood pressure
  • pulse
  • temperature
  • respiratory rate
  • oxygen saturations.
• Additional case-specific observations such as neurological assessment may be required.
• The multidisciplinary team (MDT) should be consulted about any concerns that you may have, and a review should be undertaken prior to transfer.
• Following the review by the relevant member of the MDT, any alterations in the plan of care and/or any new treatments must be implemented and their effectiveness evaluated prior to transfer.
• Ensure that any outstanding investigations or procedures are completed (e.g. 12-lead ECG, wound dressing change).
• Complete a patient moving and handling risk assessment.
• The patient must receive all prescribed medications, and this needs to be clearly documented.
• The patient must be stabilized prior to transfer. The exceptions to this would include penetrating trauma or acute ruptured aortic aneurysm.

Communication

- Discuss with the patient and their relatives the reason for transfer, the process, and timings.
- Allow the patient and their relatives the opportunity to ask questions, and provide them with reassurance.
- Following discussion with and consent from the patient, inform their next of kin of the decision to transfer if they are not already aware of this.
- Provide the next of kin with details of timings and also contact details for enquiries.
- Contact the department to which the patient is being transferred, and provide a handover using the Situation–Background–Assessment–Recommendation (SBAR) communication tool.[2]
- Inform the receiving department of the patient's expected time of arrival, clinical status, and specific equipment and monitoring requirements.
- If the patient who is being transferred has communication difficulties, a translator or signer should be available for the transfer.
- Ensure that all members of the MDT are aware of the transfer.

References

1 Jevon P. ABCDE: the assessment of the critically ill patient. *British Journal of Cardiac Nursing* 2010; 5: 268–72.

2 NHS Institute for Innovation and Improvement. *SBAR – Situation – Background – Assessment – Recommendation.* NHS Institute for Innovation and Improvement: Leeds, 2008. ℛ www.institute.nhs.uk/quality_and_service_improvement_tools/quality_and_service_improvement_tools/sbar_-_situation_-_background_-_assessment_-_recommendation.html

Equipment requirements

To ensure that a safe and effective transfer is achieved, check that:
- it is possible for the bed, staff, and equipment to get through doors, into lifts, and access corridors
- staff are trained, experienced, and competent in the transfer procedure and use of the associated equipment
- equipment is lightweight, robust, and durable, and also that it has a clear backlit display with audible alarms
- equipment is checked regularly in line with the manufacturer's instructions
- batteries are charged and spare batteries are available for longer journeys
- wherever possible equipment is mounted at or below the level of the patient
- essential fluids and drugs are administered via infusion or syringe pumps
- spare syringes and infusions are available, so that essential infusions do not run out
- if portable monitoring is required, it has the facility to record 3-lead ECG, oxygen saturation, non-invasive blood pressure, and invasive blood pressure monitoring (e.g. arterial blood pressure)
- a full portable oxygen cylinder and a spare cylinder for longer transfers are available
- an emergency transfer pack, emergency drugs, and an automated external defibrillator (AED) for the critically ill or those considered at risk of deterioration are available
- you have consulted your trust policy on the transfer of critically ill adults, which should be based on the Intensive Care Society's guidelines.[3]

Reference
3 Intensive Care Society. *Guidelines for the Transport of the Critically Ill Adult*, 3rd edn. Intensive Care Society: London, 2011.

Useful website
Intensive Care Society. ⌖ www.ics.ac.uk

Transfer staffing

All patients will be transferred to another department with a porter, and the nurse in charge or the registered nurse who is caring for the patient will need to risk assess whether an escort is also required.

Some hospital transfer policies outline those patients who would be classed as high risk and who therefore should always be transferred with a nursing or medical escort. This can include patients:

- with neurological compromise (reduced conscious level)
- with cardiovascular instability (septic shock)
- with respiratory instability (acute severe asthma)
- who are returning from an invasive procedure (cardiac catheterization)
- with severe communication difficulties (learning disability)
- with a recent history of a fresh bleed (duodenal ulcer)
- who have suffered an epileptic fit in the last 24 h
- who have chest pain.

Role of the nurse escort

The nurse escort must:

- ensure that there is meticulous planning and preparation for the transfer, in order to reduce risks
- monitor the patient's physical and mental condition throughout
- provide psychological support and answer any questions
- ensure that the patient is appropriately dressed and covered to maintain their privacy, dignity, and comfort at all times
- have knowledge of the patient's plan of care and present condition
- communicate effectively with other members of staff involved in the transfer
- be competent in the use of any equipment or monitoring that the patient requires
- ensure that items such as catheter bags, infusion lines, and monitoring equipment are securely placed in order to maintain patient safety
- complete all relevant documentation in accordance with local and national policy
- ensure that clinical notes and X-rays are delivered to the appropriate person at the destination
- at the destination hand over the patient, outlining their present condition and plan of care, their past medical history, and stating the name and contact details of their next of kin.

Pre-operative checklist

The pre-operative checklist ensures that the patient has been prepared both physically and psychologically for surgery, in order to minimize potential problems and risks that are associated with the surgical intervention, including the anaesthetic. The pre-operative checklist is the final check between the ward and the operating theatre. Each hospital will have its own policy on pre-operative checklists, but the key components are as follows.

Identification band

Identification bands play an essential part in the identification process to ensure patient safety. The National Patient Safety Agency (NPSA)[4] states that the following information is mandatory on the printed identification band:

- date of birth
- surname in capitals
- first name, with the first letter in capitals
- hospital number.

A number of hospitals have pre-operative policies which require that a patient going to theatre has two identification bands placed on different limbs. Patients with allergies should have a red allergy identification band clearly indicating the known allergy.[4] This should alert staff to the need to review the patient's prescription chart and/or notes for full details of the allergy.

In 2013, the Information Standards Board for Health and Social Care[5] made it mandatory for all patient wristbands to contain a GS1 barcode in NHS England. A GS1 barcode can be quickly scanned and used to identify a patient.

Consent

With the exception of emergency procedures, gaining consent for a surgical procedure should be a process that encompasses pre-operative education over a period of time. The patient should have been prepared well in advance of signing the consent form, and have had the opportunity to ask questions.

Nil by mouth (NBM)

Due to the risk of aspiration of gastric contents during anaesthesia, the patient is kept NBM for long enough to ensure that their stomach is empty. They should not have solid food for 6 h or clear fluids for 2 h prior to surgery.

Skin preparation and theatre gown

This may consist of washing with a chlorhexidine skin cleanser and the removal of hair from the surgical wound site, due to the risk of surgical site infections. If hair has to be removed, this is done on the day of surgery by healthcare staff using electric clippers with a single-use head.[6]

Prophylaxis for venous thromboembolism (VTE)

All adult patients who require an inpatient admission for surgery should be given prophylactic treatment to prevent VTE.[7] This may consist of low-molecular-weight heparin via subcutaneous injection, and anti-embolic stockings.

Premedication and other medication

It is essential that premedication is given as prescribed and documented on the pre-operative checklist as well as on the prescription chart. In addition, it is important to document what other medication the patient has received or has had omitted on the day of surgery.

Observations

A full set of observations should be taken and documented on the pre-operative checklist. These should include blood pressure, pulse, temperature, respiratory rate, oxygen saturations, a neurological assessment (using AVPU), blood glucose, body weight, and urinalysis.

Clinical notes and X-rays

The patient's notes should accompany the patient to theatre and include a summary of the patient's past medical history and present condition. Relevant investigation results and X-rays should be present for the anaesthetist and surgeon to review in theatre. The notes should include details of allergies, and if electronic prescribing is not being used the patient's prescription chart must be sent to theatre with the clinical notes.

The patient should have been reviewed by an anaesthetist before going to theatre, and this assessment should be documented within the notes.

References

4 National Patient Safety Agency (NPSA). *Standardising Wristbands Improves Patient Safety: guidance on implementing the Safer Practice Notice.* NPSA: London, 2007.

5 Information Standards Board for Health and Social Care. *AIDC for Patient Identification.* Department of Health: London, 2013.

6 National Institute for Health and Care Excellence (NICE). *Surgical Site Infection.* QS49. NICE: London, 2013. ℛ www.nice.org.uk/guidance/qs49

7 National Institute for Health and Care Excellence (NICE). *Venous Thromboembolism Prevention Quality Standard.* QS3. NICE: London, 2010.

Intra-operative care

The operating theatre team

The operating theatre is a highly specialized environment in which patients are cared for before, during, and after their procedure. The operating theatre is staffed by a range of medical staff (see Table 7.1) and other healthcare professionals (see Table 7.2).

Table 7.1 Medical staff roles in the operating theatre team

Team role	Qualification and experience
Consultant anaesthetist	A qualified doctor who has completed post-basic training in anaesthesia and intensive care
Anaesthetic trainee	A qualified doctor on a training programme to become a consultant anaesthetist. Training is dependent upon Fellow of the Royal College of Anaesthetists (FRCA) qualification, assessment, and ≥ 8 years' clinical experience
Consultant surgeon	A qualified doctor who has completed a post-basic training programme as a trainee in surgery. Consultant surgeons will sub-specialize during their training in the chosen field, including general surgery, trauma, orthopaedics, colorectal, breast, vascular, urology, transplant, cardiothoracic, and gynaecological surgery
Surgical trainee	A qualified doctor on a training programme to become a consultant surgeon. Training is dependent upon Fellow of the Royal College of Surgeons (FRCS) qualification, assessment, and ≥ 8 years' clinical experience

Table 7.2 Members of the operating theatre team

Team role	Qualification and experience
Nursing (scrub)	A registered nurse (RN) who has experience and skills in the support of the surgical team during the operation. They manage the surgical environment, including instruments, swabs, and sutures
Nursing (recovery)	An RN who has experience and skills in the care of patients immediately after the procedure, such as airway management and pain control
Circulating person	Operating department practitioners (ODPs) and RNs who support the surgical team during the procedure, including patient positioning, diathermy, and additional equipment
Operating department practitioner (ODP)	A registered technical practitioner who has trained in all areas of peri-operative care, including anaesthetics, scrub, and recovery
Support worker	A support to the surgical team in circulating and administration roles, similar to the support worker role on wards. Often national vocational qualification (NVQ) qualified
Assistant practitioner	An NVQ-qualified support role that is able to perform more technical roles than the support worker. This may include patient positioning, instrument counts, and scrubbing for basic surgical cases
Allied health professional (radiographer)	A qualified radiographer who provides imaging (plain film, image intensifier, and ultrasound) during procedures
Allied health professional (perfusionist)	A specialist who is qualified to manage a perfusion machine during cardiothoracic surgery
Physicians' assistant (anaesthesia) PA(A)	A specialist who is qualified to directly support the anaesthetist in the delivery of anaesthesia. They work in a team with anaesthetists, enabling one medically qualified anaesthetist to simultaneously administer anaesthesia in two places. These must be adjacent or very close together within a single operating suite

Safe site surgery checklist

A core set of safety checks has been identified in the form of a World Health Organization (WHO) Surgical Safety Checklist for use in any operating-theatre environment. The checklist is a tool to enable the relevant clinical teams to improve the safety of surgery by reducing the number of deaths and complications.

The safe site surgery checklist consists of three main elements:
- sign in (see Box 7.1)
- time out (see Box 7.2)
- sign out (see Box 7.3).

Box 7.1 Sign in (to be read aloud)

Before induction of anaesthesia

Has the patient confirmed their identity, site, procedure, and consent? Yes

Is the surgical site marked? Yes/not applicable

Is the anaesthesia machine and medication check complete? Yes

Does the patient have a:
Known allergy? Yes/No
Difficult airway/aspiration risk? No/Yes, and equipment/assistance available
Risk of > 500 mL blood loss (7 mL/kg in children)? No/Yes, and adequate IV access/fluids planned

---

Box 7.2 Time out (to be read aloud)

Before start of surgical intervention (e.g. skin incision)

Have all team members introduced themselves by name and role? Yes

Surgeon, anaesthetist, and registered practitioner verbally confirm:
- What is the patient's name?
- What procedure, site, and position are planned?

Anticipated critical events
Surgeon:
- How much blood loss is anticipated?
- Are there specific equipment requirements or special investigations?
- Are there any critical or unexpected steps you want the team to know about?

(Continued)

Box 7.2 (*Contd.*)

Anaesthetist:
- Are there any patient-specific concerns?
- What is the patient's American Society of Anesthesiologists (ASA) grade?
- What monitoring equipment and other specific levels of support are required (e.g. blood)?

Nurse/ODP:
- Has the sterility of the instrumentation been confirmed (including indicator results)?
- Are there any equipment issues or concerns?

Has the surgical site infection (SSI) bundle been undertaken?
- Yes/not applicable
- Antibiotic prophylaxis within the last 60 min
- Patient warming
- Hair removal
- Glycaemic control

Has venous thromboembolism prophylaxis been undertaken?
- Yes/not applicable

Is essential imaging displayed?
- Yes/not applicable

Box 7.3 Sign out (to be read aloud)

Before any member of the team leaves the operating room

Registered practitioner verbally confirms with the team:
- Has the name of the procedure been recorded?
- Has it been confirmed that instruments, swabs, and sharp counts are complete (or not applicable)?
- Have the specimens been labelled (including patient name)?
- Have any equipment problems been identified that need to be addressed?

Surgeon, anaesthetist, and registered practitioner:
- What are the key concerns for recovery and management of this patient?

Types of anaesthesia

Anaesthesia can be divided into the following main types of approach:
- general anaesthesia
- total intravenous anaesthesia
- regional anaesthesia
- local anaesthesia.

It is common for anaesthetists to combine approaches to ensure that patients are physiologically more stable during surgery and have better post-operative pain control. For example, general anaesthesia and regional techniques such as an epidural are used in a complex abdominal procedure, or a regional spinal block and local infiltration into the wound following knee replacement.

Anaesthetic techniques are altered depending upon the type and urgency of surgery.

Planned surgery

Planned surgery involves pre-operative assessment and the opportunity to discuss anaesthetic techniques with the patient. This will enable the anaesthesia team to discuss the use of patient-controlled analgesia (PCA), epidurals, and other techniques used during surgery. Airway management issues can be planned based upon assessment. Patients are routinely fasted to ensure that the risk of aspiration is reduced.

Emergency and trauma surgery

Emergency and trauma surgery, by its nature, reduces the time to optimize a patient's condition prior to surgery. The nature of the condition will dictate the timing of surgery. These patients still require thorough assessment and management by the anaesthesia team prior to surgery. Patients are often not fasted, and an adapted technique called rapid sequence induction (RSI) is used to protect them from the risk of aspiration.

General anaesthesia

General anaesthesia is a common technique for ensuring that the patient is sedated and pain free during a surgical procedure. It is a reversible and controlled state of unconsciousness and loss of sensation to pain or surgical stimulus following the administration of anaesthetic agents. Classically, general anaesthesia consists of three main elements, known as the 'triad of anaesthesia' (see Figure 7.1). Anaesthesia consists of the following phases:

- induction
- maintenance
- emergence and recovery.

Induction

Patients are induced using either intravenous or inhalation techniques, which are chosen based upon the urgency of surgery. Intravenous induction consists of three main elements based on the triad. Hypnosis is achieved with intravenous agents given via a cannula as a bolus dose. These agents include:

- thiopental
- propofol
- etomidate.

Potent analgesics (e.g. fentanyl, alfentanil, remifentanil) are also given at induction, to obtund the pain response to airway insertion.

Muscle relaxation is achieved with a variety of drugs depending on the requirements of the patient's clinical condition and assessment. In the emergency scenario, an RSI technique uses suxamethonium, a rapid and short-acting depolarizing muscle relaxant. For planned surgery and maintenance of muscle relaxation during surgery, other long-acting non-depolarizing agents are used (e.g. atracurium, vecuronium, pancuronium, rocuronium). They also aid mechanical ventilation and surgical access.

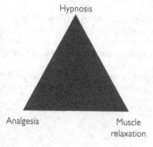

Figure 7.1 The triad of anaesthesia.

Induction precipitates a loss of consciousness and central nervous system (CNS) depression, including loss of protective airway reflexes and breathing. A device is inserted to protect the airway, and the patient requires short-term positive pressure ventilation until they are self-ventilating or, if muscle relaxants are given, until they are placed on a ventilator.

Inhalation techniques require agents that are rapidly absorbed into the circulatory system. Although many inhalation gases can be used for this, sevoflurane is preferred, due to its rapid absorbency and its reduced pungency and irritant effects on the airway.

Maintenance

Maintenance of anaesthesia requires the continued use of inhalational agents or a total intravenous anaesthesia (TIVA) technique. Inhalation agents from the following list are chosen on the basis of their characteristics:

- sevoflurane
- desflurane
- isoflurane
- halothane.

Patients are also given a mixture of oxygen (O_2) and nitrous oxide (N_2O), with continued analgesia and muscle relaxation via bolus dose or infusion.

The patient's physiological parameters are continuously monitored, and patients with comorbidity or who require complex surgery may have additional monitoring, such as central venous pressure, cardiac output studies, arterial blood pressure, and urine output.

Fluids are also given to counter insensible loss, gastrointestinal loss, and blood loss during surgery.

Emergence and recovery

Emergence from anaesthesia requires careful management of the polypharmacy to ensure that the patient wakes without residual effects of muscle relaxation, with appropriate levels of analgesia, and with return of their protective airway reflexes.

Inhaled or intravenous agents are stopped. With modern drugs and their known pharmacodynamic properties, this can take minutes, but is dependent upon dose and duration. Muscle relaxants often wear off around 20–30 min after the last dose, but can be reversed using glycopyrrolate.

Analgesia is titrated to the dose that relieves the patient's pain, with stronger opiates such as fentanyl discontinued, and morphine sulfate given by bolus, infusion, or PCA.

Total intravenous anaesthesia (TIVA)

TIVA can be defined as a technique of general anaesthesia that uses a combination of agents given solely by the intravenous route and in the absence of all inhalational agents. TIVA techniques have become increasingly common in anaesthesia due to the development of drugs such as propofol and short-acting opiates (e.g. remifentanil) with far greater refinement and control than inhalation agents. In addition, the use of target-controlled infusion (TCI) devices has enabled greater control of therapeutic levels of the drugs within the circulation.

Induction of anaesthesia is conducted in a similar way to general anaesthesia with a bolus dose of induction agent, such as propofol. After the induction phase, a continuous infusion of the agent and opiate is delivered to the patient by a TCI device. The depth of anaesthesia is controlled by manipulation of the agent by the TCI device to ensure that the patient remains sedated and pain free. On emergence from anaesthesia, the TCI rate is reduced to provide a rapid emergence.

The advantages of TIVA include rapid recovery from anaesthesia due to the short half-life of the agent and opiate. This ensures that the patient is awake, their airway is self-maintained sooner, and it often reduces drowsiness, post-operative nausea and vomiting, compared with inhalation techniques.

Regional anaesthesia

Regional anaesthesia is defined as induction of the loss of sensation of a region (e.g. the lower half) or a part (e.g. a limb) of the body using a local anaesthetic drug. Regional techniques are divided into:

• central or neuraxial blocks (epidural or spinal)
• peripheral blocks (plexus or single nerve blocks).

Detailed neuroanatomical knowledge is required in order to deliver safe and effective regional anaesthesia. Local anaesthetic agents such as bupivacaine, and lidocaine are injected adjacent to the nerve supply, to create the anaesthesia for the chosen region based on its known spinal nerve route distribution (see Figures 7.2 and 7.3).

Central blocks

Epidural block

An epidural is a technique commonly employed to provide analgesia and anaesthesia in a range of clinical scenarios, including labour, Caesarean section, and orthopaedic lower limb and abdominal procedures. It can be given as an adjunct to general anaesthesia for pain control, or on its own so that the patient remains awake, or if the patient has comorbidities that would preclude general anaesthesia.

A needle (Tuohy) is inserted into the epidural space in the posterior spine outside the dura mater. A small-gauge catheter is often inserted to provide a continuous infusion of local anaesthetic. The speed of analgesia is dependent upon the volume of drug infused and its strength, and is in the range of 2–15 min. The effect creates analgesia of the nerve roots from the point of insertion. For example, high thoracic epidurals at T5–T7 would provide cover for a thoracotomy, at T8–T10 they would do so for laparotomy, and at L2–L4 they would do so for hip and knee surgery.

Complications following the use of epidurals include:

• block height higher than intended due to local anaesthetic spread, affecting respiratory and cardiac function
• hypotension due to sympathetic blockade
• 'dural tap' or puncture of the dura mater, causing leakage of cerebrospinal fluid
• epidural haematoma
• infection
• nerve root damage
• block failure or 'patchy block' (e.g. unilateral).

Spinal (subarachnoid) block

A spinal block is the deliberate breaching of the dura mater in order to introduce local anaesthesia directly into the subarachnoid space by means of a specially adapted needle. This creates a rapid regional analgesic effect, although of limited duration (typically 1–2 h), and is used routinely for Caesarean section, total hip and knee replacement, and transurethral resection of the prostate.

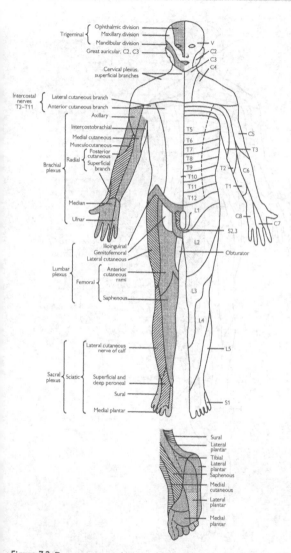

Figure 7.2 Dermatome map: front view. Reproduced from Keith Allman and Iain Wilson, *Oxford Handbook of Anaesthesia*, Third Edition, 2011, with permission from Oxford University Press.

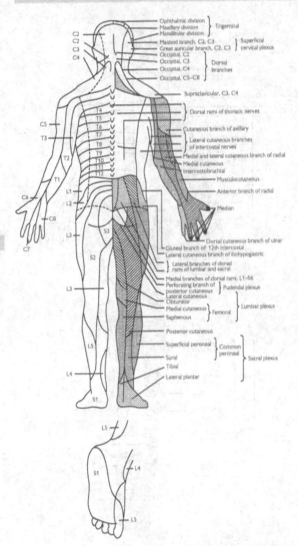

Figure 7.3 Dermatome map: back view. Reproduced from Keith Allman and Iain Wilson, *Oxford Handbook of Anaesthesia*, Third Edition, 2011, with permission from Oxford University Press.

Specific local anaesthetic is used, called Marcain Heavy® 0.5%, to prevent flow higher than the insertion point.

Complications that may occur following a spinal block include:

- block height higher than intended due to local anaesthetic spread, affecting respiratory and cardiac function
- hypotension due to sympathetic blockade
- haematoma
- infection
- nerve root damage
- block failure or 'patchy block' (e.g. unilateral).

Local anaesthesia

Local anaesthesia is a technique used to create a reversible area of loss of pain sensation by infiltration of a local anaesthetic drug.

Local anaesthetics are formulated as the hydrochloride salt to render them water soluble. Epinephrine (adrenaline) is often added in an attempt to slow down absorption from the site of injection and to prolong the duration of action.

There are two main groups of drugs:

1. Amides:
   - lidocaine
   - prilocaine
   - mepivacaine
   - bupivacaine
   - ropivacaine
   - levobupivacaine.
2. Esters:
   - cocaine
   - procaine
   - tetracaine
   - chloroprocaine.

Each drug has pharmacological benefits, such as onset time, duration, and toxicity level, which are used in clinical practice. Local anaesthetics can be administered by the following routes:

- topical (skin, mucous membranes)
- skin infiltration
- neural blockade.

Complications

- Allergy (due to vasopressors and preservatives).
- Local toxicity:
  - intraneural injection
  - neural ischaemia due to local pressure
  - radicular irritation caused by high-dose lidocaine.
- Systemic toxicity:
  - CNS depression and apnoea
  - cardiac effects (lowered heart rate, lowered blood pressure, arrhythmia, and cardiac arrest).

Airway assessment

Following the induction of anaesthesia, the loss of reflexes and respiratory function through the anaesthetic agents requires rapid control of the airway to ensure continued oxygenation and prevention of complications. Prior to anaesthesia it is important that the airway is assessed for any potential difficulties. Assessment should consider the following issues.

Patient history

- Previous history of difficult intubation.
- Tumours of the head and neck.
- Arthritis.
- Pregnancy.
- Trauma—cervical spine injury and full stomach.

Physical examination

- Tongue versus pharyngeal size.
- Atlanto-occipital joint extension:
  - cervical spine mobility (normal value is 35°).
- Anterior mandibular space and mobility:
  - thyromental distance (normal value is > 6 cm)
  - ability to sublux the jaw.
- Dental examination (loose teeth, prostheses).
- Mallampati score.

The Mallampati score is widely used and involves the patient opening their mouth wide while sitting in front of the anaesthetist. The patient is assigned a grade according to the best view obtained (see Figure 7.4). Grade 1 usually predicts an easy intubation, whereas Grade 3 or 4 suggests there is a significant likelihood that the patient will prove difficult to intubate. The results of this test are influenced by the ability to open the mouth, and by the size and mobility of the tongue and other intra-oral structures.

The type of airway selected will be based on a number of factors, including the type of surgery, its duration, and the potential for complications.

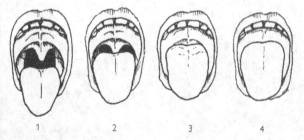

Figure 7.4 Mallampati grade 1, 2, 3, and 4. Reproduced from Keith Allman and Iain Wilson, *Oxford Handbook of Anaesthesia*, Third Edition, 2011, with permission from Oxford University Press.

Manual airway management techniques

There are a number of approaches that can be used to provide initial support of the airway of an anaesthetized patient. They include manipulation of the airway using the following techniques.

The *head tilt* and *chin lift* are used to lift the tongue from the back of the throat (see Figures 7.5 and 7.6). This technique is not advocated for patients with a potential cervical spine injury or condition.

The *jaw thrust* displaces the mandible forward, and pulls the tongue forward, thereby preventing it from occluding the tracheal opening. This technique can be used for patients with a cervical injury alongside in-line stabilization techniques or fixed collar support (see Figure 7.7).

These techniques create a patent airway, but require supplementation with additional oxygenation via a mask with intermittent positive pressure ventilation (IPPV). This is often called 'bag and mask' ventilation.

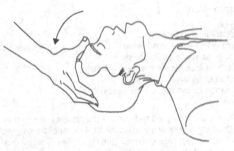

Figure 7.5 Performing a head tilt. Reproduced from James Thomas and Tanya Monaghan, *Oxford Handbook of Clinical Examination and Practical Skills*, 2007, with permission from Oxford University Press.

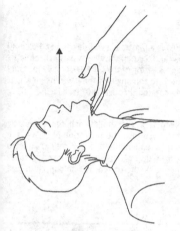

Figure 7.6 Performing a chin lift. Reproduced from James Thomas and Tanya Monaghan, *Oxford Handbook of Clinical Examination and Practical Skills*, 2007, with permission from Oxford University Press.

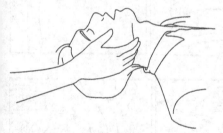

Figure 7.7 Performing a jaw thrust. Reproduced from James Thomas and Tanya Monaghan, *Oxford Handbook of Clinical Examination and Practical Skills*, 2007, with permission from Oxford University Press.

Airway adjuncts

Oropharyngeal airway

An oropharyngeal airway (OPA) is a plastic curved device used to hold the tongue away from the airway and to keep the airway patent in patients with no gag reflex. In adult patients, sizing of the OPA is done by measuring from the middle of the mouth to the angle of the jaw. The airway is inserted upside down, and then rotated through 180° (see Figure 7.8).

Nasopharyngeal airway

A nasopharyngeal airway (NPA) is a soft hollow rubber or plastic tube that is passed through the nose into the posterior pharynx (see Figure 7.9). NPAs are tolerated by patients with a gag reflex, and are easier to insert than an OPA. Insertion of a NPA is preferred in cases where the patient's jaw is clenched or the patient is semiconscious and cannot tolerate an OPA.

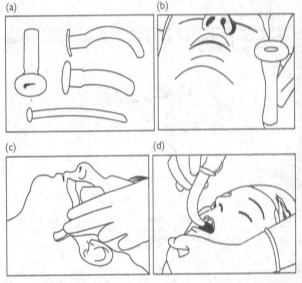

Figure 7.8 (a) Oropharyngeal and nasopharyngeal airways. (b, c) Sizing of an oropharyngeal airway. (d) Insertion of an oropharyngeal airway. Reproduced from George Castledine and Ann Close, *Oxford Handbook of Adult Nursing*, 2007, with permission from Oxford University Press.

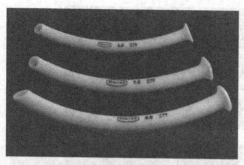

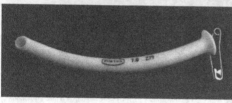

Figure 7.9 Nasopharyngeal airways. Reproduced from James Thomas and Tanya Monaghan, *Oxford Handbook of Clinical Examination and Practical Skills*, 2007, with permission from Oxford University Press.

Laryngeal mask airway (LMA)

The LMA (see Figure 7.10) consists of a tube with an inflatable cuff that is inserted into the pharynx. It is classed as a supraglottic airway, and can be used for patients who are self-ventilating or who require IPPV. LMAs are frequently used in day-case surgery and as an airway in cardiopulmonary resuscitation.

The LMA does not fully protect the trachea, and there is a risk of aspiration. Therefore it is contraindicated in the following situations:
• full stomach/significant aspiration risk (including hiatus hernia)
• morbidly obese patients
• patients with oropharyngeal pathology that is likely to result in a poor mask fit (e.g. radiotherapy for the hypopharynx or larynx)
• glottic surgery.
Caution is also needed if using the LMA:
• for a patient on positive pressure ventilation (PPV) with high airway pressures
• during very long procedures
• for a patient in a prone position.

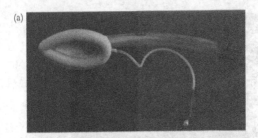

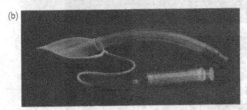

Figure 7.10 Laryngeal mask airway (LMA). (a) Inflated LMA. (b) Deflated LMA. Reproduced from James Thomas and Tanya Monaghan, *Oxford Handbook of Clinical Examination and Practical Skills*, 2007, with permission from Oxford University Press.

Endotracheal intubation

Endotracheal intubation is the placement of a tube into the trachea to maintain a patent airway in a patient who is unconscious. The tube is inserted through the vocal cords under direct visualization using a laryngoscope. The tube is placed in the trachea and a balloon cuff is inflated to ensure an air seal to allow PPV.

Complications
These include:
• oral and dental trauma
• laryngospasm
• bronchospasm
• tracheal ulceration (with longer-term intubation).

Patient positioning during surgery

The aim of optimal positioning for surgery is to provide optimum surgical access while minimizing the potential risk to the patient. The choice of position will depend on the type of procedure. Commonly adopted positions include the following:

• supine
• lithotomy
• Lloyd Davies
• lateral
• seated
• prone.

Many of these are modified with the addition of a vertical tilt (Trendelenburg or reverse Trendelenburg).

Each position carries some degree of clinical risk and physiological compromise, which are magnified in the anaesthetized patient. In addition, when anaesthetized a patient cannot make others aware of pain, discomfort, or other problems. Common problems can be summarized as follows.

Respiratory problems

Some positions, including the supine position, can restrict movement of the thorax or diaphragm and impede airflow, particularly in the case of obese patients. Obese patients must be seated upright for the duration of most procedures because of increased abdominal pressure on the chest when they are supine.

Circulatory problems

Lithotomy positions and the severe head-down positions used during some laparoscopic procedures may compromise blood flow to the lower extremities, or venous return of blood to the heart. Pressure on or obstruction of a vessel can cause the most damage to the cardiovascular system. This can be avoided by reducing the procedure time, if possible, or by moving the limbs and massaging them at regular intervals during the procedure.

Skin problems

Friction and pressure on soft tissues, especially over bony prominences, may result in changes that range from mild irritation to severe pressure-induced ischaemia.

Neurological problems

Pressure or obstruction due to faulty positioning is a common cause of nerve injury, as the case of the patient with ulnar nerve damage makes clear. Motor or sensory nerve damage can occur within minutes, and can have a long-term effect.

Inadvertent peri-operative hypothermia

Inadvertent peri-operative hypothermia (IPH) is a common but preventable complication of peri-operative procedures, and is associated with poor outcomes for patients. During the first 30–40 min of anaesthesia, a patient's temperature can drop to below 35.0°C. Reasons for this include loss of the behavioural response to cold, and the impairment of thermoregulatory heat-preserving mechanisms under general or regional anaesthesia, anaesthesia-induced peripheral vasodilation (with associated heat loss), and the patient becoming cold while waiting (on the ward or in the emergency department) for surgery. Management of IPH consists of three phases.

Pre-operative phase

Each patient should be assessed for their risk of inadvertent peri-operative hypothermia and potential adverse consequences before they are transferred to the theatre suite. The patient should be managed as higher risk if any two of the following apply:

* ASA grade II–V (the higher the grade, the greater the risk)
* the patient's pre-operative temperature is below 36.0°C, and pre-operative warming is not possible because of clinical urgency
* the patient is undergoing combined general and regional anaesthesia
* the patient is undergoing major or intermediate surgery
* the patient is at risk of cardiovascular complications.

Forced air warming should be started pre-operatively on the ward or in the emergency department, unless there is a need to expedite surgery because of clinical urgency (e.g. due to bleeding or critical limb ischaemia). Forced air warming should be maintained throughout the procedure.

Intra-operative phase

The patient's temperature should be measured and documented before induction of anaesthesia and then every 30 min until the end of surgery.

* Induction of anaesthesia should not begin unless the patient's temperature is ≥ 36.0°C, except when there is a need to expedite surgery because of clinical urgency (e.g. due to bleeding or critical limb ischaemia).
* Intravenous fluids (500 mL or more) and blood products should be warmed to 37°C using a fluid-warming device.
* Patients who are at higher risk of inadvertent peri-operative hypothermia and who are having anaesthesia for less than 30 min should be warmed intra-operatively from induction of anaesthesia, using a forced air-warming device.
* All patients who are having anaesthesia for longer than 30 min should be warmed intra-operatively from induction of anaesthesia using a forced air-warming device.

Post-operative phase

The patient's temperature should be measured and documented on admission to the recovery room and then every 15 min.
- Ward transfer should not be arranged unless the patient's temperature is ≥ 36.0°C.
- If the patient's temperature is < 36.0°C, they should be actively warmed using a forced air-warming device until they are discharged from the recovery room, or until they are comfortably warm.

Further reading

National Institute for Health and Care Excellence (NICE). *Inadvertent Perioperative Hypothermia: the management of inadvertent perioperative hypothermia in adults.* CG65. NICE: London, 2008. ℔ www.nice.org.uk/guidance/cg65

Immediate post-operative recovery

After general or regional anaesthesia, all patients should recover in a specially designated area within the operating theatre. Patients are cared for in the recovery area by appropriately trained staff on a one-to-one basis. The purpose of the post-operative recovery period is to:

- ensure that the patient has regained control of their airway, demonstrated cardiovascular stability, and is able to communicate
- monitor and manage post-operative complications (e.g. bleeding)
- achieve effective control of pain and post-operative nausea and vomiting (PONV).

Minimum standards of monitoring during post-operative recovery are:

- heart rate and rhythm
- blood pressure
- respiratory rate
- saturations
- temperature
- conscious/sedation level
- fluid management.

In addition, more complex surgery will require more detailed monitoring, including:

- invasive blood pressure (arterial)
- central venous pressure (CVP)
- urine output.

Monitoring should be commenced immediately on arrival of the patient in the recovery area, and the frequency of monitoring should be determined by the patient's clinical condition. Observations every 5 min are a minimum requirement until the patient is fully conscious.

Nursing care with regard to comfort, pressure areas, catheters, drains, wounds, and psychological support is also required.

The time period for which the patient stays in the recovery area will be dictated by the procedure time, monitoring requirements, pain and PONV management, and complications. Simple cases may require 20 min, whereas patients who have undergone more complicated surgery may need to stay in the recovery area for hours.

Handover

The following criteria must be fulfilled before a patient is discharged from the recovery unit:

- The patient is fully conscious without excessive stimulation, able to maintain a clear airway, and exhibits protective airway reflexes.
- Respiration and oxygenation are satisfactory.
- The cardiovascular system is stable, with no unexplained cardiac irregularity or persistent bleeding. The specific values of pulse and blood pressure should approximate to normal pre-operative values or be at an acceptable level, commensurate with the planned post-operative care. Peripheral perfusion should be adequate.
- Pain and emesis should be controlled, and suitable analgesic and anti-emetic regimens prescribed.
- The patient's temperature should be within acceptable limits. They should not be returned to the ward if significant hypothermia is present.
- If appropriate, oxygen and intravenous therapy should be prescribed.

Handing over to ward staff

Patients should be transferred to the ward accompanied by a suitably trained member of staff and a porter. The anaesthetic record, together with the recovery and prescription charts, must accompany the patient. The recovery nurse must ensure that full clinical details are relayed to the ward nurse, with a particular emphasis on problems and syringe pump settings.

Further reading

Whitaker DK et al. Immediate post-anaesthesia recovery 2013: Association of Anaesthetists of Great Britain and Ireland. *Anaesthesia* 2013; **68**: 288–97.

Ward post-operative care

Post-operative ward checks

Post-operative care requires a systematic and thorough approach to ensure the patient's safety, comfort, and recovery. Standardized post-operative routines should be supported by thorough and inclusive documentation (whether paper or electronically based), in order to reduce the risk of the care provider overlooking an important aspect of patient care. There are multiple reasons why these checks are so important, including how the patient is recovering from the anaesthesia and surgery, how well their pain is managed, and whether there are any potential problems that need attention. The checks cover measurable parameters (e.g. vital signs), as well as observation of the patient, including pallor and comfort.

Observation of the patient
- General colour/pallor.
- Sweating.
- Mobility of limbs.
- Confusion and/or agitation—post-operative delirium can occur in any patient group, but is common in patients with pre-existing dementia.

Physiological signs
- Respiration rate.
- Oxygen saturation.
- Pulse.
- Blood pressure.
- Temperature.
- Urine output.
- Pain score.
- Nausea and/or post-operative vomiting.
- Sedation level and responsiveness, which can be measured as AVPU in the National Early Warning Score (NEWS), or as part of the Glasgow Coma Scale (GCS) in the neurosurgical patient or the head-injured patient.
- Blood glucose levels.

Surgical intervention
- Observe the surgical wound for signs of bleeding, swelling, and the patency of dressings present. If excessive bleeding or swelling is noted there may be potential problems with wound closure which will need a surgical review by the medical team.
- Surgical drains should be observed for the colour, consistency, and amount draining, as this may indicate potential internal bleeding. The patency of the drain also needs to be checked to ensure that it is effective.
- Surgical devices (e.g. traction or pins) should be checked to ensure that they are appropriately attached and dressed according to wound care protocol.

- Catheters (peripheral, central, and urinary) should all be patent, dressed according to protocol, and accurately documented as such.
- Stomas—in colorectal surgery there may be a stoma present that needs to be observed for bleeding or herniation, and its colour monitored to ensure that appropriate perfusion is maintained. Tracheostomy sites need to be checked for bleeding and patency, as any obstruction could lead to a medical emergency.

Therapies

- Intravenous fluids—prescribed, administered, and documented accurately.
- Oxygen therapy—prescribed and delivered via the appropriate equipment at the correct flow rate, and oxygen saturation monitoring included in routine observations. As part of the oxygen prescription, target oxygenation saturation levels should be documented.
- Pain relief—prescribed, administered, and documented, including regular assessment of the patient's pain score to assess the effectiveness of the analgesia administered.
- Wound therapy (e.g. vacuum-assisted closure).
- Specific treatment regimes in place and correct.

Patient safety

- Correct pressure-relieving strategy in place.
- Pressure area checks completed as per policy.
- Use of bedside rails and/or 'high/low bed' if needed following documented risk assessment.
- Documented care of post-operative delirium.
- Nurse call-bell within reach and working.
- Accessibility of drinks and food if the patient is not NBM.
- Visibility of post-operative patient to ward staff.

Psychological care

- Give regular reassurance and explain all procedures that are being performed post-operatively.
- Provide a full explanation of the surgical procedure and allow the patient the opportunity to ask questions, once the anaesthetic has worn off sufficiently for this.
- Gain consent for procedures being carried out (e.g. blood pressure monitoring).
- Explanation of patient experiences (e.g. post-operative nausea, delirium).
- Provide relatives with the opportunity to ask questions and, with the patient's consent, keep them fully informed of the patient's condition.

Frequency of post-operative observations

This is difficult to dictate as a set routine for *all* procedures, because the level and/or frequency of observations will always be dependent on a number of factors, such as the anaesthetic used, the length and type of operation, and the physiological systems that are affected by the procedure, as well as factors specific to the patient, such as their age, comorbidities, and medication.

Baseline observations should be performed at the point of transfer of care from the theatre to the ward, so that both groups of staff are aware of the patient's condition on handover. Patients undergoing simple procedures under local anaesthesia may require no further observations. However, all patients who have received a general anaesthetic or regional anaesthesia will need repeated observations until the effects of the anaesthesia have decreased, the patient's condition has stabilized, and the risk of deterioration has lessened.

As a general guide, observations after moderate to major surgery are needed:

- every 15 min for 1 h
- every 30 min for a further 2 h
- hourly for a further 4 h
- 4-hourly thereafter until the patient is stable, or as per local policy.

This is intended as a guide, and local policy may differ. However, if the patient appears to be deteriorating or their improvement or stabilization is slower than normal, observations must be performed more frequently.

Care pathways for specific conditions and types of surgery may be in use that will guide monitoring of the patient. However, these are again a guide to the minimum observations that are needed, and if a patient's condition requires it, more frequent observations should be performed.

National Early Warning Score (NEWS)

The National Institute for Health and Care Excellence (NICE)[1] has stated that 'all adult patients in acute hospital settings should be monitored using physiological track and trigger systems. Physiological observations should be monitored at least every 12 hours, unless a decision has been made at a senior level to decrease or increase the frequency of observations for an individual patient.'

Track and trigger systems allocate points in a weighted manner based on derangements in a patient's vital signs. The sum of the allocated points is known as the 'early warning score', and it directs the patient's care.[2] In the UK, numerous early warning systems are being used in different hospitals, resulting in a lack of consistency in detecting and responding to patients' deterioration. It also leads to confusion and the potential for mistakes when healthcare staff move to work in different departments and different hospitals.

In 2012, the Royal College of Physicians led the development of the National Early Warning Score (NEWS)[3] after working in partnership with patients and a number of professional groups. The NEWS is based on the allocation of scores to six physiological parameters:

- respiratory rate
- oxygen saturation
- temperature
- systolic blood pressure
- pulse rate
- level of consciousness (AVPU).

Table 8.1 shows the NEWS score grid, with the parameter ranges and scores for each of the six physiological parameters. The patient's observations are documented on the NEWS observation chart, and the NEWS score is then calculated.

The NEWS clinical response grid provides advice on what action to take for the NEWS score calculated from the patient's observations. The action advised will include the frequency with which observations should be performed, and the clinical response required for that score (e.g. a registered nurse to assess the patient). *However, staff are reminded of the need to use clinical judgement and to summon senior help if they have any concerns about a patient, even if their NEWS score has not triggered a response.*

Blood glucose levels are not included in the NEWS score, but there is a section on the NEWS observation chart in which to record the patient's blood glucose concentration. Patients with type 1 or type 2 diabetes will need to have their blood glucose levels monitored post-operatively because they may be unstable due to the patient being NBM or having had their diabetic medication omitted prior to surgery. In addition, the stress response to surgery and the release of catecholamines can lead to raised blood glucose levels in both diabetic and non-diabetic patients. Therefore the monitoring of blood glucose levels post-operatively is important in all patients.

Table 8.1 National Early Warning Score (NEWS).[3] Reproduced from Royal College of Physicians. *National Early Warning Score (NEWS): standardising the assessment of acute-illness severity in the NHS. Report of a working party*. London: RCP, 2012.

Score	3	2	1	0	1	2	3
Respiratory rate (breaths/min)	< 8	—	9–11	12–20	—	21–24	> 25
Oxygen saturations	< 91	92–93	94–95	> 96			
Supplemental oxygen		Yes		No			
Temperature (°C)	< 35	—	35.1–36.0	36.1–38.0	38.1–39.0	> 39.0	—
Systolic blood pressure (mmHg)	< 90	91–100	101–110	111–219	—	—	> 220
Heart rate (beats/min)	< 40	—	41–50	51–90	91–110	111–130	> 131
AVPU	—	—	—	A			V, P, or U

AVPU = Alert, response to Voice, response to Pain, Unresponsive.

NEWS is not recommended for use in children or during pregnancy. The Royal College of Physicians[3] recommends that for patients with known hypercapnoeic respiratory failure due to chronic obstructive pulmonary disease (COPD), British Thoracic Society target saturations of 88–92%[4] should be used. These patients will still 'score' if their oxygen saturations are below 92%, unless the score is 'reset' by a competent clinical decision maker and patient-specific target oxygen saturations are prescribed and documented on the NEWS observation chart and in the clinical notes.

More information about the NEWS, including an e-learning package, can be found at http://tfinews.ocbmedia.com/

References

1 National Institute for Health and Care Excellence (NICE). *Acutely Ill Patients in Hospital: recognition of and response to acute illness in adults in hospital*. CG50. NICE: London, 2007. www.nice.org.uk/guidance/cg50
2 Smith G et al. The ability of the National Early Warning Score (NEWS) to discriminate patients at risk of early cardiac arrest, unanticipated intensive care unit admission and death. *Resuscitation* 2013; **84**: 465–70.
3 Royal College of Physicians. *National Early Warning Score (NEWS). Standardising the assessment of acute-illness severity in the NHS. Report of a working party*. London. Royal College of Physicians: London, 2012.
4 British Thoracic Society. *Guideline for Emergency Oxygen Use in Adult Patients*. British Thoracic Society: London, 2008.

Escalation and SBAR

When dealing with the acutely ill or deteriorating patient, communication needs to be assertive, concise, focused, and effective. The seriousness of the patient's condition needs to be imparted to colleagues, without delay to the patient's treatment, and also so that colleagues can prioritize their workload.

The NEWS score discussed earlier has a trigger tool that advises on the level of escalation needed. For example, a patient with a NEWS score of 6 will need to be escalated to a more senior colleague than a patient with a NEWS score of 3.

Escalation is always based upon patient need, and although it frequently follows hierarchical or medical experience lines, there is always the ability to 'skip' a step to escalate the more serious problems to the more senior staff. Utilizing the NEWS score allows medical staff to be confident that the patient's needs are as critical as the staff requesting assistance state they are.

To further enhance communication at this critical time, tools such as SBAR (Situation–Background–Assessment–Recommendation) (see Table 8.2) are now more commonly used. The NHS Institute for Innovation and Improvement[5] includes the SBAR tool in its quality and service improvement tools, stating that as a tool 'It enables you to clarify what information should be communicated between members of the team, and how. It can also help you to develop teamwork and foster a culture of patient safety.'

Table 8.2 SBAR tool. Reproduced with kind permission from NHS Improving Quality.

S	Situation
	• State your name and area.
	• Identify the patient (I am calling about …).
	• Describe your concerns (I am concerned because …).
B	Background
	• Diagnosis and date of admission.
	• A brief history and treatment to date.
A	Assessment
	• Vital signs.
	• Clinical impression (I think the problem is …).
R	Recommendation
	• Explain what you need, including the time span (I need you to … within … minutes).
	• Clarify expectations (What should I do now?).

Reference

5 NHS Institute for Innovation and Improvement. *SBAR – Situation – Background - Assessment – Recommendation*. NHS Institute for Innovation and Improvement: London, 2009. www.institute.nhs.uk/quality_and_service_improvement_tools/quality_and_service_improvement_tools/sbar_-_situation_-_background_-_assessment_-_recommendation.html

Post-operative oxygen therapy

Mild to moderate hypoxaemia is quite common in the first few hours after a general anaesthetic, especially following abdominal or thoracic surgery. This is attributed to a ventilation/perfusion (V/Q) mismatch. Other causes include ventilatory depression due to the residual effects of the anaesthetic and analgesics. The effects of the hypoxaemia are likely to be more severe in the presence of pre-existing risk factors such as cardiopulmonary disease and smoking.

The anaesthetist may prescribe oxygen therapy for a few hours post-operatively until the residual effects of the anaesthesia have worn off. The patient should have continuous oxygen saturation monitoring, aiming for 94–98%, and 88–92% for chronic lung conditions[6] such as chronic obstructive pulmonary disease (COPD).

If the patient requires oxygen for a prolonged period of time (> 24 h) or at high flow rates, the oxygen should be humidified to prevent dryness in the upper airways. The patient will also require regular oral fluids or oral toilet to prevent drying and cracking of their lips and oral mucosa.

Oxygen delivery systems

Oxygen delivery systems can be divided into two groups—variable performance systems and fixed performance systems. Variable performance systems provide a variable concentration of oxygen to the patient, at a low flow rate. The concentration of oxygen is variable because the patient's inspiratory flow rate is higher than the oxygen flow rate. This results in more atmospheric air being drawn in and diluting the oxygen concentration. Variable performance systems include nasal cannulae and simple face masks. They are suitable for patients who require oxygen at low concentrations and for short periods of time.[7] However, they are not appropriate for patients with high or variable respiratory rates, as this will affect the accuracy of the concentration of oxygen being delivered.

Fixed performance systems deliver oxygen at higher flow rates than normal inspiratory flow rates, and are often referred to as Venturi masks. A Venturi barrel is connected between the oxygen mask and tubing, oxygen passes through this narrow inlet, and air is entrained from the atmosphere. The concentration of oxygen is dependent upon the flow rate of oxygen via the Venturi barrel and the size of the holes in the side of the barrel, through which atmospheric air is entrained. The larger the holes in the Venturi barrel, the more air is entrained into the mask, and the lower the concentration of oxygen that is delivered.

Venturi masks can deliver between 24% and 60% oxygen, and they have different colour-coded barrels for delivering different concentrations of oxygen. On the side of each barrel is stated the percentage of oxygen that it will deliver and the flow rate at which the oxygen should be set. Fixed performance masks should be used for patients who require high or accurate concentrations of oxygen.

Respiratory failure

Respiratory failure results in inadequate levels of circulating oxygen, and can also lead to inadequate removal of carbon dioxide from the body. An arterial blood gas is required to diagnose whether a patient has type 1 or type 2 respiratory failure.

Type 1 respiratory failure is defined as a PaO_2 of < 8 kPa with a normal or low $PaCO_2$ level. Type 2 respiratory failure (hypercapnia) is present when the $PaCO_2$ is above the normal range of 4.6–6.1 kPa and the PaO_2 is low or normal.[6]

Oxygen therapy in patients with COPD

Normally a rise in the carbon dioxide level within arterial blood results in carbon dioxide crossing the blood–brain barrier into the cerebrospinal fluid (CSF). This increase in carbon dioxide level causes the pH of the CSF to fall, which stimulates the central chemoreceptors in the medulla. The central chemoreceptors in turn stimulate the respiratory centre to increase the rate and depth of breaths, in order to excrete the excess carbon dioxide.

Some patients with COPD have type 2 respiratory failure which results in blunting of the chemoreceptors, so that a rise in carbon dioxide level does not stimulate the respiratory centre, but instead a fall in the arterial oxygen level stimulates the respiratory centre. These patients are described as having a hypoxic drive, and it can be dangerous to give them high concentrations of oxygen. However, if a patient with COPD becomes acutely unwell they should be administered high-flow oxygen (100%) via a non-rebreathe mask. You should aim for oxygen saturations of 88–92% and titrate down the oxygen if the patient becomes drowsy or the saturations rise above 93–94%. The patient will also need to have regular arterial blood gases performed in order to determine their PaO_2 and $PaCO_2$ levels.[6]

References

6 British Thoracic Society. *Guideline for Emergency Oxygen Use in Adult Patients*. British Thoracic Society: London, 2008.

7 McGloin S. Administration of oxygen therapy. *Nursing Standard* 2008; **22**: 46–8.

Surgical drains

Following a surgical procedure a drain may be inserted to prevent the accumulation of fluid or air, or to drain away a collection of fluid (e.g. pus, an effusion) or air. A drain is generally inserted at the end of a surgical procedure through a separate hole to the main incision, in order to reduce the risk of a post-operative infection occurring.

The type of drain that is inserted can be either passive or active. A passive drain requires a higher pressure within the wound, in conjunction with gravity and capillary action to draw fluid out of the wound. An example of a passive drain is a stab drain attached to a reservoir drainage bag.

An active drain uses negative pressure to remove fluid from a wound, and requires the drain to be vacuumed. Vacuum drains are classified as being either high negative pressure drains (Redivac) or low negative pressure drains (Blake).

Care of surgical drains

- On return to the ward following surgery, document the volume in the drain.
- The frequency of monitoring of drainage will depend on the patient's condition, the surgical procedure, and the surgeon's instructions.
- Record the volume, colour, and consistency of drainage.
- Check that the drain is patent, observing for kinks, clots, or debris in the tubing.
- Ensure that low or high negative pressure drains are vacuumed.
- Check the drain site for signs of bleeding and swelling.
- Surgical drains can cause pain and discomfort, so assess the patient's pain score at regular intervals, and administer prescribed analgesia as required.
- Maintain asepsis when changing the drainage bottle/reservoir bag.

Equipment needed for removal of a negative pressure drain

An aseptic technique is used and the following equipment is needed:

- sterile dressing pack
- sterile gloves
- sterile stitch cutter
- normal saline
- non-adherent dressing
- disposable apron
- non-sterile gloves
- alcohol-based hand rub
- sharps bin.

Procedure for removal of a negative pressure drain

- Before removing the drain, assess the patient's pain score and administer prescribed analgesia as required.
- Explain the procedure to the patient and obtain their consent.
- Position the patient so that they are comfortable and you can gain access to the surgical drain site.
- Wash your hands, and put on a disposable apron and non-sterile gloves.
- Remove the dressing from the drain site.
- Release the vacuum on the drain according to the manufacturer's instructions.
- Remove the non-sterile gloves and clean your hands with alcohol-based hand rub.
- Open the dressing pack and all of the equipment required to remove the drain, and place on a sterile field.
- Put on sterile gloves and use the stitch cutter to remove the stitch, holding the drain *in situ*.
- Dispose of the stitch cutter in the sharps bin.
- Place a piece of dry gauze over the entry site, and then quickly and firmly remove the drain. If resistance is felt do not use undue force, but request a surgical review and ensure that the drain is safely secured.
- Clean the drain site with normal saline and gauze.
- Apply a non-adherent dressing.
- If the drain site continues to drain large volumes, apply a stoma bag.
- Check the fluid level in the drainage bottle and document this on the fluid balance chart.
- Seal the drainage bottle and dispose of it in a double clinical waste bag.
- Dispose of all waste in a clinical waste bag.
- Remove your apron and gloves and wash your hands.
- Document the care given to the patient in their notes.

Removal of sutures

Surgical sutures are classified as being absorbable or non-absorbable, depending on whether the body will naturally degrade and absorb the suture material. Depending on the material used, absorbable sutures will take from 10 days to 8 weeks to degrade.

The decision to remove non-absorbable sutures will be made by the healthcare team after they have reviewed the surgical wound site. The length of time for which sutures need to remain in place after surgery will depend on:

- the type of incision
- the location of the incision
- wound healing.

If the patient has been discharged home before the sutures have been removed, a practice nurse will remove them in the doctor's surgery, or a community nurse will remove them in the patient's home.

Equipment

An aseptic technique is used and the following equipment is needed:

- sterile dressing pack
- sterile gloves
- sterile stitch cutter
- sterile disposable forceps
- non-adherent dressing
- sharps bin
- normal saline
- disposable apron.

Procedure

- Explain the procedure to the patient and obtain their consent.
- Position the patient so that they are comfortable and you can gain access to the surgical wound site.
- Wash your hands and put on a disposable apron.
- Open the dressing pack and all of the equipment required to remove the sutures, and place on a sterile field.
- Put on the sterile gloves.
- Lift the first suture by grasping the knot with the forceps.
- Cut the suture as close to the skin as possible, using the stitch cutter and taking care not to pierce the patient's skin.
- Gently pull the suture out through the skin using the forceps. Do not use unnecessary force and risk the suture snapping inside the skin.
- This method is used to reduce the risk of infection by ensuring that the section of suture which has been lying on top of the skin does not pass through the wound.
- Repeat this procedure for all of the sutures.
- Check that all of the sutures have been completely removed.

- Dispose of the stitch cutter in the sharps bin.
- If necessary, clean the wound site using normal saline and gauze.
- If required, apply a non-adherent dressing.
- Dispose of all waste in a clinical waste bag.
- Remove your apron and gloves and wash your hands.
- Document the care given to the patient in their notes.

Removal of staples

Surgical staples are used in place of sutures to quickly close skin wounds that have fairly straight edges. The length of time for which staples remain *in situ* after surgery will depend upon:
- the size of the incision
- the location of the incision
- wound healing.

In some cases, alternate staples will be removed, and the remaining ones will be removed at a later date. If the patient has been discharged home before the staples have been removed, a practice nurse will remove them in the doctor's surgery, or a community nurse will remove them in the patient's home.

Equipment

An aseptic technique is used and the following equipment is needed:
- sterile dressing pack
- sterile gloves
- sterile disposable staple remover
- normal saline
- sharps bin
- disposable apron.

Procedure

- Explain the procedure to the patient and obtain their consent.
- Position the patient so that they are comfortable and you can gain access to the surgical wound site.
- Wash your hands and put on a disposable apron.
- Open the dressing pack and all of the equipment required to remove the staples, and place on a sterile field.
- Put on the sterile gloves.
- Holding the staple remover open, slide the lower half centrally between the staple and the skin.
- Gently close the handle of the staple remover, holding it at an angle of 90° to the skin.
- The staple should be automatically released from the skin.
- Repeat the procedure removing alternate staples, and then remove all of the staples.
- If required, clean the surgical wound site using sterile gauze and normal saline.
- Dispose of the staples and the staple remover in the sharps bin.
- Dispose of all waste in a clinical waste bag.
- Remove your apron and gloves and wash your hands.
- Document the care given to the patient in their notes.

Discharge planning

The NHS Institute for Innovation and Improvement has produced a quality and service improvement tool[8] for discharge planning, in order to improve the quality, efficiency, and productivity of patient care. Planning for discharge with clear dates and times will result in a reduction in:

- patient length of stay in hospital
- emergency readmissions to hospital
- pressure on hospital beds.

For elective surgery, discharge planning should start prior to admission during the pre-operative assessment in order to reduce unnecessary delays in the patient's pathway. Discharge planning should assess the physical, psychological, and social needs of the patient and their family.[9] This will enable healthcare staff to assess whether the patient has simple or complex discharge planning needs. Complex discharge planning needs will require additional input from other professionals, such as a social worker or an occupational therapist.

The Department of Health[10] has produced a guide outlining 10 key steps to achieving safe and timely discharge for patients. It is based on good practice that has been previously identified and evaluated. The 10 key steps are as follows:

- Start planning for discharge before or on admission.
- Identify whether the patient has simple or complex discharge needs, and involve the patient and carer(s) in your decision.
- Develop a clinical management plan within 24 h of admission.
- Coordinate the discharge, utilizing effective leadership and handover of responsibilities at ward level.
- Set an expected discharge date within 24–48 h of admission.
- Review the clinical management plan with the patient daily, taking action and updating them on progress towards the discharge date.
- Involve the patient and carer(s) in decisions to ensure a personalized care pathway.
- Plan discharges to take place over 7 days.
- Use a discharge checklist 24–48 h prior to discharge.
- Make decisions to discharge patients each day.

The Royal College of Nursing[9] has outlined the physical, psychological, and social criteria to be assessed when discharging a patient.

Physical criteria

- The patient's conscious level should be consistent with their pre-operative state.
- Cardiovascular and respiratory assessments should be stable.
- Gastrointestinal and renal input and output assessments should be undertaken.
- Pain, nausea, and vomiting should be minimal.
- The wound site should be clean and dry.
- The patient should be able to safely mobilize and climb a flight of stairs.

Psychological criteria

- Verbal and written information is provided about the patient's recovery at home in relation to the surgical procedure (e.g. when they can return to work, drive, etc.).
- Details of follow-up appointments are provided.
- Medication is provided, and it is ensured that the patient understands the administration regime.
- Contact numbers for emergency and continuing care are provided.
- A general practitioner letter is either given to the patient or posted.
- If required, referral to the district nurse or practice nurse for either dressing change or removal of sutures or staples is arranged.
- A letter, dressings, and medical supplies are provided for the district nurse or practice nurse.

Social criteria

- Transport home should be arranged.
- The home environment should be suitable for the patient following the surgery undertaken (e.g. access to a telephone and a lift if they live in a flat).
- If required, referral to a social worker or occupational therapist should be made.
- The need for any mobility support (e.g. Zimmer frame, crutches, walking stick) should be assessed.
- Arrangements should be made for the patient and/or carer(s) to take time off work.

References

8 NHS Institute for Innovation and Improvement. *Discharge Planning.* NHS Institute for Innovation and Improvement: Leeds, 2008. ℐ www.institute.nhs.uk/quality_and_service_improvement_tools/quality_and_service_improvement_tools/discharge_planning.html

9 Royal College of Nursing. *Discharge Planning.* Guideline 4 Day Surgery Information. Royal College of Nursing: London, 2013.

10 Department of Health. *Ready To Go? Planning the discharge and the transfer of patients from hospital and intermediate care.* Department of Health: London, 2010.

Documentation standards

Following the implementation of the new Nursing and Midwifery Council (NMC) Code in 2015,[11] the NMC document 'Record keeping guidance for nurses and midwives' was withdrawn from circulation. Statement 10 of the new NMC Code states that nurses and midwives must 'keep clear and accurate records relevant to their practice.' In order to do this, nurses and midwives must:

- complete records immediately or as soon as possible after an event has occurred
- document information which will provide colleagues with all of the information that they require when reading the records
- complete records accurately and without falsification
- ensure that records are signed by the person completing them, dated, timed, clearly written, and free from unnecessary abbreviations, jargon, or speculation
- ensure that all records are kept securely.

Local healthcare trusts will also have standards for documentation in locally held policies and/or procedures. All guidelines and standards are covered by the legal requirements of confidentiality and access, to ensure that the correct information is shared only among those who have both the need and the right to do this.

Reference

11 Nursing and Midwifery Council (NMC). *The Code: professional standards of practice and behaviour for nurses and midwives.* NMC: London, 2015.

Breaking bad news

The breaking of bad news can occur at many different stages in a patient's journey through healthcare, and can involve news regarding diagnosis, treatment, or prognosis. Relatives will also need to be told of bad news—for example, when being advised of a patient's death. Recent studies, such as that by Barnett and colleagues,[12] highlight the fact that although breaking bad news is a frequent event in a healthcare professional's daily work, almost 50% report that they have had little or no formal training in this area, and instead learned the majority of these skills through experience and observational exposure. The same is true of other healthcare professionals, who can learn good skills through the experiences of others.[13]

There are several factors that need to be considered when breaking bad news, including the environment in which the discussion takes place, to ensure that confidentiality, dignity, and privacy are maintained at all times. To facilitate effective communication, the seven steps to good communication should be followed:

1. Prepare for the discussion.
2. Establish what is already known by the patient and their family.
3. Determine how the information is to be handled.
4. Deliver the information.
5. Respond to emotions.
6. Establish goals and priorities for the patient's treatment and care.
7. Establish a plan.

Points for consideration when breaking bad news include the following:

- *The environment*. Is the area quiet and comfortable? Does it enable privacy and dignity to be maintained?
- *Language*. Are translators required so that the news can be delivered in the first language of the patient and carers? Medical jargon and colloquialisms should be avoided in order to prevent confusion, while at the same time maintaining professionalism.
- *Key factors*. The main points of the conversation should be reached quickly and not be hidden among less important topics. The salient points should be highlighted and repeated as necessary.
- *Audience understanding*. Asking those who have received the bad news to repeat the key factors is one way of assessing their understanding of what has been discussed.
- *Time for questions*. Provide sufficient time for questions to be asked and answered.
- *Support*. Breaking bad news can be difficult for those delivering it as well as for those receiving it, and support needs to be available for the patient, their relatives, and also the healthcare professionals. This support can be provided by clinical nurse specialists such as Macmillan nurses, the chaplaincy team, support groups such as the Kidney Association, clinical psychologists, and counselling services.

References

12 Barnett MM et al. Breaking bad news: consultants' experience, previous education and views on educational format and timing. *Medical Education* 2007; 41: 947–56.
13 Barclay JS, Blackhall LJ and Tulsky JA. Communication strategies and cultural issues in the delivery of bad news. *Journal of Palliative Medicine* 2007; 10: 958–78.

Pain management

Introduction to pain management

Pain is an intensely personal event and one that most humans have experienced. However, it is often poorly understood and may be treated inefficiently. There are many definitions of pain, each with a slightly different perspective.

The International Association for the Study of Pain suggests that pain is 'an unpleasant sensory and emotional experience associated with actual or potential tissue damage.'[1] McCaffrey proposes that pain is 'whatever the experiencing person says it is, existing wherever they say it does.'[2]

These definitions imply that pain is complicated. It is important to remember that pain is subjective. Only the person who is experiencing it can truly understand it, and there is no medical test that can establish whether or not a person is experiencing pain. Therefore the management of pain is not an easy task.

References

1 Merskey H and Bogduk N. *Classification of Chronic Pain: description of chronic pain syndromes and definitions of pain terms*, 2nd edn. IASP Press: Seattle, 1994.
2 McCaffery M. *Nursing Management of the Patient with Pain*. Lippincott Williams & Wilkins, Philadelphia, PA, 1972.

Useful website

International Association for the Study of Pain. ℗ www.iasp-pain.org

Physiology of pain

The pain experienced immediately following surgery is known as acute pain. It is a physiological response to warn that tissue damage has occurred. It usually has a defined onset and is short-lived. Nociception is the term used to describe the normal processing of pain. It consists of four processes—transduction, transmission, perception, and modulation.

Transduction of pain

Transduction occurs when free nerve endings (nociceptors) of A-delta and C fibres are stimulated by noxious stimuli (e.g. due to surgery, trauma, infection, or inflammation). Nociceptors are found in the skin, connective tissues, bones, joints, muscles, and visceral (internal) organs. A-delta fibres are fast conducting and send rapid messages to the brain, whereas C fibres are slow conducting and send slower messages.

The skin contains a large number of nociceptors, so it is easy to pinpoint where injury may have occurred. There are fewer nociceptors in bone, connective tissue, and muscle, which makes it more difficult to locate exactly where the pain is. Visceral organs have the lowest number of nociceptors, and therefore the location of pain is often vague.

Transmission of pain via the ascending pathway

Transmission occurs in three stages via three different neurons. The pain impulse is transmitted:

• from the site of transduction along nociceptor fibres to the dorsal horn of the spinal cord
• from the spinal cord to the brainstem and on to the thalamus
• from the thalamus to the sensory cortex and higher centres of the brain.

There is not a specific 'pain centre', so when impulses arrive in the thalamus they are directed to multiple areas in the brain where they are processed.

Perception of pain

Pain is perceived in the sensory cortex. However, it is a multifaceted experience that encompasses physical as well as emotional responses. These responses are controlled by different areas of the brain.

Modulation of pain

Modulation takes place when the transmission of pain impulses in the spinal cord is altered. This process occurs via the descending pathway and is intricate and complex. Pain impulses can be increased or decreased. Inhibition of messages includes the release of natural (endogenous) analgesics such as endorphins. This can help to explain the variation in pain perception that is experienced, as individuals produce different amounts of endogenous analgesics.

Figure 9.1 shows how pain is transmitted via the ascending pain pathway.

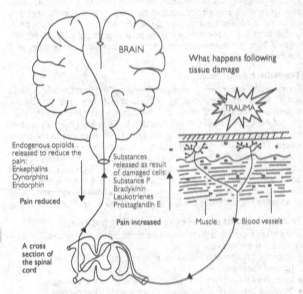

Figure 9.1 Transmission of pain via the ascending pathway.

Basic pharmacokinetics

Pharmacokinetics is fundamentally concerned with what the body does with medication once it has been administered to the patient. It includes the processes whereby the body absorbs, metabolizes, and eliminates medications.

Absorption of medication

For medication to work effectively it needs to get to the part of the body where it is needed. Medication can be administered in a variety of ways. Generally speaking, the main routes of administration for analgesia can be divided into three categories, as shown in Table 9.1.

There are some medications that do not fall within these categories. These are medications that have a systemic action but which are not given orally, via injection, or intravenously. Instead other membranes in the body are used to deliver the medication. These can include sublingual (under the tongue), rectal, and transdermal (through the skin) routes, and inhalation to the lungs.

The rate of absorption can be affected by the route of administration. Medication is absorbed most quickly when it is administered by the intravenous route.

Metabolism of medication

Substances that are absorbed by the body are metabolized by the liver. The body cannot distinguish between substances that are being given as medications and other harmful substances. The liver performs a very important role in protecting the body from toxic substances by acting as a buffer. All medications that are absorbed via the stomach and those absorbed directly into the bloodstream will pass through the liver at some point. The liver contains a family of cytochrome P450 enzymes which specialize in breaking down different substances, including medications. Medications absorbed by the digestive system pass through the liver and are metabolized by the P450 enzymes. This is known as

Table 9.1 Main routes of administration for analgesia

Route	Administration	Example
Topical	The medication is applied directly to the site of the disease or problem. This is usually via the skin in the form of creams, gels, or patches	Ibuprofen gel
Enteral	The medication is taken orally and is absorbed via the digestive system. This can be in the form of tablets, capsules, or liquids	Paracetamol tablets
Parenteral	The medication is administered directly into the body. This can be via an intramuscular injection directly into a muscle, or intravenously directly into the circulatory system via a vein	Intravenous morphine

first-pass metabolism. The amount of medication that remains active
in the circulation depends on how quickly it is metabolized. Following
metabolism there needs to be enough medication present in the circulation to have a therapeutic effect.

Elimination of medication

The kidneys are the main organ of excretion of medications. They remove
the unwanted substances from the blood but keep the useful materials
such as glucose, salts, and amino acids. The waste products are excreted
in the urine. A few medications are excreted by the liver via bile.

If a person has kidney dysfunction it can affect the rate of elimination.

Basic pharmacodynamics

Pharmacodynamics refers to the effect of the medication on the body (i.e. its pharmacological effect). It involves not only the therapeutic effects but also the adverse effects such as side effects of medications.

Medications act on different proteins which can vary widely between individuals, causing different effects. These differences can be due to disease or age.

Most medications bind to protein targets such as receptors, enzymes, carrier proteins, and ion channels. They bind because their shape matches those of particular proteins. Medications that bind to receptors are similarly shaped to the body's natural chemical agents and therefore fit in the agent's target receptor. Once in place they either stimulate or block the action of that receptor. This process is often referred to as a 'lock and key mechanism' (the medication resembling the key, and the receptor resembling the lock).

Medications that bind to receptors can be divided into two broad categories—agonists and antagonists.

- Agonist medications bind to receptors and cause a similar effect to the body's natural chemicals. For example, morphine is an agonist because it mimics the body's natural analgesics, such as endorphins. It binds to the body's opiate receptors.
- Antagonist medications bind to receptors to block them and therefore prevent any response. For example, naloxone is an antagonist, because it binds to opiate receptors and prevents natural or synthetic opiates from binding to provide pain relief.

Pain assessment in adults

Effective pain management cannot be achieved unless a thorough pain assessment is completed. It is well documented that nurses' assessment of patients' pain is often inadequate.[1] Whenever possible the patient should be included in the assessment process, as pain is subjective and only they can know exactly how their pain feels.

When to assess pain

The presence of any pain and its assessment should be documented on admission if surgery is pre-planned. This will allow a baseline observation to be documented. It is vital to remember that patients may be admitted to hospital with pre-existing pain that may have an impact on their post-surgical experience.

Pain should also be documented following any procedure, in order to ensure that adequate interventions are in place.

In addition, it is important to remember not only to ask the patient whether they have pain when they are at rest, but also to enquire whether they experience pain when carrying out activities. This is because we should be aiming for our patients to recover to a point where they are able to function as effectively as possible.

Pain should also be assessed following any intervention, such as medication administration, to ensure that the intervention has been effective.

How to assess pain

Effective communication is crucial when assessing pain. Whenever possible the patient should be given the opportunity to explain whether they have pain prior to procedures. They should be given information about the various techniques that may be utilized to help to manage their pain, as this will help to alleviate their fears and anxieties. It has been well documented that patients can experience the fear of pain as being worse than the pain itself.

It is important to show that we believe the patient's reports of pain, and then to initiate action should it be required.

Factors to include in the pain assessment

Pain assessment should be holistic and include as many aspects as possible.

Factors that should be considered include the following:

- Location. Where is the pain?
- Verbal description. What does it feel like (e.g. sharp, dull, crushing)?
- Severity or intensity. How bad is the pain?
- Duration and frequency. How long does it last and how often is it present?
- Associated symptoms (e.g. nausea, dizziness).
- Triggering and relieving factors. What makes it worse or better?
- How long has the patient had the pain?
- How does the pain affect the patient (e.g. effect on sleep)?

Assessment of these factors is dependent on the patient being able to communicate effectively. If this is not possible due to age, illness, or cognitive ability, an observational assessment must be used. These observational factors should also be assessed in patients who can communicate, as they provide valuable additional information.

Factors that should be considered include the following:
• facial expressions—grimacing, wincing
• vocalizations—moaning, crying
• guarding of body parts, limited movement, or abnormal posture
• behavioural changes—becoming withdrawn or more aggressive
• other changes may include sleep disturbance or a lack of interest in food or surroundings.

Reference

3 Mann EM and Carr ECJ. *Pain: creative approaches to effective management*, 2nd edn. Palgrave Macmillan: Basingstoke, 2009.

Pain assessment in children

Pain assessment in children can be challenging due to the wide range of ages that this group of patients encompasses. It is important when assessing children that the appropriate tool is used to ensure accurate assessment.

For children who are too young to verbalize their pain it is important to involve parents or carers who may be able to offer more information about the child's condition.

There are several approaches that can be used when assessing paediatric pain.

Self-reporting

This is considered to be the 'gold standard' of pain assessment, as only the patient can truly understand the pain that is being experienced. However, in children below the age of 4 years this method is not always accurate, as these children may not be able to express themselves accurately, nor may they understand well enough to know what is being asked. Self-reporting is usually accomplished with the aid of a pain assessment tool, such as the face rating pain assessment tool (see Figure 9.2). Self-reporting of pain is best suited to older children and adolescents.

Observational assessment

As with adult patients who are unable to verbalize, this method may be used for very young children or those who have developmental impairments. An example of an observational pain assessment tool is the Face, Legs, Activity, Cry, Consolability (FLACC) behavioural scale (see Figure 9.3). Observations that are documented may include facial expressions, crying/contentment, and physiological changes. The use of vital signs alone as a measurement of pain must be undertaken with caution, as they are susceptible to influence by homeostatic mechanisms and the condition of the patient.

The Royal College of Nursing[1] recommends that children's pain should be anticipated, assessed using a reliable assessment tool, and dealt with accordingly. Pain should be assessed, recorded, and re-evaluated at regular intervals according to the needs of the child.

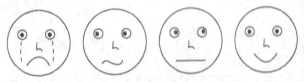

Figure 9.2 Face rating pain assessment tool. Reproduced from George Castledine and Ann Close, *Oxford Handbook of Adult Nursing*, 2007, with permission from Oxford University Press.

FLACC   Behavioural Pain Assessment

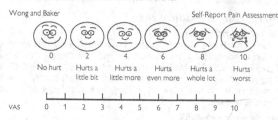

CATEGORIES	SCORING		
	0	1	2
Face	No particular expression or smile	Occasional grimace or frown, withdrawn, disinterested	Frequent to constant quivering chin, clenched jaw
Legs	Normal position or relaxed	Uneasy, restless, tense	Kicking, or legs drawn up
Activity	Lying quietly, normal position, moves easily	Squirming, shifting back and forth, tense	Arched, rigid or jerking
Cry	No crying (awake or asleep)	Moans or whimpers, occasional complaint	Crying steadily, screams or sobs, frequent complaints
Consolability	Content, relaxed	Reassured by occasional touching, hugging or being talked to, distractible	Difficult to console or comfort

Each of the five categories, (F) Face; (L) Legs; (A) Activity; (C) Cry; (C) Consolability, is scored from 0–2, which results in a total score between 0 and 10.

Wong and Baker   Self-Report Pain Assessment

0	2	4	6	8	10
No hurt	Hurts a little bit	Hurts a little more	Hurts even more	Hurts a whole lot	Hurts worst

VAS   0   1   2   3   4   5   6   7   8   9   10

Figure 9.3 Face, Legs, Activity, Cry, Consolability (FLACC) behavioural reporting tool. Reproduced from Merkel SI, Voepel-Lewis T, Shayevitz JR and Malviya S (1997). The FLACC: a behavioral scale for scoring postoperative pain in young children. *Pediatric Nursing*, 23, 293–7, with permission from Jannetti Publications Inc.

Reference

4 Royal College of Nursing. *The Recognition and Assessment of Acute Pain in Children*. Royal College of Nursing: London, 2009.

Further reading

Association of Paediatric Anaesthetists of Great Britain and Ireland (APAGBI). *Good Practice in Post-Operative and Procedural Pain Management*, 2nd edn. APAGBI: London, 2012. ℘ www.csen.com/good.pdf

Documentation of pain assessment

Assessment tools help to quantify pain and provide an objective measurement. Documenting a patient's pain enables a baseline to be established so that interventions can be evaluated. Using an appropriate pain assessment tool can allow the patient to have an active role in their pain management, help to build a therapeutic relationship, and open channels of communication. It also allows parity of assessment between members of the multidisciplinary team.

Types of assessment tools

Assessment tools fall into two main categories—self-reporting (which is classed as the gold standard) and observational. These categories can be further subdivided into unidimensional and multidimensional tools. Many self-reporting tools are unidimensional—that is, they only evaluate one aspect of the patient's pain. Often the aspect that is measured is the intensity of the pain.

Multidimensional tools may be self-reporting or observational, where several different factors are recorded. These could include pain location, severity, description, or behavioural responses (see Figure 9.4).

Self-reporting assessment tools

Visual analogue scale (VAS)

This tool consists of a drawn horizontal or vertical line with the wording 'No pain' at one end and 'Severe pain' (or similar wording) at the other end (see Figure 9.5). The patient is asked to mark the point along the line that corresponds to the severity of their pain. This tool is often used in pain research, but is rarely used in practice as patients find it difficult to understand and use.

Numerical rating scale (NRS)

Numerical rating scales use a series of numbers, from which the patient selects a number to indicate the severity of their pain. Often a scale of 0 to 10 is used, although other ranges can be utilized. A score of 0 indicates no pain, and 10 represents unbearable pain (see Figure 9.6). This tool can be used verbally or visually.

Descriptive scales

Descriptive scales use words to describe the severity of the pain that the patient is experiencing. The patient chooses the word that most accurately describes their pain (see Figure 9.7).

A. PLEASE DESCRIBE YOUR PAIN DURING THE LAST WEEK. (*Check off one box per line.*)

	None	Mild	Moderate	Severe
1. Throbbing	0 □	1 □	2 □	3 □
2. Shooting	0 □	1 □	2 □	3 □
3. Stabbing	0 □	1 □	2 □	3 □
4. Sharp	0 □	1 □	2 □	3 □
5. Cramping	0 □	1 □	2 □	3 □
6. Gnawing	0 □	1 □	2 □	3 □
7. Hot/burning	0 □	1 □	2 □	3 □
8. Aching	0 □	1 □	2 □	3 □
9. Heavy (like a weight)	0 □	1 □	2 □	3 □
10. Tender	0 □	1 □	2 □	3 □
11. Splitting	0 □	1 □	2 □	3 □
12. Tiring/exhausting	0 □	1 □	2 □	3 □
13. Sickening	0 □	1 □	2 □	3 □
14. Fear-causing	0 □	1 □	2 □	3 □
15. Punishing/cruel	0 □	1 □	2 □	3 □

B. PLEASE RATE YOUR PAIN DURING THE LAST WEEK.

The following line represents pain of increasing intensity from 'no pain' to 'worst possible pain'.
Place a vertical mark (I) across the line in the position that best describes your pain during the last week.

No
pain

Worst
possible
pain

Score in mm
(*Investigator's use only*)

C. CURRENT PAIN INTENSITY

0 □ No pain
1 □ Mild
2 □ Discomforting
3 □ Distressing
4 □ Horrible
5 □ Excruciating

Questionnaire developed by: Ronald Melzack

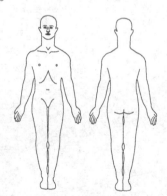

Figure 9.4 Pain questionnaire self-reporting tool. © Copyright 1970, 1987, Ronald Melzack. Reprinted with permission from Dr R Melzack.

Visual analogue scale

No pain ——————————————————— Severe pain

Figure 9.5 Visual analogue pain assessment scale. Reproduced from George Castledine and Ann Close, *Oxford Handbook of Adult Nursing*, 2007, with permission from Oxford University Press.

Numerical rating scale

0 —— 1 —— 2 —— 3 —— 4 —— 5 —— 6 —— 7 —— 8 —— 9 —— 10

Figure 9.6 Numerical rating pain assessment scale. Reproduced from George Castledine and Ann Close, *Oxford Handbook of Adult Nursing*, 2007, with permission from Oxford University Press.

Descriptive scale

No pain ———— Mild pain ———— Moderate pain ———— Severe pain

Figure 9.7 Descriptive pain assessment scale. Reproduced from George Castledine and Ann Close, *Oxford Handbook of Adult Nursing*, 2007, with permission from Oxford University Press.

Nursing care of the patient in pain

It is important to consider the nursing care required for patients who are experiencing pain. Care should not be limited to the administration of medication. The nurse has a unique role to play in supporting the patient through their acute pain experience.

The following nursing interventions may be appropriate to use to support patients in this way:
- providing information to allay the patient's fears and anxieties
- providing general comfort measures (e.g. ensuring that the patient is not too hot or too cold, and that they are supported with pillows)
- distraction techniques
- relaxation techniques.

Nursing issues

Nurses must be aware of the issues that affect patients due to pain, and should intervene appropriately. Pain affects patients in many different ways, and the following are some of the issues that may need to be considered.
- Mobility may be reduced, leading to muscle and/or joint stiffness, contractures, muscle atrophy, increased risk of deep vein thrombosis, and increased risk of pressure ulcers.
- The patient may be unable to maintain personal hygiene.
- Patient safety may be compromised (e.g. patients may fall due to pain).
- Sleep may be disturbed.
- Appetite may decrease.
- Respiration may be affected because the patient may not cough or deep breathe, which may lead to infection or hypoxia.
- Pain can affect gut motility, resulting in constipation.

World Health Organization (WHO) analgesic ladder

Originally the WHO analgesic ladder was developed for use with cancer patients. However, it is now used in many areas of pain management, including the management of acute pain.

The ladder can be used from bottom to top when the patient's pain escalates from mild to more severe, or it can be used from top to bottom when helping to reduce a patient's analgesic intake. Obviously the position on the ladder at which the patient is started will depend on the severity of their pain.

The aim of effective pain management in the post-operative period is to reduce or eliminate pain, with minimal side effects. The WHO analgesic ladder provides a useful framework to help this process, but it is not a solution for all eventualities.

Further reading

World Health Organization. *WHO's Cancer Pain Ladder for Adults.* ℛ www.who.int/cancer/palliative/painladder

Treatment strategies

Mild pain

Following the principles of the WHO analgesic ladder, the strategy to use for mild pain is to start at the bottom of the ladder with a non-upload medication along with an adjuvant medication if required.

An adjuvant medication is one that is not classed as a true analgesic, but which can provide pain relief due to its action on the complicated mechanisms of pain. The action of many adjuvants is not fully understood. For example, amitriptyline is an antidepressant drug but is widely used to help to treat neuropathic (nerve) pain.

A patient with mild pain may be prescribed paracetamol. Non-steroidal anti-inflammatory drugs (NSAIDs) may be used along with par-acetamol, if the patient is able to have them plus an adjuvant if indicated.

This approach is known as 'balanced analgesia' or a multimodal approach. Pain management can be difficult to achieve through the use of a single drug. Using several drugs with different modes of action can increase the potential effectiveness of pain management.

Moderate pain

If the patient's pain is increasing or not responding to the strategy for mild pain, a weak opioid (e.g. codeine) may be added. Non-opioids and NSAIDs plus adjuvants may still be required.

Severe pain

The final step of the WHO analgesic ladder suggests the incorporation of a strong opioid (e.g. morphine). This again would be used along with the other analgesics and adjuvants if indicated.

Paracetamol (acetaminophen)

Paracetamol is a non-anti-inflammatory, non-steroidal drug that has analgesic properties. It is used for mild to moderate pain. Its mode of action is not well understood, but it is thought to impede a type of cyclo-oxygenase enzyme that is involved in the production of prostaglandins. It has very little effect on normal prostaglandin production, and therefore its action is thought to be predominantly centrally acting rather than peripheral.

When used in combination with NSAIDs and opioids it has a synergistic effect. (Medication synergy occurs when two or more medications enhance the effects or side effects of those medications.) It has very few side effects at normal therapeutic doses. Its major disadvantage is that when taken in overdose it is extremely toxic, causing hepatic and renal failure; two to three times the therapeutic dose can cause damage. It has a ceiling effect where increasing the dosage does not improve pain relief, and therefore there is no benefit in exceeding the recommended dose. It has been found that in frail or elderly patients drug clearance is reduced.

Paracetamol also has antipyretic properties and is often used to help reduce pyrexia.

Following surgery, paracetamol is likely to be used in the short term and therefore has a high safety profile.

Formulations

Paracetamol is available in several different formulations. It can be given orally, intravenously, or rectally.

Dosage

Paracetamol is best given regularly following surgery or painful procedures. Typically in adults 1 gram is given orally four times in a 24 hour period at regular intervals.

For children, doses may be age or weight dependent.

For specific instructions on dosage regimes, the *British National Formulary (BNF)* should be consulted.

Useful website
MedicinesComplete. ♪ www.medicinescomplete.com

Non-steroidal anti-inflammatory drugs (NSAIDs)

This is a large group of medications, and it includes ibuprofen, aspirin and diclofenac. NSAIDs produce pain relief by inhibiting the production of prostaglandins, which are involved in the inflammatory process. This is achieved by inhibition of the enzyme cyclo-oxygenase, and this action is mainly at the site of injury.

NSAIDs are used for mild to moderate pain. However, they can be used in combination with opioid medications, which can help to prevent the need for large doses of opioids. The disadvantage of this group of medications relates to their side effects, which in some patients can be severe. The major side effect is gastric irritation, but these drugs should also be used with caution in patients with cardiac and renal problems. In addition, caution is needed when using NSAIDs in elderly patients, as there is a greater risk of bleeding and exacerbation of renal and cardiac conditions.

Side effects occur due to the inhibition of prostaglandin production. Prostaglandins are not only involved in the inflammatory process, but also have many other useful functions within the body. NSAIDs are not selective with regard to which prostaglandins they inhibit, and therefore have a systemic effect. There is also a risk of exacerbating asthma attacks in some asthmatic patients. Aspirin is more likely to exacerbate the condition, whereas ibuprofen is less likely to do so.

The risk of side effects occurring is greater following long-term use, so they are less likely to occur following surgery, when these medications would be used as a short-term treatment. If one type of NSAID does not provide effective pain relief it is worth trying a different type.

Formulations

NSAIDs are available in a wide range of formulations. They can be given orally, intravenously, intramuscularly, rectally, or topically. Following surgery, topical preparations are unlikely to be used.

Dosage

A regular dosage of NSAIDs is preferable following surgery. The dosage will vary depending on the specific medication that is chosen.

For children, doses may be age or weight dependent.

Two types of NSAID must never be given at the same time, as this may result in severe side effects.

For specific instructions on dosage regimes, the *British National Formulary (BNF)* should be consulted.

Useful website

MedicinesComplete. ℘ www.medicinescomplete.com

Opioids

Opioids are used for moderate to severe pain. They can be generally divided into weak opioids (e.g. codeine, dihydrocodeine) and strong opioids (e.g. morphine, diamorphine).

Opioids exert their effect by inhibiting the transmission of pain at the synapse. They mimic the body's natural analgesics, such as endorphins. Opioids bind to the opioid receptors that are found in the central nervous system. At the pre-synaptic membrane, opioids bind to the receptor and inhibit the opening of calcium channels, thereby preventing the release of neurotransmitters. At the post-synaptic membrane opioids bind to opioid receptors and thereby inhibit the transmission of pain across the synapse.

There are several important side effects to be aware of when administering opioids to patients. These include respiratory depression, nausea and vomiting, and constipation. They occur because there are receptors of a similar shape to opioid receptors throughout the body. Opioids can bind to these other receptors and thus cause unwanted side effects.

It is important to note that codeine is ineffective for some patients. For codeine to be effective within the body it must be converted into morphine. This reaction is catalysed by a specific enzyme, and 7–10% of the population are unable to convert the medication due to a deficiency or lack of this enzyme. This can result in the patient gaining no analgesic benefit but still experiencing the side effects.

There is a widespread fear of using opioids due to concerns about addiction and tolerance. When opioids are used for short-term pain management, the risks of addiction and tolerance are minimal. Tolerance occurs when a patient becomes used to a drug and the doses need to be increased in order to achieve the same analgesic effect.

Formulations

Opioids can be administered orally, intravenously, by intramuscular injection, rectally, or subcutaneously. They are also administered epidurally, but this use is unlicensed. Following surgery, opioids are most commonly administered orally, by intramuscular injection, or by the intravenous or epidural routes.

Oral preparations are available in quick-acting and long-acting (sustained-release) formulations. For acute surgical pain, quick-acting formulations are more beneficial, as they provide a fast onset of pain relief.

Dosage

There are many different dosage formulations of opioid analgesics, and the appropriate dosage regime should be used for the particular medication in use. Opioids are often used during surgery, and may be continued post-operatively. Any opioid should be introduced steadily and doses titrated according to the patient's response.

For children, doses may be age or weight dependent.

For specific instructions on dosage regimes, the *British National Formulary (BNF)* should be consulted.

Useful website

MedicinesComplete. ♒ www.medicinescomplete.com

Anti-emetics

Anti-emetic medications are used to help to control symptoms of nausea and vomiting. The use of opioid analgesics is a common cause of nausea and vomiting, which can occur in 25% of patients. A prophylactic anti-emetic should be administered concurrently to minimize the risk of the patient experiencing nausea or vomiting. This will help the patient to tolerate the analgesic medication and thus gain the benefit of its analgesic effects.

There are many different anti-emetics available, and they each have a different mode of action. If one anti-emetic is ineffective it is worth changing to another type with a different mode of action.

Formulations

Anti-emetics can be administered orally, buccally, by deep intramuscular injection, rectally, or by slow intravenous injection.

The oral route is best avoided if the patient is severely nauseous or actually vomiting, as the medication will not be absorbed.

Some anti-emetic drugs are not recommended for paediatric use.

Dosage

The dosage will depend upon the particular anti-emetic used.

For children, doses may be age or weight dependent.

For specific instructions on dosage regimes, the *British National Formulary (BNF)* should be consulted.

Useful website

MedicinesComplete. ℛ www.medicinescomplete.com

Epidural pain management

Epidural pain management is often used following abdominal, thoracic, back, or lower limb surgery. It is a useful form of pain management, especially in patients for whom a general anaesthetic is contraindicated. The use of epidural blocks, as opposed to other forms of post-operative pain management, reduces the risk of stress response and pulmonary infections, and decreases the incidence of venous thromboembolism and renal failure.

For medication to be administered epidurally, a fine catheter is inserted between the vertebrae and into the epidural space which is located between the dura mater and the spinal canal (see Figure 9.8).

This catheter is then used to deliver local anaesthetic or opioids, or a combination of both. Combined medication provides better analgesia than administration of a single drug.

Local anaesthetics produce their effect by inhibiting nervous impulses. In effect they block sodium channels in the membrane of nociceptive neurons. Small lightly myelinated and unmyelinated fibres (mainly pain-transmitting fibres) are blocked first by local anaesthetics, and large heavily myelinated fibres (motor function fibres) are blocked last. Due to this mechanism, patients who are given epidurals should experience pain management without loss of motor function. The aim of a successful epidural block is to inhibit sensory function without affecting motor function.

Opioids that are administered along with the local anaesthetic bind to opioid receptors in the spinal cord at the synapse.

Epidurals can be administered continuously or via a patient-controlled system.

Potential complications of epidural blocks

Epidural blocks are a specialized form of pain management, and therefore need to be monitored carefully. The following should be monitored closely:

- signs of local anaesthetic toxicity (e.g. tingling or numbness of the tongue or lips, drowsiness, confusion, visual disturbance, vomiting, raised blood pressure, tachycardia)
- pulse and blood pressure—use of local anaesthetic can cause hypotension
- respiratory rate and level of block—blocks can rise and inhibit respiratory function. If this happens the infusion must be stopped or reduced and the patient should be monitored
- oxygen saturation and sedation score—if opioids are being used, oxygen should be administered to ensure adequate saturation levels
- pain score—this must be assessed in order to ensure that the block is effective and is being administered at an effect level; blocks can occasionally be patchy, and this results in ineffective pain management for the patient. Sometimes this can be rectified by repositioning the patient
- epidural site—inspect for signs of leakage, catheter displacement, or signs of infection
- evidence of urinary retention—the patient's urine output should be monitored if the patient is not catheterized, as an epidural block can cause retention of urine

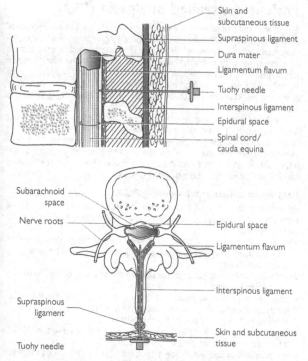

Figure 9.8 Anatomical approach to the epidural space. Reproduced from George Castledine and Ann Close, *Oxford Handbook of Adult Nursing*, 2007, with permission from Oxford University Press.

- motor blockade—occasionally patients lose motor function. This may be rectified by reducing the amount of infusion delivered
- position of limbs—if the patient has had a nerve block in a limb they may lose sensation, so care must be taken to ensure correct alignment and prevent injury to the limb.

Dosage

For specific instructions on dosage regimes, the *British National Formulary (BNF)* and local protocols should be consulted.

Useful website

MedicinesComplete. ℳ www.medicinescomplete.com

Patient-controlled analgesia (PCA)

This is a method of pain management in which the patient has control of their own pain management. Analgesia (usually morphine or a morphine-type medication) is delivered via a pump. There is a button for the patient to press when they require analgesia. The route of administration may be intravenous, subcutaneous, or epidural. The pump is programmed to deliver a small amount of medication on demand, and it has a pro-grammed 'lockout' period to prevent the patient from being given too much medication.

There are many advantages to this method of delivery. The patient feels in control of their pain and its management, as they do not have to ask a nurse for analgesia or wait for it to be administered. PCA prevents the unwanted peaks and troughs of administration associated with intramuscular injection. Peaks in administration of medication can lead to unwanted side effects, and troughs often result in pain.

Factors to consider when using PCA

As with any form of pain management, PCA use should be monitored carefully and local protocols adhered to. The following factors need to be considered:

- respiratory rate—opioids can cause respiratory depression, so when they are used, oxygen should be administered to ensure adequate saturation levels
- sedation score—opioids can cause sedation as a side effect, so this must be monitored
- pain score—this must be monitored in order to ensure that the PCA is effective; occasionally bolus doses may need to be adjusted if pain management is not adequate for the patient
- total consumption of medication and dose/demand rate—this information can be obtained from the pump
- for intravenous administration a dedicated cannula should be used, to prevent other medications from being administered in error
- anti-siphon valves should be fitted in order to prevent siphonage of the medication into the patient by backflow from the infusion
- anti-reflux or one-way valves should be fitted, to ensure that the drug enters the patient.

Dosage

The most common regime used for intravenous PCA is morphine, 1-milligram bolus, with a 5-min lock-out period. Alternatively, fentanyl, 20-microgram bolus, is used with a lock-out period.

For specific instructions on dosage regimes, the *British National Formulary (BNF)* and local protocols should be consulted.

Useful website

MedicinesComplete. ♪ www.medicinescomplete.com

Nerve blocks

Nerve blocks are increasingly being used to help to manage post-operative pain, and in some cases to help to control pain following trauma (e.g. fracture of the femur). They may be used either as the only form of pain management, or in combination with other methods.

Local anaesthetic is injected around nerves that are transmitting pain from a particular organ or body part. The local anaesthetic is absorbed slowly into the nerve, and the length of time for which the nerve will be affected will be longer for large nerves and shorter for small nerves.

Nerve blocks can be divided into proximal nerve blocks (e.g. brachial plexus) and peripheral nerve blocks (e.g. femoral nerve and ulnar nerve blocks). They can be administered either as a one-off injection or via a catheter as a continuous infusion.

Factors to consider when using nerve blocks

As with any form of pain management, nerve blocks should be monitored carefully and local protocols should be followed.

The range of possible complications associated with nerve blocks is strongly dependent on the type of nerve block in use. It is imperative that the specific issues associated with the block in use are monitored. There are some similarities to the use of epidural blocks.

- Pulse and blood pressure—use of local anaesthetic can cause hypotension.
- Pain score—this must be monitored in order to ensure that the block is effective and that it is being administered at an effect level. Nerve blocks only affect specific nerve pathways, so sometimes only part of the area is blocked (e.g. a femoral block may provide analgesia to part of the knee but not all of it).
- If a catheter is *in situ*, the insertion site should be inspected for signs of leakage, catheter displacement, or signs of infection.

Dosage

The dosage can vary depending on the technique, but 1% plain lidocaine with or without adrenaline is most commonly used. However, 0.5% bupivacaine can be used for prolonged analgesia.

For specific instructions on dosage regimes, the *British National Formulary (BNF)* and local protocols should be consulted.

Useful website

MedicinesComplete. ℘ www.medicinescomplete.com

Nutrition and hydration

Introduction to nutrition and hydration

Nurses have a basic duty to provide patients with food and fluids, which are essential for the preservation of health and prevention of complications, particularly in the surgical patient. However, for many surgical patients it is not possible to meet their fluid and nutritional requirements by oral intake alone, and they will require interventions to replace fluid and electrolyte losses and provide nutritional support.

Nutritional screening and assessment

It is important to assess and identify patients who are malnourished or at risk of worsening malnutrition on admission to hospital in order to plan effective peri-operative nutritional care and prevent surgical complications associated with poor nutritional status.

Malnutrition

Malnutrition is still prevalent in hospitals and the community, with at least one-third of patients being identified as malnourished on admission to hospital and during their hospital stay.[1] Furthermore, surgery can lead to an increased risk of malnutrition due to:

- reduced oral intake as a result of post-operative nausea and vomiting, prolonged paralytic ileus, or bowel rest following certain gastrointestinal surgical procedures
- impaired digestion and/or absorption following some gastrointestinal surgery
- increased nutritional requirements due to tissue injury and potential infection
- excess losses such as vomiting or nasogastric aspirate, diarrhoea, exudates from wounds, drains, or gastrointestinal losses from stomas or fistulae.

Nutritional screening

Nutritional screening is a process that identifies patients with or at risk of malnutrition, and is generally carried out by nurses using a valid and reliable screening tool such as the Malnutrition Universal Screening Tool (MUST).[2] A score is calculated based on objective and subjective measures within the tool which guide the nurse towards relevant nutritional care, or referral to a dietitian for a more detailed nutritional assessment, if the score is medium or high risk, respectively, or no action if the score shows the patient to be at low risk.

The National Institute for Health and Care Excellence (NICE) has recommended that screening should be carried out by appropriately trained healthcare staff at the following times:[3]

- at a first outpatient appointment and on admission to hospital
- weekly or if the patient's condition changes (e.g. following surgery).

NICE has produced a quality standard for nutritional support in adults, which includes five quality statements.[4] These relate to the following:

- screening for malnutrition
- putting management care plans in place
- documenting and communicating screening results and nutrition support goals
- providing training for people who manage their own artificial nutrition support
- offering a review for people who receive nutritional support.

Nutritional assessment

Nutritional assessment is a measure of nutritional status at a particular point in time, and should not be confused with nutritional screening, which is an indicator of malnutrition risk. Nutritional assessment should be carried out by a skilled and experienced healthcare professional, such as a dietitian, and includes a range of parameters, such as anthropometric measurements (e.g. height, weight, body mass index, percentage weight loss, triceps skinfold, mid arm muscle circumference) and grip strength (useful for predicting major post-operative complications). Clinical enquiry and observation (e.g. past medical history, dietary history, and physical assessment) are important subjective elements of nutritional assessment.

Identifying the nutritional status of the surgical patient will allow:
• evaluation of appropriate intervention and treatment in order to prevent deterioration and improve nutritional status and overall condition
• prediction of the outcome in certain patients.

In 2014, the British Association for Parenteral and Enteral Nutrition (BAPEN) launched *Malnutrition Matters: a commitment to act*,[5] an easy-to-use guide aimed at clarifying who is responsible for commissioning and delivering good nutritional care in England.

References
1 British Association for Parenteral and Enteral Nutrition (BAPEN). *Nutrition Screening Survey in the UK in 2008*. BAPEN: London, 2009.
2 British Association for Parenteral and Enteral Nutrition (BAPEN). *The 'MUST' Report. Nutritional screening of adults: a multidisciplinary responsibility. Executive summary*. BAPEN: London, 2012. ℰ www.bapen.org.uk/pdfs/must/must_exec_sum.pdf
3 National Institute for Health and Care Excellence (NICE). *Nutrition Support in Adults: oral nutrition support, enteral tube feeding and parenteral nutrition*. CG32. NICE: London, 2006. ℰ www.nice.org.uk/guidance/cg32
4 National Institute for Health and Care Excellence (NICE). *Nutrition Support in Adults*. QS24. NICE: London, 2012. ℰ www.nice.org.uk/guidance/qs24
5 British Association for Parenteral and Enteral Nutrition (BAPEN). *Malnutrition Matters: a commitment to act*. BAPEN: London, 2014.

Nutritional goals in the surgical patient

Maintaining nutritional status

Many surgical patients will not require specific nutritional interventions as part of their care while they are in hospital. However, nurses are accountable for the care that they deliver, which includes nutritional care. This involves monitoring all patients for nutritional risk, observing protected mealtimes in a suitable environment, ensuring that patients receive help in choosing their meals, and with eating and drinking as required, and monitoring intake.

One example of good peri-operative nutritional care is 'The Enhanced Recovery Programme' (ERP), which is an evidence-based model of care designed to improve patient recovery and outcome following surgery. It involves the key members of the multidisciplinary team (MDT), including nurses and the patient and their family, in recovery and care. One of the main elements of the ERP is nutrition, including reduction in fasting time and carbohydrate loading pre-operatively, nausea management, and a return to normal diet as soon as possible.[6,7]

Prevention of deterioration and improvement of nutritional status

In order to set goals for the nutritionally compromised surgical patient, a dietitian will carry out a nutritional assessment and estimate the patient's nutritional requirements before commencing the appropriate nutritional intervention and/or support.

Estimation of requirements

The following recommendations may be used to calculate a nutritional prescription or regime for most patients who are not critically ill or severely undernourished.[8]

- Total energy: 25–35 kcal/kg/day, where 25 kcal/kg/day would be recommended for a non-catabolic patient, whereas 35 kcal/kg/day would be recommended, for example, for a pyrexial post-operative trauma patient.
- Protein: 0.8–1.5 g/kg/day. A post-operative septic patient would require more protein (e.g. 1.5 g/kg/day) than a non-catabolic patient. In order to ensure that protein is utilized for tissue growth and repair, adequate energy should be provided to avoid protein being used for energy.
- Fluid: 30–35 mL/kg/day. In the post-operative patient, additional fluids may also be required to replace fluid losses.
- Sufficient micronutrients, electrolytes, minerals, and fibre based on any deficiency or losses.

Prevention of re-feeding syndrome

Over-rapid provision of nutrition and fluids in the malnourished patient can lead to severe fluid and electrolyte shifts (i.e. rapid uptake of micronutrients and electrolytes such as potassium, phosphate, and magnesium into the cells, and movement of sodium and water out of the cells). This can lead to life-threatening cardiac arrhythmias, fluid overload, and electrolyte and micronutrient deficiencies.

This highlights the importance of detecting any risk of malnutrition and the potential for re-feeding syndrome to occur pre-operatively, to allow any deficiencies to be replaced. It is recommended that nutritional support in the form of enteral or parenteral nutrition should then be given at 50% of the estimated energy and protein requirements, building up to full requirements over 24–48 h. The patient should be closely monitored for gastrointestinal disturbances, fluid imbalance, and further electrolyte, micronutrient, and vitamin deficiency, until they can tolerate a full nutritional regime.[7]

References

6 NHS Institute for Innovation and Improvement. *Enhanced Recovery Programme*. NHS Institute for Innovation and Improvement: Leeds, 2008. ℔ www.institute.nhs.uk/quality_and_service_improvement_tools/quality_and_service_improvement_tools/enhanced_recovery_programme.html

7 Enhanced Recovery Partnership Programme. *Delivering Enhanced Recovery: helping patients to get better sooner after surgery*. Department of Health: London, 2010.

8 National Institute for Health and Care Excellence (NICE). *Nutrition Support in Adults: oral nutrition support, enteral tube feeding and parenteral nutrition*. CG32. NICE: London, 2006. ℔ www.nice.org.uk/guidance/cg32

Enteral nutrition

Oral nutritional supplements (ONS)

For surgical patients who are already malnourished, peri-operative ONS should be considered so long as the patient can safely swallow and has a functional gastrointestinal tract. ONS are available in a variety of formulations depending on the manufacturer, and the standard energy content is in the range 1–1.5 kcal/mL, which may be milk, fruit, or yoghurt based. A wide range of specialist ONS are available, such as those with a higher protein content or added fibre. ONS are generally prescribed by a dietitian, but can be administered by nurses as a meal replacement. To aid compliance, the patient should be involved in choosing the flavour and formulation.

Indications for enteral tube feeding (ETF)

Surgical patients who are malnourished or at risk of this, or who have an inadequate or unsafe oral intake but still have a functional and accessible gastrointestinal tract, should be considered for ETF. Pre-operative ETF may be considered for malnourished patients who are due to undergo major abdominal surgery. The potential benefits of ETF are that it maintains gut barrier function, increases blood flow to the gut, and stimulates gastrointestinal function and immunity.

Routes of ETF

Nasogastric feeding

A fine-bore tube is inserted via the nose and oesophagus into the stomach. This is used for short-term feeding, usually for less than 4 weeks.

Gastrostomy feeding

A tube is passed through the abdominal wall into the stomach. This is used for longer-term feeding, usually for more than 4 weeks.

Percutaneous endoscopic gastrostomy (PEG)

This is an endoscopic procedure in which an insertion site is created via the gastric wall, and the tube is pulled into position by thread via the mouth and secured by an internal bumper and external fixation device.

Radiologically inserted gastrostomy (RIG)

A gastrostomy tube is inserted directly via the stomach wall and secured with a pigtail device.

Replacement gastrostomy

This is retained by a water-filled balloon or soft bumper and inserted at the bedside via an established gastrostomy tract (at least 4–6 weeks after initial tube insertion).

Upper gastrointestinal tract dysfunction

Nasojejunal tube

A fine-bore enteral tube is passed via the nose into the jejunum, preferably past the ligament of Treitz.

Percutaneous endoscopic jejunostomy (PEJ)
A fine-bore jejunal tube is passed through a gastrostomy tube into the jejunum.

Jejunostomy
A fine-bore tube is inserted directly into the jejunum.

Commencement of feed

A feed regime is provided by a dietitian based on an estimation of nutritional requirements as set out on ➔ p. 197. The feed is usually delivered via an enteral feeding pump in the acute hospital setting over a set period of time in 24 h depending on the patient's clinical condition, the nutritional regime, the route of ETF, and patient choice.

Specific care issues

- The position of all nasogastric tubes should be confirmed after placement *and before each use* by aspiration and pH indicator strips. If the pH is in the range 1–5.5, commence the feed. If the pH is ≥ 5.5 or there is no aspirate, do not commence the feed, and request X-ray confirmation.[9]
- Position the patient at an angle of at least 30–45° during feeding and for 45–60 min afterwards, to prevent aspiration.
- Using an aseptic technique, flush the tube with at least 30 mL of freshly drawn tap water using a 50-mL enteral syringe before and after feed and drug administration. Sterile water should be used when feeding into the jejunum or if the patient is immunocompromised.
- Use sterile, pre-packaged feed and enteral feeding systems, where the hang time should not exceed 24 h.
- Use aseptic technique to dress gastrostomy and jejunostomy stoma sites for the first 3 days, then soap and water and dry thoroughly thereafter.

Reference

9 National Patient Safety Agency (NPSA). *Reducing the Harm Caused by Misplaced Nasogastric Feeding Tubes in Adults, Children and Infants.* NPSA: London, 2011. ℛ www.nrls.npsa.nhs.uk/alerts/?entryid45=129640

Further reading

Bowling T (ed.) *Nutritional Support for Adults and Children: a handbook for hospital practice.* Radcliffe Medical Press: Oxford, 2004.

British Association for Parenteral and Enteral Nutrition (BAPEN). *Administering Drugs via Enteral Feeding Tubes: a practical guide.* BAPEN: London, 2004. ℛ www.bapen.org.uk/pdfs/d_and_e/de_pract_guide.pdf

Department of Health. *High Impact Intervention: enteral feeding care bundle.* Department of Health: London, 2010. ℛ http://webarchive.nationalarchives.gov.uk/20120118164404/hcai.dh.gov.uk/files/2011/03/2011-03-14-HII-Enteral-Feeding-Care-Bundle-FINAL.pdf

National Institute for Health and Care Excellence (NICE). *Nutrition Support in Adults: oral nutrition support, enteral tube feeding and parenteral nutrition.* CG32. London: NICE, 2006. ℛ www.nice.org.uk/guidance/cg32

Parenteral nutrition

Indications for parenteral nutrition (PN)

Surgical patients should be considered for PN according to the criteria for ETF on ⮕ p. 199, but when the gastrointestinal tract is non-functional, inaccessible, or perforated or fistulated. Peri-operative supplementary PN can be considered in the malnourished surgical patient and where intolerance prevents the patient's nutritional requirements from being met by the enteral route alone.[10]

Legal and ethical considerations

The decision to commence nutritional support (ETF or PN) should be made by the consultant in conjunction with the patient, their family, and the healthcare team. Informed consent of a competent adult patient is essential before commencement of ETF or PN, as this is deemed a medical treatment as opposed to basic care. In the case of an incompetent patient, the consultant makes the final decision based on the best interests of the patient, although others may be involved in this decision, such as a Lasting Power of Attorney and Independent Mental Capacity Advocate.[11]

Routes of access

The route of access will depend on several factors:
• nutritional requirements and the osmolality of the feed
• other intravenous therapies
• the estimated duration of feeding
• the patency of suitable veins
• staff availability and expertise
• patient preference.

Peripheral
• Recommended for less than 2 weeks using low-osmolality feed.
• A specific insertion kit and long line are needed.
• The tip usually sits in the upper arm region of the cephalic or basilic vein. Good peripheral veins are needed for access.
• There is a risk of chemical and mechanical phlebitis.
• There is a low risk of infection.

Central: untunnelled
• Recommended for less than 30 days using higher-osmolality feed.
• *Peripherally inserted central catheter* is inserted via a peripheral vein, but the tip sits in the superior vena cava.
• *Centrally inserted catheter* is usually inserted into the subclavian vein using a single-lumen catheter for PN, but jugular or femoral access may be used via a multiple-lumen line in critically ill patients where one lumen is dedicated for PN use.
• There is a higher risk of mechanical and septic complications.

Central: tunnelled
- Recommended for more than 30 days.
- Subclavian access and catheter tunnelled under the skin away from the insertion site.

All procedures for IV catheter insertion require a strict aseptic non-touch technique (ANTT) and use of an appropriate skin cleansing agent (e.g. 2% chlorhexidine in 70% alcohol) according to local hospital policy.

Specific care issues

In 2010, the National Confidential Enquiry into Patient Outcome and Death (NCEPOD)[12] identified some key deficiencies in relation to PN care in hospital patients, and has recommended that the following aspects of care are undertaken in accordance with local hospital policy for surgical patients who are receiving PN:
- initial assessment of indications for PN, nutritional status, and clinical status by specialist healthcare practitioners or the nutrition team
- insertion of PN catheter by a skilled operator
- management of catheter interventions by a competent nurse or healthcare practitioner
- monitoring of temperature, pulse, blood pressure, and respiration rate 4- to 6-hourly to identify potential infection
- inspection of the catheter insertion site daily for redness, swelling, pain, and exudate
- 6-hourly blood glucose monitoring
- daily weight monitoring to detect fluid retention or overload
- accurate documentation of monitoring, catheter interventions, and complications.

References

10 National Institute for Health and Care Excellence (NICE). *Nutrition Support in Adults: oral nutrition support, enteral tube feeding and parenteral nutrition.* CG32. London: NICE, 2006. ℘ www.nice.org.uk/guidance/cg32

11 Department of Health. *Reference Guide to Consent for Examination or Treatment,* 2nd edn. Department of Health: London, 2009. ℘ www.gov.uk/government/uploads/system/uploads/attachment_data/file/138296/dh_103653__1_.pdf

12 National Confidential Enquiry into Patient Outcome and Death (NCEPOD). *Parenteral Nutrition: a mixed bag.* NCEPOD: London, 2010. ℘ www.ncepod.org.uk/2010pn.htm

Further reading

Department of Health. *High Impact Intervention: central venous catheter care bundle.* Department of Health: London, 2010. ℘ http://webarchive.nationalarchives.gov.uk/20120118164404/hcai.dh.gov.uk/files/2011/03/2011-03-14-HII-Central-Venous-Catheter-Care-Bundle-FINAL.pdf

Fluid balance

Understanding fluid compartments

The human body contains approximately 60% water, depending on age, gender, and body fat. Total body water (TBW) is about 45 L, and it is compartmented as follows:

- *Extracellular fluid (ECF)*, which represents approximately one-third of TBW, is contained within the vascular (plasma) and interstitial compartments, which are separated by the semipermeable capillary wall. *Transcellular fluids* are also part of the ECF, and include cerebrospinal fluid, and secretions from the gastrointestinal tract, the respiratory tract, and the kidneys. In healthy individuals, gastrointestinal secretions are reabsorbed within the body, and only approximately 150 mL/day are excreted in the faeces. However, they can be a major cause of fluid volume deficit in some patients following gastrointestinal surgery.
- *Intracellular fluid (ICF)*, which represents approximately two-thirds of TBW, is contained within the cells.

Body water contains a range of positively and negatively charged electrolytes, of which sodium (Na^+), potassium (K^+), chloride (Cl^-), bicarbonate (HCO_3^-), calcium (Ca^{2+}), and magnesium (Mg^{2+}) are among the most common.

- Sodium and chloride are the main extracellular electrolytes.
- Potassium and phosphate are the main intracellular electrolytes.

Overview of fluid balance

Movement of body fluids

In healthy individuals the ICF remains constant, whereas the ECF moves around the body as follows:

- The ECF is forced out of the capillaries into the interstitial fluid by the hydrostatic pressure created by the force of the cardiac output. At the venous end of the capillary, the colloid oncotic pressure created by protein molecules (mainly albumin) within the plasma exceeds the hydrostatic pressure where the fluid moves from an area of low solute (albumin) concentration in the interstitial space to an area of high solute concentration. This results in fluid re-entering the capillaries, thereby preventing the development of tissue oedema and maintaining blood pressure.
- *Osmosis*—osmotic pressure is created by electrolytes. For example, water will move from an area of low sodium concentration to an area of high sodium concentration to maintain the osmolality (ideal concentration) of body fluids (approximately 285 mOsm).
- Electrolytes can move through the body by diffusion from a high concentration to a low concentration. Therefore, in order to regulate the concentration of sodium in the ECF and the concentration of potassium in the ICF, the sodium–potassium pump actively moves sodium against the concentration gradient from the ICF to the ECF, and the opposite situation occurs for potassium.

- The kidney has a vital role in regulating fluid and electrolyte balance, and normally excretes urine at a rate of around 1 mL/kg/h (approximately 1500–2000 mL/day) for the average adult. Other factors that are involved in fluid and electrolyte regulation include antidiuretic hormone (ADH), the renin–angiotensin–aldosterone system, and atrial natriuretic peptide.
- *Dehydration*—this refers to loss of water alone, whereas *fluid volume deficit (FVD)* refers to loss of water and electrolytes, which is a common cause of hypovolaemia in the post-operative patient.
- *Overhydration/fluid overload*—this refers to an excess of body water, and is more common in patients with impaired cardiac, renal, or liver function, or as a result of steroid use.

Further reading

Metheny NM. *Fluid and Electrolyte Balance: nursing considerations*, 5th edn. Jones & Bartlett Learning: Sudbury, MA, 2012.
Scales K and Pilsworth J. The importance of fluid balance in clinical practice. *Nursing Standard* 2008; 22: 50–57.

Fluid balance and the surgical patient

Specific factors relating to the surgical patient

Risk factors for peri-operative fluid and/or electrolyte disturbance include:

- the surgical condition
- pre-existing medical problems (e.g. renal, cardiac, or hepatic disease)
- medication (e.g. diuretics)
- peri-operative myocardial infarction
- large peri-operative fluid losses, which may be due to:
  - prolonged pre-operative fasting or periods when the patient is nil by mouth (NBM) for investigations
  - mechanical bowel preparation
  - vomiting and nasogastric drainage
  - stoma and fistula losses, particularly in the jejunum and ileum
  - drains
  - wound exudate
  - loose stool and/or diarrhoea
  - insensible losses—from respiration, sweating, or faecal loss
  - third-space losses—movement of fluid from the ECF into another body cavity (e.g. ascites in the peritoneal cavity, or oedema). The fluid is still within the body, but is not functional.

Fluid overload—increased production of aldosterone and ADH is common after surgery, due to intra-operative fluid losses resulting in conservation of water and sodium for approximately 12–24 h. Excessive fluid infusion leading to sodium and water overload is recognized as a major cause of post-operative morbidity.[13]

Oedema can occur due to increased interstitial fluid volume, but also as a result of hypoalbuminaemia, which reduces the colloid oncotic pressure in approximately 20–40% of post-operative patients.[14]

Assessment of the surgical patient

Clinical assessment of fluid balance

- Respiratory rate—this may increase due to hypovolaemia and reduced oxygen delivery to the cells. Increased respiration is also a sign of fluid overload associated with shortness of breath, cough, and production of pink frothy sputum.
- Changes in pulse rate and blood pressure—a decrease in the patient's baseline blood pressure of 25% or systolic blood pressure below 100 mmHg and an increase in the pulse rate (> 100 beats/min) is an indication of hypovolaemia. Any blood loss and other fluid losses should be recorded. Septic shock should also be considered if there are signs of infection.
- Capillary refill time—this is normally less than 2 s, but can be increased due to vasoconstriction of the peripheral blood vessels to maintain pulse and blood pressure.

- Urine output—hypovolaemia is indicated if urine output falls below 0.5 mL/kg/h (approximately 20–30 mL/h) for 2 consecutive hours. Alternatively, polyuria may result from hyperglycaemia in poorly controlled diabetes or with overuse of diuretics.
- Monitoring of the patient's conscious level—AVPU should be used to determine conscious level and response, as moderate ECF loss may result in confusion and irritability.
- Temperature—pyrexia and sweating can increase fluid loss.
- Thirst—this is the first clinical indicator of dehydration. If the patient is NBM or unconscious, prevention of dehydration by using alternative non-oral routes is essential.
- Assessment of the mouth and tongue—for dry and cracked mucous membranes resulting from dehydration.
- Elasticity of skin—dehydrated patients may have loose inelastic skin, whereas oedema can be identified by applying fingertip pressure over a bony area for a few seconds, which leaves an indentation that does not disappear after 30 s.
- Blood tests—to determine serum concentrations of electrolytes, urea, and creatinine in order to assess renal function.
- Daily weight measurements—to detect excessive fluid loss or retention.

References

13 Powell-Tuck J et al. *British Consensus Guidelines on Intravenous Fluid Therapy for Adult Surgical Patients*. GIFTASUP. British Association for Parenteral and Enteral Nutrition (BAPEN): London, 2011. www.bapen.org.uk/pdfs/bapen_pubs/giftasup.pdf
14 Redelmeier DA. New thinking about postoperative hypoalbuminaemia: a hypothesis of occult protein-losing enteropathy. *Open Medicine* 2009; 3: e215–19.

Intravenous fluid regimes

Solutions that are used for intravenous (IV) fluid replacement therapy can be divided into two main categories.

Crystalloids

Crystalloids are solutions that contain small molecules of salts or sugars which dissolve completely in water and can move easily between intra-vascular, interstitial, and intracellular fluid compartments.

Crystalloids are available in a variety of concentrations:

- *Isotonic* fluids have similar concentrations of sodium and chloride to those of the fluids in the body, with osmolality in the range 240–340 mOsm/kg.
- *Hypotonic* fluids have an osmolality of less than 240 mOsm/kg (e.g. 0.45% normal saline). Osmotic pressure draws water into the cells from the ECF, causing the cells to swell. This type of fluid should not be given to patients who are at increased risk of raised intracranial pressure (e.g. following head trauma or neurosurgery).
- *Hypertonic* fluids have an osmolality greater than 340 mOsm/kg (e.g. glucose 5% in 0.45% normal saline). They draw fluid from the cells into the extracellular space, and they can cause fluid overload and pulmonary oedema, particularly in cardiac or renal disease.

Common compositions of IV fluids are shown in Table 10.1.

Recommendations for surgical patients[16]

- Hartmann's solution or Ringer's solution should be used in preference to 0.9% normal saline except when there is vomiting or gastric drainage, due to the potential risk of hypochloraemia.
- Sodium chloride (0.18%) and 4% glucose are important for free water maintenance in fluid regimes, but excessive amounts may cause hyponatraemia, particularly in the elderly.

Table 10.1 Composition of intravenous fluids

Intravenous fluid	Electrolyte	Amount
4% Glucose	None	None
Normal saline 0.9%	Sodium and chloride	150 mmol/L of each
Hartmann's solution	Sodium	147 mmol/L
	Chloride	156 mmol/L
	Potassium	4 mmol/L
	Calcium	2.2 mmol/L
Ringer's solution	Sodium	131 mmol/L
	Chloride	111 mmol/L
	Potassium	5 mmol/L
	Lactate	29 mmol/L
	Calcium	2 mmol/L

Colloids

Colloid solutions (plasma expanders) contain larger molecules that do not completely dissolve in solution, and remain in the ECF longer than crystalloids.

Colloids have been widely used for fluid resuscitation in hypovolaemic shock. The National Institute for Health and Care Excellence (NICE)[17] has produced new guidelines on the use of intravenous fluids in adults. For patients who require fluid resuscitation they recommend the use of crystalloids, and they state that tetrastarch should not be used. For patients with severe sepsis who require significant fluid resuscitation, they recommend considering the use of 4–5% human albumin.

For patients in hypovolaemic shock due to haemorrhage, the use of blood, platelets, and fresh frozen plasma (FFP) should be considered based upon the patient's blood results and physiological signs.

References

15 Willis L (ed.). *Fluids and Electrolytes Made Incredibly Easy!* 6th edn. Wolters Kluwer Health: Philadelphia, PA, 2015.

16 Powell-Tuck J et al. *British Consensus Guidelines on Intravenous Fluid Therapy for Adult Surgical Patients.* GIFTASUP. British Association for Parenteral and Enteral Nutrition (BAPEN): London, 2011. ℬ www.bapen.org.uk/pdfs/bapen_pubs/giftasup.pdf

17 National Institute for Health and Care Excellence (NICE). *Intravenous Fluid Therapy in Adults in Hospital.* CG174. NICE: London, 2013. ℬ www.nice.org.uk/guidance/cg174

Peri-operative fluid regimes

To meet maintenance requirements, patients should receive 25–30 mL/kg/day of water, 1 mmol/kg/day of potassium, sodium, and chloride, and 50–100 g of glucose by the oral, enteral, or parenteral routes (or a combination of these).[18] Therefore fluid requirements should be assessed on an individual basis by considering patient history, clinical examination, and investigation results. IV fluids are usually prescribed by a doctor, but can be prescribed or adjusted in specified circumstances by other healthcare practitioners, including senior or specialist nurses as part of patient group directions (PGDs) in some hospital trusts.

GIFTASUP[19] has identified the following standard principles of fluid balance in the peri-operative period:

- Oral fluids should not be withheld for more than 2 h prior to the anaesthetic, with administration of a carbohydrate-rich drink 2–3 h before the anaesthetic.
- Routine use of pre-operative mechanical bowel preparation is not recommended, and any fluid and electrolyte imbalance as a result of bowel preparation should be corrected using IV fluid therapy.
- *Use the oral route* where possible to avoid a delay in commencing oral intake. For example, use of the ERP programme supports an early return to fluid and dietary intake.
- *Correct any pre-existing fluid deficit* (e.g. prolonged pre-operative fasting and/or use of bowel preparation).
- *Replace fluid losses.* For example:
  - For peri-operative gastric aspirate or vomiting, 0.9% normal saline with an appropriate potassium supplement is indicated in hypochloraemia while monitoring for sodium overload.
  - Other fluid losses, such as those due to diarrhoea, jejunostomy, ileostomy, or small bowel fistula, should be replaced with equal volumes of IV Hartmann's solution or Ringer's solution.
  - Patients with a high-output stoma with ongoing losses of more than 1200 mL/24 h will develop fluid and electrolyte depletion. In addition to IV replacement, oral hypotonic fluids such as water, tea, squash, etc. should be restricted to 500–1500 mL/day, as they dilute sodium in the jejunum, which results in sodium moving into the gut by diffusion and then being excreted via the stoma or fistula. Oral rehydration solution containing 90 mmol/L of sodium plus glucose is recommended to avoid this movement and loss of sodium. To enhance the palatability of this solution it should be served cold, with the addition of squash or lime cordial as required by the patient.[20]

- *Post-operative oedema* is a result of accumulation of salt and water in the interstitial space, and is a cause of positive fluid balance. In addition, critically ill patients may also have intravascular hypovolaemia, which should be treated using IV fluid therapy. Improvement in nutritional intake will also help to restore the normal fluid and electrolyte compartments.

References

18 National Institute for Health and Care Excellence (NICE). *Intravenous Fluid Therapy in Adults in Hospital.* CG174. NICE: London, 2013. ℐⓇ www.nice.org.uk/guidance/cg174
19 Powell-Tuck J et al. *British Consensus Guidelines on Intravenous Fluid Therapy for Adult Surgical Patients.* GIFTASUP. British Association for Parenteral and Enteral Nutrition (BAPEN): London, 2011. ℐⓇ www.bapen.org.uk/pdfs/bapen_pubs/giftasup.pdf
20 Medlin S. Nutritional and fluid requirements: high-output stomas. *British Journal of Nursing* 2012; 21: S22–5.

Monitoring fluid balance

Fluid balance charts

The aim of a fluid balance chart is to provide an accurate record of a patient's fluid input and output in order to identify any fluid deficits or overload. Each chart is kept over a 24 hour period, and is then totalled (usually at midnight) to give the daily fluid balance. A positive fluid balance indicates fluid overload, and a negative fluid balance indicates a fluid deficit. Cumulative totals of fluid balance charts are particularly important in surgical patients for identifying peri-operative trends in fluid balance and facilitating prescription of individual patients' fluid regimes. Cumulative totals may be reviewed on a 24 hour basis or over longer periods of 7 days or more.

Indications for a fluid balance chart in the surgical patient

- Prolonged NBM.
- Subcutaneous or intravenous infusions.
- Enteral or parenteral feeding.
- Underlying medical conditions that affect fluid balance, such as cardiac, renal, or hepatic disease, and pre-existing malnutrition.
- Nasogastric tube for aspiration of gastric contents or vomiting.
- Diarrhoea or rectal tube.
- Urinary catheterization.
- Wound drains.
- Newly formed stomas, particularly jejunostomy and ileostomy.
- Abdominal fistulae.
- Chest drain.

Measurement of input

- *Oral* input—all oral fluids, including soups and fluid added to food (e.g. milk on cereal) and any oral nutritional supplements. Accurate cup or glass volumes should be available.
- *Subcutaneous and intravenous fluids*, including parenteral nutrition, medication administered in IV fluids, blood and blood products, and flushes. Nurses should ensure that subcutaneous and IV fluids are kept to rota at the correct drop rate or pump rate, and that the start time, volume, hourly rate, completion rate, and volume are documented accurately and totalled on the fluid balance chart.
- Ensure that enteral feed is kept to rota at the correct pump rate, and that the start time, volume, hourly rate, completion rate, and volume are documented accurately and totalled on the fluid balance chart. Also include any medication that is dissolved or mixed in water, flushes, and supplementary water given via the enteral tube.

Measurement of output

- Record all measurable losses in the appropriate columns on the fluid balance chart.
- Patients with a urinary catheter who are acutely unwell may require measurement and monitoring of hourly urine output.

- If fluid output cannot be measured due to incontinence, this should be indicated on the fluid balance chart.
- Calculate and record insensible losses, particularly in patients who are pyrexial and sweating.

Problems with accurate completion of fluid balance charts

Maintaining and interpreting accurate fluid balance charts and cumulative totals is a crucial aspect of ongoing assessment and care of the surgical patient. The Care Quality Commission[21] has identified that the fluid balance of patients is not always well monitored. Therefore it is imperative that surgical nurses understand the mechanisms of fluid balance, fluid regimes in the peri-operative patient, and the risks, signs, and symptoms of fluid imbalance in the surgical patient, so that they appreciate the importance of accurate completion of fluid balance charts.

Reference

21 Care Quality Commission. *Review of Compliance.* Care Quality Commission: Newcastle upon Tyne, 2012.

Transfusion of blood products

Basic physiology of blood production

Blood is the only liquid tissue in the body, and consists of living blood cells suspended in a non-living fluid called plasma. The formed elements of blood are red blood cells (erythrocytes), white blood cells (leucocytes), and platelets. Blood represents 8% of body weight, and the body of a healthy male contains around 5 L of blood.

Plasma

Around 90% of plasma consists of water, with over 100 substances dissolved in it, including nutrients, electrolytes, respiratory gases, hormones, plasma proteins, waste products of metabolism, and products of cell metabolism.

Plasma proteins are the main solute in plasma. One of these proteins, albumin, contributes to the osmotic pressure of blood, keeping water in the bloodstream. Clotting proteins stem bleeding when a blood vessel is damaged, and antibodies help to protect the body from pathogens.

Red blood cells

Red blood cells contribute to the viscosity of blood, and their main function is to transport oxygen to all the cells of the body. They differ from other cells of the body in that they do not have a nucleus. They contain haemoglobin (Hb), an iron-bearing protein that carries the majority of oxygen within the blood and also binds with a small amount of carbon dioxide. Each red blood cell contains 250 million haemoglobin molecules, each of which is capable of carrying four molecules of oxygen.

Normal blood contains 12–18 g of Hb per 100 mL of blood. Anaemia is characterized by a decrease in the oxygen-carrying capacity of the blood, which may be due to a reduced number of red blood cells, or abnormal or insufficient Hb in the red blood cells.

The rate of red blood cell formation is fairly constant, and is controlled by the hormone erythropoietin, which is produced by the kidneys. When blood levels of oxygen decline due to decreased red blood cells, decreased haemoglobin levels, or hypoxia, erythropoietin is released, which stimulates the bone marrow to produce red blood cells. Healthy red blood cells have a lifespan of 120 days in the circulatory system.

White blood cells

Blood contains significantly fewer leucocytes than erythrocytes, but they are crucial as they defend the body against disease (e.g. bacteria, viruses, parasites, tumour cells). They are also capable of moving in and out of blood vessels by a process called diapedesis. They travel via the circulatory system to areas of the body where they are required for an inflammatory or immune response.

White blood cells are classified into two main groups, called granulocytes and agranulocytes, depending on whether or not they contain visible granules in their cytoplasm.

Granulocytes consist of:
- neutrophils, which act as phagocytes, engulfing and destroying bacteria and fungi at the site of acute infection
- eosinophils, which increase in number when a person is infected by parasitic worms
- basophils, which contain histamine, an inflammatory mediator that is released into the bloodstream and causes blood vessels to become leaky, so that white blood cells can travel to the site of inflammation.

Agranulocytes consist of:
- lymphocytes, which play an important role in the immune response and are found in lymphatic tissue
- monocytes, which become macrophages when they migrate into tissue and clean up the debris from infections, especially chronic infections.

Platelets

Platelets are fragments of multinucleate cells called megakaryocytes. They are needed for the clotting process when blood vessels are ruptured or damaged. They are always present in the blood, but are only activated when a blood vessel wall is damaged. Platelets adhere to the damaged blood vessel wall, forming a plug, to which the clotting factor fibrin also adheres, forming a clot. Platelets are formed in the bone marrow and in the circulatory system, and have a lifespan of 10 days.

Further reading

Marieb E. *Essentials of Human Anatomy and Physiology*, 10th edn. Pearson Education, Inc.: San Francisco, CA, 2012.

ABO compatibility and rhesus status

People belong to one of four main blood groups—A, B, AB, or O—and need to be transfused the correct red blood cells. Receiving incompatible blood exposes an individual to the risk of serious injury or even death.

The plasma membranes of red blood cells contain genetically determined proteins known as antigens. Most antigens are foreign proteins, which stimulate the immune system to produce antibodies as a defence reaction to the antigen. We tolerate our own cellular antigens, but if we were to receive a transfusion of red blood cells from another person who had different red blood cell antigens, this would stimulate an immune response.

Antibodies present in the plasma of the blood recipient attach to the red blood cells bearing surface antigens different from those of the blood recipient. This binding by the antibodies causes the foreign (donor) red blood cells to clump together in a process known as agglutination. Small blood vessels become blocked and the 'foreign' red blood cells are ruptured by the process of lysis. Their haemoglobin is released into the bloodstream, causing blockage of the renal tubules, which results in renal failure and death.

There are over 30 common red blood cell antigens in humans. However, the antigens of the ABO and rhesus groups cause the most severe reactions.

ABO system

The ABO system is based on two inherited antigens called type A and type B. If neither antigen is present on the red blood cell, a person belongs to blood group O. If both antigens are present, they belong to blood group AB. If they have only antigen A or only antigen B, they belong to blood group A or blood group B, respectively.

If a person belongs to blood group AB, they have surface antigens A and B on their red blood cells but do not have anti-A or anti-B immunoglobulin M (IgM) antibodies in their serum. This means that they can receive blood from any of the other blood groups (A, B, O, and AB), as they do not produce antibodies to them, so they are known as the 'universal recipient.' However, they can only donate blood to a recipient with blood group AB, as the other blood groups will produce antibodies to AB blood.

If a person belongs to blood group O, they have no surface antigens on their red blood cells, and have anti-A and anti-B IgM in their serum. This means that they can only receive blood group O, as they produce antibodies to the other blood groups. However, they can donate blood to all of the other blood groups (A, B, AB, and O), so they are known as the 'universal donor.'

If a person belongs to blood group A, they have surface antigen A on their red blood cells and anti-B IgM in their serum. This means that they can receive blood from groups A and O, and they can donate blood to a recipient belonging to blood group A or AB.

Table 11.1 ABO blood group compatibility

Blood group	Red blood cell antigens	Serum antibodies	Donor blood group that they can receive
	ABO blood groups		
AB	A and B	None	A, B, O, and AB
B	B	Anti-A	B and O
A	A	Anti-B	A and O
O	None	Anti-A and anti-B	O

If a person belongs to blood group B, they have surface antigen B on their red blood cells and anti-A IgM in their serum. This means that they can receive blood from groups B and O, and they can donate blood to a recipient belonging to blood group B or AB.

Table 11.1 provides a summary of ABO blood group compatibility.

Rhesus status

There are two rhesus (Rh) blood groups which are inherited—rhesus positive and rhesus negative. If the Rh antigen is present on the surface of a person's red blood cells, they are Rh positive. If a person does not have the Rh antigen on their red blood cells, they are Rh negative.

Rh-positive people cannot form Rh antibodies, so can receive Rh-positive or Rh-negative blood. An Rh-negative person can form Rh antibodies, so can only receive Rh-negative blood.

Therefore, taking into consideration both blood group and Rh factor:
• The universal donor is O Rh-negative.
• The universal recipient is AB Rh-positive.

Further reading

Marieb E. *Essentials of Human Anatomy and Physiology*, 10th edn. Pearson Education, Inc.: San Francisco, CA, 2012.

Blood products

Blood donation in the UK is a voluntary process, which aims to protect the donor from any harm caused by the process and also to protect the recipient of blood products from incompatible or contaminated donated blood. Assessment of fitness to donate blood consists of a questionnaire relating to health, lifestyle, medication, and past medical history. Donors are also screened for exposure to transmissible infectious diseases such as hepatitis and human immunodeficiency virus (HIV).

The blood products produced from blood donations are red blood cells, platelets, fresh frozen plasma (FFP), cryoprecipitate, and human albumin (4.5% and 20% solution).

Red blood cells

A unit of red blood cells is produced from a single whole blood donation, with the majority of plasma removed from the blood. The red blood cells are preserved in a solution of saline, adenine, glucose, and mannitol (SAG-M). The saline is isotonic with blood, the adenine maintains adenosine triphosphate (ATP) for red cell viability, the glucose supports red cell metabolism, and mannitol helps to reduce red cell lysis (breakdown).

An adult unit of red blood cells has a shelf life of 35 days from donation, has a volume of 220–340 mL, and must be stored in a blood fridge at 4°C with continuous temperature regulation. Administration should be commenced via a standard blood transfusion set within 30 min of the unit of red blood cells being removed from the fridge, and the transfusion should be completed within 4 h.

Platelets

An adult unit of platelets requires the pooling of platelets from four blood donations, and thus exposes the recipient to four donors. The more donors a recipient is exposed to, the more likely it is that they will produce antibodies to any antigens that are present in the donor blood.

Platelets can be collected directly from one donor using a process called apheresis. This involves attaching the donor to a cell separator machine which extracts specific blood components (i.e. platelets) from the blood. The blood transfusion service is establishing dedicated platelet donors who can donate platelets more regularly than blood. It has set a target of 80% of platelets to be produced in this way.[1] A unit of platelets should preferably be ABO identical or compatible, and rhesus compatibility is required if the recipient is a woman of childbearing age, in order to prevent haemolytic disease of the newborn.

A unit of platelets will expire 5 days after donation. It should be stored at 22°C on an agitator to prevent clumping, and should never be placed in a fridge, as this causes clumping. An adult unit of platelets has a volume of 200–300 mL. It should be administered rapidly via a platelet giving set.

Fresh frozen plasma (FFP)

Within 6 h of a blood donation, the plasma is removed from the donated blood and is rapidly frozen to −30°C, in order to maintain the coagulation factors. An adult unit of FFP has a shelf life of 1 year when stored at −30°C, and has a volume of approximately 250 mL. FFP needs to be ABO compatible but not rhesus compatible, as there are insufficient red blood cells present to cause an antibody response.

Prior to administration, FFP must be thawed by the blood bank, and it should then be administered within 30 min of thawing. FFP should be transfused using a standard blood transfusion set, and the transfusion should be completed within 4 h.

Cryoprecipitate

This is the cold insoluble portion of plasma which is formed when plasma is rapidly frozen into FFP. Cryoprecipitate is rich in factor XIII, von Willebrand factor, and fibrinogen, which is suspended in a small amount of plasma. A unit of cryoprecipitate has a shelf life of 1 year when stored at −30°C, and has a volume of 20–40 mL. Cryoprecipitate needs to be ABO compatible but not rhesus compatible, as there are insufficient red blood cells present to cause an antibody response.

Prior to administration, cryoprecipitate must be thawed by the blood bank. Administration must be commenced immediately after thawing, via a syringe pump or a standard blood transfusion set over 15–30 min.

Human albumin solution 4.5% and 20%

This is a solution of albumin which is produced from pooled plasma (i.e. from more than one donor) and diluted with buffered, stabilized 0.9% sodium chloride. Human albumin does not have to be ABO or rhesus compatible.

It is produced as human albumin 4.5% in 250-mL and 500-mL bottles, whereas human albumin 20% is produced in 100-mL bottles. It is administered over 30–60 min, or more slowly if a cardiac disorder is present, in order to prevent fluid overload. These solutions are stored in the dark at room temperature and have a shelf life of 5 years.

Reference

1 NHS Blood and Transplant (NHSBT). *Apheresis Collection Systems Framework Agreement Extension*. NHSBT: Watford, 2014.

Useful website

NHS Blood and Transplant (NHSBT). ♫ www.nhsbt.nhs.uk

Serious Hazards of Transfusion (SHOT)

In 1996, the Serious Hazards of Transfusion (SHOT) scheme was established in the UK as an independent and professionally led confidential enquiry into the serious hazards of blood transfusion. Its remit is to:

- work collaboratively with other regulatory bodies involved in transfusion, to ensure compliance with regulations
- promote safety in the transfusion process
- conduct research studies
- audit all stages of the transfusion process, from donor to recipient.

SHOT collects information on transfusion reactions and adverse events from healthcare providers who are involved in blood transfusion. These data are used to identify where areas of laboratory and clinical practice need to be improved, while supporting the production of clinical guidelines on blood transfusion.

During 2014, a total of 3668 reports were made to SHOT, of which 3017 were analysed for the 2014 Annual Report[2] (incomplete and withdrawn reports were not analysed). In 77.8% of cases the underlying cause of adverse events was errors (a similar finding to the 2013 figures). The Medicines and Healthcare products Regulatory Agency (MHRA) received 1110 reports, of which 764 were classed as serious adverse events (97.8% were errors) and 346 as serious adverse reactions. The majority of the reports received by SHOT and the MHRA related to errors in the transfusion process. SHOT emphasized the need to identify the factors involved in order to promptly correct them and prevent the occurrence of these incidents.

SHOT have revised their guidelines for transfusion at night because some patients were being denied essential transfusions in the night-time. The key revisions to their 'Transfusion at night' recommendations are as follows:

- Patient observations during transfusion should be given the same amount of attention regardless of the time of day or night.
- Transfusions must be given at night if there is a clear clinical indication and there is sufficient staffing to comply with the standards defined by the British Committee for Standards in Haematology (BCSH).[3]
- Decisions to transfuse should take into consideration the patient's full medical history, their current medical condition, and the patient's wishes.

In their review of errors that had led to the wrong blood component being transfused, SHOT stated that 'the pre-administration bedside check is a fundamental step, as it is the final opportunity to detect errors made earlier in the process and prevent a wrong transfusion.'

In 2014, SHOT received 122 reports relating to patients under the age of 18 years and, following the review of these reports, the key recommendations from SHOT are as follows:

- In children, blood component volumes should be prescribed based on the child's weight, but should not exceed the standard accepted dose for an adult.
- There has been an increase in the number of reported severe allergic reactions across all blood component types in paediatrics, but not in the neonatal/infant group.

Finally, SHOT stated in their 2014 Annual Report that all ABO-incompatible red cell transfusions should be included as 'never events.'[2]

References
2 Serious Hazards of Transfusion (SHOT). *Annual SHOT Report 2014*. SHOT: Manchester, 2015.
3 British Committee for Standards in Haematology (BCSH). *Guideline on the Administration of Blood Components*. BCSH: London, 2009.

Indications for transfusion

As there is not an unlimited supply of blood donations available, and there are inherent risks associated with blood transfusion, patients should only receive a transfusion when it is necessary.

Red blood cells

When a person is anaemic their haemoglobin level is below the expected level, and in certain circumstances this may need to be corrected with a transfusion of red blood cells. It is difficult to set a transfusion threshold, due to variability in patients' tolerance of anaemia and their associated comorbidities (e.g. cardiac disease). For chronic conditions the decision to transfuse will be made on an individual basis, once alternative treatment options have been explored.

Red blood cell transfusion is used following major surgery, trauma, and acute bleeds, in order to maintain the oxygen-carrying capacity of the blood.

Platelets

Platelet transfusion may be required due to a low platelet count caused by major haemorrhage or a bone marrow failure. It is used to treat significant bleeding following major surgery, trauma, and bleeding from the gastrointestinal tract. Platelets are also used to prevent bleeding in patients with bone marrow dysfunction, such as aplastic anaemia and leukaemia.

Fresh frozen plasma (FFP)

FFP is used to treat coagulation disorders and in major haemorrhage to prevent the dilutional effect of massive red blood cell transfusion.

Cryoprecipitate

Cryoprecipitate is used as a source of fibrinogen in disseminated intravascular coagulopathy (DIC) and in massive red blood cell transfusion, when the fibrinogen level is less than 1 g/L.

Human albumin solution (4.5% and 20%)

Human albumin solution is used to treat hypovolaemic shock due to burns, trauma, surgery, or infection. It is also used in liver disease for individuals with low serum albumin levels.

Blood sampling for blood transfusion

The information on a blood request form and blood sample bottles is the only communication between a clinical area and the blood bank. Therefore it is imperative that local and national policies are adhered to, so that the right patient receives the right blood. Receiving incompatible blood exposes an individual to the risk of serious injury or even death.

The cross-match request form should include details of why the request is being made, the component required, and the quantity. It should provide details of the recipient's medical history, including any previous obstetric or transfusion history and any specific requirements such as cytomegalovirus (CMV)-negative or irradiated red blood cells. The form should also state the date and time when the blood products are required.

The person who is requesting the blood should sign and print their name on the request form. This should also be done by the person taking the blood samples for cross-matching or group and save.

Group and save, and cross-matching

A group and save is performed by the blood bank to ascertain the patient's blood group and rhesus status, and also to identify any irregular antibodies. In an emergency, 2 units of emergency O Rh negative red blood cells can be given while the blood bank is sampling the recipient's blood.

A cross-match ensures that the red blood cells selected from donated stocks are compatible with the patient's blood. The patient will be cross-matched for a certain number of units of red blood cells. Once all of these units have been given to the patient, or some of them have been given over a set time period, the patient will need to be cross-matched again.

If an irregular antibody is identified during cross-matching, the patient should be issued with an antibody card that they must carry with them at all times.

Sampling procedure

Essential equipment

- Antimicrobial skin cleanser.
- Non-sterile gloves.
- Disposable apron.
- Blood sampling device.
- Cross-match/group and save blood sampling bottles.
- Gauze and hypoallergenic tape.
- Sharps container.
- Completed cross-match/group and save request forms.

Pre-procedure

- Explain the procedure to the patient and obtain their consent.
- Take blood samples from one patient at a time.
- Ensure that all equipment and packaging is intact and in date, before opening it and preparing to take blood samples.

Procedure
- Ask the patient to state their first name, surname, and date of birth. If they are unable to answer these questions due to confusion or unconsciousness, another member of staff can verify their identity.
- Cross-check this information with the patient's identification band.
- Check that the details on the patient's identification band correspond to the information on the blood request form. This should include the patient's hospital number.
- All stages of the checking procedure must be completed in full.
- Obtain the blood sample as per local or national policy.
- Do not take blood samples from the arm through which intravenous fluids are being administered, in order to prevent haemodilution of the blood sample.

Post-procedure
Hand write the following patient details on the blood bottles:
- first name
- surname (written in capital letters)
- date of birth
- hospital number
- ward or department
- gender
- date and time when the sample was taken
- signature of the person who took the blood sample.

Printed labels should only be used on blood sampling bottles if the 'red label' transfusion system is in operation or patient labels are printed at the bedside using the bar code system of patient identification wristbands.

Pre-transfusion checks

Pre-transfusion checks should consist of pre-procedure checks, which take place before requesting the blood products to be collected from the blood bank, and pre-administration checks, which take place once the blood product is available to administer to the patient.

Pre-procedure checks

- Is the transfusion prescribed correctly?
- Why does the patient require a transfusion?
- Is the reason for a transfusion still valid (e.g. is the haemoglobin level below 8 g/dL)?
- Does the patient have venous access which is patent?
- Are the correct blood administration sets available?
- If infusion devices (pumps) are to be used, check that they are compatible with the blood administration sets.
- Is a blood-warming device required?
- Has the collection of the blood products from the blood bank been requested as per local policy? This should include completion of the relevant request form.

Pre-administration checks

- All staff involved in blood administration must have completed core blood competencies as outlined by the National Patient Safety Agency (NPSA).[4]
- Visually inspect the blood bag for damage, discoloration, clumping, and the expiry date.
- Ensure that the patient understands the reason for the transfusion, and answer any questions that they may have.
- Check the prescription, including any specific requirements (e.g. furosemide to be administered with red blood cell transfusion).
- Perform baseline observations of blood pressure, pulse, respiration rate, oxygen saturation, urine output, and temperature.
- Positively identify the patient at the bedside. This should include checking their first name, surname, and date of birth.
- If the patient is unable to answer these questions due to confusion or unconsciousness, another member of staff can verify the patient's identity.
- Check the patient's identification band against the blood compatibility label. This should include their first name, surname, date of birth, and hospital number (see Figure 11.1).
- Check the blood unit number on the blood compatibility label against the blood unit number on the blood bag label.

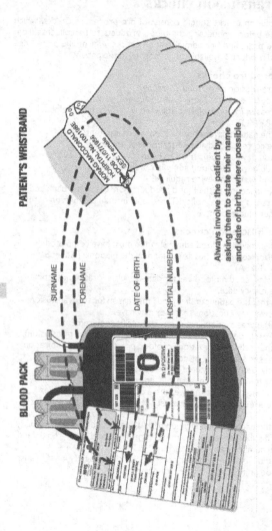

Always involve the patient by asking them to state their name and date of birth, where possible

PATIENT'S WRISTBAND

HORACE MACDONALD
HOSPITAL No. 10708E
DOB 11/07/1965
SEX: Female

BLOOD PACK

SURNAME

FORENAME

DATE OF BIRTH

HOSPITAL NUMBER

Figure 11.1 Checking the laboratory-generated compatibility label or tie-on tag against the patient's identity wristband. Reproduced with permission from *Handbook of Transfusion Medicine*, 5th edition, Figure 4.1. UK Blood Tissue Transplant Services, London. Available at: % www.transfusionguidelines.org.uk

- Check the blood group and rhesus status of the blood donor on the blood bag.
- Check the blood group and rhesus status of the recipient (patient) on the blood compatibility form. Are the blood groups and rhesus status of the donor and recipient compatible?
- Check the expiry date on the blood bag label.
- All stages of the checking procedure must be completed in full.
- If there are any discrepancies, *do not administer the blood product.*

Reference

4 National Patient Safety Agency (NPSA). *Right Patient, Right Blood; advice for safer blood transfusions. Action 1: competencies and competency assessment framework.* NPSA: London, 2006.

Administration of blood products

Always follow local and national policies when administering blood products.

Pre-procedure
- Wash your hands, and put on a disposable apron and non-sterile gloves.
- Obtain the patient's verbal consent for the procedure.
- Open the pack containing the blood administration set, and close the roller clamp so that the line is occluded.
- On the unit of red blood cells pull the tabs to expose the outlet port, and using the aseptic non-touch technique (ANTT) insert the spike on the blood administration set into the outlet port of the bag of red blood cells.
- Prime the blood administration line with blood, ensuring that all air is expelled.

Procedure
- Using the ANTT, attach the blood administration set to the patient's cannula, ensuring that both the cannula and the giving set are secure.
- If delivering the transfusion via a volumetric infusion pump, set the infusion rate as stated on the prescription.
- If delivering the transfusion via gravity using a standard blood administration set, first set and then monitor the drops per minute required (see Box 11.1).
- Sign the prescription and complete the relevant transfusion documentation according to local and national policy.
- Measure and record the patient's pulse, blood pressure, respiration rate, and temperature 15 min after each new unit has been commenced.
- Observe the patient for any signs of an adverse reaction, especially during the first 15 min after commencing the transfusion.
- If there are any concerns, perform additional observations as required.

Post-procedure
- On completion of the transfusion, perform and record the patient's observations.
- Dispose of the empty transfusion bag according to local policy.
- Blood administration sets should be changed at least 12-hourly and after every second unit has been transfused.
- Return all unused blood products to the blood bank.

Box 11.1 Calculating the drop rate per minute for a unit of blood delivered via a gravity blood administration set

In order to calculate the drop rate for a 350-mL bag of blood to be administered over 2 h, the drop rate for blood is 15 drops/min. This means that in a standard blood administration set there will be 15 drops in 1 mL of blood.

The calculation for working out the drop rate is as follows:

$$\frac{\text{volume to be infused (mL)}}{\text{time (h)}} \times \frac{\text{drop rate}}{60 \text{ min}} = \text{drops/min}$$

$$\frac{350}{2} \times \frac{15}{60} = \text{drops/min}$$

Cancel these fractions down to:

$$\frac{175}{1} \times \frac{1}{4} = \text{drops/min}$$

$$\frac{175}{4} = 43.75 \text{ drops/min}$$

Therefore, rounding up to the nearest whole number, the drop rate is 44 drops/min.

Blood warming

The routine use of blood-warming devices when delivering blood products is not recommended. These devices are used when caring for patients who are hypothermic, and also when giving massive rapid transfusion during a severe haemorrhage. In rapid transfusion there is a risk of cooling cardiac tissue, which can lead to cardiac dysrhythmias and even cardiac arrest. The risk is greatest when blood products are transfused through a central venous catheter, which terminates in or near the right atrium.

The National Institute for Health and Care Excellence (NICE) now recommends that all adults undergoing elective or emergency surgery should have intravenous fluids and blood products warmed to 37°C.[5]

There are two types of blood warmer available—water baths and dry heat blood warmers. With both types, the temperature should be below 38°C to reduce the risk of bacterial infections and damage to red blood cells and plasma proteins.

Only products designed as blood warmers should be used. Hot water, radiators, or microwave ovens should never be used to warm blood products.

When using water baths, the following safety measures must be adhered to due to the risk of bacterial contamination:

- Always follow the manufacturer's instructions.
- Before use, fill the water bath with sterile water.
- After use, drain the water bath and store it dry.
- Ensure that the blood warmer is given annual safety checks.

Reference

5 National Institute for Health and Care Excellence (NICE). *Inadvertent Perioperative Hypothermia: the management of inadvertent perioperative hypothermia in adults.* CG65. NICE: London, 2008. Jℵ www.nice.org.uk/guidance/cg65

Monitoring and documentation

All documentation relating to transfusion must comply with the Medicines and Healthcare products Regulatory Agency (MHRA) Blood Safety and Quality Regulations,[6] to ensure the traceability of donors and recipients of blood products for a minimum period of 30 years.

Nurses must ensure that all documentation complies with the Nursing and Midwifery Council's Code, Statement 10—'Keep clear and accurate records relevant to your practice.'[7]

Annual reports from SHOT have confirmed that errors in the transfusion process are often due to communication breakdown.[8] SHOT advise that, wherever possible, written or electronic communication should be utilized, as verbal communication is very susceptible to errors or misinterpretation. A key component of written communication is ensuring that all staff involved in the transfusion process have undergone training and competency assessment.

The NPSA has developed competencies[9] with which all organizations responsible for administering blood transfusions in England and Wales must comply. They relate to the following stages of the transfusion pathway:
• blood sampling
• organizing the receipt of blood
• collecting blood
• administering blood.

NHS Blood and Transplant (NHSBT) encourages the use of transfusion care pathways. However, as a minimum, documentation in the patient's notes should include the following.

Pre-transfusion

• The reason for the transfusion, the date and time requested, and when the transfusion is to be administered.
• Any relevant clinical information (e.g. blood results).
• The blood product required, the number of units to be administered, and any specific requirements (e.g. CMV negative).

Administration

• The date and time when the unit was commenced.
• The signature of the person who commenced the transfusion.
• The volume infused and the unique donation number of the blood product.
• The observations performed before, during, and after the transfusion.
• The date and time when the unit was completed.

Post-transfusion

- Complete any additional transfusion records.
- State whether the transfusion has corrected the haemoglobin level, platelet count, and/or clotting.
- State whether the patient's condition has stabilized if they were haemorrhaging.
- Outline the management and outcome of any adverse reactions or adverse events.

References

6 Medicines and Healthcare products Regulatory Agency (MHRA). *The Blood Safety and Quality Regulations Number 50.* MHRA: London, 2005.
7 Nursing and Midwifery Council (NMC). *The Code: professional standards of practice and behaviour for nurses and midwives.* NMC: London, 2015.
8 Serious Hazards of Transfusion (SHOT). *Annual Report 2012.* SHOT: Manchester, 2013.
9 National Patient Safety Agency (NPSA). *Right Patient, Right Blood; advice for safer blood transfusions. Action 1; competencies and competency assessment framework.* NPSA: London, 2006.

Useful website

NHS Blood and Transplant (NHSBT). ℘ www.nhsbt.nhs.uk

Transfusion reactions

The Medicines and Healthcare products Regulatory Agency (MHRA) is a government agency that has produced blood safety and quality regulations in which it defines a serious adverse reaction as 'an unintended response in a donor or recipient associated with the collection or transfusion of blood components that is fatal, life-threatening, disabling or incapacitating for the individual.'[10]

A transfusion reaction can be classified as being either minor or major, but it is important to remember that a minor reaction may be the precursor to a major reaction. A minor reaction may be due to immunological reactions to the blood product, whereas a major reaction may result in anaphylaxis or haemolysis.

Transfusion reactions generally occur within 15 min of commencing a transfusion, but can occur at any time, including after a transfusion has been completed.

Symptoms of a minor transfusion reaction
- A temperature increase of up to 1.5°C.
- Rash (but not systemic).
- Tachycardia.
- Blood pressure within normal range.

Treatment of a minor transfusion reaction
- Perform a full set of observations.
- Confirm the patient's identity and recheck their details against the blood compatibility label.
- Stop the transfusion and seek a medical review.
- Give prescribed medication (e.g. antihistamine and antipyretic).
- Reassure the patient and answer any questions they may have.
- The transfusion may be recommenced at a slower rate with close observation.
- Document the reaction in the patient's notes.

Symptoms of a major transfusion reaction
- Pyrexia greater than 38.5°C.
- Tachycardia.
- Hypotension.
- Tachypnoea and/or respiratory distress.
- Chest or abdominal pain.
- Nausea.
- Urticaria.
- Anaphylaxis.

Treatment of a major transfusion reaction
- Stop the transfusion and seek urgent medical assistance.
- In the event of suspected anaphylaxis, call the emergency medical team and follow the Resuscitation Council (UK) anaphylaxis guidelines.[11]
- Confirm the patient's identity and recheck their details against the blood compatibility label.

- Perform a baseline set of observations and repeat them based on the patient's condition.
- Remain with the patient, providing them with reassurance and keeping them informed of progress.
- Commence oxygen therapy and continuous saturation monitoring.
- Commence a strict fluid balance chart if this is not already in place.
- Take down the transfusion and ensure that the cannula remains patent, drawing back before flushing with saline.
- Inform the blood bank immediately, return the blood product with a completed reaction form, and send new blood samples taken from the opposite arm to that through which the transfusion was being given.
- Complete the patient documentation, including reporting of the adverse reaction.
- If an adverse event (e.g. ABO incompatibility) has caused the transfusion reaction, an incident form should be completed.

In 2011, NICE produced guidance on anaphylaxis,[12] and stated within their recommendations that following a suspected anaphylactic reaction in adults or in young people aged 16 years or over, blood samples should be taken for mast cell tryptase at the following times:

- as soon as possible after emergency treatment has commenced
- a second sample should be taken within 1–2 h, but no later than 4 h after the onset of the symptoms.

For children under the age of 16 years, NICE state that it is important to consider taking blood samples for mast cell tryptase if the cause of the anaphylactic reaction is thought to be venom related, drug related, or idiopathic.[12]

References

10 Medicines and Healthcare products Regulatory Agency (MHRA). *The Blood Safety and Quality Regulations Number 50.* MHRA: London, 2005.
11 Resuscitation Council (UK). *Emergency Treatment of Anaphylactic Reactions.* Resuscitation Council (UK): London, 2008.
12 National Institute for Health and Care Excellence (NICE). *Anaphylaxis: assessment to confirm an anaphylactic episode and the decision to refer after emergency treatment for a suspected anaphylactic episode.* CG134. NICE: London, 2011. ☞ www.nice.org.uk/guidance/cg134

Major haemorrhage

A major haemorrhage can be defined as the loss of the body's blood volume within 24 h, leading to hypovolaemic shock which is characterized by a reduced venous return and cardiac output. If the haemorrhage is not halted and circulatory volume restored, the body's compensatory mechanisms will fail. This will result in the hypovolaemic shock progressing to the refractory stage, leading to multi-organ failure and ultimately death.

The aim of massive transfusion is to rapidly and effectively restore an adequate circulatory volume in order to maintain homeostasis and the oxygen-carrying capacity of the blood.

In 2010, the NPSA issued a rapid response report on the transfusion of blood products in an emergency.[13] This was in response to reports of delays in providing blood components for life-threatening haemorrhages, resulting in serious incidents and even the death of patients. The NPSA advised that all hospitals should have a major haemorrhage protocol in place and ensure that staff receive training.

Causes of major haemorrhage

- Trauma.
- Gastrointestinal bleed.
- Acute or chronic liver disease.
- Obstetric haemorrhage.
- Surgical intervention.
- Coagulation disorders.
- Bone marrow dysfunction.

Treatment and protocols

- Positively identify the patient, or if this is not possible, issue an emergency hospital number.
- Initiate the hospital's major haemorrhage protocol.
- Request expert assistance (e.g. surgeon) to halt the haemorrhage.
- Use the ABCDE approach to assessment.[14]
- Perform a full set of observations and repeat as required by the hospital policy and the patient's condition.
- Administer oxygen therapy to maintain saturations of 95–100%.
- Insert two wide-bore cannulae in order to give fluid resuscitation.
- Take bloods for group and save, cross-match, full blood count, clotting, and renal and liver function tests.
- Contact the blood bank to request urgent cross-match, group and save, and blood products.
- Give 2 units of O Rh negative emergency blood, using a blood warmer, if ABO and Rh compatible blood is not available.
- Maintain a strict fluid balance chart.

The major haemorrhage protocol is summarized in Figure 11.2.

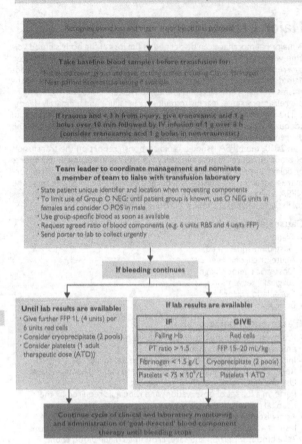

Figure 11.2 Major haemorrhage protocol. Reproduced with permission from *Handbook of Transfusion Medicine*, 5th edition, Figure 7.2, UK Blood Tissue Transplant Services, London. Available at ℗ www.transfusionguidelines.org.uk. Adapted from the *BCSH Practical Guideline for the Management of Those With, or at Risk of, Major Haemorrhage* (2014). This information is licensed under the terms of the Open Government Licence (www.nationalarchives.gov.uk/doc/open-government-licence/version/2).

Complications of massive transfusion

- Circulatory overload, especially if the patient has a history of cardiac and/or renal insufficiency.
- Coagulopathy caused by the depletion of clotting factors, due to haemorrhage and the dilutional effect of red blood cell transfusion.
- Electrolyte imbalance, because the infusion of blood products can lead to elevated potassium levels and low calcium levels.
- Acid–base disturbance due to the lactic acid content of transfused red blood cells.
- Hypothermia if a blood warmer is not used to infuse all blood products.
- Transfusion-related acute lung injury (TRALI) due to anti-leucocyte antibody reaction.

References

13 National Patient Safety Agency (NPSA). *Rapid Response Report: the transfusion of blood and blood components in an emergency.* NPSA: London, 2010.
14 Jevon P. ABCDE: the assessment of the critically ill patient. *British Journal of Cardiac Nursing* 2010; 5: 268–72.

Circumstances in which individuals may refuse blood products

Healthcare professionals need to be sensitive to the personal, cultural, and religious beliefs of the patient and their relatives, as these may lead them to refuse blood products either during a routine procedure or in the event of a massive haemorrhage.

Law and consent

Under British law (Mental Capacity Act 2005)[15] a competent adult has the right to refuse medical treatment or choose an alternative treatment. A competent person is able to:

- understand and retain the information required to make a decision about their care
- use this information in order to decide whether to consent to the treatment being offered
- communicate their wishes.

Ethically their decision should be respected, once they have been fully informed of the consequences of not receiving the treatment. For example, an individual may not wish to receive blood products because of the potential risk of transmissible infections. Healthcare professionals should consider alternative therapies, whilst also informing them of the potential risks associated with not receiving blood products, when this is considered to be in their best interest.

An advance directive or decision enables a person with mental capacity to refuse healthcare in the future. For an advance directive to be valid, the person must:

- be aged 18 years or over
- have full mental capacity when the advance directive is made
- state what treatments they do not want to receive and under what circumstances
- sign and date the advance directive in the presence of two adults who have mental capacity.

The Court of Protection deals with all financial and health issues relating to people who lack mental capacity. They will look at cases where the person's carer, healthcare worker, or social worker disagrees as to what is in their best interest.

Jehovah's Witnesses

Jehovah's Witnesses are from a Christian background, but have some differing theological viewpoints from the Church of England and the Catholic Church. They believe that Jesus Christ's loss of blood on the cross is highly symbolic and that receiving another person's blood is sinful, as it contains their soul.

Most Jehovah's Witnesses carry a 'No Blood' card, and others have advance directives lodged in their medical notes or held by their general practitioner and/or family. In the event of an individual being unconscious and their status as a Jehovah's Witness being unknown or unclear, healthcare professionals are expected to provide care to the best of their ability and 'do good', even if this includes giving blood. Advice can be obtained from the Hospital Liaison Committee for Jehovah's Witnesses 24 hours a day (tel. 020 8906 2211).

Prior to planned admission for surgery it is important to ascertain the patient's status as a Jehovah's Witness and obtain informed consent for the procedure. The patient should be made aware of the blood products available and decide which of these are acceptable. This will enable a plan of care to be drawn up and clearly documented in the patient's medical notes.[16] The patient should be checked for clotting disorders and signs of anaemia, and anaemia should be treated using oral iron therapy and/or erythropoietin. Non-steroidal anti-inflammatory drugs and anticoagulant medication should be stopped prior to surgery.

The surgery should be undertaken by a surgeon whose seniority is appropriate to the risk associated with the procedure. In the event of an emergency, the healthcare professional must comply with the wishes of the Jehovah's Witness.

Young people
Young people should be involved as much as possible in decisions about their care, even if they are not able to make decisions on their own. All young people aged 16–18 years are presumed in law to have the capacity to consent to treatment. However, if they are deemed not to be competent, consent should be obtained from an adult with parental responsibility.

References
15 *Mental Capacity Act 2005. Chapter 9.* London: The Stationery Office.
16 Effa-Heap G. Blood transfusion: implications for treating a Jehovah's Witness patient. *British Journal of Nursing* 2009; **18**: 174–7.

Wound care

Physiology of wound healing

The process of wound healing is a dynamic one, and involves the body repairing its largest organ—the skin. This process can be divided into the following stages.

Haemostasis

- This stage commences at the time of injury, and in the case of surgery this is usually due to an incision.
- The action of injury causes chemicals to be released which initiate the clotting cascade. This includes the activation of platelets from within the blood circulation at the point of injury. Degranulation of the platelets allows them to clump together to form a clot.
- Fibrinogen is also released, and forms a fibrin mesh which helps to support the clot. The purpose of the clot is to stem blood flow and help to prevent bacteria from gaining entry into the body.
- The damaged blood vessels at the site of injury vasoconstrict to help to reduce blood loss.

Inflammation

- Blood vessels near the point of injury start to dilate due to the release of histamine.
- This allows the capillaries to widen their spaces to facilitate the passage of the first white blood cells (the neutrophils) from the circulating blood out into the injured tissue. The neutrophils start to clear any dead and devitalized tissue together with bacteria from the site of injury.
- Around 24 h later, the larger white blood cells (the monocytes) arrive at the area of injury and exit the blood supply in the same manner as the neutrophils. The monocytes are activated by this process and mature into macrophages. The macrophages are able to ingest larger pieces of material than the neutrophils, together with bacteria and the dying neutrophils.
- Both neutrophils and monocytes are summoned to the area of injury until the wound has been cleared of dead and devitalized tissue together with bacteria.
- The macrophages then help to coordinate the next stage of wound healing.

Proliferation

- This stage involves the creation of new tissue called granulation tissue, which is needed to fill the wound with new connective tissue and finally seal it with new epithelial cells.
- The proliferative phase requires an increased blood supply. This is achieved by angiogenesis—that is, the creation of new capillary loops which develop and grow from existing capillaries.
- This new blood supply is needed to create the granulation tissue. The latter is mainly composed of the protein collagen, and is laid down to fill any void in the dermis or below it that has been created by the injury. This is termed the granulation process.

- When the granulation process has filled the void, epithelial cells will start to replicate and migrate from the edges of the wound and from hair follicles (if these are still present) to cover the wound. The process stops when these epithelial cells make contact with epithelial cells that are replicating and migrating in the opposite direction.
- At this stage the wound has sealed but it lacks tensile strength.

Maturation

- This phase can last for up to 2 years.
- The tissue is refined and the blood vessels that are no longer required are reabsorbed by the body.
- The strength of the wound increases, reaching up to 70–90% of the original strength of the body tissue.
- This process creates scar tissue which is not the same as normal body tissue, although it is refined over time. The body cannot heal without scarring.

Prevention of surgical site infection

Pre-operative assessment

- Routine blood tests to detect anaemia and malnutrition should be undertaken, and anaemia should be corrected if possible.
- The patient should be advised to eat a well-balanced diet to ensure adequate intake of essential vitamins and minerals for wound healing. If this is not physically possible, the dietitian should be involved prior to surgery.
- Smoking cessation should be advised. If the patient is not able to stop smoking, nicotine replacement therapy for the inpatient stay should be discussed. Smoking decreases oxygen saturation, which can delay wound healing.
- If the patient is obese, weight loss in the period while they are waiting for surgery should be encouraged, as obese patients tend to have more complications related to wound healing. However, in the last few weeks before surgery they should be advised to eat a balanced diet to ensure intake of essential vitamins and minerals together with adequate protein and carbohydrate to facilitate wound healing.
- Screening for MRSA should be undertaken according to local policy, providing details of how eradication treatment will be obtained if required.
- Explain to the patient the admission process and what to expect during their stay, in order to reduce patient anxiety. Anxiety can affect wound repair, as the stress hormones that are released slow down the rate of wound healing.

Pre-operative stage

- The patient should be instructed to bathe or shower on either the day before or the day of surgery in order to reduce the bacterial skin burden.
- If hair has to be removed, this is done on the day of surgery by healthcare staff using electric clippers with a single-use head.[1]

Intra-operative stage

- Use povidone iodine or chlorhexidine to prepare the skin for incision immediately before surgery.
- Apply an appropriate interactive dressing to cover the wound and to meet the likely needs of the wound. Interactive dressings promote a moist environment, maintain the wound temperature as close to body temperature as possible, and prevent bacteria from entering the wound.
- For wound healing by primary intention (i.e. using sutures, clips, etc.), a wound dressing that will absorb blood and exudate is required— for example, a non-adherent absorbent dressing covered by a film dressing, an alginate dressing covered by a film dressing, or a foam dressing.

- The aim is to have a dressing that can be disturbed as little as possible, but which will facilitate examination of the wound margins and the nature and amount (usually minimal) of fluid that is being released from the wound.
- Cavity wounds should be dressed as dictated by the wound assessment. Frequently topical negative pressure is applied to wounds that are healing by secondary intention following surgery, to enhance the rate of production of granulation tissue (see section on topical negative pressure on ➔ p. 252).

Post-operative stage

Wound healing by primary intention (using clips, sutures, etc.)
- If the dressing needs to be changed in the first 48 h post-operatively, an aseptic technique using saline to cleanse the wound is required.
- After 48 h the dressing can be removed and the patient will be able to shower.

Wound healing by secondary intention (cavity wounds)
- Dress as dictated by the wound assessment. Immediately post-operatively, alginates which act as a haemostat to help to stop bleeding, with a film dressing to hold them in place, may be useful (for further information, see dressings section on ➔ p. 250).

Reference

1 National Institute for Health and Care Excellence (NICE). *Surgical Site Infection.* QS49. London. NICE: London, 2013. ℛ www.nice.org.uk/guidance/qs49

Wound assessment

Types of wound closure

Wound healing by primary intention
- In this type of wound closure the wound edges can be realigned and closed by using sutures, clips, skin closure strips, or glue.
- The wound usually seals within 48–72 h, and after this time will not necessarily require a dressing unless it is oozing.
- However, patients usually prefer to have a dressing in place for comfort and cosmetic reasons.
- In this type of wound closure the essential checks would involve observing for redness and inflammation. If this extends from the wound edges by more than 1–2 cm, it could be a sign of infection.
- There should be minimal discharge or oozing from the wound once the bleeding has stopped (this should have occurred prior to return from surgery). If there is more than slight blood loss this must be reviewed medically.
- If there is discharge (known as exudate) from the wound, the colour, thickness, and amount must be noted and reported. Discharge of pus (thick and green/brown in colour) could indicate infection below the suture line.
- If the wound starts to separate due to infection, discussions should take place with medical staff regarding the viability of the suture line and the need to remove the sutures. It is usually easier to manage an open wound than a wound held together by sutures. Specialist help from the tissue viability team may be required to manage such a wound in order to determine whether debridement is needed and, if so, which method would be most appropriate. When the wound has been debrided, specialist techniques such as topical negative pressure may be indicated to help to speed up the healing process. If sutures are removed, the wound needs to be managed in the same way as any cavity wound healing by secondary intention (see section on dressings for secondary intention wound healing on → p. 250).

Wound healing by secondary intention
- In this type of wound the extent of tissue destruction means that the wound edges cannot be realigned.
- The wound needs to heal from its base, filling with new granulating tissue first, before epithelialization from the wound edges completes the sealing of the wound with new skin.
- This process will be impaired in the presence of dead or devitalized tissue, which therefore needs to be debrided.
- The following methods of debridement are most commonly used:
  - *Autolytic debridement* involves keeping the wound under ideal conditions to allow the body to clear the devitalized tissue. This can be achieved by using dressings that facilitate a moist wound environment. This method is slow but gentle.

- *Mechanical debridement* can be achieved by irrigation under pressure, or by applying a physical mechanical force using a debriding pad such as Debrisoft®. This method is relatively fast and gentle.
- *Biosurgery* involves the application of larvae, usually for a 3-day period. This method is relatively fast.
- *Conservative sharp debridement* involves the removal of dead tissue with a scalpel or scissors. Competencies are required to undertake this procedure. This method is fairly fast.
- *Surgical debridement* is the removal of dead and devitalized tissue by surgeons, and requires a theatre and anaesthetic.

- When the wound has been debrided, material must be placed in the wound to create a moist environment.
- The amount of exudate produced by the wound will determine the choice of dressing. If the wound is producing low levels of exudate, a dressing that provides hydration is required. If the wound is producing moderate or high levels of exudate, an absorptive product is needed.
- The dressing material must be in contact with the whole of the base and sides of the wound.

The choice of dressings for different wound types is summarized in Table 12.1.

Table 12.1 Choice of wound dressing according to wound type

Type of dressing	Amount of exudate	Primary intention wound healing	Secondary intention wound healing
Traditional gauze	None/dry	Yes	No
Tulle	None/dry	Yes	No
Film/post-operative film dressing	None/dry	Yes	Only used as a secondary dressing
Hydrogel	None/dry	No	Yes, with secondary dressing (e.g. film)
Hydrocolloid	None/dry	Yes	No, unless shallow cavity wound
Alginate	Moderate	Yes, with secondary dressing	Yes, with secondary dressing
Foam	Moderate to high	Yes	Yes, cavity filler with secondary dressing
Hydrofibre	Moderate to high	Yes, with secondary dressing	Yes, cavity filler with secondary dressing
Capillary dressing	High	Yes, with secondary dressing	Yes, cavity filler with secondary dressing
Superabsorbent	High	Yes	As a secondary dressing

Dressings for primary intention wounds

Primary intention wounds are wounds that have been closed by means of sutures, clips, skin closure strips, or glue.

Dressings can be divided into two types. Primary dressings come into direct contact with the wound bed, whereas secondary dressings cover the primary dressings. Not all primary dressings require a secondary dressing.

Traditional dressings
- Gauze-type material.
- Absorbency rate is minimal. Fluid will 'strike through' to the outer dressing, thus providing a route for infection into and from the wound. When wet the wound is cooled, and then the material dries out, adhering to the wound as it does so. This can cause trauma on removal.
- The wound needs to be redressed when 'strike through' occurs.
- This type of dressing is only advocated for dry wounds.

Tulles
- Open-weave gauze impregnated with paraffin.
- Absorbency rate is minimal. As with gauze dressings, fluid will 'strike through' to the outer dressing, thus providing a route for infection into and from the wound. When wet the wound is cooled, and then the material dries out, adhering to the wound as it does so. This can cause trauma on removal. Granulating tissue can hook through the openings in the tulle, causing trauma on removal.
- The wound needs to be redressed when 'strike through' occurs.
- This type of dressing is only advocated for dry wounds, and will need a secondary dressing to cover it.

Modern dressings
- Surgical dressings.
- These dressings are the kind traditionally used to cover primary intention wounds. There are several different types:
    - dressing pad alone
    - dressing pad with adhesive covering
    - dressing pad with shower-proof adhesive covering
    - dressing pad with film.
- The choice of dressing needs to be based on patient requirements. For example, if the patient is likely to shower, the last two types will be more useful.
- Absorbency of these products is limited. If the wound is likely to produce exudate, a more absorbent dressing type will be more effective.

Alginate dressings
- These are available in flat sheet, fleece, and ribbon form.
- They absorb exudate by ion exchange, with sodium being absorbed and calcium donated.
- They can be used in flat wounds and cavity wounds.
- The dressing needs to be replaced at least weekly.
- Fleece and ribbon dressings require a secondary dressing (e.g. film dressing).
- Flat dressings with a backing do not require a secondary dressing.

Antimicrobial dressings
- These dressings should only be used to treat wounds that are heavily colonized with bacteria, or infected wounds. The benefits of their prophylactic use in at-risk patients have yet to be demonstrated.
- Antimicrobial substances can damage the bacterial cell wall, causing cell death. The pH of the wound may also be altered to inhibit bacterial proliferation.
- The following types of antimicrobial dressings are available:
  - silver
  - honey
  - povidone iodine or cadexomer iodine
  - oxygen-releasing.
- The choice of dressing needs to be based on the amount of exudate, to facilitate a moist environment.
- At present there is no evidence to suggest that any one antimicrobial dressing is preferable to another.

Dressings for secondary intention wounds

Secondary intention wounds are wounds that cannot be closed with sutures, clips, skin closure strips, or glue, but which need to heal by granulation and epithelialization.

For this type of wound, the dressing material needs to be in contact with the wound bed.

Traditional dressing types are not recommended, as they lack absorbency and cause pain on removal.

Hydrogel dressings
- These are available in gel form or as a sheet.
- They donate fluid to the wound to create a moist environment.
- A dressing is needed to hold them in place. A film dressing is a cheap and effective secondary dressing option.
- Redressing is required after 2–3 days.

Hydrocolloid dressings
- These are available as a sheet dressing that is self-adhesive, so do not require a secondary dressing. They are only suitable for flat or very shallow wounds.
- They donate fluid to the wound and have some limited absorbency properties.
- The dressing can remain in place for up to 1 week.
- At least a 2 cm overlap from the edge of the wound is required all around the wound.
- They can be used as a secondary dressing.

Foam dressings
- These are available as flat dressings or as cavity fillers.
- They absorb exudate, and the manufacturers produce a range of absorbency levels.
- Cavity fillers will require a secondary dressing (e.g. film dressing).
- Flat dressings are either self-adhesive or non-adhesive.
- Non-adhesive flat dressings are attached by taping around the edge of the dressing like a picture frame.
- Foam dressings need to be changed at least weekly.

Hydrofibre dressings
- These are available in flat sheet and ribbon form.
- They absorb exudate.
- They are suitable for wounds with a moderate to high level of exudate.
- They can be used for flat wounds and cavity wounds.
- Dressings need to be replaced at least weekly.
- Flat sheet and ribbon dressings require a secondary dressing (e.g. film dressing).

Capillary dressings

- These are available in flat sheet or spiral form.
- They absorb large amounts of exudate, and can transport exudate by capillary action to another dressing or into a bag.
- They can be used in cavity wounds or sinus-type wounds.
- Dressings need to be replaced at least weekly.

Superabsorbent pads

- These are available as flat dressings.
- The dressing is impregnated with crystals that absorb the exudate and form a gel, in a similar manner to nappy technology.
- They can absorb large amounts of exudate.
- At least a 2 cm overlap from the edge of the wound is required all around the wound.
- Dressings need to be changed at least weekly.

Further reading

Dealey C. *The Care of Wounds: a guide for nurses.* Wiley-Blackwell: Chichester, 2012.
Slachta PA (ed.). *Wound Care Made Incredibly Easy!* 3rd edn. Lippincott Williams & Wilkins: Philadelphia, PA, 2015.

Useful website

World Wide Wounds. 🔗 www.worldwidewounds.com

Topical negative pressure therapy

Topical negative pressure (TNP) therapy involves the application of suction to a wound. The main aim of its use is to stimulate the proliferation of granulation tissue. TNP therapy is also used to enhance the attachment process in skin grafts and some sutured wounds.

- The therapy works by stimulating granulation tissue to proliferate at a faster rate.
- It does this by reducing oedema, stimulating blood flow, and promoting cell division.
- The system is sealed, so exogenous bacteria are less likely to enter the wound. Infrequent dressing changes can also be helpful in this respect.
- The suction removes exudate, but the foam or gauze that is used under the film dressing provides a moist environment.
- The therapy also draws in the wound, so that the wound edges are brought closer together.

These instructions are only a general guide. Always consult the manufacturer's instructions, and only undertake TNP therapy if you are competent in the use of this procedure.

Open cavity wounds

- Open, less dense foam, or else gauze, is usually used for TNP. The foam or gauze needs to be the correct type for the specific TNP machine being used, as the foam and gauze vary between manufacturers. Only the consumables specified by the manufacturer of the machine should be used.
- Foam is cut to the shape of the wound cavity. It can consist of one piece or several pieces (all of which must be in contact with each other). Do not place small foam chips inside the wound, as they may become embedded in the granulation tissue and be difficult to remove. Some practitioners prefer to place a perforated film or a silicone-coated gauze dressing across the wound bed and then place foam or gauze for TNP on top of it.
- Next apply film dressing over the foam and onto the skin to seal the foam in place. Ensure that the skin is dry and that no gaps are present when applying the film, otherwise the suction will not work. Apply the suction tubing to the dressing according to the manufacturer's instructions.
- Connect the tubing to the suction device at the setting indicated by the manufacturer or the specialist nurse. Turn on the machine. The foam should shrink and become harder and the machine should reach the optimum suction level. If this does not happen, check for air leaks and re-patch with foam as necessary.
- The dressing needs to be changed every 3 days or as specified in the manufacturer's instructions.

Shallow wounds, skin grafts, or incisional wounds at risk of complications

- Some practitioners use a denser type of foam, or else gauze, for these wounds.
- The foam or gauze should be cut to the size of the wound, allowing some extra for shrinkage.
- Follow the procedure described in the section on open cavity wounds on ◑ p. 252.

Contraindications to TNP therapy

- Wounds at risk of bleeding (i.e. with exposed blood vessels).
- Patients with clotting disorders or on anticoagulants.
- Malignant wounds and unexplored fistulae.

Further reading

European Wound Management Association (EWMA). *Topical Negative Pressure in Wound Management*. EWMA: London, 2007. ℘ www.woundsinternational.com/media/issues/84/files/content_46.pdf

Common wound infections and treatment

The intact skin is a barrier to infection, whereas a breach in the integrity of the skin caused by surgical incision or cannulation provides a route for bacteria to enter the body. If the patient is not able to mount an effective host response to clear the bacteria, there is an increased risk of an infection developing.

In order to avoid overprescribing of antibiotics it is important to know the differences between normal inflammation and infection. Wounds should be assessed regularly, and any signs of infection noted (see Table 12.2).

The different types of infection can be classified as follows.

Cellulitis

- A spreading inflammation of the tissues, characterized by redness, heat, and tenderness.
- Pus may be present.
- Tissue necrosis may ensue.
- Lymph glands near to the area may become enlarged.
- Analysis of a wound swab or aspirated wound fluid may aid microbial type classification and antibiotic prescribing.
- In the early stages, oral antibiotics may be sufficient, but in more advanced cases intravenous (IV) antibiotics will be required.
- The standard antibiotic treatment is amoxicillin and flucloxacillin, or cefuroxime or erythromycin.
- Topical antimicrobial dressings should be used.
- The increase or reduction in inflammation can be monitored by marking the outline of the inflammation with a fine marker pen, with the patient's consent.

Table 12.2 Assessment of a wound for signs of infection

Sign	Inflammation	Infection
Redness of skin	Present but not more than 2 cm from the wound margin	Present, usually more than 2 cm from the wound margin and spreading
Heat		
Swelling		
Exudate	Minimal clear fluid	Thick, increasing amount, and yellow, green, or rust coloured
Pain	Decreasing	Persistent or increasing
Malodour	Absent	Present
Tissue	Well adhered	Fragile, pocketing, and breaking down

Necrotizing infections of skin and soft tissues
- Usually caused by Gram-negative bacteria.
- Inflammation is usually present and gas formation may occur.
- Tissue necrosis is present.
- Analysis of a wound swab, aspirated wound fluid, or tissue biopsy may aid microbial type classification and antibiotic prescribing.
- Oral antibiotic treatment: amoxicillin, co-amoxicillin, and metronidazole.
- IV antibiotic treatment: amoxicillin, piperacillin/tazobactam, ciprofloxacin, and clindamycin.
- Topical antimicrobial dressings should be used.

Necrotizing fasciitis
- This is a rapidly spreading infection of tissues and the subcutaneous layer. It spreads along the muscle fascia, and the tissues first appear bruised and then liquefy.
- Rapid radical debridement surgery is required to remove devitalized tissue and a substantial margin of unaffected tissue, the aim being to remove any tissue that may be infected but which is not yet demonstrating signs. Several surgical visits may be needed to clear the bacteria.
- Analysis of tissue samples can aid bacterial identification.
- Multi-organ failure can occur.
- IV antibiotics are urgently required, with multiple antibiotic prescribing, as this is usually a mixed bacterial infection.
- Antimicrobial dressings should be used.
- When all of the infected tissue has been completely removed, TNP therapy can be used to help to increase the rate of new tissue formation by the body.

Further reading

Bannister B, Gillespie S and Jones J. *Infection: microbiology and management*, 3rd edn. Wiley-Blackwell: Chichester, 2006.
European Wound Management Association (EWMA). *Identifying Criteria for Wound Infection*. EWMA: London, 2005. http://ewma.org/fileadmin/user_upload/EWMA/pdf/Position_Documents/2005__Wound_Infection_/English_pos_doc_final.pdf

Useful website

World Wide Wounds. www.worldwidewounds.com

Skin assessment

Skin assessment

As soon as a patient is admitted to the area, a top-to-toe examination of the skin should take place in order to identify the condition of the skin and any existing pressure damage.

Skin assessment is both visual and tactile.

Pressure damage in adults usually occurs over bony prominences (see Figure 13.1).

On smaller areas, such as the nose and fingers, masks, tubing, or devices may cause pressure damage.

Visual assessment

- Red areas need to be assessed for blanching. Light finger pressure should be applied to the tissues and then removed. If the area turns from red to white, and then turns red again on removal of pressure, it indicates a normal physiological reaction with a normal microcirculation, so the red area is not due to pressure damage.
- If the area remains red and does not turn white when pressure is applied, this indicates stage 1 pressure damage. This should be identified in the notes by stating the precise area, and measurements of the extent of the damage. This should prompt instigation of a repositioning schedule (see ➔ p. 262).
- In darkly pigmented skin the blanching test does not apply, as the tissues do not produce a red hue. Instead the area should be palpated to determine any sogginess, bogginess, and whether the area is hotter or cooler than the surrounding tissues. Again this indicates stage 1 pressure damage which needs to be reported in line with local policy, and appropriate action instigated.
- Blue or purple hues occur in all skin tones, and usually indicate deeper tissue damage. Again the position of the colour change must be stated in the notes, together with measurements of the extent of the area. Photographs of the area could also be taken, with the patient's consent, as per local guidelines. This should prompt instigation of methods of managing deeper tissue damage, the most important element of which is to reposition the patient off the area if possible (for treatment guidance, see ➔ p. 264).
- The visual assessment should also include identification of the condition of the skin. Dry skin needs to be moisturized regularly to make its function more efficient. The buttocks and genital areas need to be assessed for any damage caused by incontinence. Wet soggy skin will not withstand pressure well, and the area should be protected from excoriation by using barrier products and addressing continence problems. If there is profound incontinence, use of a shaped pad is recommended.
- Any other skin lesions (e.g. eczema) should be recorded and the normal management methods discussed with the patient.
- Any old pressure ulceration areas which have healed also need to be noted and considered when care planning for repositioning. These areas only attain 70–90% of their pre-ulceration strength, so are at higher risk of breaking down.

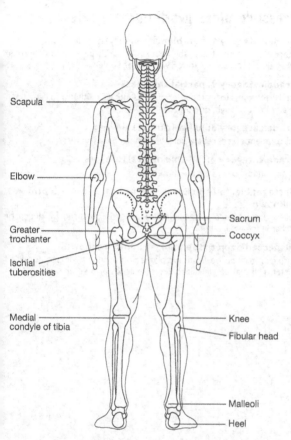

Figure 13.1 Bony prominences that are the main sites of pressure ulcers.
Reproduced from George Castledine and Ann Close, *Oxford Handbook of Adult Nursing*, 2007, with permission from Oxford University Press.

Pressure ulcer grading/categories

Grade/category 1: non-blanchable erythema
Intact skin with non-blanchable redness, in darkly pigmented skin, could be a painful area, firmer, softer, warmer, or cooler.

Grade/category 2: partial thickness
Partial-thickness loss of the dermis presenting as either a shallow open ulcer without slough, or a blister.

Grade/category 3: full-thickness skin loss
Subcutaneous fat may be visible, but not deeper structures.

Grade/category 4: full-thickness tissue loss
Bone, tendon, or muscle is exposed.

Unstageable: full-thickness skin or tissue loss—depth unknown
Full-thickness tissue loss, but actual depth is obscured by slough or eschar in the wound bed.

Suspected deep tissue injury—depth unknown
Purple or maroon localized area of discoloured intact skin or blood-filled blister. This may be difficult to detect in darkly pigmented skin.

Useful websites
European Pressure Ulcer Advisory Panel (EPUAP). ♪ www.epuap.org
Stop the Pressure. ♪ nhs.stopthepressure.co.uk

Pressure ulcer risk assessment

Patients should be assessed for pressure ulcer risk within 6 h of admission.[1] The facts gathered during the risk assessment process should aid care planning. The risk assessment should be used to aid clinical judgement, not to replace it.

The most widely used risk assessment tool for pressure ulceration in the UK is the Waterlow Scale, but other tools are also used, such as the Braden Scale, Norton Scale, Walsall Scale, and Maelor Scale.

Risk assessment tools look at intrinsic and extrinsic factors that may contribute to pressure damage. The tools are not predictive, but provide an assessment of risk of damage, and are designed to guide care. They are useful if they are completed accurately and care is then planned to protect the patient from their specific risks.

- *Mobility.* This is the main risk factor. If the patient is not able to walk or move him- or herself, appropriate care needs to be planned.
  For the patient who is undergoing surgery, issues to be considered include how long they are likely to be sedated prior to theatre and on the theatre table, how long they are likely to be immobile following surgery, and whether this factor increases their overall risk score.
- *Sensation and neuropathic feedback.* If the patient is usually able to respond to the body's messages to move or reposition him- or herself, will sedation and pain relief dull the body's ability to perceive these messages? If so, care needs to be planned to take into account this risk factor.
- *Nutrition.* How long will it be before the patient resumes a normal diet? This question needs to be considered in terms of both the potential pressure ulcer risk and the body's ability to heal itself. Does the patient need other forms of nutrition until they are able to resume normal diet?
- *Pain.* This can make patients reluctant to move, or in some cases may cause them to thrash about, generating friction and shear forces. Pain relief is important both in terms of comfort and in enabling the patient to move adequately.
- *Moisture.* Anything that causes the patient's tissues to become moist can contribute to pressure damage, so it is important to ensure that the patient is kept clean and dry.

Pressure ulcer risk assessment needs to be reviewed, usually on a daily basis, in the surgical setting. Any additional risk factors relating to surgery can usually be removed from the risk assessment after 48 h.

Reference

1 National Institute for Health and Care Excellence (NICE). *Pressure Ulcers; prevention and management of pressure ulcers.* CG179. NICE: London, 2014. ℀ www.nice.org.uk/guidance/cg179

Pressure ulcer prevention

Pressure ulcer prevention is based on optimal management of the patient.

- If the patient is unable to reposition him- or herself, a repositioning schedule must be instigated. The frequency of repositioning should be based on the individual's response to pressure.
- To determine the optimum frequency, 2-hourly repositioning is a good place to start, then either shortening or prolonging the frequency as determined by the reaction of the patient's skin.
- If the patient is at high risk of pressure ulceration, a high-specification mattress may be appropriate to aid pressure relief. The increased risk that surgery will incur should be considered prior to surgery so that the correct equipment can be obtained and placed beneath the patient before they attend theatre.
- The position in which the patient can be placed will depend on their individual circumstances. For example, they may be uncomfortable if placed on the site of surgery.
- The 30° tilt is advocated, with the patient placed on a fatty pad rather than a bony prominence. Five pillows are required for placing the patient in this position.
- If the patient is diabetic or has peripheral vascular disease and is immobile, their heels should be elevated from the mattress by means of pillows or another heel-raising device. Heel condition should be monitored at each positional change.
- Skin assessment should be performed at each positional change, and the findings must be documented.
- The patient's skin must be kept clean and dry. The patient should be changed on return from theatre to ensure that they are not lying on damp sheets or clothing.
- Urine output and drainage from wounds and drain sites should be monitored, as these could also cause the skin to become moist and contribute to pressure damage.
- Ensure that clothing is smooth and not rolled under the patient.
- If the patient is not able to mobilize independently, they should not be allowed to sit out for longer than 2 h before being returned to bed to rest. This aspect needs to be considered when planning their daily care (e.g. to ensure that they are sitting out of bed for meals).
- If the patient is at risk of pressure ulceration, a cushion should be provided to offer pressure relief when they are sitting out of bed. The width, depth, and height of the chair all need to be considered, to ensure that it is the right size for the patient.
- If the patient is to be transported to other areas by wheelchair, ensure that a cushion appropriate to the patient's needs is used.
- Remember that sitting the patient out of bed is not the same as mobilizing them, unless the patient can and does mobilize independently. Sitting out of bed puts 75% of the pressure load on the buttocks, whereas when the patient is in bed the load is spread over a much larger area.

• Patients who will be at risk of developing pressure ulcers on and after discharge should be taught together with their carer how to prevent pressure ulcers at home, as well as how to identify the early signs of pressure damage. The patient and their carer should also be informed how to contact the community nursing team if any early signs develop. Patient and carer information leaflets are available free from NICE, and most hospitals also produce their own leaflets. These resources should form the basis for educating the patient and their carer about pressure ulcers.

Pressure ulcer treatment

Once a pressure ulcer has developed, the local policy with regard to notification of pressure ulceration should be followed.

- The pressure ulcer may or may not be gradable. It is usual for deep pressure ulcers to be covered with tissue, in the form of either a blister or necrotic tissue. It is impossible to make more than an educated guess about grading until all of the devitalized tissue has been removed.
- The area where the pressure ulcer forms will dictate the mode of wound care treatment. Any area other than the heel should be debrided according to local policy, in line with the competencies of those providing care (see section on wound management on ➔ p. 246).
- The heel should be kept clean and dry, and the necrotic eschar that forms should be left intact unless it starts to separate naturally. The area should be monitored for signs of excessive inflammation or infection, and treated according to wound care guidelines if this occurs. Otherwise the consensus of expert opinion is that the eschar should be left intact, as it will act as a 'natural' sticking plaster, and the heel will heal under the eschar.
- The area that has been damaged by pressure should become and remain pressure free.
- If the patient develops pressure damage to the buttocks, sitting out of bed on a suitable cushion in a suitably sized chair should be restricted to a maximum of 1 h before returning to bed. Again the timing of sitting out should be taken into consideration when planning the patient's day (e.g. so that they are able to sit out for meals).
- The patient should be nursed on a high-specification mattress if the pressure ulcer is grade 3 or above. Repositioning should still take place on such mattresses.
- A dietitian should be involved in the care of all patients with a pressure ulcer of grade 3 or above. Nutritional intake should be monitored, and the patient should be given a high-protein diet if possible.
- Patient education should be provided as described on ➔ p. 262. If the pressure ulcer is grade 3 or above and requires debridement, the patient and their carer should be informed that the wound will get larger before it gets better, because dead tissue is being removed, and that this is not a sign of deterioration.
- If the pressure ulcer is extensive, a surgical opinion may be useful for either debridement or reconstructive surgery.

Further reading

National Institute for Health and Care Excellence (NICE). *Pressure Ulcers; prevention and management of pressure ulcers.* CG179. NICE: London, 2014. ⅏ www.nice.org.uk/guidance/cg179

National Pressure Ulcer Advisory Panel, European Pressure Ulcer Advisory Panel and Pan Pacific Pressure Injury Alliance. *Prevention and Treatment of Pressure Ulcers: quick reference guide,* 2nd edn. Cambridge Media: Perth, Australia, 2014. ⅏ www.epuap.org/wp-content/uploads/2010/10/Quick-Reference-Guide-DIGITAL-NPUAP-EPUAP-PPPIA-16Oct2014.pdf

Wounds International. *International Guidelines. Pressure ulcer prevention: prevalence and incidence in context. A consensus document.* Medical Education Partnership (MEP) Ltd: London, 2009. ⅏ www.woundsinternational.com/media/issues/64/files/content_24.pdf

Infection: prevention, control, and treatment

The Hygiene Code

- The 'Hygiene Code' is more formally known as the *Health and Social Care Act 2008: Code of Practice on the prevention and control of infections and related guidance.*[1]
- It applies to all registered providers of healthcare and adult social care in England.
- If a registered healthcare provider does not meet the requirements of the Hygiene Code, the Care Quality Commission (CQC) may use its enforcement powers if it decides that the provider is not meeting its legal obligation to provide a safe environment for its users.

The 10 compliance criteria of the Hygiene Code, with examples of evidence of compliance

1. Systems to manage and monitor the prevention and control of infection. These systems use risk assessments and consider how susceptible service users are and any risks that their environment and other users may pose to them.

- Infection prevention and control (IPC) policies and procedures are evidence based, regularly reviewed, and audited against compliance (e.g. *Saving Lives: reducing infection, delivering clean and safe care*[2]).
- An IPC team is available to provide advice.

2. Provide and maintain a clean and appropriate environment in managed premises that facilitates the prevention and control of infections.

- The person identified as being in charge of a clinical area has the responsibility to ensure that both environmental and equipment cleanliness standards are met throughout their shift.
- A schedule of cleaning frequency is available for anyone (e.g. visitors, relatives) to see.
- There is adequate provision of hand-wash facilities/antimicrobial hand rubs where appropriate.

3. Provide suitable accurate information on infections to service users and their visitors.

- Patient leaflets are available and provided, giving advice on specific infections (e.g. MRSA, *Clostridium difficile*, Norovirus).

4. Provide suitable accurate information on infections to any person concerned with providing further support or nursing/medical care in a timely fashion.

- Patient transfer letters should inform other healthcare providers of any infections the patient has had, and any special care required (e.g. isolation, ongoing treatment).

5. Ensure that people who have or develop an infection are identified promptly and receive the appropriate treatment and care to reduce the risk of passing on the infection to other people.

- Outbreaks of infection are identified promptly, and managed efficiently and appropriately.

6. Ensure that all staff and those employed to provide care in all settings are fully involved in the process of preventing and controlling infection.

- IPC is included in all job descriptions, staff induction, and training.

7. Provide or secure adequate isolation facilities.

- Isolation policies and isolation facilities for nursing infections such as MRSA, *Clostridium difficile*, and tuberculosis should be available, and all staff are accountable for ensuring that these policies are followed.

8. Secure adequate access to laboratory support as appropriate.

- Microbiology laboratories must have appropriate policies and protocols.

9. Have and adhere to policies, designed for the individual's care and provider organizations, that will help to prevent and control infections.

- A series of evidence-based policies, protocols and/or guidelines are provided for all staff.
- IPC policies, protocols and/or guidelines are audited against and actioned (e.g. hand hygiene, personal protective equipment, aseptic technique, decontamination, antimicrobial prescribing, MRSA, *C. difficile*, and immunization of staff).
- All staff are accountable for ensuring that these are complied with.

10. Ensure, so far as is reasonably practicable, that care workers are free of and are protected from exposure to infections that can be caught at work, and that all staff are suitably educated in the prevention and control of infection associated with the provision of health and social care.

- All staff have access to an occupational health team.
- IPC is included in staff induction, updates, and training.

References

1 Department of Health. *The Health and Social Care Act 2008: Code of Practice on the prevention and control of infections and related guidance.* Department of Health: London, 2015. ℜ www.gov.uk/government/uploads/system/uploads/attachment_data/file/400105/code_of_practice_14_Jan_15.pdf
2 Department of Health. *Saving Lives: reducing infection, delivering clean and safe care.* Department of Health: London, 2007.

The Care Quality Commission (CQC)

- The CQC is the independent regulator of health and adult social care services in England.
- The NHS is a service provider. If any of its regulated activities are carried out in England, it must be registered with the CQC and comply with the Health and Social Care Act 2008 (Regulated Activities) Regulations 2010,[3] and the Care Quality Commission (Registration) Regulations 2009.[4]
- These regulations are part of a wider framework which also incorporates the regulation of professionals such as nurses, doctors, and social workers.
- The framework defines the essential standards of quality and safety to ensure that the people who use health and adult social care services are protected and receive the care, treatment, and support that they have a right to expect.
- The CQC assessment is based around six themes and incorporates 28 outcome measures:
  - Theme 3, Safeguarding and Safety, includes Outcome 8: Cleanliness and Infection Control, which states that providers of services must comply with the requirements of Regulation 12, with regard to the *Code of Practice on the prevention and control of infections and related guidance*, or 'Hygiene Code.'[5]
- There are 15 regulated activities in the CQC (Registration) Regulations that were published in 2013.[6] The seventh of these is 'Surgical procedures.'

Description of surgical procedures that are required to be registered with the CQC

- Surgical procedures are defined as being for the purpose of treating disease, disorder, or injury, or cosmetic surgery, or for religious observance (e.g. circumcision), and carried out by a healthcare professional.
- Minor surgical procedures are not included, such as curettage, cautery or cryocautery of skin lesions, nail bed procedures, and those which involve the use of local anaesthesia (or no anaesthesia).

The key points of the surgical procedures which are covered by the CQC regulations

- The 'surgical procedure' covers all pre- and post-operative care associated with the procedure, such as pre-procedure assessment by an anaesthetist once the procedure has been decided upon, pre-operative check, post-operative recovery, follow-up in an intensive care unit, and rehabilitation when it is part of the planned care package.
- Surgical procedures carried out for religious reasons (e.g. circumcision) are included where carried out by a healthcare professional.

References

3 UK Parliament. *Health and Social Care Act 2008 (Regulated Activities) Regulations 2014.* ℘ www.cqc.org.uk/sites/default/files/20150510_hsca_2008_regulated_activities_regs_2104_current.pdf

4 Secretary of State. *Care Quality Commission (Registration) Regulations 2009.* ℘ www.cqc.org.uk/sites/default/files/2009_3112s-care-quality-commission-regulations-2009.pdf

5 Department of Health. *The Health and Social Care Act 2008: Code of Practice on the prevention and control of infections and related guidance.* Department of Health: London, 2015. ℘ www.gov.uk/government/uploads/system/uploads/attachment_data/file/400105/code_of_practice_14_Jan_15.pdf

6 Care Quality Commission. *Registration under the Health and Social Care Act 2008: the scope of registration.* Care Quality Commission: Newcastle upon Tyne, 2013. ℘ www.cqc.org.uk/sites/default/files/documents/20130717_100001_v5_0_scope_of_registration_guidance.pdf

Basic microbiology

Types of microorganisms

- Bacteria are unicellular microorganisms without nuclei.
- Like human cells, fungi and parasites have nuclei and complex cell structures. They are larger than bacteria, and although some are unicellular, they include many multicellular species.
- Viruses and prions are non-cellular and are smaller than bacteria.

Bacterial growth and identification

An understanding of bacterial anatomy and physiology allows us to grow, classify, and identify most pathogenic bacteria in the microbiology laboratory. The accurate identification of bacteria and determination of their sensitivity to various antibiotics is compulsory for optimal directed antibiotic therapy.

Growth

- When optimal growth conditions are present, bacterial cells divide into two daughter cells which are identical to the parent cell.
- Most pathogenic bacteria require:
  - carbon
  - nitrogen
  - inorganic salts
  - water
  - a source of energy.
- Different bacteria have specific oxygen requirements.
  - Obligate (strict) aerobes require oxygen for growth (e.g. *Pseudomonas aeruginosa*).
  - Obligate anaerobes require the absence of oxygen (e.g. *Clostridium difficile*).
  - Facultative anaerobes grow better in the presence of oxygen, but also grow when it is absent (e.g. *Staphylococcus aureus*).
  - Microaerophilic bacteria require a reduced oxygen level (e.g. *Campylobacter jejuni*).
- Carbon dioxide (which is present in the air) is required for bacterial growth. However, some bacteria require additional carbon dioxide.
- Many pathogenic bacteria grow best at 37°C. However, some can grow at lower temperatures and others at higher ones.
- Most bacteria grow best at a mildly alkaline pH. However, some require acidic conditions.
- Bacteria multiply to produce visible colonies on agar plates. The morphology of these colonies can be used to aid identification.

Microscopic appearance
- Bacteria can be either Gram-positive or Gram-negative. This refers to the microscopic appearance of bacteria following Gram staining. This stain can be performed on cells taken from colonies on agar plates or directly from clinical specimens, and this differentiation is based on the composition of the cell wall. After a series of steps in the staining process:
  - Gram-positive bacteria appear purple (e.g. *Staphylococcus aureus*)
  - Gram-negative bacteria appear pink (e.g. *Escherichia coli*).
- Bacteria can be of various shapes, including the following:
  - rods (bacilli) (e.g. *Escherichia coli*)
  - spheres (cocci) (e.g. *Staphylococcus aureus*)
  - curves (e.g. *Vibrio cholerae*)
  - spirals (e.g. *Treponema pallidum*).

These shapes and the arrangement of these cells (e.g. chains, clusters, etc.) are fundamental to the classification and identification of bacteria.

Staphylococcus aureus: MRSA and MSSA

Staphylococcus aureus

- This is a Gram-positive bacterium.
- It is observed under the microscope as grape-like clusters of cocci.
- Colonies are cream-yellow, and the bacteria are non-motile, non-spore-forming, and catalase-positive.
- It lives on (colonizes) the human skin and mucosa (e.g. inside the nose) without causing any problems.
- Approximately 30% of the general population are colonized with *S. aureus*.[7]
- It may enter the body via cuts, scratching, ingestion, or procedures.
- It may cause a range of infections, such as skin infections (abscesses, impetigo, pimples, boils, etc.), wound infections, surgical site infections, pneumonia, and bacteraemias (bloodstream infections).
- It can produce toxins which, if they contaminate food, cause acute diarrhoea and vomiting 2–6 h after ingestion.
- Some strains may also produce a toxin called Panton–Valentine leukocidin (PVL), which can cause more severe infections.

Antibiotic resistance

- Many strains of *S. aureus* are sensitive to most antibiotics, and therefore infections are easy to treat.
- Resistance to penicillin was noted as early as 1942.
- When *S. aureus* is identified in the laboratory as being resistant to meticillin/flucloxacillin (β-lactam antibiotics) it is called meticillin-resistant *S. aureus* (MRSA).
- Those strains that are sensitive to meticillin/flucloxacillin are termed meticillin-sensitive *S. aureus* (MSSA). The only real difference between MRSA and MSSA is their resistance patterns.
- Resistance to meticillin was first noted in 1961.
- There are now a number of different epidemic strains of MRSA.
- Vancomycin is one of the common antibiotics used to treat infections caused by MRSA.
- Vancomycin-resistant *S. aureus* has been noted a few times in the USA. This has raised serious concerns due to the increasing resistance pattern of a common bacterial infection.

MRSA

- Approximately 3% of the population are colonized with MRSA.[8]
- People who are colonized with MRSA do not have any symptoms. Therefore screening for MRSA is undertaken if they are admitted to hospital.
- MRSA does not usually affect healthy people, pregnant women, babies, children, or elderly people (although they may be colonized).
- MRSA may affect people who have serious health problems, and those with serious skin conditions (e.g. eczema) or open wounds.

MRSA colonization and infection

- Colonization occurs when a person carries a particular microorganism but shows no clinical signs or symptoms of infection.
- Infection occurs when a harmful microbe enters the body and then multiplies within the body tissue.
- If a patient is identified as being colonized with MRSA they may be prescribed an antimicrobial shampoo/body wash and a nasal cream in order to reduce the bacterial load.
- A patient who is infected with MRSA will be prescribed appropriate antibiotic therapy.

Infection prevention and control

- MRSA may be spread from person to person via contaminated hands and equipment and/or environment.
- Scrupulous hand hygiene between patients is essential.
- Patients who are identified as being either colonized or infected with MRSA will require appropriate infection prevention and control precautions according to local and national policy.
- Hospital visitors are requested to help to reduce the risk of spreading MRSA by not sitting on the beds, and by washing their hands at the end of the visit. Casual contact, such as kissing, hugging, and touching, is usually acceptable. However, the touching of catheters or wound sites should be discouraged.
- 'Terminal cleaning' of the isolation room and all equipment must be undertaken on patient discharge or transfer.

Surveillance of MRSA bloodstream infections

- NHS hospitals in England are required to send information about MRSA bloodstream infections to the Health Protection Agency (HPA), which is now part of Public Health England. These figures are published for individual NHS trusts, for regions, and for England.

References

7 Department of Health. *A Simple Guide to MRSA*. Department of Health: London, 2007.
8 Coia JE et al. Guidelines for the control and prevention of meticillin-resistant *Staphylococcus aureus* (MRSA) in healthcare facilities. *Journal of Hospital Infection* 2006: 63: S1–44.

Clostridium difficile

- This is a Gram-positive, anaerobic bacterium.
- Its vegetative bacilli can form spores, which confer resistance to heat, chemicals, and drying, thus enabling the microorganism to survive most environments.
- The Health Protection Agency (now part of Public Health England) has reported that *C. difficile* asymptomatically colonizes about 3% of adults and 66% of babies.[9]
- *C. difficile* can cause disease when the normal bacteria in the gut, with which it competes, are disadvantaged. This is usually a result of a person taking antibiotics. Antibiotics can disturb the normal gut flora, which then allows the *C. difficile* to grow to abnormally high levels, and the toxin that *C. difficile* produces reaches levels at which it can then attack the intestine and cause symptoms of disease—diarrhoea (mild to severe) and, rarely, life-threatening inflammation of the intestines, known as pseudomembranous colitis (PMC).
- Risk factors for acquiring *C. difficile* include antibiotic therapy, age over 65 years, cancer, surgery, tube feeding, and proton pump inhibitors.

Antibiotic resistance

- *C. difficile* is commonly treated with oral vancomycin and/or intravenous metronidazole.

Infection prevention and control

- *C. difficile* may be spread from person to person via ingestion of the bacterium from contaminated hands and equipment or the environment.
- Scrupulous hand hygiene is essential. Hand washing using soap and water rather than alcohol-based hand rubs is recommended after contact with a patient with *C. difficile* and their environment, as alcohol hand rubs will not destroy the spores.
- Patients with suspected but as yet unconfirmed *C. difficile* infection should be isolated in a single room until laboratory confirmation has been received.
- Patients who are identified as being infected with *C. difficile* will require appropriate infection prevention and control precautions, such as isolation/cohort nursing with enteric precautions undertaken until they have been free of symptoms of diarrhoea for a minimum of 48 h.
- 'Terminal cleaning' of the isolation room and all equipment must be undertaken on patient discharge or transfer.
- Restrictive antibiotic policies and effective antibiotic stewardship are essential, as antibiotics such as cephalosporins (e.g. cefotaxime, cefalexin) are implicated in the development of *C. difficile*-associated diarrhoea.
- Hospital visitors should be requested to help to reduce the risk of spreading *C. difficile* by not sitting on the beds, and by washing their hands at the end of the visit.

Monitoring of *C. difficile* infection

- All NHS trusts in England are required to participate in the Department of Health's mandatory *C. difficile* infection-reporting system, and to report all cases of *C. difficile* toxin-positive diarrhoea in patients over 2 years of age. These figures are published for individual NHS trusts, for regions, and nationally.
- Doctors have a legal duty to mention *C. difficile* infection on a death certificate if it was part of the sequence of events that directly led to death, or if it contributed in some way.

Case definitions

- *C. difficile* infection[10]: one episode of diarrhoea, defined either as stool loose enough to take the shape of a container used to sample it or as Bristol Stool Chart[11] types 5–7, that is not attributable to any other cause and that occurs at the same time as a positive toxin assay and/or endoscopic evidence of PMC.
- A period of increased incidence (PII) of *C. difficile* infection: two or more new cases (occurring more than 48 h post admission, not relapses) in a 28-day period on a ward.
- An outbreak of *C. difficile* infection: two or more cases caused by the same strain related in time and place over a defined period that is based on the date of onset of the first case. An outbreak must be reported as a serious incident, and must be fully investigated by undertaking, at the very minimum, a root cause analysis (RCA), audits of environmental cleanliness, audits of antibiotic stewardship, and hand hygiene compliance.

References

9 Public Health England. *Updated Guidance on the Management and Treatment of* Clostridium difficile *Infection*. Public Health England: London, 2013.
10 Department of Health and Health Protection Agency. *Clostridium difficile Infection: how to deal with the problem*. Department of Health: London, 2008.
11 Lewis SJ and Heaton KW. Stool form scale as a useful guide to intestinal transit time. *Scandinavian Journal of Gastroenterology* 1997; 32: 920–24.

Further reading

Public Health England. Clostridium difficile: *guidance, data and analysis*. Public Health England: London, 2014. www.hpa.org.uk/Topics/InfectiousDiseases/InfectionsAZ/ClostridiumDifficile

Extended-spectrum β-lactamase (ESBL)-producing Gram-negative bacilli

β-lactams
β-lactam antibiotics have a common element in their structure, namely a β-lactam ring that contains four atoms.

β-lactamases
- β-lactamases are enzymes produced by bacteria which hydrolyse the β-lactam ring, thus inactivating the antibiotic and causing resistance.
- Resistance to older antibiotics caused by the production of β-lactamases has been documented for some decades.
- Some of the newer antibiotics, such as third-generation cephalosporins (extended-spectrum β-lactams), were developed to overcome such β-lactamases.
- However, these extended-spectrum β-lactamases (ESBLs) are now present in some bacteria.
- Bacteria that produce ESBLs are often resistant to other antibiotics, such as aminoglycosides and fluoroquinolones, making front-line antibiotics ineffective for the treatment of infections caused by ESBL-producing bacteria.
- This in turn has led to dependence on carbapenems and the subsequent development of resistance to these antibiotics.

Infections caused by ESBL-producing bacteria
- ESBL-producing bacteria cause the same type of infections as susceptible Gram-negative bacilli.
- *Escherichia coli* often causes endogenous urinary tract and abdominal infections.
- Other Gram-negative bacilli, such as *Klebsiella* and *Acinetobacter baumannii*, can cause outbreaks in hospitals.

Treatment
- ESBL-producing bacteria are not more virulent than susceptible strains, but they are more difficult to treat.
- As with all infections, treatment is dependent on infection type, severity, antibiotic susceptibility of the causative isolate, and local policy.
- A relatively new antibiotic, tigecycline, may be used for more minor infections. In severe infections (for isolates which are still susceptible), carbapenems are used.
- For severe infection caused by carbapenem-resistant isolates, colistimethate sodium can be used.

Prevention

Implementation of standard infection control precautions can control the spread of most ESBL-producing bacteria.

A toolkit for acute trusts for the early detection and management of carbapenemase-producing Enterobacteriaceae has been produced to provide expert advice, as there has been a rapid increase in the number of multi-drug-resistant carbapenemase-producing organisms in recent years.[12]

Reference

12 Public Health England. *Acute Trust Toolkit for the Early Detection, Management and Control of Carbapenemase-Producing Enterobacteriaceae.* Public Health England: London, 2013. http://webarchive.nationalarchives.gov.uk/20140714084352/ http://www.hpa.org.uk/webc/HPAwebFile/HPAweb_C/1317140378646

Carbapenemase-producing Enterobacteriaceae (CPE)

Enterobacteriaceae
- Enterobacteriaceae are aerobic Gram-negative bacteria that inhabit the gut of humans and animals.
- They are a common cause of urinary tract infections, surgical site infections, and bloodstream infections.
- Enterobacteriaceae include species such as *Escherichia coli*, *Enterobacter* species and *Klebsiella* species.

Carbapenems
- Carbapenems are a powerful group of β-lactam antibiotics that are usually reserved for drug-resistant Gram-negative bacteria. Examples include meropenem, ertapenem, and imipenem.
- Concern is increasing because of the emergence of carbapenem-resistant bacteria.

Carbapenemases
- Carbapenemases are enzymes that destroy carbapenem antibiotics, leading to resistance.
- The most common types of carbapenemases are KPC, OXA-48, VIM, and NDM.

Countries where healthcare-associated CPE is prevalent
- These include Bangladesh, Greece, India, Ireland, Israel, Turkey, and the USA.
- CPE has also been noted in Manchester and London in the UK.

Infection prevention and control
- All patients being admitted to hospital should be assessed for CPE.
- CPE should be suspected if; during the last 12 months, the patient has been in hospital abroad, or in the UK where CPE has been identified, or if they have been previously CPE positive.
- Laboratory confirmation of CPE carriage is made from either a rectal swab or a stool sample.
- Patients who are suspected of being either colonized or infected with CPE will require appropriate infection prevention and control precautions, such as immediate isolation and cohort nursing.
- If the patient is confirmed as being CPE positive they should remain in isolation or cohorted until discharge.
- Compliance with the following standard precautions is essential:
  - hand hygiene
  - personal protective equipment (PPE)
  - aseptic technique
  - waste management, including faeces
  - safe sharps.

- The utilization of single-use equipment is encouraged where possible.
- 'Terminal cleaning' of the isolation room and all equipment must be undertaken on patient discharge or transfer.
- Screening of household contacts and healthcare staff is not required.

Further reading

Public Health England. *Acute Trust Toolkit for the Early Detection, Management and Control of Carbapenemase-Producing Enterobacteriaceae.* Public Health England: London, 2013. ℘ http://webarchive.nationalarchives.gov.uk/20140714084352/ http://www.hpa.org.uk/webc/HPAwebFile/HPAweb_C/1317140378646
Public Health England. *Acute Trust Toolkit for the Early Detection, Management and Control of Carbapenemase-Producing Enterobacteriaceae: frequently asked questions for health professionals.* Public Health England: London, 2014. ℘ www.gov.uk/government/uploads/system/uploads/attachment_data/file/329229/CPE_Acute_Trust_Toolkit_FAQs_for_Health_Professionals.pdf

Blood-borne viruses

HIV

The virus
- The human immunodeficiency virus (HIV) is an enveloped RNA virus of the Retroviridae family.
- It infects white blood cells that express the CD4 antigen, leading to a reduction in function and then in numbers of these cells.

Epidemiology
- Since the early 1980s there has been a worldwide spread of HIV. Indeed it is thought that 20 million people have died of HIV-related illnesses and up to 60 million people are currently living with the infection.
- Transmission from person to person is via sexual intercourse, exposure to infected blood or blood products, or from mother to baby.

Clinical symptoms
Acute infection lasts for about 10 weeks after exposure, and is characterized by non-specific symptoms such as lymphadenopathy, fever, and pharyngitis. Following this, the patient remains asymptomatic for approximately 10 years, after which time viral replication increases and the patient's CD4 counts decline. At this stage the patient is severely immunocompromised, and if they do not receive treatment may develop acquired immunodeficiency syndrome (AIDS)-defining illnesses, which include specific types of malignancy and opportunistic bacterial, fungal, protozoal, and viral infections.

Laboratory diagnosis
Diagnosis is based on the detection of HIV antigen and antibody, or on the detection of HIV RNA.

Treatment
There are several different types of antiretroviral drugs available, and the combined use of three drugs, known as highly active antiretroviral therapy (HAART), has revolutionized the treatment of patients infected with HIV. HAART should be taken indefinitely, with the continuous monitoring of CD4 and viral counts and monitoring of resistance to antiretroviral agents.

Prevention
- Use of condoms and needle-exchange programmes.
- Post-exposure prophylaxis with HAART.
- For infected pregnant female patients: HAART, Caesarean section, and avoidance of breastfeeding.
- Standard infection control precautions should be employed when caring for any patient, regardless of their HIV status. If a healthcare worker is exposed to bodily fluids (e.g. via a needlestick or splash injury) they should contact the occupational health department immediately, whether or not the patient's HIV status is known.

Hepatitis

Hepatitis A virus (HAV)

- HAV is a non-enveloped RNA virus.
- It is transmitted via the faecal–oral route.
- Infection is endemic in the developing world.
- It causes acute hepatitis characterized by fever, malaise, pain, and jaundice.
- It is diagnosed by the detection of HAV-specific antibodies in serum.
- There is no treatment, just symptomatic care.
- A vaccine is available for high-risk groups.

Hepatitis B virus (HBV)

- HBV is an enveloped DNA virus.
- It is transmitted via exposure to infected blood, sexual intercourse, and from mother to baby.
- It has a worldwide distribution.
- It causes acute and chronic hepatitis, cirrhosis, and hepatocellular carcinoma.
- It is diagnosed by the detection of HBV-specific antigen and antibodies.
- Treatment includes antiviral agents such as lamivudine and tenofovir.
- Healthcare workers should employ standard infection control precautions.
- A vaccine is available for high-risk groups, including healthcare workers who may be exposed to the virus (e.g. via needlestick injury).

Hepatitis C virus (HCV)

- HCV is an enveloped RNA virus.
- It is transmitted via exposure to infected blood and, to a lesser extent, by sexual intercourse and from mother to baby.
- It has a worldwide distribution.
- It causes acute and chronic hepatitis, cirrhosis, and hepatocellular carcinoma.
- It is diagnosed by the detection of HCV-specific antigen and antibodies.
- Treatment is with pegylated interferon and ribavirin.
- Healthcare workers should adopt standard infection control precautions.
- No vaccine is available, but all blood and transplant donors are screened.

Hepatitis D virus (HDV) (delta agent)

- HDV is a defective, incomplete RNA virus.
- It is transmitted in a similar way to HBV, and in fact only infects individuals who are infected with or are carriers of HBV.
- It causes aggravation of HBV infection.
- It is diagnosed by the detection of HDV-specific antigen and antibodies.
- It can be treated and prevented by controlling HBV infection.

Hepatitis E virus (HEV)
- HEV is a non-enveloped RNA virus.
- It is transmitted via the faecal–oral route.
- Infection is endemic in the developing world.
- It causes acute hepatitis, which has a high mortality rate, particularly in pregnancy.
- It is diagnosed by the detection of HEV-specific antibodies in serum.
- There is no treatment, only symptomatic care.
- No vaccine is available.

Creutzfeldt–Jakob disease (CJD)

Transmissible spongiform encephalopathies

- These are degenerative neurological disorders caused by prions.
- Prions are proteinaceous agents which are isoforms of normal cellular proteins.
- A range of diseases are caused by prions, including scrapie (in sheep), bovine spongiform encephalopathy (BSE, also known as 'mad cow disease') and CJD (in humans).
- CJD is a rare disease. It affects approximately one person per million members of the population.

Types of CJD

- Sporadic CJD (sCJD), which occurs spontaneously, is the most common form (approximately 85% of cases), and is normally characterized by onset in the later years of life.
- Familial CJD (fCJD) is an inherited form of the disease which is normally characterized by a younger age of onset than sCJD. This form accounts for 5–10% of cases.
- Iatrogenic CJD (iCJD) occurs when contaminated CJD tissue is inadvertently inoculated into another patient (e.g. as a result of using contaminated neurosurgical instruments). This form affects younger individuals.
- Variant CJD (vCJD) is caused by exposure such as eating contaminated meat from cattle with BSE. In the mid-1980s an epidemic of BSE was identified. This was caused by feeding ruminant offal to cows. vCJD typically affects younger people.

Clinical symptoms of vCJD

- The onset of disease is characterized by sensory and psychiatric symptoms followed by ataxia and myoclonus (involuntary muscle jerks).
- As the disease progresses, dementia develops.
- Symptoms are caused by brain cell death, which creates small holes in the brain, giving it a sponge-like appearance.

Diagnosis

- CJD is normally diagnosed by ruling out other diseases.
- Cerebral biopsies are infrequently undertaken.
- Laboratory tests that utilize a protein marker in cerebrospinal fluid are being developed.

Treatment

At present no treatment for CJD is available, and the disease is fatal.

Prevention

- The feeding of ruminant offal to cattle and the use of bovine offal for human consumption are now banned.
- Prions are resistant to inactivation by conventional methods such as autoclaving at 121°C.
- For patients with definite, probable, or possible CJD, medical items are incinerated after use.
- The Department of Health has produced guidance to minimize the risk of transmission of CJD and vCJD in healthcare settings.[13]

Reference

13 Department of Health. *Minimise Transmission Risk of CJD and vCJD in Healthcare Settings*. Department of Health: London, 2013. http://webarchive.nationalarchives.gov.uk/20140714084352/ https://www.gov.uk/government/publications/guidance- from-the-acdp-tse-risk-management-subgroup-formerly-tse-working-group

Meticillin-resistant *Staphylococcus aureus* (MRSA) screening and decolonization

- MRSA is a Gram-positive bacterium.
- Approximately 3% of the population are colonized with MRSA.[14]
- MRSA is resistant to several antibiotics.
- People who are colonized with MRSA do not have any symptoms. Therefore the infection is difficult to detect.
- MRSA does not usually affect healthy people, pregnant women, babies, children, or elderly people (although they may be colonized).

Screening

- MRSA screening involves the testing of patients for the presence of MRSA on common body sites either on, or prior to, admission.
- It aims to identify carriers of MRSA and enable appropriate precautions to be taken in order to minimize the risk of spread, such as:
  - hand and environmental decontamination
  - patient decolonization
  - isolation
  - terminal cleaning.
- MRSA screening should be performed according to national guidelines.[15–17]
- It should include the anterior nares (the nasal region is the most common site of MRSA colonization).
- Local policy will determine other sites, which may include:
  - axilla
  - groin and perineum
  - lesions
  - exfoliating skin conditions
  - urine, if a catheter is present
  - sputum, if a productive cough is present
  - insertion sites of foreign bodies
  - the umbilicus in neonates.
- Patients who are at high risk for MRSA colonization include those who are:
  - known to be previous carriers
  - frequent admissions to healthcare facilities
  - direct inter-hospital transfers
  - transfers from establishments that have a high prevalence of MRSA.

Staff screening

The routine screening of healthcare staff for MRSA is not recommended. However, screening may be advised if there are potential epidemiological indications that staff may be linked to the source of MRSA infection.

Decolonization

- Decolonization is the attempt to eradicate the carriage of MRSA.
- Local and national decolonization advice should be followed. This generally includes the following:
  - Nasal decolonization is generally achieved by the application of 2% mupirocin to each nostril three times a day for 5 days.
  - Skin decolonization is generally achieved using 4% (w/v) chlorhexidine body wash daily for 5 days and shampoo as required.
  - Advice should be sought from dermatologists and microbiologists for patients with known skin conditions (e.g. eczema, psoriasis).
- Decolonization should start immediately after a patient has been identified as a carrier.
- If a patient is confirmed as being MRSA positive during a pre-operative assessment screen, decolonization therapy should commence 5 days prior to surgery.

References

14 Department of Health. *A Simple Guide to MRSA*. Department of Health: London, 2007.
15 Department of Health. *MRSA Screening: operational guidance 2*. Department of Health: London, 2008.
16 Department of Health. *Screening Elective Patients for MRSA: FAQs*. Department of Health: London, 2009.
17 Coia JE et al. Guidelines for the control and prevention of meticillin-resistant *Staphylococcus aureus* (MRSA) in healthcare facilities. *Journal of Hospital Infection* 2006; 63: S1–44.

Control of infection

- Standard Infection Control Precautions (SICP)[18] (see Table 14.1) are implemented to prevent cross-transmission from recognized and unrecognized sources of potential infection, blood and other body fluids, secretions or excretions (excluding sweat), non-intact skin or mucous membranes, and any equipment or items in the care environment that are likely to become contaminated.
- SICP must underpin all healthcare activities.
- SICP cannot prevent transmission of infection from all infectious agents. Therefore when specific infectious agents are suspected or known, additional Transmission-Based Precautions (TBP) are required.

Table 14.1 Standard Infection Control Precautions (SICP)

SICP	Examples of practice
Provision of care in the most appropriate place	Undertake risk assessments of the individual, the environment, and the suspected/actual infection before placement
Hand washing	Five Moments for Hand Hygiene[19]
Personal protective equipment (PPE)	Assess risk of procedure and wear appropriate PPE.
	Seek advice from Infection Prevention Control for patients with suspected or confirmed infections such as TB or MRSA
Sharps safety	Use equipment with safety features where possible.
	Dispose of sharps at point of care
Safe handling of clinical waste	Wear suitable PPE to handle and dispose of waste.
	Appropriately segregate waste according to national guidelines
Safe handling of linen	Wear suitable PPE to handle and dispose of linen.
	Appropriately segregate used or contaminated linen according to local and national guidelines
Decontamination of equipment	Wear suitable PPE to appropriately decontaminate equipment following use
Decontamination of environment	Keep the environment tidy and clean.
	Appropriately decontaminate spills of body fluids
Occupational exposure management	Cover cuts with a waterproof dressing.
	Provide hepatitis B vaccination for at-risk staff.
	Provide occupational healthcare following exposure to blood and body fluids (e.g. needlestick injury)
Cough etiquette	Cover nose and mouth with disposable single-use tissues when sneezing, coughing, or blowing nose

Transmission-Based Precautions (TBP)

- There are three categories of TBP—airborne, droplet, and contact—which are utilized in addition to SICP for a limited period of time dependent upon the risk of spread of infection.
- There may be more than one route of transmission of infectious pathogens.

Airborne precautions

- These aim to prevent the transmission of infectious agents via small particles (≤ 5 μm in diameter) which enter the respiratory tract of individuals without there necessarily being close contact with another individual.
- Patients should be placed in a specialized isolation room or negative pressure isolation room (with anteroom), with hand-washing and en suite facilities, as soon as possible. The door to these rooms must be kept closed.
- Examples of infections for which airborne precautions are required include pulmonary tuberculosis and chickenpox.

Droplet precautions

- These aim to prevent the transmission of infectious agents via large droplets (> 5 μm in diameter) from the respiratory tract of an infected individual directly onto a mucosal surface or the conjunctivae of another individual.
- It is accepted that when droplets are dispelled (by coughing, sneezing, intubation, or suctioning) they only travel relatively short distances through the air (e.g. less than 1 m).
- Patients with known or suspected infections that require droplet precautions should be placed in single rooms with en suite facilities as soon as possible. The door should be kept closed.
- Examples of infections for which droplet precautions are required include group A streptococcal disease, meningococcal disease (meningitis and septicaemia), and influenza.

Contact precautions

- These are required to prevent the transmission of infectious agents via direct and indirect contact.
  - Direct contact transmission occurs when an infectious agent is transferred directly from one person to another.
  - Indirect contact transmission occurs when an infectious agent is transferred to an individual from an object and/or another person.
- If possible, single rooms with hand-washing facilities and en suite toilets are preferred. The requirement to keep the door closed will depend on the risk assessment, but it is considered good practice.
- Examples of infections for which contact precautions are required include MRSA and *Clostridium difficile*.

References

18 Siegel JD et al. *Guideline for Isolation Precautions: preventing transmission of infectious agents in healthcare settings*. Centers for Disease Control and Prevention: Atlanta, GA, 2007. www.cdc.gov/hicpac/pdf/isolation/Isolation2007.pdf

19 World Health Organization and Patient Safety. *WHO Guidelines on Hand Hygiene in Health Care: a summary. First global patient safety challenge: clean care is safer care*. World Health Organization: Geneva, 2009. http://whqlibdoc.who.int/hq/2009/WHO_IER_PSP_2009.07_eng.pdf

The environment

Definition

The environment includes any frequently touched surfaces, such as (but not limited to) the following:

- beds
- lockers
- tables
- toilets
- commodes
- sinks
- basins
- baths
- showers
- door handles
- walls
- curtains
- screens
- window blinds
- light switches
- horizontal surfaces.

Why should the environment be controlled?

Potentially pathogenic microorganisms may be transferred from environmental surfaces to patients via direct (hand) contact with contaminated surfaces.

- The state of repair of the environment, and items contained within it, is also important, as surfaces that are not smooth and intact can harbour bacteria.
- To facilitate environmental decontamination, a tidy, clutter-free environment is also important.

How to control the environment

- A routine cleaning schedule should be available in the local area.
- Ensure that equipment is decontaminated if it is visibly dirty.
- Whenever a patient is discharged from their care environment, appropriate decontamination of their environment and equipment should be undertaken.
- When purchasing equipment such as chairs and lockers, ensure that they facilitate effective decontamination.
- Items that are damaged should be removed, repaired, and replaced as soon as it is practicable to do so.
- Liaise with the estates department to ensure that environmental structures such as ventilation ducts are decontaminated and maintained according to local and national guidelines.
- Environmental decontamination should always take into account national guidelines.[20,21]
- Involve infection prevention and control teams when planning new-build projects or refurbishments.

Examples of key factors to consider when planning the environment

- Bed centres should be a minimum of 3.6 m apart.[22]
- There should be hands-free operation of utilities (e.g. sensor taps and toilet flush).
- Clinical hand-wash basins should not have overflows, as these are difficult to clean.
- Policies should be in place to ensure that clinical hand-wash basins are not used for other purposes (e.g. emptying of patient bathing water).
- It is recommended that there are wall-mounted soap dispensers and paper towel dispensers at each clinical hand-wash sink.
- The use of carpets is not advised in any clinical areas.
- Any soft furnishings, such as chairs, should be covered in impervious material to reduce the risk of internal contamination.
- All surfaces should be designed to be easily accessible and easily cleaned.
- There should be sufficient storage for both patient use and the clinical area to enable the ward area to be clutter free.
- There should be separate storage areas for clean linen and dirty linen.
- Ventilation and heating units should be designed to ensure that they do not trap dust and are easy to clean.

References

20 National Patient Safety Agency (NPSA). *The National Specifications for Cleanliness in the NHS: a framework for setting and measuring performance outcomes*. NPSA: London, 2007.
21 British Standards Institution (BSI). *PAS 5748:2014: specification for the planning, application, measurement and review of cleanliness services in hospitals*. BSI: London, 2014.
22 Department of Health. *Health Building Note 00-09. Infection Control in the Built Environment*. Department of Health: London, 2013.

Cleanliness standards

There is clear evidence that transmission of many healthcare-associated infections (HCAI) is related to contamination of the environment and equipment. Therefore it is essential that hospitals provide and maintain a clean and appropriate environment to facilitate the prevention and control of infections.

Specification for the planning, application, measurement and review of cleanliness services in hospitals: PAS 5748:2014[23]
This Publicly Available Specification (PAS) provides guidance on the provision of cleaning services within a hospital.

The Health and Social Care Act 2008: Code of Practice on the prevention and control of infections and related guidance[24]
Criterion 2 states that 'Matrons are responsible and accountable for delivering a clean environment.' A Matron's Charter: an action plan for cleaner hospitals[25] identified 10 commitments which include, but are not limited to, the following:
- The patient environment will be well maintained, clean, and safe.
- Matrons will establish a cleanliness culture across their wards/units.
- The nurse in charge is responsible for ensuring that standards of cleanliness are maintained throughout that shift.

Standards for Better Health[26]
These standards describe the level of quality that healthcare organizations are expected to achieve in terms of safety, clinical and cost-effectiveness, governance, patient focus, accessible and responsive care, care environment and amenities, and public health.
There are two standards that relate to cleanliness:
- Core Standard C4a: 'Healthcare organizations keep patients, staff and visitors safe by having systems to ensure that the risk of healthcare-acquired infection to patients is reduced, with particular emphasis on high standards of hygiene and cleanliness.'
- Core Standard C21: 'Healthcare services are provided in environments which promote effective care and optimize health outcomes by being well designed and well maintained with cleanliness levels in clinical and non-clinical areas that meet the national specification for clean NHS premises.'

The National Specifications for Cleanliness in the NHS: a framework for setting and measuring performance outcomes[27]

- The cleanliness standards are a range of 49 elements which include, but are not limited to:
  - commodes
  - intravenous pumps and drip stands
  - gel dispensers
  - beds
  - microwave ovens.
- Each element has a standard of cleanliness; the element should be visibly clean, with no blood, body substances, dust, dirt, debris, or spillages.
- NHS trusts should produce a schedule of cleaning frequencies.

Colour coding system for hospital cleaning materials and equipment[28]

The following colour coding system for all hospital cleaning materials and equipment ensures that the items are not used in multiple areas:
- *Red*: bathrooms, washrooms, showers, toilets, basins, and bathroom floors.
- *Blue*: general areas including wards, departments, offices, and basins in public areas.
- *Green*: catering departments, ward kitchen areas, and patient food service at ward level.
- *Yellow*: isolation areas.

Patient-led assessments of the care environment (PLACE)

- PLACE is an annual self-assessment that uses a standard benchmarking tool to evaluate four key areas from the patient's perspective:
  - privacy and dignity
  - well-being
  - food
  - cleanliness
  - general maintenance.
- PLACE scores will be reported publicly.

References

23 British Standards Institution (BSI). *Specification for the planning, application, measurement and review of cleanliness services in hospitals. PAS 5748:2014.* BSI: London, 2014.

24 Department of Health. *The Health and Social Care Act 2008: code of practice on the prevention and control of infections and related guidance.* Department of Health: London, 2015.

25 Jones E. *A Matron's Charter: an action plan for cleaner hospitals.* Department of Health: London, 2004.

26 Department of Health. *Standards for Better Health.* Department of Health: London, 2006.

27 National Patient Safety Agency (NPSA). *The National Specifications for Cleanliness in the NHS: a framework for setting and measuring performance outcomes.* NPSA: London, 2007.

28 National Patient Safety Agency (NPSA). *Safer Practice Notice; colour coding hospital cleaning materials and equipment.* NPSA: London, 2007.

Environmental decontamination

- Effective decontamination of healthcare equipment reduces the risk of transmission of infection.
- Decontamination is a general term used to describe the removal of microbial contamination, which can be achieved by:
  - cleaning
  - disinfection
  - sterilization.
- Decontamination should be carried out immediately after use of the equipment by the patient or staff member.
- Systematic decontamination of equipment should be carried out in line with local policy if this is available. Where local policy is not available, it should be carried out according to the manufacturer's guidance.
- Healthcare workers who are undertaking the decontamination of any equipment must be trained in the correct procedures.

Responsibilities

Criterion 2 in *The Health and Social Care Act 2008: Code of Practice on the prevention and control of infections and related guidance*[29] states that:
- Matrons are responsible and accountable for delivering a clean environment.
- The nurse in charge is responsible for ensuring that standards of cleanliness are maintained throughout that shift.

Assurance

Patients and healthcare staff require assurance that healthcare equipment has been decontaminated before they use it. Therefore healthcare facilities should determine how assurance that safe care in a clean environment has been provided.

The three levels of decontamination

Cleaning
- This is the physical removal of contaminants such as organic matter, dust, dirt, and microorganisms, using detergent and water and thorough drying.
- It is used for items that either only come into contact with intact skin or do not come into contact with the patient.
- Cleaning is a necessary process before disinfection or sterilization.
- *Example of practice*: using a neutral detergent to clean a mattress after it has been used for a patient not known to have an infection.

Disinfection
- This is the use of chemicals or heat to reduce the number of microorganisms to a level that is not harmful to health.
- Disinfection does not usually remove or reduce the number of bacterial spores.

- It is used for items which come into contact with intact mucous membranes or which may be contaminated with particularly virulent or readily transmissible microorganisms.
- *Examples of practice*:
  - disinfection of a commode following use by a patient with *Clostridium difficile*, utilizing a 1000 parts per million (ppm) bleach solution
  - disinfection of a dressing trolley with an alcohol-based wipe
  - disinfection of the hands with an alcohol-based hand rub.

Sterilization

- This process is used to render an object free from microorganisms and spores. It is used on items which penetrate skin or mucous membranes, or enter the vascular system, or sterile spaces.
- Where disinfection or sterilization of equipment is required, ideally the Hospital Sterilization and Disinfection Unit (HSDU) or single-use disposables should be used.
- *Example of practice*: sterilizing a piece of equipment before undertaking a surgical procedure.

Risk assessment

The choice of procedure for decontaminating equipment depends on the following factors:

- the type of equipment
- the microorganism involved
- the time required for processing
- the risk to patients and staff
- the manufacturer's written instructions.

Decontamination and storage of decontaminated equipment

- Equipment should be decontaminated in a designated area, or away from clean items.
- Decontaminated equipment should be stored separately from used items, and away from areas where cleaning is taking place, in order to reduce the risk of recontamination.

Reference

29 Department of Health. *The Health and Social Care Act 2008: Code of Practice on the prevention and control of infections and related guidance*. Department of Health: London, 2015.

Terminal cleaning and hydrogen peroxide vaporization

Terminal cleaning

- 'Terminal cleaning' is not a standardized term, and this process should correctly be called 'terminal decontamination' in order to reflect the fact that not only cleaning but a variety of other methods of decontamination may be used.
- Local policies should be followed.
- Decontamination of the environment contributes to infection prevention and control by decreasing the number of microorganisms and thus reducing their potential spread.
- Specific local guidance may be in place regarding the steps to take at the time of patient discharge to ensure that the environment is safe to receive the next patient. This will include decontaminating equipment such as:
  - beds
  - lockers
  - tables
  - chairs, etc.
- In addition, if the patient who is being discharged had an infection, the environment will need to be decontaminated with an appropriate disinfectant, and items such as curtains may have to be changed before the next patient is admitted.

Hydrogen peroxide vapour bio-decontamination and disinfection systems

- The use of a hydrogen peroxide vapour disinfection system is dependent upon local choice.
- Hydrogen peroxide vapour disinfection systems are used to eradicate pathogens that cause healthcare-associated infections (HCAIs) from the hospital environment and medical equipment.
- Hydrogen peroxide vapour disinfection systems use a vapour generator to vaporize aqueous hydrogen peroxide so that in its gaseous state it can permeate all surface areas to ensure thorough bio-decontamination and disinfection.
- Hydrogen peroxide vapour decomposes to form oxygen and water vapour, so the process is residue-free.
- It has been shown that hydrogen peroxide vapour not only reduces the acquisition of pathogens but also kills a wide range of microorganisms, including bacteria, viruses, and fungi. It is highly effective against pathogens such as *C. difficile* spores, MRSA, and Norovirus that cause HCAIs.[30]
- When hydrogen peroxide vapour comes into contact with microorganisms it uses a variety of methods to inactivate them, including rupture of the cell wall, destruction of cell contents, and damage to the genetic material (i.e. cellular DNA).
- Hydrogen peroxide vapour disinfection is used in addition to standard cleaning, not as a substitute for it.

- All surfaces must be visibly clean before hydrogen peroxide vapour is used, to ensure complete surface coverage.
- Hydrogen peroxide vapour is hazardous to human health if it is not controlled and managed correctly. It must only be used in areas where no patients and staff are present. The rooms should be adequately sealed, and appropriate monitoring equipment used to ensure that:
  - the optimum levels of hydrogen peroxide vapour have been reached and are maintained to maximize microbial killing power
  - there is no leakage
  - the level of hydrogen peroxide vapour has returned to safe levels before re-entry.

HCAI technology innovation programme

The Department of Health has set up a Rapid Review Panel (RRP) to assess new and novel technologies and consider their potential for reducing hospital infections. The BIOQUELL® hydrogen peroxide vapour disinfection system (see Figure 14.1) was awarded a Department of Health RRP recommendation 1 in 2007.[31]

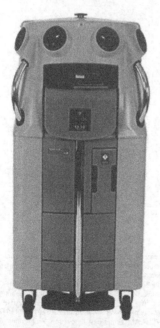

Figure 14.1 The BIOQUELL® Q-10-room/suite bio-decontamination system.
Reproduced with permission from www.bioquell.com/products/bioquell-q-10

References

30 Boyce JM et al. Impact of hydrogen peroxide vapor room decontamination on *Clostridium difficile* environmental contamination and transmission in a healthcare setting. *Infection Control and Hospital Epidemiology* 2008; 29: 723–9.

31 Department of Health and the NHS Purchasing and Supply Agency. *The Results: using technology to help fight infection.* HCAI Technology Innovation Programme: Showcase Hospitals Report Number 3. The Bioquell hydrogen peroxide vapour (HPV) disinfection system. ℘ http://webarchive.nationalarchives.gov.uk/20120118164404/hcai.dh.gov.uk/files/2011/03/090817_HCAI_Technology_Innovation_Programme_Showcase_Hospitals_Report_3_The_Bioquell_Hydrogen_Peroxide_Vapour_HPV_Disinfection_System.pdf

Hand hygiene

- Hand hygiene is essential for preventing the transmission of infection. Hands can acquire and then transfer microorganisms following contact with a patient, equipment, or the environment.
- National evidence-based guidelines associated with hand hygiene were identified in the epic3 guidelines.[32]

Hand decontamination

Liquid soap

- If the hands are visibly soiled it is recommended that effective washing with liquid detergent soap is undertaken to render the hands socially clean.
- Liquid detergent soap prevents the carriage of transient microorganisms (see Figure 14.2).

Alcohol-based hand rub

- Alcohol-based hand rub is recommended for all other situations in which hand hygiene is required during patient care, as it is more effective, better tolerated by the skin, and its action is faster (see Figure 14.3).
- Alcohol-based hand rubs remove transient microorganisms and reduce the resident flora. However, it must be noted that:
  - they are not effective against *C. difficile*
  - some of them are not effective against Norovirus
  - they are only effective on visibly clean hands
  - the hands should be washed with liquid detergent soap after several consecutive applications of alcohol-based hand rub.

Moisturizers

- Frequent use of hand-decontaminating products can lead to healthcare workers developing sore or damaged skin. To reduce this risk it is important that:
  - soap products are applied to wet hands and not directly onto dry skin
  - hands are rinsed and then dried thoroughly after washing with liquid soap.
- Healthcare workers should regularly moisturize their hands to prevent drying and excoriation.
- It is important that the moisturizer is stored appropriately so that it does not become contaminated and thus a source of cross-transmission of infection.

Hand decontamination facilities

- Alcohol-based hand rub should be available at the point of care (e.g. the patient's bed space, the treatment room, personal dispensers).
- Placement at other sites should be risk assessed by the healthcare facility.
- Hand-wash basins should be appropriately positioned to allow easy access, and be equipped with a liquid soap dispenser, paper towel dispenser, and waste bin.

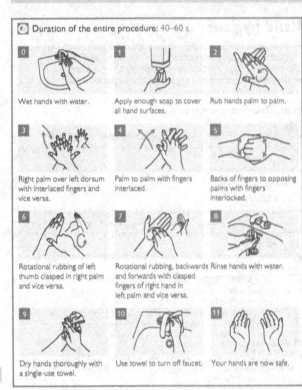

⏱ Duration of the entire procedure: 40–60 s

0	1	2
Wet hands with water.	Apply enough soap to cover all hand surfaces.	Rub hands palm to palm.

3	4	5
Right palm over left dorsum with interlaced fingers and vice versa.	Palm to palm with fingers interlaced.	Backs of fingers to opposing palms with fingers interlocked.

6	7	8
Rotational rubbing of left thumb clasped in right palm and vice versa.	Rotational rubbing, backwards and forwards with clasped fingers of right hand in left palm and vice versa.	Rinse hands with water.

9	10	11
Dry hands thoroughly with a single-use towel.	Use towel to turn off faucet.	Your hands are now safe.

Figure 14.2 How to hand wash: hand hygiene technique with soap and water. Reproduced from the WHO Guidelines on Hand Hygiene in Healthcare (2009), http://whqlibdoc.who.int/publications/2009/9789241597906_eng.pdf, with kind permission of the WHO.

Indications for effective hand decontamination
The 'Five Moments for Hand Hygiene'[33]
- Before touching a patient.
- Before a clean aseptic procedure.
- After body fluid exposure risk.
- After touching a patient.
- After touching a patient's surroundings.

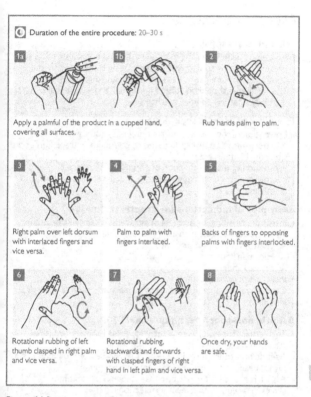

Figure 14.3 How to hand rub: hand hygiene technique with alcohol-based formulation. Reproduced from the WHO Guidelines on Hand Hygiene in Healthcare (2009), http://whqlibdoc.who.int/publications/2009/9789241597906_eng.pdf, with kind permission of the WHO.

References

32 Loveday HP et al. epic3: national evidence-based guidelines for preventing healthcare associated infections in NHS hospitals in England. *Journal of Hospital Infection* 2014; **86**: S1–70.

33 World Health Organization and Patient Safety. *WHO Guidelines on Hand Hygiene in Health Care. First global patient safety challenge: clean care is safer care.* World Health Organization: Geneva, 2009. http://whqlibdoc.who.int/publications/2009/9789241597906_eng.pdf

Aseptic technique

Principles of asepsis
- An aseptic technique aims to prevent the microorganisms that are present on hands and equipment from being transferred to and potentially contaminating a susceptible site, leading to infection.
- The technique should be utilized during any procedure that bypasses the body's natural defence mechanisms.

The aims of aseptic technique
- Prevention of the transmission of potentially pathogenic microorganisms to susceptible sites (e.g. wounds, intravenous access sites, the bladder, etc.).
- Prevention of the transmission of potentially pathogenic microorganisms from patient to patient, from staff to patient, and from patient to staff.

Examples of indications for aseptic technique
- Insertion, re-siting, or dressing of intravenous cannulae or other intravascular devices, such as:
  - central venous pressure lines
  - Hickman lines
  - arterial lines.
- Insertion of urinary catheters.
- Care of wounds that are healing by primary intention (e.g. surgical incisions).

Aseptic non-touch technique (ANTT)
- The actual process of aseptic technique was for many years not standardized.
- Aseptic non-touch technique (ANTT)[14] was devised to introduce a logical practice framework for aseptic technique.
- ANTT is based on the premise that asepsis is the common aim of all clinical procedures that incur an infection risk.
- The underlying principles of ANTT are as follows:
  - Always wash your hands effectively.
  - Never contaminate key parts.
  - Touch non-key parts with confidence.
  - Take appropriate infective precautions.

Standard ANTT
This includes simple procedures that are of short duration, involving smaller key sites and key parts (e.g. intravenous therapy, simple dressings).

Surgical ANTT
This includes complex procedures that take place over extended periods of time, involving large open key sites and/or large or numerous key parts (e.g. central venous catheter insertion, surgery, large complex dressings).

Key parts and key sites

These are those parts or sites that, if contaminated with microorganisms, provide a direct route for the transmission of pathogenic microorganisms (e.g. syringe tip, needleless connectors, urinary catheter tip, rubber tops of vials containing medication, patient's wounds, insertion sites).

Glove choice

- If it is necessary to touch key parts, sterile gloves should be used. Otherwise, non-sterile gloves are usually the glove of choice.

Hand decontamination

- Hand decontamination is an essential component of aseptic technique and ANTT.
- When undertaking standard ANTT, the WHO guidelines on how to hand wash and how to hand rub[35] should be followed.
- When undertaking surgical ANTT, a surgical hand scrub with an antiseptic soap should be used. The procedure takes 2–3 min, and covers all areas of the forearms and hands.[36]

References

34 Rowley S et al. ANTT v2: an updated practice framework for aseptic technique. *British Journal of Nursing* 2010; 19: S5–11.
35 World Health Organization and Patient Safety. *WHO Guidelines on Hand Hygiene in Health Care. First global patient safety challenge: clean care is safer care.* World Health Organization: Geneva, 2009. http://whqlibdoc.who.int/publications/2009/9789241597906_eng.pdf
36 Fraise AP and Bradley C (eds). *Ayliffe's Control of Healthcare-Associated Infection*, 5th edn. CRC Press: Boca Raton, FL, 2009.

Principles of antibiotic therapy

Antibiotic modes of action
- The basis of antibiotic therapy is that antibiotics have targets that are present in bacteria but not in mammalian cells (or the target is different in nature).
- There are four main modes of action:
  - inhibition of cell wall synthesis—the cell wall is required for bacterial survival, whereas mammalian cells do not have a cell wall
  - disruption of the cell membrane—causes leakage of cell contents
  - inhibition of protein synthesis
  - inhibition of nucleic acid synthesis and function.

Types of antibiotics
- Antibiotics have either a narrow or broad spectrum of activity. This refers to the range of bacteria against which the antibiotic is active.
- Bactericidal agents kill microorganisms, whereas bacteriostatic agents simply inhibit microbial multiplication. The host immune system then kills these bacteria. Therefore bacteriostatic agents should not be used in patients who are immunosuppressed.

Types of antibiotic regimens
- Monotherapy is the use of one agent alone.
- Combination therapy is the use of two or more agents. This may have an additive or synergistic effect (or an antagonistic effect if inappropriate combinations of agents are selected).
- Antimicrobial prophylaxis refers to the use of antimicrobial agents to prevent infection from occurring (e.g. during surgery) when there is a significant risk of acquiring an infection.
- Empirical therapy refers to the use of antibiotics before microbiological results are available, because a delay in therapy is likely to be detrimental (microbiological specimens should be collected before antibiotics are administered).
- Directed therapy can then be used to target specific pathogens when microbiological data are available.

Routes of antibiotic administration
The main routes of administration of antibiotics are oral and intravenous. However, some agents can be given intramuscularly (IM), topically, per rectum, or via nebulization. The chosen route of administration depends on a number of factors, including the type, location, and severity of infection.

Other factors to consider in antibiotic therapy
- A number of factors should be taken into consideration when selecting an antimicrobial agent for use. These include:
  - penetration into the infected site
  - half-life
  - toxicity
  - drug interactions
  - allergies.

- The levels of certain antibiotics in the blood are monitored for one of two reasons:
  - to ensure that therapeutic levels are reached (e.g. vancomycin)
  - to avoid toxic levels being reached (e.g. gentamicin).
- Local antibiotic guidelines should be developed and used, as antibiotic resistance can vary geographically and over time.

Resistance to antibiotics

- There are a number of mechanisms by which bacteria become resistant to antibiotics.
  - The target site in the bacterium can be altered or protected.
  - The antibiotic may be destroyed or inactivated by the bacteria.
  - The bacteria may interfere with transportation of the antibiotic to the cell.
- The emergence of resistance is related to the level of use of antibiotics. Therefore it is important that antibiotics are prescribed carefully. In response to this, guidance on antimicrobial stewardship[37] and a 5-year strategy to help to combat this emerging problem[38] have been developed.

References

37 Public Health England. *Start Smart – Then Focus. Antimicrobial stewardship toolkit for English hospitals.* Public Health England: London, 2015. ℗ www.gov.uk/government/uploads/system/uploads/attachment_data/file/417032/Start_Smart_Then_Focus_FINAL.PDF
38 Department of Health and Department for Environment, Food and Rural Affairs. *UK Five Year Antimicrobial Resistance Strategy: 2013 to 2018.* Department of Health: London, 2013. ℗ www.gov.uk/government/uploads/system/uploads/attachment_data/file/244058/20130902_UK_5_year_AMR_strategy.pdf

Antibiotics that inhibit bacterial cell wall synthesis

The penicillins, cephalosporins, carbapenems, and monobactams all belong to a group of antibiotics known as the β-lactams, which are so called because they all contain a β-lactam ring in their chemical structure. These antibiotics are bactericidal.

Penicillins

This is the largest group of antibiotics. Most of them are semi-synthetic, and some range from a narrow spectrum of activity (e.g. benzylpenicillin) to an extended spectrum (e.g. piperacillin). Some of these antibiotics are inactivated by β-lactamases.

- Benzylpenicillin is commonly used to treat streptococcal and meningococcal infections, and is normally given intravenously (IV) or IM, as it is destroyed by acid in the stomach. Most strains of *Staphylococcus aureus* are resistant to benzylpenicillin.
- Amoxicillin and ampicillin have a broader spectrum of activity than benzylpenicillin, and are often used to treat respiratory tract infections. They can be given by the oral, IM, or IV route.
- Amoxicillin can be used in combination with clavulanic acid (or co-amoxiclav) to inhibit β-lactamases. This antibiotic can also be given orally or IV, and is often used for bites and surgical prophylaxis.
- Flucloxacillin is active against most β-lactamase-producing Gram-positive bacteria, and is used to treat staphylococcal infections (but not those caused by MRSA). It can be given orally, IM, or IV.
- Piperacillin is active against a broad range of bacteria. This antibiotic is normally used in combination with tazobactam (a β-lactamase inhibitor). It is often used for treatment of severe intra-abdominal infections and pneumonia, and is normally given by the IV route.

Cephalosporins

There are four 'generations' of cephalosporins.

- First-generation cephalosporins, such as cefalexin, have good activity against staphylococci and some Gram-negative species.
- Second-generation cephalosporins are resistant to some β-lactamases and have good Gram-negative activity. An example is cefuroxime, which can be given orally, IM, or IV. It is often used to treat intra-abdominal infections and pneumonia, and as prophylaxis for some surgical procedures.
- Third-generation cephalosporins have enhanced activity against Gram-negative bacteria but reduced activity against Gram-positive bacteria. Examples of commonly used agents are ceftazidime and cefotaxime, which both have anti-pseudomonal activity. These agents are given IV or IM, mainly for hospital-acquired infections. They cross the blood–brain barrier, and this makes them particularly useful for the treatment of bacterial meningitis.
- Fourth-generation cephalosporins, such as cefepime, have enhanced Gram-positive activity as well as maintaining Gram-negative activity.

Cephalosporins have a tendency to cause *Clostridium difficile*-associated diarrhoea. Therefore their use should be avoided where possible, particularly on medical wards.

Carbapenems

- Carbapenems have a very broad spectrum of antimicrobial activity, and are resistant to most β-lactamases.
- They are all given by the IV route, and are used for empirical treatment of severe hospital infections, including intra-abdominal infections, meningitis, pneumonia, necrotizing fasciitis, and febrile neutropenia, and for directed therapy of resistant Gram-negative infections.
- Imipenem is given with cilastatin to prevent breakdown of the imipenem and toxicity in the kidneys. At high doses it can cause seizures, whereas meropenem does not have this side effect.
- Ertapenem is not anti-pseudomonal. It has a longer half-life than the other carbapenems, so it only needs to be administered once daily.

Monobactams

Aztreonam is active against certain Gram-negative bacteria, including *Pseudomonas* species, and can be given IV or IM. It can be used for patients who have penicillin allergies, and in a nebulized form in cystic fibrosis patients with pulmonary *Pseudomonas aeruginosa* infection.

Glycopeptides

- Vancomycin and teicoplanin are commonly used glycopeptide antibiotics.
- They are bactericidal.
- Vancomycin and teicoplanin can both be given IV, IM, or orally.
- They are active against Gram-positive bacteria. For a long time vancomycin has been known as the drug of last resort, as it can be used to treat resistant pathogens. The glycopeptides, and vancomycin in particular, are often used to treat severe resistant staphylococcal and enterococcal infections.
- Vancomycin is administered orally to treat severe *C. difficile* infections.
- Resistance has been observed in enterococci, known as vancomycin-resistant enterococci (VRE). Reduced susceptibility to vancomycin has been reported among strains of *Staphylococcus aureus*. However, full resistance to vancomycin in this group is extremely rare. New antibiotics to treat such resistant bacteria have been developed.
- Serum levels of vancomycin must be monitored, as it can cause nephrotoxicity. Teicoplanin is associated with a reduced level of toxicity.

Useful website

MedicinesComplete. ♫ www.medicinescomplete.com

Antibiotics that disrupt bacterial cell membranes

Polymyxins

- One example of a polymyxin is colistimethate sodium.
- These antibiotics disrupt the cell membranes of some Gram-negative bacteria.
- Polymyxins are bactericidal.
- They are nephrotoxic, so are commonly used topically. They can be used in a nebulized form to treat cystic fibrosis patients who are infected with *Pseudomonas aeruginosa*, or administered by the IV route as a last resort to treat severe infection with multi-resistant Gram-negative bacilli.

Daptomycin

- Daptomycin is a relatively new antibiotic. It is a novel lipopeptide.
- It works by disrupting the cell membrane of Gram-positive bacteria.
- It is bactericidal.
- It is administered by the IV route, and was developed to combat increasingly resistant Gram-positive bacteria.
- Its indicated uses are:
  - complicated skin and soft tissue infections
  - right-sided endocarditis
  - bloodstream infection (caused by *Staphylococcus aureus*).
- Reported side effects include rhabdomyolysis.

Useful website

MedicinesComplete. ♪ www.medicinescomplete.com

Antibiotics that inhibit bacterial protein synthesis

Aminoglycosides

- Examples of commonly used aminoglycosides include gentamicin (intrathecally or IV), tobramycin (IM, IV, or via inhalation), and amikacin (IV and IM).
- They are bactericidal.
- They are active against Gram-negative bacteria (including *Pseudomonas* species), and are used in combination with other antibiotics for severe staphylococcal and streptococcal infections. Indeed, they enhance the effect of some other antibiotics, such as vancomycin.
- Aminoglycosides are nephrotoxic and ototoxic, so serum levels must be monitored.

Tetracyclines

- Examples of commonly used tetracyclines include tetracycline, doxycycline, and minocycline.
- Tetracyclines can be given orally or IV, but must not be given to children or women during pregnancy, as the drug is deposited in developing bones and teeth.
- They are bacteriostatic.
- They have a broad spectrum of activity against Gram-positive and Gram-negative bacteria, and are often used to treat infection with atypical bacteria (i.e. chlamydial and rickettsial infections) as well as brucellosis and Lyme disease.

Tigecycline

- Tigecycline is a glycylcycline antibiotic that is a derivative of minocycline.
- It is given by the IV route.
- It is bacteriostatic.
- It is a relatively new antibiotic that has been developed to treat bacteria which are resistant to other antibiotics. Unlike other new antibiotics, tigecycline is active against many Gram-positive and Gram-negative bacteria. However, it has no activity against *Pseudomonas* species.
- It is licensed for use in complicated skin and skin structure infections, complicated intra-abdominal infections, and community-acquired bacterial pneumonia.

Macrolides

- Examples of commonly used macrolides include clarithromycin, erythromycin, and azithromycin.
- They can be given orally or by the IV route.
- They are bacteriostatic.
- The macrolides have activity against some Gram-positive bacteria, Gram-negative bacteria, anaerobes, and atypical bacteria. They are sometimes used to treat respiratory and soft tissue infections. Erythromycin is sometimes used in patients who have penicillin allergies.
- Macrolides are occasionally hepatotoxic.

Lincosamides
- An example of a commonly used lincosamide is clindamycin.
- It can be given orally, IV, or IM.
- It is bacteriostatic.
- It has a similar spectrum of activity to the macrolides, but it has greater activity against anaerobes.
- It is used in the treatment of bone and joint infections and cellulitis.

Oxazolidinones
- An example of an oxazolidinone is linezolid.
- It can be given orally or IV.
- It is bacteriostatic.
- Linezolid is a relatively new antibiotic. It is active against a wide range of Gram-positive bacteria, including resistant microorganisms such as MRSA and VRE.
- It is therefore used to treat infections caused by such resistant bacteria. These include skin and soft tissue infections and pneumonia.
- Blood counts must be monitored, as prolonged use of linezolid can result in anaemia.

Chloramphenicol
- Chloramphenicol can be given orally, IV, or topically.
- It is bacteriostatic.
- It has a wide spectrum of activity against Gram-positive, Gram-negative, and atypical bacteria.
- It is used topically to treat eye infections. However, systemic use is reserved for life-threatening infections, as it can cause aplastic anaemia, which can be fatal.

Fusidic acid
- Fusidic acid is available in oral, IV, and topical formulations.
- It is bacteriostatic.
- It has activity against a range of bacteria. However, it is used as an anti-staphylococcal agent, mostly in combination with other agents (e.g. flucloxacillin) for treatment of serious infections such as osteomyelitis.

Mupirocin
- Mupirocin is available as a topical agent.
- It is bactericidal at high concentrations.
- Its spectrum of activity includes staphylococci and streptococci.
- It is used to treat skin infections, and for decolonization of nasal carriage of MRSA.
- Resistance develops quickly if mupirocin is used continuously.

Useful website
MedicinesComplete. ♪ www.medicinescomplete.com

Antibiotics that inhibit bacterial nucleic acid synthesis and function

Trimethoprim

- Trimethoprim is a diaminopyrimidine that is administered orally.
- It is bacteriostatic.
- It has a broad spectrum of activity against Gram-positive and Gram-negative bacteria, and is used to treat urinary tract infections.

Co-trimoxazole

- Co-trimoxazole is a combination of trimethoprim and sulfamethoxazole (a sulfonamide).
- Sulfonamides are broad-spectrum agents, but due to their toxicity and resistance they are rarely used alone.
- Co-trimoxazole is bactericidal.
- It can be given orally or by the IV route.
- It is often used for the prophylaxis and treatment of *Pneumocystis jirovecii* pneumonia.

Quinolones

Nalidixic acid

Nalidixic acid is an oral bacteriostatic agent with activity against many members of the Enterobacteriaceae. It is used predominantly to treat urinary tract infections.

Fluoroquinolones

- Examples of fluoroquinolones include ciprofloxacin, levofloxacin, and moxifloxacin.
- They are available in both oral and IV formulations.
- They are bactericidal.
- Ciprofloxacin has a wider spectrum of activity against Gram-negative bacteria than nalidixic acid. It is the only oral antibiotic with activity against *Pseudomonas* species. Levofloxacin and moxifloxacin have better Gram-positive activity.
- Resistance to fluoroquinolones is increasingly prevalent due to their overuse.
- The quinolones have a tendency to cause *C. difficile*-associated diarrhoea, so their use should be avoided where possible, particularly on medical wards.

Metronidazole

- Metronidazole is a nitroimidazole antibiotic.
- It can be given orally, IV, or topically.
- It is bactericidal.
- It has activity against a range of anaerobic bacteria, and also protozoa, and is therefore commonly used to treat infections caused by anaerobic bacteria such as *C. difficile*.

Rifampicin

- Rifampicin is a rifamycin, and can be given orally or IV.
- It is bactericidal.
- It is active against a range of Gram-positive and Gram-negative bacteria.
- Resistance emerges during therapy, so rifampicin is given in combination with other agents to prevent this.
- It is often used to treat tuberculosis and severe infections such as osteomyelitis, endocarditis, and meningitis.
- Rifampicin can cause liver function abnormalities, so liver function tests must be monitored.
- It also interacts with many drugs.
- It can give a red-orange tint to the patient's urine, sweat, sputum, and tears.

Useful website
MedicinesComplete. ℐ www.medicinescomplete.com

Post-operative complications

Airway problems

Compromise of the airway during the immediate post-operative period can occur for the following reasons:

- inadequate metabolism and/or elimination of general anaesthetic agents or reversal of muscle relaxants
- inappropriate use of the supine position when the conscious level is compromised, leading to tongue and/or denture obstruction (tongue obstruction is more common in patients who are obese, pregnant, or have a very short or large neck)
- substance obstructions (e.g. the presence of blood clots or mucus); the risk of this is increased by a difficult intubation process and surgery involving the head and neck
- aspiration of gastric contents:
  - this can occur either by active vomiting or passively as a result of silent regurgitation
  - the presence of gastric contents in the airway can cause bronchospasm and airway closure
- laryngeal obstruction—in patients with a history of smoking, asthma, or chronic obstructive pulmonary disease (COPD) there is a higher risk of the muscles of the larynx going into spasm when irritated by the presence of an endotracheal tube.

Recognition of airway compromise

The airway should be constantly monitored for signs of compromise during the immediate post-operative period. This should be done by making frequent attempts at verbal communication with the patient. If the patient can talk, their airway is clear.

The patient should be continually observed for the following:

- stridor—this is a high-pitched musical sound:
  - if it is inspiratory it indicates partial airway obstruction above the vocal cords
  - if it is biphasic it indicates obstruction in the trachea or subglottis
  - if it is present on expiration it indicates small airway obstruction (e.g. asthma)
- an unusual degree of restlessness or dyspnoea
- increased use of the accessory muscles around the neck and abdomen
- the presence of noisy or unusual upper airway sounds (e.g. crowing, snoring, gurgling)
- the absence of breath sounds
- the presence of cyanosis.

Response of airway compromise

If the airway is completely obstructed, immediate intervention is required. Consider the following:

- simple airway manoeuvres, such as head tilt, chin lift, and jaw thrust (see Figure 15.1)
- insertion of airway adjuncts, such as oropharyngeal or nasopharyngeal airways

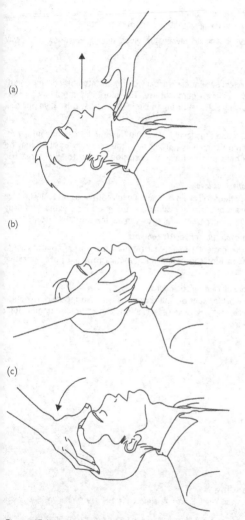

Figure 15.1 (a) Performing a chin lift. (b) Performing a jaw thrust. (c) Performing a head tilt. Reproduced from Suzanne Hughes and Andy Mardell, *Oxford Handbook of Perioperative Practice*, 2009, with permission from Oxford University Press.

- suctioning of oral secretions
- intubation via a laryngeal mask or endotracheal tube.

High-flow oxygen should always be given during episodes of airway compromise.

Prevention

Even if the surgical patient can verbally communicate, it is still important to act to prevent airway compromise. Therefore it is important to consider the following actions during the immediate post-operative period.

Patient position

If the patient's conscious level is or could become imminently impaired, positioning them sitting fully upright or in the recovery position may be important to help to avoid airway occlusion by the tongue or gastric secretions.

Maximizing conscious level

Assisting the patient to regain or maintain full consciousness may involve frequent interaction, critical evaluation, and good management of drug therapy that has depressant effects on the central nervous system.

Preventing the aspiration of gastric contents

Ensure that the patient remains nil by mouth until full consciousness is regained. Consider the use of anti-emetics to avoid post-operative vomiting.

Keeping the airway clear of secretions

Ensure that a working suction unit is close by with the appropriate equipment to ensure that any clots or secretions can be voided immediately from the airway.

Further reading

Adam S, Odell M and Welch J. *Rapid Assessment of the Acutely Ill Adult*. Wiley-Blackwell: Chichester, 2010.
Smith S, Price A and Challiner A. *Ward-Based Critical Care: a guide for health professionals*. M&K Publishing: Keswick, 2009.

Useful website

Resuscitation Council (UK). ∾ www.resus.org.uk

Respiratory problems

Respiratory compromise during the immediate post-operative period can occur for the following reasons:

- The *respiratory depressant effect* of many general anaesthetic agents and opioid-based analgesics.
- *Acute post-operative pain*. This can cause shallow breathing which may lead to basal atelectasis (collapse of the alveoli) and pneumonia. Abdominal distension increases this risk.
- *Bronchospasm*. Spasmodic contractions of the bronchial tubes may occur as a result of local irritation caused by anaesthesia. The likelihood of this is increased if the lung tissue itself has been involved in the surgery, or if the lower airways have been directly stimulated by procedures such as bronchoscopy. If the patient has a history of smoking, chronic bronchitis, asthma, or recent chest infection there is also an increased risk.
- *Bronchial obstruction with secretions*. The presence of a foreign body and unnatural flow of gas in the airway stimulates an increased level of bronchial secretions. If pain control is inadequate and this results in an ineffective cough, bronchial obstructions can occur.
- *Pulmonary oedema*. If fluid balance is not carefully controlled post-operatively, a build-up of fluid can occur that can cause oedema to develop in the lungs. This is particularly likely if the excretory capacity of the kidneys is diminished and/or the cardiac muscle is in some way impaired.
- *Pneumothorax/haemothorax*. Excessive pressures utilized during peri-operative ventilation or the opportunity for air or blood to enter the pleural space may result in the collapse of lung tissue.
- *Pulmonary embolus*. This may reduce gas exchange due to compromised blood flow to the lungs (see ⮕ p. 331).
- *Aspiration pneumonitis*. Inflammation of the lungs can occur as a result of inhalation of gastric contents (see ⮕ p. 314).
- *Acute respiratory distress syndrome*. A rapid, shallow breathing pattern accompanied by severe hypoxaemia with scattered crepitations (but no cough or chest pain) can develop 24–28 h after surgery, particularly if there has been a direct insult (e.g. stab wound) or systemic insult (e.g. sepsis) to the lungs.

Respiratory failure

Respiratory failure is considered to have occurred if the blood gas exchange values are as follows:

- PaO_2 < 8 kPa with PCO_2 < 6.6 kPa (type 1 respiratory failure)
- PaO_2 < 8 kPa with PCO_2 > 6.6 kPa (type 2 respiratory failure).[1]

Recognition of respiratory compromise

The respiratory system should be constantly monitored for signs of compromise during the immediate post-operative period. This should be done by:

- observing the respiratory rate, pattern, and depth
- use of pulse oximetry

- observing for evidence of hypoxia (peripheral or central cyanosis) or hypercarbia (flushed skin and/or headache)
- assessing conscious level (this could be affected by hypoxia, hypercarbia, and/or a disturbance in acid–base balance)
- considering arterial blood gas analysis to establish CO_2 levels as well as other useful parameters of respiratory function
- considering taking a chest X-ray to look for evidence of lung collapse or obstruction, or a CT scan to assess for pulmonary embolism.

The development of respiratory compromise should be suspected if the patient develops:
- a respiratory rate of < 10 breaths/min or > 25 breaths/min
- a pulse rate of > 100 beats/min
- a reduced conscious level.[1]

It is also important to be vigilant for other indicators of respiratory compromise. These include:
- the presence of wheeze—a high-pitched musical sound which if present on expiration can indicate small airway obstruction
- an unusual degree of restlessness, or patient reports of dyspnoea
- increased use of the accessory muscles in the chest
- the presence of unusual secretions (e.g. pink frothy expectorated secretions may indicate pulmonary oedema).

Response to respiratory compromise

If respiration is adversely affected in any of the ways listed earlier under the initial indicators of respiratory compromise, immediate action is required. Consider the following:
- oxygen therapy[2]
- optimization of analgesia
- mobilization, breathing exercises, and chest physiotherapy to prevent and treat atelectesis
- bronchodilators, which may be useful for bronchospasm
- optimization of fluid balance.

Prevention

Even if the post-operative patient shows no initial signs of respiratory compromise, it is still important to act to prevent this by attending to the following:
- patient position
- maximizing conscious level
- preventing the aspiration of gastric contents
- keeping the airway clear of secretions.

References

1 Scottish Intercollegiate Guidelines Network (SIGN). *Postoperative Management in Adults*. Guideline No. 77. SIGN: Edinburgh, 2004.
2 British Thoracic Society (BTS). *Guideline for Emergency Oxygen Use in Adult Patients*. BTS: London, 2008.

Cardiovascular problems

Compromise of the cardiovascular system during the immediate post-operative period can occur for the following reasons.

- *Myocardial ischaemia.* This can occur silently peri-operatively or post-operatively with non-specific ECG changes, or with classical presentation. It can result from a decrease in myocardial blood flow that may be secondary to atherosclerosis, vasospasm, or hypotension. The physiological stress of surgery can also cause myocardial ischaemia, and there is an increased risk in patients with a high pre-operative systolic blood pressure or with known coronary artery disease.

- *Arrhythmias.* Cardiac arrhythmias can result from pain, anxiety, hypoxia, hypovolaemia, anaesthetic agents, and electrolyte imbalances. The degree to which they cause compromise to the post-operative patient will depend on their rate, electrophysiological pathway, and type (e.g. fibrillation, block). Increased release of endogenous catecholamines causes an increase in sinus and atrioventricular (AV) node rates as well as atrial and ventricular irritability.

- *Hypotension.* This can occur when the intravascular volume is depleted due to inadequate replacement of blood loss, inadequate hydration regimes, third-space fluid loss, or polyuria. It may also result from pulmonary embolus or depressed myocardial contractility. Vasodilation in conditions such as sepsis and hyperthermia or as a result of medication (e.g. propofol) is another cause.

- *Hypertension.* Pain, anxiety, interrupted anti-hypertensive medication, fluid overload, hypothermia (with shivering), urine retention, and the physiological stress response can all be causes of hypertension in the immediate post-operative period. It can also result from an acute cerebral event.

- *Depressed myocardial muscle function.* Some anaesthetic agents (e.g. halothane, enflurane, isoflurane, and ketamine) can cause a reduction in myocardial muscle contractility. The effects of these drugs may last for up to 6 h after surgery. Opioids and benzodiazepines have a similar effect, although to a lesser degree.

- *Pulmonary embolus.* This can have a direct impact on cardiac performance by blocking the flow of blood to the left side of the heart.

- *Cardiac tamponade.* Blood or fluid accumulating in the mediastinal space (with no exit point) can cause impairment of myocardial contraction and eventual cardiac arrest.

- *Cardiac arrest.* This is a possibility during the immediate post-operative period if any of the above compromises of the cardiovascular system are sustained.

Recognition of cardiovascular compromise

The cardiovascular system should be constantly monitored for signs of compromise during the immediate post-operative period. This should be done by:

- assessing heart rate, rhythm, and cardiac output to the peripheries—the manual pulse method measures all of these parameters, in contrast to electronic devices, which only measure heart rate
- assessing blood pressure—manual methods of recording blood pressure provide the most accurate readings when physiological stress is present
- continuous cardiac monitoring of patients with a high risk of cardiac complications—a 12-lead ECG should be performed routinely for these patients after surgery and whenever any irregularities in pulse or heart rhythm occur
- regularly assessing circulatory volume by interpreting vital signs, blood results, skin turgor, and capillary refill testing, and by examining the skin and mucous membranes.

If cardiac compromise is detected, the following procedures may be indicated to further clarify the cause of the compromise:

- echocardiogram
- chest X-ray
- central venous pressure monitoring
- continuous invasive blood pressure monitoring (via an arterial line)
- measurement of cardiac output and vascular tone (via oesophageal Doppler or alternative methods).

Response to cardiovascular compromise

If the cardiovascular system is adversely affected in any of the ways listed earlier under the initial indicators of respiratory compromise, immediate action is required. Consider:

- increasing the preload with fluid and/or elevation of the legs if the compromise is due to myocardial depression caused by anaesthetic agents
- timely and accurate identification of arrhythmias so that the correct therapeutic intervention can be employed (e.g. cardioversion, anticoagulation). Patients with implanted pacemakers or defibrillators should have their device checked before and after surgery[1]
- treating the underlying cause of hypotension or hypertension. Pharmacological treatment of hypertension may include vasodilators, adrenergic inhibitors, and calcium-channel blockers
- if myocardial ischaemia is present, a normal treatment course for this should be followed, except for thrombolysis, which is contraindicated
- anticoagulation for embolus—thrombolysis for pulmonary embolism should only be considered in exceptionally life-threatening circumstances
- basic and advanced life support algorithms to guide the response to cardiac arrest should it occur.[4]

Prevention

Even if the post-operative patient shows no initial signs of cardiovascular compromise, it is still important to act to prevent this, by considering the following actions:

- regular and accurate monitoring of cardiovascular parameters
- accurate and effective post-operative fluid management.

References

3 Scottish Intercollegiate Guidelines Network (SIGN). *Postoperative Management in Adults.* Guideline No. 77. SIGN: Edinburgh, 2004.
4 Resuscitation Council (UK). *Advanced Life Support: algorithm.* Resuscitation Council (UK): London, 2010. ♫ https://lms.resus.org.uk/modules/m25-v2-als-algorithm/11118/resources/chapter_6.pdf

Renal and urological problems

Compromise of the renal and urological system during the immediate post-operative period can occur for the following reasons:

- *Acute kidney injury (AKI).* Sustained periods of hypoxia, reduced circulatory volume, or reduced cardiac output (due to alterations in vessel tone or impaired myocardial performance) can result in a sudden decline in renal function. Typically in post-operative patients the episode of AKI is initially pre-renal in nature,[5] and therefore reversible.
- *Nephrotoxic medication.* An abrupt decline in renal function (AKI) of an intrinsic type may be caused by nephrotoxic medications (e.g. contrast dyes, non-steroidal anti-inflammatory drugs, gentamicin), particularly in older adults.
- *Urinary retention.* Post-operative pain may cause a self-voiding patient to incompletely empty their bladder. Pre-existing bladder problems or obstructions can exacerbate this. Urological surgery can also result in tissue injury and inflammation that can provide an obstruction to urine flow. Regional blocks such as spinal and epidural anaesthesia can affect bladder tone and may cause difficulty in micturition.
- *Urinary tract infections (UTIs).* Urinary retention can lead to UTI, which is a common cause of post-operative infection, as residual urine provides an environment conducive to bacterial growth. Indwelling urinary catheters can also provide an infection source.

Recognition of renal and/or urological compromise

The renal and urological systems should be constantly monitored for signs of compromise during the immediate post-operative period. This should involve the following:

- Accurate, hourly monitoring of urine output. Normal urine output is 0.5–1 mL/kg/h. The cause of low urine output (oliguria) should be immediately investigated and acted upon. AKI should be considered to be the cause of oliguria in a well-hydrated patient.
- Accurate fluid balance documentation. The volume and type of fluids given peri-operatively should be reviewed and compared with fluid losses in theatre, including urine and insensible losses and any bowel preparation fluid losses at the start of the post-operative period.[6] Any fluid intake or output should then continue to be accurately documented in the post-operative period.
- Urinalysis. This can provide an indication of hydration, infection, or the presence of glucose, which may affect urine output values. The colour and clarity of urine should be observed, and pain or difficulty during micturition should be assessed.
- Close observations should be made for evidence of bladder distension. Discomfort may be present, and a full bladder may be externally palpable. Small amounts of urine may be passed as overflow. Bladder scans should be used to confirm and quantify retained urine volume.
- Close observations should be made for developing electrolyte, acid–base and/or fluid imbalances. Serum metabolic waste product levels should also be monitored.

Response to renal or urological compromise

If the renal or urological system is adversely affected in any of the ways listed earlier, consider the following:

- Intravenous fluid challenge may be necessary in the hypovolaemic patient or in the patient with clinical signs of hypoperfusion. Fluid replacement should be appropriate to the type of fluid deficit. Fluid optimization is particularly important for surgical patients because they may have fasted for long periods and lost large amounts of fluid during surgery. Details of all fluid administered must be clearly recorded and easily accessible.[6]
- Diuretics should not be used to treat oliguria. They should only be indicated for fluid overload.
- Monitoring and recording of mean arterial pressure (MAP). A single episode of hypotension can result in acute tubular necrosis of renal cells.
- In the event of hydration not being the cause of AKI, pharmacological strategies such as vasopressors to increase renal perfusion may be considered.
- Invasive monitoring of central venous pressure (CVP) can help to provide an accurate assessment of fluid balance.
- Older adults or those with complex medical histories and/or long histories of nephrotoxic medication groups should be vigilantly monitored for AKI during the post-operative period. Nephrotoxic drugs and their doses should be reviewed and altered as necessary.
- Low serum electrolyte levels (e.g. hypokalaemia and hypomagnesaemia) can delay post-operative recovery, so supplementation may be required.
- Renal replacement therapy (RRT) may be indicated if life-threatening acidosis or fluid or electrolyte imbalance occurs.

Prevention

Even if the post-operative patient shows no initial signs of renal or urological compromise, it is still important to act to prevent this by considering accurate and effective post-operative fluid management and accurate fluid balance documentation. Both excessive and inadequate intravenous fluid administration during the post-operative period can be harmful, particularly in the elderly.[7]

References

5 National Confidential Enquiry into Patient Outcome and Death (NCEPOD). *Acute Kidney Injury: adding insult to injury.* NCEPOD: London, 2009.

6 Powell-Tuck J et al. *British Consensus Guidelines on Intravenous Fluid Therapy for Adult Surgical Patients. GIFTASUP.* British Association for Parenteral and Enteral Nutrition (BAPEN): London, 2011. ℘ www.bapen.org.uk/pdfs/bapen_pubs/giftasup.pdf

7 Royal College of Surgeons of England and the Department of Health. *The Higher Risk General Surgical Patient: towards improved care for a forgotten group.* Royal College of Surgeons of England: London, 2011.

Gastrointestinal problems

Compromise of the gastrointestinal system during the immediate post-operative period can occur for the following reasons.

- *Nausea and vomiting.* In addition to being an unpleasant experience, nausea and vomiting can have life-threatening consequences during the post-operative period. Aspiration of emesis, dehydration, disordered electrolyte balance and/or post-operative bleeding (as a result of physical exertion and disruption of suture lines) can occur. Common causes in the immediate post-operative period are listed in Table 15.1.

   The prevalence of post-operative nausea and vomiting is higher in females, older adults, patients with a history of travel sickness, and those with inadequate pre-operative fasting, alcohol or drug intoxication, or increased intracranial pressure.

- *Ileus.* Reduced motor activity in the gastrointestinal tract can cause a temporary disruption in peristalsis during the immediate post-operative period. This may occur selectively in the stomach, small intestine, or colon. It is prevalent after bowel surgery, but can also occur after other types of surgery as a result of medications (e.g. opiates), inflammation, long surgery times and/or administration of large volumes of intravenous fluid. It is a non-mechanical cause of bowel obstruction, and can lead to nausea and vomiting, abdominal pain, poor absorption of oral medication, delayed nutritional intake and, if prolonged, bacterial translocation, aspiration, and venous thromboembolism.

- *Mechanical bowel obstruction.* This can occur as a result of twisted or trapped loops of bowel after lower gastrointestinal surgery.

- *Anastomotic leakage or breakdown of surgical sites in the bowel.* These can cause localized abscesses that delay the recovery of bowel function and may lead to sepsis as a result of the development of peritonitis. The use of laxatives as bowel preparation prior to colorectal surgery may increase this risk.

Table 15.1 Causes of nausea and vomiting during the post-operative period

Anaesthetic agents	Nitrous oxide and many anaesthetic, opioid, and sedative medications can cause nausea and vomiting as side effects
Gastric distension	Distension caused by manual ventilation methods used during the induction of anaesthesia can cause nausea and vomiting by direct stimulation of the cerebral vomiting centre
Gastric irritation	Air, blood, or diagnostic instruments (e.g. endoscope) in the gastric cavity can cause gastric irritation and vomiting, as can specific conditions (e.g. acute appendicitis) or bowel obstruction
Pain	Pain triggers nausea and vomiting in many patients

Recognition of gastrointestinal compromise

The gastrointestinal system should be constantly monitored for signs of compromise during the immediate post-operative period. This should include regular assessment of the following:

- The return of gastrointestinal motility, which may be indicated by the return of bowel sounds. It may be evidenced by passage of flatus, auscultated from the lower abdomen, tolerance of oral intake, and bowel movement. Tolerance of oral intake without gastric distension, nausea, or vomiting is proof that normal gastric motility has resumed.
- Nausea and vomiting must be accurately assessed and documented. Fluid losses from vomiting should be estimated and recorded on fluid balance charts.
- Abdominal pain. As mechanical bowel obstruction or the breakdown of bowel surgical sites is likely to be accompanied by abdominal pain, any pain in the abdomen that does not appear to be specifically related to a surgical wound should be investigated further.

Response to gastrointestinal compromise

If the gastrointestinal system is adversely affected in any of the ways listed earlier under initial indicators of gastrointestinal problems, consider the following:

- A nasogastric tube may be useful to empty fluids and gases from the stomach.
- Routine anti-emetic prophylaxis should be provided for all patients at medium to high risk of post-operative nausea and vomiting.
- Early post-operative feeding is thought to expedite the recovery of peristaltic motion in the gastrointestinal tract. Oral nutrition should therefore be commenced as soon as possible post-operatively.[a]
- The administration of high levels of oxygen to patients whose systolic blood pressure falls below 80 mmHg during spinal anaesthesia has been shown to significantly decrease the development of emesis.
- Prokinetic drugs such as metoclopramide and erythromycin have been shown to reduce gastroparesis.
- Intravenous fluids and electrolyte replacement may be needed to compensate for gastrointestinal fluid losses.
- Opioids should not be withheld from the nauseated patient, as pain itself may be the cause of the nausea.

Prevention

Even if the post-operative patient shows no initial signs of gastrointestinal compromise, it is still important to act to prevent this by considering the following actions:

- Remove oropharyngeal airways at the first indication of gagging.
- Communicate regularly with the patient to ensure that early signs and symptoms of gastrointestinal compromise are recognized.

Reference

8 Scottish Intercollegiate Guidelines Network (SIGN). *Postoperative Management in Adults.* Guideline No. 77. SIGN: Edinburgh, 2004.

Further reading

Manley K and Bellman L. *Surgical Nursing: advancing practice.* Churchill Livingstone: Edinburgh, 2000.

Neurological problems and confusional states

Compromise of the neurological system can occur during the immediate post-operative period for the following reasons:

- *Hypoxia.* Whether it is a result of hypovolaemia, sepsis, the hypoventilating effects of anaesthesia, or other causes of reduced cardiac output, hypoxia can quickly have an impact on neurological function.
- *Hypercapnia.* High CO_2 levels can lead to significant narcosis. This can potentiate the depressive effects of anaesthetics. Acidosis also leads to depression of central nervous system function.
- *Anaesthetic and analgesic drugs.* High concentrations of inhaled anaesthetic agents can cause hypoventilation, which prolongs their elimination. Opiates that are used as adjuncts to anaesthesia or in post-operative pain management can also cause hypoventilation and have an impact on conscious level through their sedative effects.
- *Pre-medication.* The use of some drugs (e.g. narcotics, benzodiazepines) can delay arousal following anaesthesia.
- *Nerve damage.* Unavoidable damage to nerves may occur during some episodes of surgery (e.g. impotence following prostate surgery).
- *Neurological injury.* This may result from an unsuspected peri-operative cerebrovascular accident (stroke). Intracranial haemorrhage can occur as a result of hypertensive responses to anaesthetic or surgical intervention, especially in patients who are receiving anticoagulants. Uncontrolled intra-operative hypotension may result in ischaemia, particularly in patients with hypertension or carotid vessel disease. Emboli can also be a cause of neurological injury.
- *Seizures.* Sudden abnormal electrical activity in the brain can result from hypoxia, hypoglycaemia, disordered electrolyte balance, or direct irritation of brain tissue as a result of surgical intervention.
- *Disordered electrolyte balance.* Excessive water absorption can occur in some types of surgery (e.g. during transurethral prostate surgery). The resulting dilutional hyponatraemia can manifest as sedation, coma, or hemiparesis. Hypocalcaemia can result in delayed wakening, and high magnesium levels can cause prolonged sedation.
- *Blood glucose mismanagement.* Post-operative hypoglycaemia or hyperglycaemia can impair conscious level because the cerebral cells have an inadequate glucose supply.

Confusional states

Confusional states can arise during the immediate post-operative period. It is not uncommon for patients to emerge from anaesthesia in a delirious state, with restlessness, disorientation, crying, moaning, or irrational talking. In extreme cases, patients may scream, shout, and flail unpredictably, posing a safety risk to themselves and others. It is important to be aware that patients with significant pre-operative anxiety, a history of alcoholism, insomnia and/or depression are at increased risk of post-operative confusion and/or delirium.

Recognition of neurological/confusional state compromise

The neurological system should be constantly monitored for signs of compromise during the immediate post-operative period. This should involve regular assessment of the following:

- *The patient's psychosocial well-being.* Anxiety and confusion can have physiological consequences, such as tachycardia, hypertension, hyperventilation, increased muscle tone, restlessness, agitation, and dilated pupils. Accurate assessment of psychosocial well-being is important to enable differentiation between physical and psychological causes of changes in vital signs.
- *Level of consciousness.* A tool such as the Glasgow Coma Scale (GCS) should be used regularly during the post-operative period to assess changes in conscious level. If neurological injury is suspected, regular recording of wider neurological observations should be undertaken.
- *Respiratory function.* The effectiveness of respiration should be regularly and holistically assessed in order to detect potential hypoxia and/or hypercarbia as causes of neurological deterioration.
- *Serum electrolyte and glucose levels* should be analysed regularly.
- If direct neurological injury is suspected, CT scanning or an MRI scan may be required for an accurate assessment of the cause.

Response to neurological compromise

If the neurological system is adversely affected in any of the ways listed earlier under initial indicators of neurological problems, consider the following:

- Residual opioids can be reversed by naloxone, anticholinergic CNS depression can be reversed by physostigmine, and benzodiazepines can be reversed by flumazenil.
- It is important to maintain effective ventilation.
- Effective management of serum electrolyte and glucose levels is required.
- Hypoxia, pain, discomfort caused by bladder or gastric distension, and the effects of medications (e.g. anticholinergic agents, ketamine, neuroleptics) are all common causes of a new onset of post-operative confusion. Their prompt identification and treatment can have a positive impact on reducing confusion.
- Small intravenous doses of short-acting benzodiazepines may be warranted if patient safety (or that of others) is at risk during an episode of acute confusion.

Prevention

Even if the post-operative patient shows no initial signs of neurological compromise, it is still important to act to prevent this. Consider the importance to cerebral perfusion and the metabolism of anaesthetic and analgesic agents of an adequate mean arterial pressure (MAP).

Further reading

Manley K and Bellman L. *Surgical Nursing: advancing practice*. Churchill Livingstone: Edinburgh, 2000.
Pudner R (ed.). *Nursing the Surgical Patient*, 3rd edn. Baillière Tindall: Edinburgh, 2001.

Thermoregulatory problems

Compromise of the thermoregulatory system can occur during the immediate post-operative period for the following reasons:

- *Effects of anaesthesia.* Some anaesthetic agents inhibit the body's heat-generating mechanisms and enhance its heat loss mechanisms.
- Hyperthermia can be caused by accidental overwarming of the patient during surgery. Infection, sepsis, and transfusion reactions are also potential causes.
- *Malignant hyperthermia.* In some individuals, certain general inhalational anaesthetics, muscle relaxants, local anaesthetics, and episodes of stress can induce a sudden increase in skeletal muscle metabolism that overwhelms the body's ability to supply oxygen, eliminate carbon dioxide, and regulate body temperature, resulting in a rapidly developing hyperthermia.
- *Pre-operative medications.* Anticholinergic drugs can increase body temperature due to the metabolic effects of interrupting parasympathetic innervation.
- *Patient age.* Baseline core temperature often decreases with advancing age. Thermoregulatory control mechanisms may also be less effective at extremes of age.
- *Site and temperature of intravenous fluids.* Hypothermia can result when significant quantities of IV fluids and/or blood are given that have not been pre-warmed to body temperature. This also applies to fluids used for irrigation purposes.[9]
- *Body surface exposure.* Increased body surface exposure peri-operatively can lead to hypothermia. This risk is increased if the environmental temperature is suboptimal.
- *Vessel tone.* This changes as a result of medications, epidural analgesia, or physiological stress, which can thus all cause core and peripheral temperature changes.

Effects of hypothermia and hyperthermia

Both hypothermia (core temperature below 36°C) and hyperthermia (core temperature above 38°C) can have a negative impact on post-operative recovery. Hypothermia with shivering causes discomfort and a significant increase in metabolic rate, which results in increased demands on the respiratory and cardiovascular system. In the later stages, hypothermia can suppress myocardial function and lead to arrhythmias, reduced drug metabolism, and impaired renal function.

Recognition of thermoregulatory compromise

The patient should be constantly monitored for signs of thermoregulatory compromise during the immediate post-operative period. This should involve close observation for the following physiological responses to altered body temperature:

- Sweating, peripheral vasodilation, and a lowering of the basal metabolic rate indicate that the body is hyperthermic and attempting to lose heat and reduce heat production.

- Shivering, an increased muscle tone, vasoconstriction, and an increase in basal metabolic rate indicate that the body is hypothermic and attempting to gain and conserve heat.
- In addition there should be:
  - frequent monitoring of the core temperature by axilla, tympanic, or invasive methods. The core temperature should initially be recorded every 15 min post surgery[9]
  - frequent monitoring of peripheral temperature. This may be assessed by hand, but on occasion a temperature probe attached to the foot can provide a useful assessment of the progression of vessel tone alterations in conditions such as sepsis or hypovolaemia
  - observation for muscle rigidity, as this often occurs before the steady rise in temperature of malignant hyperthermia.

Response to thermoregulatory compromise

If the thermoregulatory system is adversely affected in any of the ways listed earlier under initial indicators of thermoregulatory problems, consider the following:

- Hypothermia that is mild may be effectively treated by covering the patient adequately, the application of blankets, and the maintenance of a warm environment. If the core temperature falls below 36°C, more severe hypothermia requires active rewarming. A forced air blanket should be applied and the temperature monitored every 30 min.[9] Strategies such as the application of convective warming devices, intravenous fluid or blood warming, and environmental warming may also be used for patients with persistent or severe hypothermia.
- Supplemental oxygen must be administered to shivering patients to meet the increased metabolic demand.
- Hyperthermia may respond to cooling via evaporative or direct external methods such as ice packs, cooling blankets, and a cool environment. Antipyretics can be useful, as they prevent prostaglandin synthesis in the hypothalamus. However, caution must be exercised in the management of hyperthermia that is infection related, as the immune response is more effective in mild hyperthermia.
- It is also important to reduce thermogenesis in the hyperthermic patient.

Prevention

Even if the post-operative patient shows no initial signs of thermoregulatory or infection compromise, it is still important to act to prevent this. It is important to consider the following actions:

- Ensure that the patient's temperature is recorded by accurate methods. Clinical staff should be aware of any adjustments that need to be made in order to obtain an accurate core temperature estimate from a particular recording site.[10]

References

9 National Institute for Health and Care Excellence (NICE). *Inadvertent Perioperative Hypothermia: the management of inadvertent perioperative hypothermia in adults*. CG65 NICE: London, 2008. www.nice.org.uk/guidance/cg65

10 National Institute for Health and Care Excellence (NICE). *Surgical Site Infection: prevention and treatment of surgical site infection*. CG74. NICE: London, 2008. www.nice.org.uk/guidance/cg74

Haematological problems

Compromise of the haematological system during the immediate post-operative period can occur for the following reasons:

- *Haemorrhage*. This can occur during or after surgery, and most commonly results from inadequate haemostasis for injured blood vessels.
- *Coagulopathy*. This can occur in patients with existing coagulation disorders (e.g. haemophilia) or in those receiving anticoagulant therapy (e.g. heparin or warfarin). Multiple transfusions can lead to consumption coagulopathy, which can then exacerbate and make it more difficult to manage an existing site of haemorrhage.
- *Disseminated intravascular coagulopathy (DIC)*. This systemic condition, in which a generalized coagulation in small blood vessels occurs at the same time as bleeding, can be a life-threatening complication of severe trauma, sepsis, blood transfusion, and hypoxia.
- *Thromboembolus*. Patients undergoing surgery are at increased risk of clot formation because of the nature of surgery and the impact of surgery on the body's clotting mechanisms. It is often predicted that 20–30% of patients will routinely develop a deep vein thrombosis or pulmonary embolus if they do not receive appropriate thromboprophylaxis.
- *Deep vein thrombosis (DVT)*. This remains a major cause of post-surgery complications and mortality. The deep veins of the leg are the most common sites of DVT.
- *Pulmonary embolus*. When an embolus forms and enters the pulmonary circulation, sudden dyspnoea with cardiovascular collapse, pleuritic chest pain, pleural rub, and haemoptysis may occur. Around 80–90% of pulmonary emboli are thought to result from DVTs.

Recognition of haematological compromise

The patient should be constantly monitored in the immediate post-operative period for signs of haematological compromise. This should be done by close observation for the following signs:

- *Signs of bleeding*. Internal bleeding may by recognized by hypovolaemia from vital sign changes and peripheral cooling. External bleeding may be identified from surgical wound, invasive line, and drain sites. Observations for bleeding should be particularly vigilant in patients who are receiving anticoagulant therapy.
- *Full blood count and clotting screen tests*. It is particularly important to analyse the results of these tests regularly if the patient has received a blood transfusion, as stored blood is deficient in many of the factors that are necessary for normal coagulation. Monitoring of the white cell count (WCC) will help to identify leucocytosis and infection. A reduced haemoglobin or haematocrit level may indicate a shift in extracellular fluid volume status due to the haemodilutional effects of IV fluid administration.
- *Signs of DVT*. Some cases present silently, but many are associated with swelling of the leg and/or increased tenderness and warmth of the calf muscle. Doppler ultrasound or venography may be used to identify DVT.

- *Signs of pulmonary embolus.* Patients with smaller pulmonary emboli may present with confusion, breathlessness, and chest pain. Those with larger pulmonary emboli may present as described in the section on respiratory compromise (see p. 314). Ventilation/perfusion scanning, dynamic CT scanning, or pulmonary angiography should be used to identify pulmonary emboli.
- *Signs of an adverse blood transfusion reaction.* Sudden discomfort, flushing, rash, fever, and nausea may all be early indications of this.

Response to haematological compromise

If the haematological system is adversely affected in any of the ways listed earlier under initial indicators of haematological problems, consider the following:

- Post-operative haemorrhage may require a return to theatre for wound exploration and ligation of bleeding vessels. External sources of bleeding may respond to the application of pressure.
- Administration of blood or blood products. Whole blood or packed red blood cell transfusion may be indicated to increase oxygen-carrying capacity in patients with anaemia. Fresh frozen plasma may be indicated to increase clotting factor levels in patients with deficiencies of these factors. Platelets may be used to treat bleeding associated with deficiencies in platelet number or function.
- The use of appropriate blood-administering devices with microfilters effectively prevents the microaggregate load that develops in stored blood transfusing into the patient. Equally vigilant patient and blood group checking is essential in order to avoid adverse transfusion reactions.
- Regular monitoring of electrolyte levels is required after blood transfusion, especially in patients with cardiac and renal dysfunction, who may not respond well to the increase in sodium and potassium levels that transfused blood can incur.
- Anticoagulation agents may be used to prevent the formation of venous thrombus associated with prolonged bed rest and haemostasis.
- If DVT or pulmonary embolus is diagnosed, anticoagulation therapy remains important, and commonly involves the administration of intravenous heparin or subcutaneous low-molecular-weight heparin for 5 days. Oral warfarin may be required in addition to this. Thrombolytic agents should only be considered in patients with life-threatening pulmonary embolus.
- If heparin is thought to have resulted in a coagulopathy, the use of protamine can be considered.

Prevention

Even if the post-operative patient shows no initial signs of compromise of the haematological system, it is still important to act to prevent this. Thromboembolus prophylaxis using mechanical and pharmacological approaches is essential.

Further reading

British Committee for Standards in Haematology (BCSH). *Guideline on the Assessment of Bleeding Risk Prior to Surgery or Invasive Procedures.* BCSH: London, 2008.

Sepsis

Infections in the surgical patient are common and treatable. However, in some cases infection can trigger a systemic response distant to the site of infection. This is known as systemic inflammatory response syndrome (SIRS). Pathogens that cause such infections release exogenous toxins and increase production of endogenous pyrogens, including cytokinin, giving rise to immune activation and changes in the circulation. Sepsis is defined as the presence of SIRS that has developed as a result of an infection. It causes a range of physiological changes in the patient that must be actively monitored by the nurse. If the sepsis worsens and affects organ function, this is defined as severe sepsis. Without treatment, severe sepsis will lead to septic shock, which is characterized by profound cardio-vascular instability and multi-organ dysfunction.

Sepsis most commonly occurs in surgical patients who have:
- traumatic or surgical wound infections
- tissue infections (e.g. peri-anal, pilonidal, breast abscess)
- acute organ dysfunction or infections (e.g. acute pancreatitis, mesenteric infarction, cholecystitis)
- post-operative surgical complications (e.g. adhesions, anastomotic leakage, pelvic abscess)
- non-surgical comorbidity (e.g. lower respiratory tract infection, urinary tract infection, cellulitis, endocarditis).

Screening tools have been developed to assist healthcare practitioners in identifying patients at risk of sepsis (see Figure 15.2).

Early indications of sepsis in the surgical patient include the following clinical signs and investigations:
- body temperature > 38.3°C or < 36.0°C
- heart rate > 90 beats/min
- respiratory rate > 20 breaths/min
- hypotension (systolic pressure < 90 mmHg, mean arterial pressure < 65 mmHg or a fall of 40 mmHg relative to the patient's normal systolic blood pressure)
- oliguria (< 0.5 mL/kg/h; for example, 40 mL urine/h for an 80 kg adult)
- white cell count < 4.0 or > 12 x 10^9/L
- altered mental status
- hyperglycaemia (7.7 mmol/L), unless the patient is diabetic.

The speed and appropriateness of therapy in the early hours after sepsis diagnosis significantly influence the likelihood of survival. If the criteria for sepsis have been met, ideally the following treatments, known as the Sepsis Six (see Box 15.1), should be initiated within 1 h.

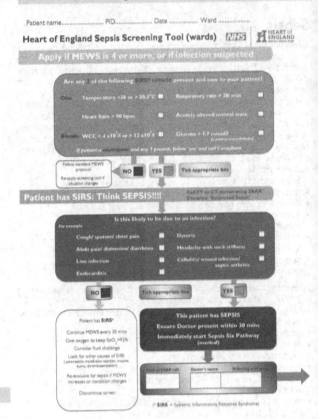

Patient name.................... PID.............. Date .... Ward ....

Heart of England Sepsis Screening Tool (wards) NHS / HEART of ENGLAND

Apply if MEWS is 4 or more, or if infection suspected

Are any 2 of the following SIRS criteria present and new to your patient?

Obs: Temperature <36 or > 38.3°C ☐   Respiratory rate > 20/min ☐

Heart Rate > 90 bpm ☐   Acutely altered mental state ☐

Bloods: WCC < 4 x10⁹/l or > 12 x10⁹/l ☐   Glucose > 7.7 mmol/l ☐ (if patient not diabetic)

If patient is neutropenic and any 1 present, follow 'yes' and call Consultant

NO ☐ | YES ☐ | Tick appropriate box

Follow standard MEWS protocol / Re-apply screening tool if situation changes

Patient has SIRS: Think SEPSIS!!!! Call FY or CT doctor using SBAR Situation 'Suspected Sepsis'

Is this likely to be due to an infection?

For example:
Cough/ sputum/ chest pain ☐   Dysuria ☐
Abdo pain/ distension/ diarrhoea ☐   Headache with neck stiffness ☐
Line infection ☐   Cellulitis/ wound infection/ septic arthritis ☐
Endocarditis ☐

NO ☐ | Tick appropriate box | YES ☐

Patient has SIRS*
Continue MEWS every 30 mins
Give oxygen to keep SpO₂ >92%
Consider fluid challenge
Look for other causes of SIRS (pancreatitis, transfusion reaction, trauma, burns, thromboembolism)
Re-evaluate for sepsis if MEWS increases or condition changes
Discontinue screen

This patient has SEPSIS
Ensure Doctor present within 30 mins
Immediately start Sepsis Six Pathway (overleaf)

Time of SBAR call | Doctor's name | Referring staff member

(* SIRS = Systemic Inflammatory Response Syndrome)

Figure 15.2 Heart of England Sepsis Screening Tool (wards). Reproduced with permission from Ron Daniels (2010), UK Sepsis Trust.

Box 15.1 The Sepsis Six
- Give high-flow oxygen (15 L/min via a non-rebreathe bag).
- Take blood cultures.
- Give antibiotics (broad spectrum unless contraindicated).
- Initiate fluid resuscitation (fluid challenge of 250–500 mL of crystalloid).
- Measure serum lactate concentration.
- Monitor urine output hourly (consider catheterization).

Surgical nursing procedures

Phlebotomy

Phlebotomy is the process of making an incision into a vein. The main purpose of this is to draw blood for laboratory testing.

Site selection

In order to draw blood safely, effectively, and with minimum discomfort, the three veins that can be found in the antecubital fossa are most commonly used for phlebotomy (see Figure 16.1). If these are not accessible, the metacarpal veins may be used.

Complications and their prevention

Haematoma

- This occurs due to either the needle puncturing the posterior wall of the vein, or inadequate pressure being applied after withdrawal of the needle.
- It can be avoided by selecting appropriate phlebotomy equipment and removing the tourniquet before removing the needle. Elevation of the limb and the effective application of pressure to the site until the bleeding has stopped is also effective.

Arterial puncture

- If this occurs, the blood drawn will be bright red and fill receiving containers quickly. If this happens the needle should be removed quickly and firm pressure applied for more than 5 min.
- Arterial puncture can be avoided by thorough visual inspection and physical palpation of the site prior to venepuncture.

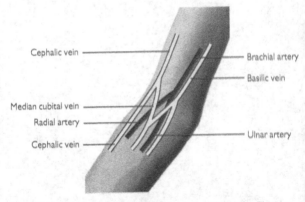

Cephalic vein — Brachial artery

— Basilic vein

Median cubital vein —
Radial artery —
Cephalic vein —

— Ulnar artery

Figure 16.1 Veins in the antecubital fossa. Reproduced from James Thomas and Tanya Monaghan, *Oxford Handbook of Clinical Examination and Practical Skills*, 2007, with permission from Oxford University Press.

Infection
- Infection of the site can occur if the standard of hand washing and site cleansing is poor.
- Cross-infection can be avoided if universal precautions are followed. Needle insertion sites should be cleaned with a 70% alcohol preparation and allowed to dry prior to puncture.

Fear of needles and vasovagal reaction
- Patients who have a fear of needles can feel unwell or faint.
- Phlebotomy should be performed in a calm and reassuring manner.
- If the patient feels unwell or faints, they should be encouraged to put their head down between their knees, or else supported to lie down with their legs raised.

Pain
- If the patient experiences sharp pain that moves along the arm and fingers, a nerve or artery may have been touched. The needle should immediately be removed. Some patients who are sensitive to phlebotomy may benefit from the application of local anaesthetic cream.

Mechanical phlebitis
- Inflammation of the vein can occur when needles are repositioned under the skin or when multiple venepuncture attempts are made in one area.
- Incisions should not be made into injured or thrombosed veins. If an unsuccessful draw occurs, one further attempt may be made above that site. After that alternative sites should be sought.

Haemoconcentration
- Incorrect phlebotomy technique can lead to an increase in viscosity of the blood sample, which can affect the laboratory results.
- To avoid this, tourniquets should not be used for more than 1 min, and excessive manipulation of the site prior to venepuncture should be avoided.

Blood collection tubes

Clinical blood collection tubes are most often glass and/or plastic and contain some degree of vacuum which assists the filling of the tube with drawn blood. A rubber top allows penetration of the needle from the venepuncture device. Different tubes are used for different types of laboratory testing, and may contain different types of additives. Common additives include an anticoagulant or clot activator.

Order of draw

In order to avoid cross-contamination of these additives, if multiple blood samples are to be taken then consideration has to be given to the order in which blood is drawn into the tubes.

Improving venous access

The following interventions may help to facilitate successful phlebotomy:

- use of a tourniquet
- positioning of the arm below heart level
- light tapping of the vein prior to venepuncture
- the patient clenching (but not pumping) their fist to facilitate venous distension
- exposing the arm to mild heat (e.g. in a bowl of warm water) for 10 min
- local application of small amounts of glyceryl trinitrate.

Further reading

Dougherty L and Lister S (eds), *The Royal Marsden Hospital Manual of Clinical Nursing Procedures*, 8th edn, Wiley-Blackwell: Oxford, 2011.

Endacott R, Jevon P and Cooper S (eds). *Clinical Nursing Skills: core and advanced*, Oxford University Press: Oxford, 2009.

Blood cultures

A blood culture is a laboratory test that aims to identify the presence of bacteria or other microorganisms in a sample of blood.

Purpose of the investigation

The identification of microorganisms in the blood that are either present in abnormal amounts or have migrated there from other body sites can be an effective guide to the treatment of infection. Antibiotic susceptibility testing can be performed on some microorganisms, and this can enable clinicians to prescribe the antibiotics that are likely to be most effective. Prompt and accurate blood culture analysis can significantly reduce morbidity and mortality from sepsis.[1]

Indications

Blood cultures should not be taken routinely, but only when there is a clinical need to do so. Potential indications include:

- core temperature outside the normal range
- focal signs of infection
- raised heart rate, raised respiratory rate, raised blood pressure, or low blood pressure
- chills or rigors
- raised or very low white blood cell count
- new or worsening confusion.[2]

Blood sampling for culture

It is possible for a blood culture to give negative results for the presence of microorganisms when the patient's symptoms persist and microorganisms are indeed present in the bloodstream. In order to minimize the risk of this and increase the accuracy of the result, the following procedural factors should be considered.

Correct volume

It is vital that the manufacturer's instructions are followed and the collecting vial is filled with the correct amount of blood. The correct ratio of blood volume to vial additives is also necessary in order to optimize the conditions for growth of microorganisms.

Timing of the sample

Bacteraemias can be intermittent. Therefore the accuracy of the test can be increased by taking the blood sample when signs of infection are present. It is also important to take the sample before administering antibiotics, otherwise the growth of bacteria in the sample can be inhibited.

Asepsis during the drawing of blood samples

To avoid contamination of the culture by microorganisms that are present on the skin (or elsewhere), a strict aseptic technique should be used when drawing and transferring the blood sample. Vacuumed blood-drawing systems that avoid the need to transfer samples into a vial via a needle can reduce the risk of sample contamination.

Laboratory results

In the laboratory, blood cultures are incubated in a supportive environment for several days to promote the growth and multiplication of any microorganisms present. Therefore the results are not available immediately. Repeat blood cultures may be requested if a false-positive result from a contamination source is suspected. If two consecutive blood culture samples give negative results, it is unlikely that bacteria or fungi are present in the bloodstream. Different collection vials and tests are required to establish the presence of viruses. Blood culture results should be interpreted alongside other blood tests that may indicate whether infection is present, such as white cell count (WCC), complement protein C3, and C-reactive protein (CRP).

References

1 Dellinger RP et al. Surviving sepsis campaign: international guidelines for management of severe sepsis and septic shock: 2012. *Critical Care Medicine* 2013; **41**: 580–637.
2 Department of Health. *Taking Blood Cultures: a summary of best practice*. Department of Health: London, 2007.

Cannulation

The process of cannulation refers to the insertion of a cannula or tube for the purpose of administering medication or draining blood or other fluids. Cannulae are most commonly inserted into vessels.

Peripheral cannulae

A peripheral cannula is a short catheter that is inserted through the skin into a peripheral vessel. Peripheral venous cannulae are usually inserted for the purpose of intravenous drug administration. Peripheral arteries can be cannulated for accurate blood pressure monitoring and regular arterial blood gas analysis.

Central cannulae

A central cannula is a long catheter that is inserted through the skin into a central vessel. Central venous cannulae are inserted for the purpose of monitoring central venous pressure (CVP) and/or administering intravenous drugs or fluids that might cause local damage to peripheral veins. Central arteries are rarely cannulated, due to the high risk of exsanguination. However, they may be cannulated during specialized cardiothoracic procedures.

Site selection

Peripheral cannulae are typically inserted into the lower arm or, only if access is difficult, the lower limbs. When selecting a site, comfort, ease of access, and visibility must be optimized. This is important because a peripheral cannula may remain *in situ* for up to 72 h (or longer if there are no signs of infection and vascular access is limited).[3]

Central cannulae are usually inserted via the internal jugular, subclavian, or femoral veins using the Seldinger technique. Considerations with regard to site selection are similar to those for peripheral cannulae. Many patients find subclavian or femoral cannulae more comfortable to tolerate, but this has to be weighed against the fact that these routes are associated with slightly higher risks of pneumothorax and infection, respectively.

Peripherally inserted central catheters (PICCs)

Central cannulae that are to be used for the medium- to long-term administration of medication or nutrition may be inserted via a peripheral vein. These are known as peripherally inserted central catheters (PICCs).

Types of cannula

It is possible to select from a wide range of different types of cannula, depending on the purpose for which it is needed. Peripheral cannulae are available in different gauge (G) sizes (e.g. 14G, 16G), which enable different rates of fluid flow. They can be winged, non-winged, or ported. Central cannulae are available in different lengths, with different coatings (e.g. antimicrobial or heparin) and/or single, dual, or multiple lumens. Cannulae are made from a range of different materials (e.g. Teflon, Vialon, silicone, polyurethane).

Principles of care

The following universal principles apply to the care of cannulae, irrespective of the location or type of cannula.

Prevention of infection

When inserting or using a cannula, strict aseptic and universal precaution procedures should be adhered to throughout, due to the high risk of blood-borne infection. Needle-free devices should be used if they are available. A new cannula should be used for each cannulation attempt and flushed in line with local policy.[3,4] A solution of 2% chlorhexidine gluconate in 70% isopropyl alcohol is recommended as the most effective means of decontaminating ports and the surrounding area of vascular access devices. However, this solution needs to be allowed to dry for at least 30 s. The period of time for which ports are open should be minimized. A sterile semipermeable transparent dressing should be used to allow observation of the site, and documented review of the cannula site, by determining the Visual Infusion Phlebitis (VIP) score, should take place at least daily.[3,4]

Maintenance of the device

To ensure that the cannula remains fit for purpose, it must remain patent. Flushes of 0.9% sodium chloride should be utilized to establish cannula patency before and immediately after the administration of drugs or fluids. On occasion, in order to further prevent clot or precipitate formation, a continuous flush infusion of 0.9% sodium chloride via a volumetric pump may be indicated, or the use of an anticoagulant-coated device. Excessive force should never be used when flushing a cannula. Care should also be taken to ensure that the device is not kinked or clamped, as this could cause damage to and fragmentation of the device.

Complications

Many of the complications of cannulation are similar to those associated with the procedure of phlebotomy (see ➲ p. 336). However, cannulation poses a greater risk of blood-borne infection. For this reason, in addition to following the principles of care described in the previous section, cannulae should be removed as soon as they are no longer required.

References

3 Department of Health. *High Impact Intervention: peripheral intravenous cannula care bundle*. Department of Health: London, 2010.
4 Department of Health. *High Impact Intervention: central venous catheter care bundle*. Department of Health: London, 2010.

Further reading

Dougherty L and Lister S (eds). *The Royal Marsden Hospital Manual of Clinical Nursing Procedures*, 8th edn. Wiley-Blackwell: Oxford, 2011.
Endacott R, Jevon P and Cooper S (eds). *Clinical Nursing Skills: core and advanced*. Oxford University Press: Oxford, 2009.

Arterial blood gas analysis

Arterial blood gas analysis is a blood test that is performed on arterial blood to determine the partial pressures of O_2 and CO_2 and the concentration of hydrogen ions and bicarbonate ions (among other values) in arterial blood.

Purpose of the investigation

Interpretation of these values can be used to evaluate respiratory and acid–base conditions in the body.

Indications

An arterial blood gas test is often performed for one or more of the following reasons:

* when there is an acute deterioration in the condition of the patient
* when there are signs of respiratory dysfunction (e.g. altered respiratory rate or pattern, decline in pulse oximetry values)
* when there are signs of metabolic dysfunction (e.g. diabetic ketoacidosis (DKA), hyperosmolar hyperglycaemic state (HHS), poisoning)
* to assist titration of mechanical ventilation
* to evaluate the effects of treatment intervention (e.g. IV fluids, oxygen, inotropic therapy)
* when there is an altered conscious level (see p. 153).

Blood sampling

In order to obtain an arterial blood gas sample, percutaneous puncture of the radial, brachial, or femoral artery is required, or alternatively a sample can be drawn from an arterial line. Prior to puncture of the radial artery, a peripheral circulation check known as the Allen's test should take place. Arterial puncture can be very painful, so a local anaesthetic may be used. The blood sample should be drawn into a specialized syringe that contains an anticoagulant.

After the sample has been collected by arterial puncture, a gauze pad should be placed firmly over the puncture site for at least 5 min to ensure that bleeding does not occur. It may need to remain in place for longer if the patient is receiving anticoagulant therapy or has a haematological disorder. Monitoring should then be commenced for bleeding or symptoms of circulatory impairment distal to the puncture site, such as altered sensation (e.g. numbness), swelling, or discoloration.

Processing the sample

The sample should be analysed as soon as possible after it has been drawn. Therefore it is important to identify the location of the nearest available working arterial blood gas analysis machine before drawing blood samples. Information will need to be entered into the machine about parameters such as the amount of oxygen the patient is currently receiving and their core body temperature. These values should also be recorded in the patient's notes next to the results, together with the time when the measurements were taken.

Sample analysis

An understanding of the following values will help nurses to evaluate patients' pre- and post-operative respiratory and metabolic function.

pH (normal range, 7.35–7.45)

The pH of the blood sample indicates the number of hydrogen (H^+) ions present and therefore the acidity (or alkalinity) of the blood. Acidic and alkalotic blood conditions have a wide range of detrimental effects on cellular and body organ function.

Partial pressure of CO_2 ($PaCO_2$) (normal range, 4.5–6 kPa)

$PaCO_2$ indicates how effectively the removal of the waste product CO_2 is being achieved by the respiratory system. When in solution, CO_2 forms carbonic acid, so a high $PaCO_2$ level can cause respiratory acidosis.

Partial pressure of O_2 (PaO_2) (normal range, 10–13 kPa)

The amount of oxygen that is bound to haemoglobin is strongly dependent on the PaO_2 of oxygen in the blood. A low PaO_2 can indicate respiratory dysfunction, and could lead to acidosis as a result of lactic acid production from anaerobic cellular respiration. A high PaO_2 indicates that it is now possible to begin to decrease the amount of supplementary oxygen that is being delivered.

Standard bicarbonate concentration (SBC) (normal range, 22–26 mmol/L)

Bicarbonates are alkaline substances that can buffer (or neutralize) acidity by combining with H^+ ions as part of the carbonic acid–bicarbonate compensatory system. Low bicarbonate levels may indicate that many bicarbonate ions have been used up and therefore metabolic acidosis is present. High levels are less common, but may be iatrogenically induced or indicate abnormal renal function.

Base excess (BE) (normal range, –2.5 to +2.5 mmol/L)

Base excess is a measure of the amount of acid or base that is needed to return the blood pH to normal.

Additional values

Arterial blood gas analysis will typically also provide values for oxygen saturation, and for haemoglobin, lactate, glucose, potassium, sodium, calcium, and magnesium levels.

Further reading

Hastings M. *Clinical Skills Made Incredibly Easy!* Lippincott Williams & Wilkins: London, 2009.
Hatchett R. Interpreting arterial blood gas results. *British Journal of Cardiac Nursing* 2007; 2: 520–23.

Nasogastric tubes

A nasogastric tube is a plastic tube that is inserted through the nose and down the oesophagus into the stomach.

Indications

Nasogastric tubes may be inserted for one or more of the following reasons:

- to administer nutrition (short-term enteral feeding)
- to administer medications
- to prevent vomiting after major surgery by decompressing the stomach
- for the aspiration of gastric secretions
- for the analysis of gastric secretions
- for the assessment and treatment of upper gastrointestinal bleeding.

Nasogastric tubes may not be appropriate for patients with any of the following conditions:

- gastro-oesophageal reflux[5]
- new basal skull fracture
- poor gastric emptying, intestinal obstruction, or ileus[5]
- a high risk of aspiration.

Types of nasogastric tube

A wide range of different types of nasogastric tube are available. They vary in material, length, size (Fr) of internal lumen, cost, and number of ports. Two common types of nasogastric tube are described here.

Ryles tube

Ryles tubes have a wide bore and are used for the aspiration of gastric secretions and for decompression purposes. They should be used for the minimum duration possible, as they are uncomfortable and are associated with a higher risk of rhinitis, pharyngitis, and oesophageal erosion than are fine-bore tubes.

Fine-bore tube

Fine-bore tubes are predominantly used for the administration of enteral feeds. PVC fine-bore tubes can be used for up to 10 days, but they can then become brittle. A polyurethane tube may be more appropriate for feeding that is required for several weeks.

Insertion of a nasogastric tube

Nasogastric tubes are inserted as a clean procedure, ideally with the patient in an upright position. The length of tube required should be estimated by holding the distal end of the tube at the patient's nose and extending it via the ear lobe down to the xiphoid process.[6] A note should be made of the measurement marking on the tube, so that the distance for which it will be necessary to advance the tube is established.

Successful insertion is aided by the following considerations:

- Add lubricant or activate existing lubricant (by placing it in warm water) at the insertion end of the tube.
- Gently and steadily insert the tube, taking into account the anatomical angle of the pharynx and oesophageal opening.
- If possible, ask the patient to swallow during insertion, by taking a small amount of water.
- Ask the patient to lean their head slightly forward, as this can help to direct the tube towards the oesophagus and away from the trachea.

Complications of nasogastric tube insertion

- Tube placement in the bronchi.
- Nasal trauma.
- Oesophageal or pharyngeal pouch perforation.
- Precipitation of a variceal bleed.
- Intracranial insertion.[5]

Confirmation of tube position

After insertion, and before any drugs or fluids are administered, it is vital to confirm that the nasogastric tube is in the correct position, because of the risk of pulmonary aspiration if the tube is placed in the bronchi.

The position of the tube should be confirmed by at least one of the following methods.

Testing of gastric aspirate

It is possible to obtain gastric aspirate from all types of nasogastric tubes. Smaller syringes may be more effective in smaller, shorter tubes. A sample of 1 mL is sufficient to check the pH of gastric aspirate.[7] A pH of 1–5.5 indicates that the tube is safely in the stomach. Due to the difficulty of differentiating pH values between 5 and 6 it is recommended that a second competent healthcare professional checks the readings that fall within this range.[8] If the pH of the aspirate is 6.0–8.0, bronchial placement should be suspected.

X-ray

All nasogastric tubes that are used in the clinical environment should be radiopaque. X-ray confirmation of correct placement of the tube should only be used if no aspirate can be obtained, or if pH indicator paper has failed to confirm the location of the nasogastric tube.[8]

References

5 National Institute for Health and Care Excellence (NICE). *Nutrition Support in Adults: oral nutrition support, enteral tube feeding and parenteral nutrition.* CG32. NICE: London, 2006. Ⓝ www.nice.org.uk/guidance/cg32

6 Best C. Nasogastric insertion in adults who require enteral feeding. *Nursing Standard* 2007 21: 39–43.

7 National Patient Safety Agency (NPSA). *Patient Safety Alert 05. Reducing harm caused by the misplacement of nasogastric feeding tubes.* NPSA: London, 2005.

8 National Patient Safety Agency (NPSA). *Patient Safety Alert NPSA/2011/PSA002. Reducing the harm caused by misplaced nasogastric feeding tubes in adults, children and infants.* NPSA: London, 2011.

Urinary catheterization

Urinary catheterization is the aseptic insertion of a tube into the bladder to enable the drainage of urine or the instillation of drugs or fluids.

Urethral catheterization

Urethral catheterization involves the insertion of a Foley catheter, which is a flexible tube with two separate inner tubes. One of the tubes is open at both ends to allow the drainage of urine. The other tube links a closed port to a balloon which, when inflated with sterile water, helps to keep the catheter *in situ*.

Suprapubic catheterization

Suprapubic catheterization involves making a surgical connection between the bladder and the skin and then inserting a tube to allow the drainage of urine. It is indicated for specialist urological trauma or conditions in which it is advantageous to bypass the urethra.

Indications

Urinary catheterization should only be undertaken when it is medically required, and the catheter should remain *in situ* for the shortest time possible. Urethral catheterization is the most common route. It may be indicated for one or more of the following reasons:

- for accurate measurement of urine output during an acute deterioration in the patient's condition
- in acute or chronic urine retention
- to bypass an obstruction (e.g. swelling following urological surgery, stricture, tumour)
- in intractable incontinence, when excoriated skin needs to heal
- for administration of drug(s) into the bladder (e.g. cytotoxic drugs)
- for bladder irrigation
- for bladder investigations (e.g. urodynamic studies).

Types of catheter

A wide range of urinary catheters are available. Consideration of the following factors will aid selection of the correct type of catheter.

Time duration and catheter material

If the catheter is likely to remain *in situ* for a short time (e.g. less than 7 days), a plastic-based catheter can be used. If it is likely to be in place for up to 28 days, a catheter made of uncoated latex, polytetrafluoroethylene (PTFE), or that is Teflon-coated may be appropriate. For long-term use (up to 12 weeks), 100% silicone catheters or silicone-coated latex catheters may be used.

Catheter length

Female and male urinary catheters are typically 20–26 cm and 40–45 cm in length, respectively. However, variations from this may occur. For example, an obese or female wheelchair user may benefit from a longer catheter (i.e. male catheter), which can help to avoid soreness from rubbing of the inflation valve or discomfort from the catheter pulling.

Catheter size

The optimal size should be chosen for the purpose of the catheterization (e.g., for irrigation and the removal of blood clots, larger sizes should be chosen, whereas to maximize comfort and facilitate adequate drainage, a catheter of size 14–16 Ch (Charrière) (also known as French gauge, or F) may be most appropriate).

Catheter type

Foley catheters usually contain two channels, but can have three channels, the additional one being for irrigation purposes. Some urinary catheters do not have a balloon, as they are designed for short, intermittent episodes of bladder emptying, or for inserting drugs or fluids into the bladder.

Catheter balloon infill volume

Infill volumes vary according to the purpose of the catheter. Standard drainage catheters require 10–30 mL volumes of sterile water. Some larger urology catheters may require 20–80 mL volumes of sterile water. For long-term catheters made of 100% silicone, 5% aqueous glycerin in 10 mL of sterile water helps to reduce catheter balloon diffusion.

Catheter insertion

Detailed procedural guidelines on urinary catheter insertion should be consulted before performing this procedure. The following key principles may increase the likelihood of successful urethral catheterization.

- *Adequate equipment assembly.* This procedure must be undertaken using strict aseptic technique. Therefore preparation of the patient, the equipment, and the environment before catheter insertion is vital.
- Good lighting is needed so that the urethra can be visualized.
- A local anaesthetic gel should be applied prior to catheter insertion. This ensures that there is minimal trauma to the urethra, and it minimizes patient discomfort during the procedure.
- After successful catheterization, the most appropriate drainage device should be connected immediately in order to avoid further disconnections in the tubing.
- The residual volume of urine, the date and time of catheterization, the brand and size of catheter, the amount and type of fluid in the balloon, the type of local anaesthetic used, and any difficulties encountered should all be documented.

Further reading

Dougherty L and Lister S (eds). *The Royal Marsden Hospital Manual of Clinical Nursing Procedures* 8th edn. Wiley-Blackwell: Oxford, 2011.
Endacott R, Jevon P and Cooper S (eds). *Clinical Nursing Skills: core and advanced.* Oxford University Press: Oxford, 2009.

Male and female catheterization

The previously described principles of urinary catheterization are applicable to male and female patients. However, there are some gender-specific differences that need to be considered.

Female catheterization

Examples of specific indications for female urinary catheterization include the following:
• during childbirth
• to avoid complications during the insertion of radioactive material into the cervix or uterus.

Insertion of the catheter in female patients
The female urethra in particular can be difficult to visualize. In addition to good lighting, placing the patient in the supine position with their knees bent, hips flexed, and feet resting apart may best facilitate the procedure. Local anaesthetic gel can help to locate the female urethra, as it causes the urethra to open slightly.

Male catheterization

Examples of specific indications for male urinary catheterization include the following:
• to bypass a prostrate obstruction
• to facilitate recovery after prostrate surgery.

Insertion of the catheter in male patients
Advanced training for male catheterization is required in the majority of clinical areas, due to the increased potential for trauma in the male patient. The male urethra bends, thus presenting an anatomical obstruction to the passing of the catheter. This can be exacerbated by an enlarged prostrate.

Potential complications of male and female catheterization

Infection
Urinary catheter-related infections are the most common hospital-acquired infection, and can lead to death from blood-borne infection. It is therefore of paramount importance that strict aseptic technique is adhered to when inserting and managing any tube changes in the urethral catheter. In addition, urine must be regularly observed for signs of infection, and samples sent for laboratory investigation when appropriate.

Urethral and bladder trauma
It is important that the catheter is never forced during insertion, and that urgent medical review is sought if bleeding occurs or blood becomes evident in the urine. The use of leg straps can be beneficial, to help to immobilize the catheter and reduce trauma to the bladder neck and urethra.

Bladder spasms

The presence of a catheter in the bladder can cause irritation and inter-mittent spasm. The patient should be informed that they may experience a sudden urge to pass urine, and some discomfort, and that they may pass some urine around the sides of the catheter when this occurs. In order to avoid this, there should be adequate fluid intake, the appro-priate type of catheter should be selected, and the patient should be encouraged to relax.

Crustation

Crustation can occur around the urethral meatus as a result of increased production of urethral secretions in response to the presence of the catheter. Regular catheter toilet is important to prevent this.

Further reading

Dougherty L and Lister S (eds). *The Royal Marsden Hospital Manual of Clinical Nursing Procedures* 8th edn. Wiley-Blackwell: Oxford, 2011.

Endacott R, Jevon P and Cooper S (eds). *Clinical Nursing Skills: core and advanced*. Oxford University Press: Oxford, 2009.

Robinson J. Female urethral catheterisation. *Nursing Standard* 2007; 22: 48–56.

Intravenous drug mixing

Intravenous (IV) drug preparation should only be undertaken by those who have been trained to do this and who are competent in IV drug administration. When preparing drugs that are going to be administered via this route, local IV drug policy should be adhered to. However, the following is a summary of the key steps.

- All equipment and drugs required should be assembled in a designated clean area with an injection tray and a sharps box present to reduce the risk of needlestick injury.
- Disposable gloves should be worn to reduce the risk of skin irritation and/or sensitization. Some medications can cause dermatitis after contact.
- All equipment should be checked to ensure that it is sterile and in date, including any diluents, syringes, or needles. Glass ampoules should be checked for cracks, and all fluids should be visually checked for cloudiness or precipitation.[9]
- All IV fluid containers that have been opened should be labelled with the date and time when they were opened, and discarded within 24 h.
- Hand-washing procedure should follow local guidelines.

Some hospitals in the UK use filling needles with integral filters or medication in prefilled syringes. However, where this is not the case, the following procedure should be used.

- Needles up to 21G (green) should be used to draw up medicines. This reduces the risk of drawing up any foreign bodies into the syringe.[10]
- Medication should be drawn up in the smallest possible size of syringe that will accommodate the given volume of fluid or medication.
- A non-touch technique should be employed when opening the needle and syringe packets and connecting the needle to the syringe.
- Draw up the fluid by inserting the tip of the needle into the ampoule, and pull back the plunger of the syringe.
- After the appropriate amount of fluid has been drawn, expel any bubbles by either a single flick of the syringe or gently pushing the syringe plunger. Recheck that the required volume is present.
- The needle should not be resheathed, but gently removed at its base and disposed of immediately into a sharps box.
- The prepared IV medication should be placed in a clean injection tray alongside any other flushes or fluids that are required. These should then be administered as soon as possible.

Before preparing medications for IV administration (as with any route of administration), the 5 R's should be checked alongside other guidance on correct administration of medication:[11]

- the right patient
- the right medicine
- the right dose
- the right route
- the right date and time.

References

9 National Patient Safety Agency (NPSA). *Patient Safety Alert 20: promoting safer use of injectable medicines.* NPSA: London, 2007.

10 Department of Health. *Saving Lives: reducing infection, delivering clean and safe care.* Department of Health: London, 2007.

11 Nursing and Midwifery Council (NMC). *Standards for Medicines Management.* NMC: London, 2010.

Intravenous drug administration

IV drug administration involves injecting a drug directly into a vein. This can be done via peripheral or central venous access devices (VADs). It should only be undertaken by nurses who have completed appropriate training.

Indications

IV drug administration is associated with significant risks, ranging from localized phlebitis to sepsis and severe anaphylaxis. Therefore this route should only be used in the following situations:

• if the medicinal effect of the drug is needed urgently
• if the drug is not licensed or able to be given by any other route
• if it is most appropriate to the part of the body that is being treated
• if the patient is sufficiently ill that absorption from other routes may be impaired.

Methods

Drugs may be administered intravenously by bolus, intermittent, or continuous infusion methods. Most drugs can be given by peripheral or central routes. However, different routes may require different dilutional concentrations and/or speeds of delivery. Therefore detailed attention must be given to the pharmacological information that is supplied with the medicine.

Bolus IV injections

Bolus IV injections achieve a high blood concentration of a drug with minimal fluid administered. They should be given at the correct speed (usually over 3–5 min), and should always be preceded and followed by a 0.9% saline flush to ensure that the drug is fully delivered to the circulatory system.

Intermittent infusion

Intermittent infusions, in which a drug is given over a period ranging from more than 5 min to several hours, with a break occurring before the next dose, are used for drugs that require slow delivery or large dilutional volumes. Delivery should normally be controlled by an infusion pump.

Continuous infusion

Continuous infusions ensure that a constant blood concentration of a drug is achieved. This is important when administering drugs such as inotropes and vasodilators, particularly as they may have a short half-life. IV fluids and parenteral nutrition are most commonly delivered in this way. Again an infusion pump is required for accuracy in delivery.

Infusion giving sets

When administering drugs or fluids as intermittent or continuous infusions, the correct giving set should be used. All IV administration sets should be labelled with the date and time when their use commenced. Crystalloid or colloid clear fluids and pre-prepared medications such as metronidazole and paracetamol should be given through a solution giving set that incorporates a 5–15 micron filter. These can be used for up to 72 h.[12] Blood and fresh frozen plasma should be administered through a blood transfusion set which has a 170–200 micron filter. These can be used for up to 12 h (or in accordance with the manufacturer's instructions).[13] A new infusion set should be used if another infusion is to continue after the transfusion.[13] Platelets can be given in a standard blood transfusion set or platelet giving set. Any IV giving set that has been disconnected from the patient should then be discarded.

Avoiding infection

The following practice pointers will help to reduce the risk of infection via IV drug administration:

- Hands should be washed, gloves used, and aseptic non-touch technique employed for all aspects of IV therapy.
- Every additional piece of equipment in an infusion system is a portal for entry of infection, so the number of connections should be minimized.
- The use of premixed solutions avoids the need to use additives in the clinical area.
- Before and after use, all administration ports should be cleaned with a solution of 2% chlorhexidine gluconate in 70% isopropyl alcohol, and allowed to dry.[14]
- VAD sites should be regularly inspected for signs of infection. Dressings should be changed when loose, wet, or soiled, and local policy followed.[12]
- Needle-free devices should be used wherever possible.

References

12 Scales K. Intravenous therapy: a guide to good practice. *British Journal of Nursing* 2008; 17: S4–12.
13 British Committee for Standards in Haematology (BCSH). *Guideline on the Administration of Blood Components.* BCSH: London, 2009.
14 Department of Health. *High Impact Intervention: peripheral intravenous cannula care bundle.* Department of Health: London, 2010.

Further reading

Dougherty L and Lister S (eds). *The Royal Marsden Hospital Manual of Clinical Nursing Procedures* 8th edn. Wiley-Blackwell: Oxford, 2011.

Intramuscular injection

Intramuscular (IM) injection involves the injection of a fluid directly into muscle.

Indications

The IM route for administering medication may be chosen for one or more of the following reasons:
- if it is not possible to give medication via the oral route
- if reasonably fast (within 15–20 min) systemic uptake of a drug is required with relatively prolonged action
- if a larger fluid volume of medication (1–5 mL) needs to be given than can be injected into subcutaneous tissue (< 1 mL)
- if a medication needs to be injected that could be irritant to subcutaneous tissue.

IM injection technique

If the correct technique is used, IM injections can be less painful than subcutaneous injections, as skeletal muscles have fewer pain-sensing nerves. Uptake of the injected drug into the systemic circulation is also faster than uptake via the subcutaneous route, due to the active nature of the muscle fibres.

Needle selection

To ensure that the medication is injected directly into the muscle, a sterile 21G green needle or 23G blue needle should be used. A thinner (higher-gauge) needle may increase patient discomfort due to the additional pressure required to inject the medication through it. The length of the needle should be taken into consideration. In an emaciated or frail patient the needle should be inserted less far. In an obese patient, the maximum 35 mm reach of the standard 21G green needle may not be sufficient to reach deeper muscles, and an extra long needle may be required.

Site selection

IM injections should be given into the densest part of the muscle. There are five potential sites for IM injection. Factors that may help to inform the choice of site are listed in Table 16.1.

Deep muscle and Z-track injection techniques

There are two methods of administering an IM injection to the quadriceps or gluteal muscle sites.
- The deep muscle technique involves using the non-dominant hand to stretch the skin over the chosen injection site so as to displace the underlying subcutaneous tissue. With the dominant hand the needle is quickly and firmly inserted at an angle of 90°, using a dart-like hold until approximately 1 cm of the needle is left outside.[15]
- The Z-track technique aims to minimize discomfort and prevent leakage from the needle site. The method of needle entry remains the same, but in order to 'lock in' and prevent the leakage of

Table 16.1 Site selection for IM injection

Muscle	Considerations	Injection volume
Mid-deltoid	This site is easily accessible, although the small muscle mass dictates that only small fluid volumes can be injected	< 1 mL
Rectus femoris	A large well-defined muscle, which facilitates self-administration of IM injections	1–5 mL
Vastus lateralis	An accessible large muscle that is not close to major blood vessels or significant nerve structures	≤ 5 mL
Dorsogluteal	This has the lowest drug absorption rate of the five sites, and is close to the superior gluteal artery and sciatic nerve	≤ 4 mL
Ventrogluteal	The gluteus medius muscle can be more difficult to access than the dorsogluteal muscle, but this site has been suggested to be the IM injection site of choice. There is very effective uptake of drugs from it, and minimal risk of site injury	≤ 2.5 mL

medication into subcutaneous tissue the non-dominant hand initially pulls the skin 2–3 cm sideways or downwards from the injection site. The medication is then slowly injected at a rate of approximately 1 mL per 10 s. After this the needle is held in place for 10 s. It is then quickly withdrawn and the tension on the skin is released, allowing the tissues to return to their normal position.[16]

Site cleansing

There is conflicting evidence about skin preparation prior to IM injection. Cleansing the injection site with an alcohol swab prior to injecting is known to reduce the number of bacteria on the skin. However, if the drying time is inadequate, injection with alcohol present on the skin can cause pain and local irritation that could encourage the entry of bacteria. For this reason, some hospitals in the UK no longer advocate specific skin cleansing if the patient's skin is clean. However, standard universal precautions should always be followed.

Complications of poor IM injection technique

Poor injection technique and/or inappropriate site selection can lead to:
- inadequate medication delivery
- pain
- local tissue injury and/or haematoma
- nerve injury
- inadvertent IV drug administration
- sterile abscesses (caused by repeated injections in one site with poor blood flow).

References

15 Corben V. Administration of medicines. In: L Baillie (ed.) *Developing Practical Nursing Skills*, 2nd edn. Hodder Education: London, 2005. pp. 114–54.
16 Hunter J. Intramuscular injection techniques. *Nursing Standard* 2008; 22: 35–40.

Further reading

Dougherty L and Lister S (eds). *The Royal Marsden Hospital Manual of Clinical Nursing Procedures*, 8th edn. Wiley-Blackwell: Oxford, 2011.

Measurement for and fitting of VTE stockings

Patients should be assessed in hospital for the individual risk factors for venous thromboembolism (VTE) when hospitalized, in order to determine the most appropriate thromboprophylaxis.[17] VTE (or anti-embolic) stockings achieve thromboprophylaxis by promoting venous flow and reducing venous stasis in the legs, inferior vena cava, and pelvic veins. Anti-embolism stockings are recommended for all surgical patients in the absence of any contraindications.[18] Examples of contraindications to their use include diabetic neuropathy, peripheral artery disease, and skin conditions such as dermatitis. Unusual limb sizes and shapes can also prevent the stockings from working correctly.

If VTE stockings are indicated, it is imperative that they fit correctly. Poorly fitted stockings can result in compromised lower limb perfusion and/or skin or tissue injury, and therefore in fact increase the risk of VTE.

Three measurements need to be taken to determine the correct size of VTE stocking for a patient:
- thigh circumference (at its widest point)
- calf circumference (at its widest point)
- leg length (measure from the gluteal fold to the heel for thigh length, and from the popliteal fold to the heel for knee length).

Manufacturers of anti-embolic stockings supply a size chart on the packing, so that these measurements can be used to determine the correct size for the patient to wear. It is important to note that if the patient's thigh circumference is larger than the manufacturer's largest size, knee-length stockings should be supplied.

Fitting the VTE stocking

Once the correct size has been selected it is important to fit the stocking properly. The following points may help to facilitate this:
- After removal from the packaging turn the stocking inside out.
- Ask or help the patient to place their foot in the foot part of the stocking.
- Ensure that the heel section is under their heel and that the toes are not protruding from the hole. The hole should be situated underneath the foot to allow inspection for any skin discoloration that may indicate circulatory compromise.
- Gently pull the stocking up to its full length, ensuring that it is smooth and any wrinkles are pulled out.
- The patient should be instructed not to roll or fold down the top of the stocking. They should also be advised that if they need to remove the stockings they should put them back on again as soon as possible. If they want to wash any part of the stocking, only warm water should be used, as hot water can impair the effectiveness of the fabric.

Thigh length or knee length

The National Institute for Health and Care Excellence (NICE)[17] advocates that thigh-length VTE stockings should be fitted from the time of admission to hospital until the patient has returned to their normal level of activity. However, thigh-length VTEs are more difficult to put on than knee-length ones and are prone to rolling down, potentially creating a tourniquet-type effect. Patient compliance can be poorer for these reasons. In situations where this makes thigh-length stockings inappropriate, knee-length stockings are a suitable alternative.

References

17 National Institute for Health and Care Excellence (NICE). *Venous Thromboembolism Prevention Quality Standard.* QS3. NICE: London, 2010. ℛ www.nice.org.uk/guidance/qs3

18 Scottish Intercollegiate Guidelines Network (SIGN). *Prevention and Management of Venous Thromboembolism.* Guideline No. 122. SIGN: Edinburgh, 2010.

Useful website

ℛ www.rcn.org.uk/development/practice/cpd_online_learning/nice_care_preventing_venousthromboembolism/preventing_vte

Ophthalmology

External anatomy of the eye

The eyes are situated on the face and enclosed in their own bony orbits, separated by the nose. The eyes work together, receiving similar but different perspectives which are fused together as one image. This ability to fuse two images together is called binocular vision.

The initial analysis of images is relatively crude. Light is transformed into electrical potentials which then travel via the optic nerve and visual pathway system. The sophisticated analysis of the visual world occurs in the primary visual cortex, and this is where colour depth contrast occurs.

The orbit

The eye is located within the orbit, and in the average adult it measures approximately 24 mm in diameter. The optic nerve leaves the eye at the optic disc and transports the entire visual image to the brain. The globe (eyeball) is protected by the orbit in which it sits. As shown in Figure 17.1, the orbit consists of seven bones:

• frontal
• maxillary
• zygomatic
• sphenoid
• ethmoid
• lacrimal
• palatine.

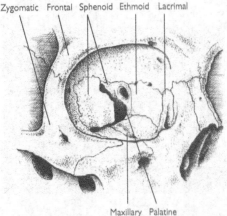

Figure 17.1 Anatomy of the skull and orbit. Reproduced from Alastair Denniston and Philip Murray, *Oxford Handbook of Ophthalmology*, Third Edition, 2014, with permission from Oxford University Press.

The orbit consists of four walls—the roof, lateral wall, orbital floor, and medial wall. The orbit is pyramid shaped, and the highest tip, which is called the optic foramen, is the opening to the optic canal. Both the optic nerve and the ophthalmic artery pass through the optic foramen.

Eyelids

- They provide protection to the eye (blinking).
- They secrete the oily component of the tear film.
- They help to spread the tear film over the eye.
- They prevent the eye from drying out.
- They contain the puncta, through which tears drain into the lacrimal system.
- The eyelid is opened by the levator muscle.
- The eyelid is closed by the orbicularis muscle.

Internal anatomy of the eye

Cornea

The cornea (see Figure 17.2) is a transparent avascular structure, which is convex in shape (often likened to a watch-glass cover) and 0.5 mm in thickness. It allows light rays through, and its shape allows light rays to bend. It is highly sensitive and protects the front of the eyeball. The cornea consists of five layers:

- epithelium
- Bowman's membrane
- stroma
- Descemet's membrane
- endothelium.

The epithelium is the only layer that can regenerate if it is damaged. For example, if it is scratched by a fingernail, resulting in a corneal abrasion, it will heal within 24–48 h.

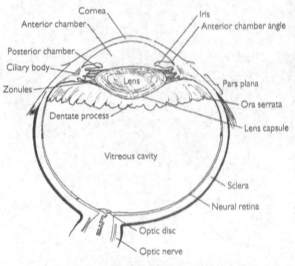

Figure 17.2 Anatomy of the eye. Reproduced from PM Dodson, Oxford Diabetes Library, *Diabetic Retinopathy: screening to treatment*, 2008, with permission from Oxford University Press.

Anterior and posterior chamber

The anterior chamber (see Figure 17.2) is the area between the posterior surface of the cornea and the anterior surface of the iris. When the eye is inflamed, cells may be visible on examination with a slit-lamp microscope.

The posterior chamber is the area between the posterior surface of the iris and the anterior surface of the lens and suspensory ligaments.

The anterior and posterior chambers are both filled with aqueous fluid that provides nourishment to the lens and maintains the eye's intra-ocular pressure.

Ciliary body

This is a triangular structure lying between the choroid and the iris. It consists of the ciliary processes and the ciliary muscle.

Iris

This is the coloured circular diaphragm that lies behind the cornea and in front of the lens. It forms the pupil centrally, and is attached peripherally to the ciliary body. There are two muscles responsible for constricting and dilating the pupil.

- The sphincter muscle constricts the pupil, restricting the amount of light that enters the eye. It is the more powerful muscle of the two.
- The dilater muscle dilates the pupil.

Lens

This is the focusing mechanism of the eye, and it is held in place by sus-pensory ligaments known as zonules.

Vitreous

The vitreous is transparent and fills the posterior segment of the eye, between the lens and the retina. It consists of 98–99% water and 1–2% hyaluronic acid and collagen fibres. The vitreous maintains the eye shape and aids the refraction of light.

Sclera

The sclera extends from the cornea (limbal area) to the optic nerve, and is composed of dense, white, non-uniform collagen fibres. It is often described as the hard protective coating of the eye.

Choroid

The choroid lies between the sclera and the retina, and its function is to provide nourishment to the underlying retina. It contains blood vessels that supply the underlying retina.

Retina

The retina consists of ten layers. The first layer contains pigmented epi-thelium, and the other nine layers contain neural layers. It is transparent (its colour comes from the choroid's blood supply) and contains rods and cones. The rods are important for night vision and the cones are responsible for daytime vision.

Optic disc

This is the area where the retinal fibres leave the eyeball as the optic nerve.

The visually impaired patient

Patients may present with either acute or chronic visual impairment. It may be either slight (images slightly blurred) or severe (total blindness). In any of these scenarios the patient may be very anxious, as many patients attending with visual impairment, especially in an emergency situation, will fear that they are going to lose their vision.

Many patients have a fear of having their eyes touched. Some feel physically nauseous, and others feel faint or do faint while they are having their eye examined or having an eye procedure performed.

Ophthalmic patients can be from any age group across the lifespan. With the growing size of the ageing population there are now many more patients who are experiencing age-related eye problems.

It is essential that the nurse is sympathetic to the patient's needs—for example, by making effective communication with the patient a priority. The website of the Royal National Institute of Blind People (RNIB) includes many useful resources for healthcare professionals. However, the following points are of paramount importance when caring for visually impaired patients.

- When greeting the visually impaired person for the first time it is essential to introduce yourself and explain what you are going to be doing, as the patient may have very limited vision and it can be very disconcerting to hear movement but not know what is happening.
- Ensure that the nurse call-bell is readily to hand so that the patient can summon help easily.
- Do not move items without informing the patient (e.g. items in a cupboard), or leave a door open that was closed, or vice versa. Visually impaired patients have set places for where they keep household items so that they can easily find them. It could also be dangerous to change them (e.g. the patient could walk into a door they thought was open).
- Do not just leave food at the patient's bedside and expect them to find it. Tell them where exactly you have left it.
- Try using coloured drinking glasses so that the patient can see the water being poured into the glass. Use lipped plates so that the food stays on the plate.
- Provide large-print menus and patient information.
- Inform the patient tactfully if they have food on their clothing or are wearing a garment inside out.

Useful website

Royal National Institute of Blind People (RNIB). ♫ www.rnib.org.uk

Principles of ophthalmic history taking

It is important to take a thorough history from the ophthalmic patient in order to:

- identify the problem
- ascertain a visual history
- determine the severity of the symptoms and whether more urgent treatment is required (e.g. in the case of a chemical injury)
- determine whether any treatment has already been used (this may have been prescribed or bought over the counter)
- develop a rapport with the patient
- identify any medico-legal issues associated with possible work-related injury or following an assault.

As mentioned earlier, patients with an ophthalmic complaint may well present with considerable anxiety, as there is often a fear of blindness. Walsh[1] suggests that when patients attend, nurses should exercise tact and understanding when the patient is describing their symptoms. For patients with eye problems, extra time and careful questioning may be needed to obtain all of the information that is required. In addition, a professional and friendly manner is essential. The patient may not express their concerns to an interviewer who does not demonstrate a professional approach and genuine interest.[2]

References

1 Walsh M. *Nurse Practitioners: clinical skills and professional issues*. Butterworth–Heinemann: Edinburgh, 2006.
2 Goldblum K. Obtaining a complete and pertinent patient history. *Insight* 2004; **29**: 17–20.

Ophthalmic history taking guide

Presenting complaint

It is important to ascertain why the patient is attending and which eye is causing a problem.

Duration of symptoms

- How long have the symptoms been present? Are they there all the time or do they come and go?
- Did the symptoms come on suddenly or were they gradual? Identify what the patient was doing at the time. This is very important if there is any suspicion of a foreign body which could be a penetrating injury.
- Was the patient drilling, chiselling, hammering, or carrying out a task that could have caused a high-speed injury? If the answer is yes, there should be a high level of suspicion of penetrating injury.
- If a chemical injury splash has occurred, does the patient have information on the ingredients of the chemical, and has the eye been irrigated?
- Was the patient wearing eye protection? If they were, how old was the eye protection and was it a good fit?
- Has the patient tried any treatments at home? If the answer is yes, what have they tried and has there been any improvement?
- If they have a discharge, ask whether the patient has had a recent cough or cold.
- If the patient has a red eye, is photophobic, and has a foreign body sensation that came on gradually, ask whether they suffer from cold sores. It could be a herpes simplex condition.
- If the patient is complaining of a headache, find out where it is located. The location can indicate whether the headache is due to eye strain or some other condition. Does the patient suffer from migraine? If the headache is temporal, does the patient have jaw claudication or general malaise?
- Ask whether the patient is experiencing any nausea.
- If the patient is complaining of vision loss, ask whether their vision is blurred.
- Did the vision deteriorate suddenly, or gradually over a course of weeks? Was it like a shutter closing over the eye, and can they identify out shapes?
- Ask whether there is any distortion in the vision. Sometimes it is better to ask the patient to describe their vision. For example, if you simply ask them whether it is blurred they may give a yes or no response that can compromise the examination.

Previous ocular history

- Has the patient ever experienced anything similar before? If the answer is yes, do they know what condition they had and what made the condition better?
- Do they have a history of any of the following?
  - Iritis.
  - Episcleritis or scleritis.
  - Previous eye injury.
  - Diabetic eye disease.
  - Corneal abrasion.
- Do they wear glasses for short- or long-sightedness?
- Do they wear contact lenses? If the answer is yes, what type do they use, how do they disinfect them, and what is the average length of time for which the lenses are worn?

Family ocular history

Is there a family ocular history of glaucoma, diabetic eye disease, iritis, cataract, or retinal detachment?

General medical health problems

It is important to ask about the following:
- diabetes—type, duration, and how it is controlled
- hypertension
- thyroid disorders
- heart problems
- eczema
- asthma.

Medication and allergies

- Record any medication that the patient is taking, including prescribed, over-the-counter, and complementary medicines. It is vital that all medications are noted, including any complementary therapies, as some herbal medications interact with prescribed medications.
- Record all drug-related, food-related, and other allergies (e.g. latex).

Occupation

Consider the patient's occupation in order to determine whether there is a need to advise them to refrain from work or use eye protection.

Vision assessment

Prior to a formal ophthalmic examination, it is an essential requirement that a formal visual acuity measurement is performed and documented. However, in cases of chemical injury it is vital that the patient has their eye irrigated thoroughly before the visual acuity measurement.

The standard tool for measuring visual acuity is a Snellen chart, with acuity measured at a distance of 6 m. Some charts are designed for use at shorter distances. For example, if using a reverse Snellen chart with a mirror, the vision will be measured at 3 m but recorded as 6 m. It is not acceptable practice to record vision as 'normal' or 'not affected.'

The Snellen chart

- It consists of nine rows of letters that get progressively smaller.
- The letters are heavy block letters, numbers, or symbols, printed in black on a white background.
- The top letter can be read by a normal eye at a distance of 60 m, and the smallest letter can be read by a normal eye at 4 m.
- The vision is recorded as a fraction—that is, distance from chart/line read on the chart. For example, if the patient is seated at a distance of 6 m from the chart and they read the line that the normal eye would see at 6 m, the fraction would be 6/6.

Method of assessment

- Ask the patient to use their distance glasses, or contact lenses if appropriate.
- Ask them to cover their eye with a tissue, starting with the right eye.
- Ask them to read down the letters from the top, starting at the left and reading across to the right, to the lowest line they can see.
- If the patient does not reach the 6/9 line, use a pinhole to establish whether the decreased vision is correctable or not. In some cases the cause of loss of vision is refractive error.
- If the patient cannot read any of the letters, move them closer to the chart by 1 m at a time until they can read the top letter.
- If they are still unable to read the top letter, stand in front of the patient at a distance of 1 m and hold your fingers up. Ask the patient to count the number of fingers you are holding up. If they can see your fingers, record this as CF (counting fingers).
- If the patient is unable to see the number of fingers you are holding up, wave your hand in front of their eye at a distance of 30 cm and ask whether they can see your hand. If they can see it, record this as HM (hand movements vision).
- If the patient cannot see your hand, shine a bright light and ask them to tell you from which direction the light came. If they can see the light, this should be recorded as PL (perception of light). If no light is seen, this should be recorded as NPL (no perception of light).

The Sheridan–Gardiner method

This test can be used in illiterate or young patients. The examiner holds a card at a distance of 6 m and the patient is asked to match the corresponding letter on their card. This provides a Snellen chart recording.

LogMAR vision testing

- Although this is a more complex test, it is well documented as being more accurate.
- The main advantage of the LogMAR chart is that there are five letters on each line, and each letter is scored, giving the patient a fairer chance of being able to read letters on the chart.
- The main disadvantage is that the test is time-consuming, because each letter is given a score.
- The LogMAR is the chart of choice in the medical retina and glaucoma clinic, where a very accurate assessment of vision is essential.

Near vision

Near vision is tested with a specifically designed reading card, using different sizes of ordinary print types.

Colour vision assessment

- Colour vision should be assessed in any patient who presents with painful loss of vision, or if requested (e.g. for employment purposes).
- The standard method of assessing colour vision involves the use of pseudoisochromatic plates such as Ishihara colour plates, which test for red–green colour blindness.

Testing central vision with an Amsler grid

- This test is performed on all patients who complain of distortion in their vision, and regularly on patients at medical retina clinics.
- The test uses an A5 sheet of paper with a grid of black lines. In the centre of each grid there is a black dot.
- Each eye is tested at a distance of 25 cm.
- The patient looks at the central spot and marks on the chart any areas of blurring, distortion, or missing parts.
- In cases of macular disease the patient would see the straight lines as distorted, wavy, or completely absent.

Testing eye movements

- This test must be done on all patients who complain of double vision.
- The examiner sits in front of the patient at the same height as them.
- The patient is required to follow the direction of a red hat pin with their eyes, not their head.
- Ask the patient to cover their left eye, and then move the target slowly up and down, left and right, asking the patient to report any pain on movement, or double vision. Repeat for the other eye.
- Observe for full eye movements in all directions.

Cataracts

A cataract is an opacity (clouding) of the lens of the eye. It occurs with increasing age, and is one of the leading causes of blindness worldwide.

Types of cataract

- Senile—occurs over the age of 60 years, and is caused by sclerosis of the lens.
- Traumatic—occurs as a direct result of injury, such as blunt trauma or a penetrating injury.
- Toxic—caused by substances (e.g. steroids) affecting the metabolism of the lens.
- Secondary to systemic disease—patients with conditions such as diabetes are more likely to develop cataracts.
- Congenital—caused by abnormal development of the eye in the fetus as a result of the mother contracting rubella during the first trimester of pregnancy.

Presenting symptoms

- Reduction in vision.
- Change in colour vision.
- Change in refractive prescription.
- Monocular diplopia.
- Problems with night driving.

Surgery

Cataract surgery involves removing the opacified lens and replacing it with an artificial intra-ocular lens (IOL). Most cataract surgery in the UK is now performed under local anaesthetic as a day case.

Indications for surgery

- When the visual acuity is having an impact on the patient's daily life.
- When there is a need to visualize other structures in the eye (e.g. the retina in diabetic patients).
- To improve the cosmetic appearance of a blind eye.

Benefits

Cataract surgery improves the quality of vision and also improves the view of the eye (for visualizing the ocular structures).

Risks

- The risk of blindness is 1 in 1000.
- Infection such as endophthalmitis after 0.1% of cataract procedures.
- Retinal detachment.
- Cystoid macular oedema.
- Dropped nucleus.
- Wound leakage.
- Posterior capsule opacification.

Nursing pre-operative assessment

Patients need to attend the service provider for a pre-operative assessment to ensure that they are fully prepared for their surgery, and that any extra needs that the patient may have are identified (e.g. a patient who needs to have a special IOL ordered, or who will require extra time to be positioned for the surgery due to a physical disability).

The patient should be informed that they will still need to wear glasses for reading, as the majority of patients wish to have their new IOL prescription set for distance vision.

Investigations required

- Best corrected visual acuity and pinhole visual acuity.
- Blood pressure.
- Blood glucose levels if the patient is diabetic.
- INR to be arranged to ensure up-to-date measurement prior to surgery.
- Medical history.
- Autorefraction if no up-to-date refraction has been performed.
- Slit-lamp examination to exclude infection or blepharitis that will require treatment pre-operatively.
- Biometry—scan the lens selection printout, to be available to the consultant at all times.

Day of surgery

- On arrival at the eye unit the patient's details are checked.
- The consent form is checked.
- The eye to be operated on will be marked with an arrow.
- Lens power is selected by the operating consultant.
- The pupil is dilated with cyclopentolate 1%, phenylephrine 2.5% given three times at 15-min intervals.
- The patient is escorted to theatre.

Post-operative care

- Steroid and antibiotic eye drops will be required for up to 1 month.
- Cleansing of the eye is important.
- Post-operative appointments will vary from unit to unit.

Post-operative complications

- The patients should be instructed that if they experience increasing pain, increasing sticky discharge, or a reduction in vision they must contact the unit where they had their surgery to ask for advice. Most units provide a contact telephone number and instructions about what to do out of hours for the first 2 weeks post-operatively.
- Long-term visual acuity may be reduced due to thickening of the posterior capsule.

Glaucoma

Glaucoma refers to a group of conditions that affect the optic nerve and can be associated with raised intra-ocular eye pressure (IOP), although this is not always the case. The normal IOP is in the range 15–21 mmHg.

Primary open-angle glaucoma

Primary open-angle glaucoma can occur in either men or women aged over 45 years, and the risk increases with age.

Risk factors
- Family history of first-degree relative with glaucoma.
- High myopia.
- Black or Afro-Caribbean descent.

Investigations
- Visual acuity.
- IOP using Goldmann applanation tonometry.
- Open angle with a normal appearance (gonioscopy).
- Visual field (Humphrey visual field analysis).
- Pachymetry (to measure the corneal thickness).
- Heidelberg retina tomograph.
- Scanning laser polarimeter (GDx, short for glaucoma diagnosis) test.
- Optic disc photography.

Treatment and follow-up
- Pressure-lowering eye drops are the first line of treatment.
- Surgical treatment with a trabeculectomy should be performed if drop therapy is unsuccessful.
- A clinic appointment is needed every 6 months once the eye is stable.
- Visual field testing should be performed on a yearly basis.

Angle-closure glaucoma

This condition is considered to be an ophthalmic emergency. It occurs when the iris moves forward and blocks the trabecular meshwork, obstructing the flow of aqueous humour and thus causing a rise in pressure.

Risk factors
- Female gender (female:male ratio is 4:1).
- Family history of the disorder.
- Hypermetropia (long sight).
- South East Asian, Chinese, or Inuit descent.
- Shallow anterior chambers.
- Narrow angles.

Symptoms
- Visual loss.
- Severe eye pain.
- Nausea and vomiting.
- Headache.
- The patient may complain of previous intermittent blurred vision, possibly with halos around bright lights.

Signs on examination
- Red eye.
- Corneal oedema, which resembles frosted glass.
- Fixed mid-dilated pupil (slow reaction) may be oval in shape.
- IOP higher than 40 mmHg.
- Occluded angle on gonioscopy.

Treatment required
▶▶ Immediate
- Acetazolamide, 500 mg intravenously (IV).
- Acetazolamide, 500 mg orally (*not* slow release).
- Pilocarpine 2%, 2 drops to both eyes.
- Dexamethasone, 1 drop to affected eye.
- Beta-blocking drops may or may not be required. Do not use them if the patient has asthma or heart problems.
▶▶ One hour
- IOP check.
- Pilocarpine 2%, four times a day.
- 1–2 h from IV acetazolamide.
- Check IOP. If it is less than 35 mmHg the patient may require oral glycerin 50% (1 g/kg). *Note that this may make the patient vomit* and is very sweet tasting. If the patient cannot be administered glycerin, they may require IV mannitol 20% (1 g/kg).

When there has been a reduction in IOP
- Laser iridotomy should be performed. This successfully treats 75% of cases. However, if it is unsuccessful a trabeculectomy may be required.
- The other eye can be treated at a later date.

Follow-up
- The patient should attend for a clinic appointment daily until the IOP is stable.
- Recheck gonioscopy.

Secondary glaucoma

Secondary glaucoma is glaucoma resulting from any other identifiable pathology, including the following:

- pseudoexfoliation—deposits of grey flecks of amyloid-like fibrillar material on the lens capsule
- pigment dispersion syndrome—shedding of pigment from the iris epithelium onto ocular structures
- inflammatory changes
- neovascular glaucoma—caused by new blood vessels crossing into the trabecular meshwork
- uveitic glaucoma—10% of patients with uveitis develop secondary glaucoma
- steroid-induced glaucoma—usually caused by topical steroids
- lens-induced glaucoma—disorders of the lens (e.g. cataract) may cause patients to develop a secondary glaucoma
- traumatic glaucoma—this may lead to an early or late rise in IOP, often caused by hyphaema reducing the aqueous flow
- surgery—a temporary rise in IOP after surgery is common.

Treatment of the underlying cause may be sufficient.

Glaucoma drops

- These are prostaglandin analogues.
- They lower IOP by increasing uveoscleral flow.
- They are very effective.
- They are usually prescribed once daily, which can aid compliance.
- They can cause hyperaemia (redness).
- They may cause a dry sensation.
- They may cause the eyelashes to lengthen.

Beta blockers

- These decrease IOP by reducing the secretion of aqueous humour by blocking the beta receptors in the ciliary body.
- They are usually prescribed twice daily.
- They should not be used in patients with asthma.
- They can induce bradycardia.

Alpha-2 receptors

- These decrease aqueous humour formation by stimulating alpha receptors. This prevents the release of noradrenaline, which in turn reduces the formation of aqueous humour.
- They are a good alternative to beta blockers.
- Apraclonidine has an immediate effect.
- They may cause allergic reactions in patients.
- They need to be administered two to three times a day, which can reduce compliance.

Carbonic anhydrase inhibitors

- These powerful drugs for lowering IOP can also be used systemically (e.g. acetazolamide).
- They reduce the flow of aqueous humour production by blocking the enzyme carbonic anhydrase in the ciliary epithelial cells.
- They cannot be used in patients with compromised endothelium or in those who have had recent corneal grafts, as they can impair the pump function of the endothelium.[3]
- They may cause allergic reactions in patients.

Combination drops

- These may increase compliance by reducing the number of bottles, as there are two medications in one bottle.
- They are useful when IOP control is not achieved using a single product.
- They reduce the number of preservatives to which the eye is exposed.

Miotics

- These stimulate the muscarinic receptors in the ciliary smooth muscle, thereby opening up the trabecular meshwork and increasing the flow of aqueous humour.
- They can cause headaches and blurred vision.

Reference

3 Hopkins G and Pearson R. Ophthalmic Drugs: diagnostic and therapeutic uses, 5th edn. Elsevier: Edinburgh, 2007.

Retinal detachment

The retina has ten layers:
- epithelial layer
- receptor layer (containing the rods and cones)
- external limiting membrane
- outer nuclear layer
- outer plexiform layer
- inner nuclear layer
- inner plexiform layer
- ganglion cell layer
- nerve fibre layer
- internal limiting membrane.

Retinal detachment is a separation of the epithelial layer in the retina from the neural layers. Retinal detachments may be:
- pushed off (e.g. by a lesion behind the retina)
- pulled off (e.g. the neural layer can be pulled off by vitreous traction)
- floated off (if a tear or hole appears, subretinal fluid can pass into the tear and cause the neural layers to detach).

Symptoms
- The perception of flashing lights (photopsia), caused by the separating layers stimulating the rods and cones.
- A sudden onset of increasing showers of floaters. Many people suffer from floaters on an everyday basis, and the occasional floater is harmless.
- The patient may complain of a dark curtain in their field of vision.
- They may describe their vision as like looking through a net curtain.

Risk factors
- Age—with advancing age the vitreous undergoes a benign change called syneresis, which causes it to liquefy and shrink.
- Myopia.
- Trauma.
- History of ocular surgery, particularly cataract surgery involving vitreous loss.
- Lattice degeneration—people with this condition are more likely to suffer a retinal tear.

Diagnosis
- Visual acuity may be severely reduced.
- If a large detachment is present, the red reflex may appear grey.
- A relative afferent pupillary defect (RAPD) may be present if the macula is detached.
- Dilation is required for detailed fundoscopy.
- A macula-on detachment is considered more urgent than a macula-off detachment, and is usually operated on within 24 h.[4]

▶▶ Treatment

Retinal tears

• Retinopexy with either an argon laser or cryotherapy.

Retinal detachment

• Cryobuckle surgery, in which a silicone explant is sutured externally to the sclera. Retinopexy is used to seal the tear in the retina, and sulphur hexafluoride (SF6) gas is sometimes inserted.
• Vitrectomy, in which the vitreous is removed and then retinopexy is performed and either SF6 gas or octafluoropropane (C3F8) is applied as tamponade to the retina (in some cases silicone oil is used).

▶ Post-operative care

Day 1

• Posturing will be needed for patients who have had gas inserted. This is usually right cheek to pillow if the right eye was operated on, and vice versa, for 50 min in every hour for a period of 10 days.
• The eye dressing should be removed and the eye bathed.
• Slit-lamp examination.
• Measurement of IOP.
• Antibiotic eye drops four times a day for 2 weeks.
• Steroid eye drops four times a day for 2 weeks, then gradually reduced over 3 weeks.
• Dilating drops (e.g. atropine 1%) twice a day for 1 week.
• Regular outpatient follow-up according to the surgeon's preference.

Reference

4 Jackson TL (ed.). *Moorfields Manual of Ophthalmology*, 2nd edn. JP Medical Ltd: London, 2014.

Corneal graft (keratoplasty)

A corneal graft is a surgical procedure in which a damaged cornea is replaced with a healthy donor cornea, and it is one of the most successful human organ transplantations. A partial-thickness graft is called a lamellar keratoplasty, and a full-thickness graft is called a penetrating keratoplasty.

Penetrating keratoplasty

- This is the most common type of graft performed.
- It is used to correct conditions such as keratoconus, bullous keratopathy, scarring, injury, and corneal dystrophies.
- It can be used to remove dead tissue (e.g. in microbial keratitis that has not responded to medical treatment).
- It can be used to replace either a thinning cornea or a cornea that has become perforated due to injury or a corneal ulcer.
- Surgery can be performed under a local or general anaesthetic.
- The patient will need careful pre-operative assessment and must be fully informed that they are to receive a cornea from a human donor. Some patients may become very distressed when given this information, and it is vital to carefully explain that the donor will have given their consent to this, and that the donor material is carefully screened to ensure it is free of disease.
- The patient must be given a full explanation of the risks of rejection and be informed that they should get in urgent contact with an eye department if they experience reduced vision, pain, or redness.
- The patient may suffer double vision and astigmatism initially post-operatively, due to the sutures.
- The patient will need to have miotic drops instilled to prevent damage to the intra-ocular lens during surgery.

Lamellar keratoplasty

- This procedure is used in patients who do not require a full-thickness graft because the disease has not penetrated all of the layers of the cornea.
- It has a shorter rehabilitation time than a full-thickness graft.
- There is a reduced risk of rejection.
- It is a more complex operation to perform.

Complications of surgery

- Damage to the iris or the lens during surgery.
- Aqueous leakage from the graft causing a shallow or flat anterior chamber.
- Infection.
- Rejection, although the risk is lower than in other human transplants, due to the cornea being avascular.
- Astigmatism.
- The graft may require re-suturing if the sutures are loose.

Post-operative care

- Topical steroids should be applied 1- to 2-hourly for the first 2–3 days, and then four times a day for several weeks. Thereafter the dose is very slowly reduced to once daily for at least 1 year.
- Antibiotic drops should be given four times a day for 2–3 weeks post-operatively.
- Patients with a previous history of herpes simplex keratitis may require oral aciclovir.

Follow-up

- On day 1.
- At 1 week.
- At 2 weeks.
- At 4 weeks.
- Thereafter monthly until the patient is stable, and then every 2–3 months until the surgeon feels that this frequency can be reduced.

Temporal arteritis

Temporal arteritis is a condition that results from inflammation of the large arteries in the head and neck. It most commonly affects the temporal artery, but several arteries may be affected at the same time. It usually affects women more often than men, and individuals aged over 60 years. It is rare before the age of 50 years.

Symptoms

- Temporal headache.
- Pain on chewing or talking due to jaw claudication.
- Pain on brushing the hair, due to generalized scalp tenderness.
- General malaise and fatigue.
- Weight loss.
- Loss of appetite.
- There may be sudden transient loss of vision or blurred vision.

Signs

- The temporal arteries at the sides of the forehead may be tender if touched.
- The scalp is tender if touched.
- The patient may look unwell.

Management

- Urgent erythrocyte sedimentation rate (ESR) (usually > 50 mm/h) and C-reactive protein (CRP) (> 3 mg/L).
- Baseline blood pressure measurement.
- Urinalysis.
- Urgent ophthalmology review is needed if visual symptoms are present. If there are no visual symptoms, urgent referral to the rheumatologist is required.

If a diagnosis of temporal arteritis is confirmed, the patient will require:
- high-dose steroids to protect their vision, reducing the dose over a period of approximately 1 year
- temporal artery biopsy to confirm the diagnosis.

Complications

- Blindness in one or both eyes.
- Cerebrovascular accident (CVA).

Red eye

Conjunctivitis

Conjunctivitis is an inflammation of the conjunctiva which can be caused by a bacterial infection, a viral infection, an allergic reaction, or an irritant such as chlorinated water.

Signs and symptoms
- Generalized redness of the conjunctiva and the posterior surface of the eyelid. The top lid will need to be everted to visualize this.
- Discomfort, may be itchy.
- Discharge can be either watery or purulent.
- Crusty eyelids which are stuck down in the morning.
- General flu-like symptoms and/or a history of recent cough or cold which are consistent with viral conjunctivitis.
- The patient may have eczema or hay fever if it is allergic conjunctivitis.
- Conjunctival chemosis may be present if the patient has allergic or viral conjunctivitis.
- History of contact with an individual with red eyes, or sharing make-up with a person with a red eye.
- Lymph nodes may be palpable (viral infection).

Treatment
- Provide hygiene advice—no towel sharing, advice on hand washing after touching the eye, no sharing of make-up, use of disposable tissues (not handkerchiefs) to wipe the eyes.
- In cases of purulent conjunctivitis, antibiotic drops may be prescribed.
- In cases of viral conjunctivitis, no treatment is required unless other ocular signs are present.
- In cases of allergic conjunctivitis, topical antihistamines are required.

Chlamydial infection
- This should be suspected in patients who have persistent conjunctivitis and are sexually active.
- It typically occurs in young adults.
- Large conjunctival follicles are present in the conjunctiva.
- Chlamydial swabs will need to be taken to confirm the diagnosis (the patient's verbal consent will be required for this).
- If the results are positive, the patient must be referred to the sexual health clinic.
- Topical tetracycline ointment should be applied four times a day for 6 weeks.

Episcleritis
This is an inflammatory condition of the episcleral blood vessels.

Signs and symptoms
- Redness of the eye which may be sectoral.
- Mild ache.
- Normal vision.
- No discharge.

Treatment
- Oral ibuprofen unless contraindicated.
- Ocular lubricants.
- In severe cases, mild steroid eye drops.

Scleritis

This is inflammation of the sclera.

Signs and symptoms
- Deep redness of the scleral and episcleral blood vessels.
- The eye is tender when touched.
- Intense pain that causes sleep loss.
- Throbbing head pain.
- The patient may have blurred vision.
- They may be photophobic due to pain.

Treatment
- Rule out systemic causes such as rheumatoid arthritis.
- Give oral flurbiprofen 100 mg three times a day.
- Administer steroid eye drops.

Subconjunctival haemorrhage

This is caused by bleeding under the conjunctiva as a result of rupture o
the subconjunctival blood vessels.

Signs and symptoms
- Sudden onset of painless red eye which the patient may have been
  unaware of but someone else has noticed.
- Occasionally the patient will experience a sensation like a small pop ir
  their eye, and then on inspection will notice a red eye.
- An otherwise 'quiet' eye.
- The patient may have a cough. Also ask them whether they have had
  any recent vomiting or straining, or performed any heavy lifting.

Treatment
- Check the blood pressure, as the haemorrhage may have been
  caused by high blood pressure.
- Reassure the patient that it is just like a bruise and will disperse
  slowly.
- Ocular lubricants may be required.

Corneal disorders

Corneal abrasion

There is generally a history of trauma to the surface of the eye, such as a scratch caused by a child's fingernail, the corner of a piece of paper, or part of a plant.

Signs and symptoms
- Severe pain.
- Watery eye.
- Red eye.
- A visible scratch or abrasion when blue light is shone on fluorescein.
- Photophobia.

Treatment
- Antibiotic ointment applied four times a day for 5 days.
- In the case of abrasions caused by sharp objects, or diabetics who may be at risk of corneal erosion syndrome, lubricants will need to be applied to the eye for 2–3 months.
- If the patient is in severe pain, cyclopentolate 1% should be administered in order to dilate the pupil and stop the muscle spasm, thereby reducing the pain.
- Eye pads are no longer recommended, as they do not aid healing.

Corneal ulcer

A corneal ulcer is an open sore on the cornea. It can be caused by bacterial, viral, or fungal infections, or by injury to the cornea.

Signs and symptoms
- Painful red eye.
- Photophobia.
- There may be a purulent discharge.
- History of wearing contact lenses.
- Visual acuity may be reduced.
- A white ulcer may be visible.
- Fluorescein staining identifies an epithelial defect.

Treatment
- The patient needs to be seen by the eye unit.
- They may need a corneal scrape to confirm the bacteria to be treated.
- Intensive topical antibiotics may need to be applied every 30 min, depending on the severity of the ulcer.
- The patient will require regular follow-ups to check that the ulcer is healing.

Corneal foreign body

The patient may have a history of having felt something entering their eye. Check whether there is any history of working with high-speed equipment (e.g. nail gun) prior to injury.

Signs and symptoms
- The sensation of something in the eye, especially on blinking.
- Watering eye.
- Red eye.
- May be sensitive to light.
- A corneal foreign body firmly embedded in the cornea.

Treatment
- Evert the eyelid to ensure that no other foreign body is visible.
- Instil one drop of local anaesthetic eye drops.
- Try to flick the corneal foreign body off with a cotton bud that has been moistened with a drop of normal saline. If it is impossible to remove it in this way, refer the patient to the eye unit.
- Antibiotic ointment should be applied four times a day for 5 days.

Trauma to the eyelid and orbit

▶ Blunt trauma

This is usually caused by direct blows (e.g. from a fist or squash ball).

Examination

The aim of this is to exclude:
- trauma to the globe or orbit
- corneal abrasion
- subconjunctival haemorrhage
- raised IOP
- hyphaema (blood in the anterior chamber).

Dilated fundoscopy

The aim of this is to exclude:
- cataract
- vitreous detachment
- retinal detachment
- commotio retinae.

Treatment

This will depend on the extent of the injury, but the patient may require surgical intervention.

Partial- or full-thickness lid laceration

Lacerations involving the eyelid are common. They require a thorough examination to ensure that no foreign bodies remain *in situ* and that there is good anatomical closure, especially around the lacrimal area.

Treatment
- Check the patient's tetanus status.
- Complex lacerations should be repaired by an oculoplastic specialist.
- The patient will require antibiotic ointment to prevent wound infection.
- Arrange suture removal within 7 days.

▶▶ Penetrating injury

This can range from a small injury (e.g. from a dart) to larger injuries (e.g. from a drill bit). *Do not attempt to remove a penetrating foreign body.*
- Always obtain an opinion from an eye department.
- The patient may require magnetic resonance imaging (MRI), X-ray, or a computed tomography (CT) scan to confirm the diagnosis.

Treatment
- The patient will require emergency surgery to remove any intra-ocular foreign body and repair the eye as soon as possible.
- Intravenous antibiotics should be administered.
- The patient's tetanus status should be checked.
- Antibiotic eye drops should be applied.
- Dilating eye drops should be applied.
- Steroid eye drops should be applied.
- It may not always be possible to save the eye, depending on the severity of the injury.

Orbital floor fracture (blowout fracture)

This is usually caused by an object larger than the orbit (e.g. tennis ball, fist) hitting the face with force. This force produces a sudden rise in pressure within the maxillary bone which fractures, causing the eye to sink into the gap.

Signs and symptoms
- Sunken eye (enophthalmos).
- Bruising and swelling of the eye.
- Pain on eye movement.
- The patient may have double vision.
- Numbness of the lower lid and cheek.
- Inability to move the eye in all fields of vision, as the muscle has been caught in the fractured bone.

Treatment
- Admit the patient, and check for head injury.
- Perform a CT scan of the orbit.
- Refer the patient to the maxillofacial team for surgery.

Management of chemical eye injuries

▶▶ Chemical injury

Serious chemical injuries are considered to be among the most urgent ocular emergency conditions requiring immediate attention. Patients attending with such conditions require immediate irrigation, as this will improve their prognosis.

Chemical injuries can range from very mild (e.g. shampoo) to severely sight-threatening alkali burns (e.g. plaster, oven cleaner). Alkali burns tend to be more severe than acid burns, with the exception of concentrated acid.

Signs and symptoms
- Pain.
- Blurred vision.
- Photophobia.
- The sensation of a foreign body in the eye.
- Red eye, although caution is needed, as in severe alkali burns the conjunctiva will appear white due to the conjunctival blood vessels being damaged.
- Decreased visual acuity.
- Epithelial defect shown on fluorescein staining.
- Hazy cornea.

Management

- Check the pH of both eyes, even if the patient states that the chemical only entered one eye. Normal pH is 7.4.
- Document the time and nature of the chemical injury, and ask to see the container if this is available. If there is any uncertainty about the nature of the substance, contact the National Poisons Information Service for further information.
- Instil local anaesthetic eye drops as per local policy to the affected eye to ensure that irrigation will be tolerated.
- Irrigate the eye copiously with at least 1 L of normal saline 0.9% solution delivered via an intravenous giving set. The eye needs to be everted, and irrigation should be delivered for 15–30 min. Ask the patient to move their eye from left to right and up and down, to ensure that all areas of the eye are irrigated.
- When irrigation is complete, wait 5 min before retesting the pH of the eye. If the pH remains abnormal, recommence irrigation.

Useful website

TOXBASE®. ℛ www.toxbase.org

Ocular tumours

A tumour is a swelling of a part of the body caused by an abnormal growth of tissue. A neoplastic tumour is a growth consisting of abnormal new tissue, which may be either benign or malignant. Malignant tumours can spread to various parts of the eye as well as other parts of the body.

Conjunctival tumours

Conjunctival tumours grow on the surface of the eye and may be pigmented or non-pigmented. They are usually benign, but can be malignant.

Non-pigmented conjunctival tumours
- Benign papilloma.
- Benign (pre-malignant).
- Squamous-cell carcinoma (malignant).

Pigmented conjunctival tumours
- Naevus (benign).
- Benign (pre-malignant).
- Malignant melanoma.
- Conjunctival lymphoma.

Haemangioma

This is a benign tumour that consists of abnormal blood vessels. Fluid can leak from the tumour, causing distorted and blurred vision.

Treatment
- Photodynamic therapy.
- Radiotherapy.

Choroidal naevus

These tumours are typically asymptomatic, flat, and pigmented. They can cause retinal detachment.

Low-risk naevus
- Small in size (< 1 mm in height).
- Retinal photography should be performed every 4–6 months to monitor the tumour.

High-risk naevus
- Larger than low-risk naevus (> 2 mm in height).
- Contains lipofuscin pigment granules.
- May be associated with retinal detachment.
- Refer the patient to the ocular oncology unit for investigation.

Choroidal melanoma

Choroidal melanoma accounts for the majority of uveal melanomas. Patients are usually Caucasian and aged 55–75 years.

Signs and symptoms
- Vision loss.
- Floaters.
- Conjunctival and episcleral vessels will be dilated.
- Posterior malignant melanomas are elevated.
- Brown lesions will be seen.

Classification
- Small (< 2 mm in thickness and < 8 mm in diameter).
- Medium (> 2.5 mm in thickness and 8–16 mm in diameter).
- Large (> 8 mm in thickness and > 16 mm in diameter).

Investigations
- Colour photography.
- Ultrasound scan.
- Liver function tests.
- Liver ultrasound scan.
- If metastases are present, refer the patient to an oncologist.

Treatment
- Referral to ocular oncology unit.
- Brachytherapy for tumours up to 7 mm in height.
- Local tumour resection.
- Enucleation for large tumours.
- The patient will require lifelong follow-up, initially 6-monthly and then annually.
- The patient should be told to contact the eye unit if their vision deteriorates.
- The patient will need to be offered counselling.

Iris melanoma

Iris melanoma accounts for 5–10% of all uveal tract melanomas.[5] It is usually well differentiated, and rarely metastasizes.

Signs and symptoms
- If the tumour is large there may be visual symptoms.
- IOP may be elevated.
- The patient may be symptom free.
- The melanoma will be raised.
- It will appear dark brown in colour.
- It usually grows from the pupil margin.

Treatment
- Treat any raised IOP.
- Observation may be sufficient if the melanoma is small.
- Tumour resection.
- Radiation therapy.

Reference

5 Jackson TL (ed.). *Moorfields Manual of Ophthalmology*, 2nd edn. JP Medical Ltd: London, 2014.

Conditions of the eyelid

Entropion
This is a condition in which the eyelid turns inward. It more commonly affects the lower lid, and usually occurs in old age.

Signs and symptoms
- Watery eye.
- Red eye.
- The sensation of a foreign body in the eye, caused by the eyelashes rubbing the eye.
- Inverted lid.
- Punctate epithelial keratopathy.
- Skin laxity.

Treatment
- The patient will require surgery to repair entropion.
- The lid can be taped outward to prevent it from rolling inward. Use a thin strip of Transpore™ tape, but tell the patient to change the site of the tape regularly to prevent soreness of the skin.
- A botulinum toxin A injection may offer a solution for those who are unable to tolerate surgery.[6]

Ectropion
This is a condition in which the eyelid is turned outward.

Signs and symptoms
- Watery eye.
- Red eye.
- Mucous discharge.
- Part or all of the lower lid is everted.
- The lid fails to return to the normal position when pulled away from the eye.

Treatment
- Careful examination to exclude a lower lid mass.
- Temporary taping of the lid horizontally.
- Surgical repair.

Trichiasis
This condition is caused by misdirection of an eyelash growing inward toward the eye.

Signs and symptoms
- The sensation of a foreign body in the eye.
- Watery eye.
- Ingrowing eyelash rubbing on the conjunctiva and cornea.
- Mild conjunctival redness where the eyelash is rubbing.

Treatment
- Epilation.
- If the condition is persistent, electrolysis may be required.
- The patient may need ocular lubricants.

Chalazion

A cyst in the eyelid that is formed as a result of blockage of one of the meibomian glands in the eyelid.

Signs and symptoms
- Mild discomfort.
- Redness and swelling of the lid, which may sometimes be as large as a pea.
- On eversion a yellow area may be seen.
- If the cyst is large, vision may be distorted due to pressure on the cornea.

Treatment
- Warm compressions several times a day.
- If this does not resolve the condition after several weeks, the patient may need a referral for incision and drainage.
- Advise the patient to seek medical advice if they develop a temperature, or if the lid becomes swollen or hot to touch.

Herpes zoster

In patients who have previously had chicken pox, herpes zoster occurs when the virus becomes reactivated in the ophthalmic division of the trigeminal nerve. This is often due to age or a compromised immune system.

Signs and symptoms
- Flu-like symptoms.
- A burning or needle-pricking sensation around the eye, followed by a rash on the upper eyelid following the fifth cranial nerve.
- The patient may have a red conjunctiva. This is more likely if the rash extends to the tip of the nose.
- The patient may have blurred vision if there is corneal involvement.
- Pain.
- Usually occurs in individuals over 60 years of age.
- Punctate keratitis.

Treatment
- Oral aciclovir five times a day for 5 days.
- The patient may require ocular lubricants.
- If there is corneal involvement, the patient may require steroid eye drops.
- They may need to see their GP regarding neuralgia pain.
- If the patient is employed, they will need to be on sick leave by either self-certification or a sickness certification.

Reference

6 Jackson TL (ed.). *Moorfields Manual of Ophthalmology*, 2nd edn. JP Medical Ltd: London, 2014.

Upper gastrointestinal and hepatobiliary surgery

Acute upper gastrointestinal bleed

Upper gastrointestinal bleeds arise from above the ligament of Treitz, which connects the fourth portion of the duodenum to the diaphragm. Haematemesis is the vomiting of blood, and is indicative of an acute upper gastrointestinal bleed. Melaena is predominantly due to an upper gastrointestinal bleed, and is the passing of black 'tarry' faeces. The black appearance is due to the oxidation of the iron in haemoglobin, as blood passes through the ileum and colon.

Causes

- Duodenal ulcer is the most common cause of acute upper gastrointestinal bleed, and is due to *Helicobactor pylori* (*H. pylori*) infection or non-steroidal anti-inflammatory drugs (NSAIDs).
- Gastric ulcer is common in the elderly, and is mainly caused by *H. pylori* or NSAIDs.
- Gastric erosion is inflammation of the mucous membrane of the stomach due to NSAIDs, excessive alcohol consumption, or stress following trauma or major surgery.
- Mallory–Weiss tear of the gastric or oesophageal mucosa is caused by forceful vomiting.
- Oesophageal varices develop as a result of portal hypertension, which is mainly caused by liver cirrhosis.
- Oesophagitis is an acute or chronic inflammation of the oesophagus due to gastro-oesophageal reflux disease (GORD), infection, or excessive alcohol consumption.

►► Initial management

- Assessment of the severity of haemorrhage and haemodynamic state.
- Fluid replacement to restore blood volume, in order to ensure that tissue perfusion and oxygen delivery are not compromised.
- Assess whether the airway is at risk due to altered mental or respiratory status or ongoing haematemesis, as this may require intubation.

Endoscopy

After fluid resuscitation and stabilization, endoscopy is the preferred procedure for diagnosis and treatment of an upper gastrointestinal bleed. Endoscopic therapy can be broadly categorized into injection therapy, thermal coagulation, and mechanical haemostasis.

- Injection therapy involves injecting a solution of diluted epinephrine into the bleeding ulcer, causing vasoconstriction and compression.
- Thermal coagulation involves the heating of tissue and the compression of the blood vessel during heating.
- Mechanical methods include the use of a haemoclip, which is similar in principle to applying a surgical ligature.

Pharmacological therapies

- Intravenous proton pump inhibitors (omeprazole or pantoprazole) reduce the risk of re-bleeding and the need for surgery on peptic ulcers.
- Somatostatin and octreotide injections for the treatment of oesophageal and gastric variceal bleeding.

Surgical interventions

Urgent surgery is undertaken if a large haemorrhage is not stopped by endoscopic treatment, or if the patient re-bleeds after endoscopic treatment. The type of surgery can vary depending on the site of the bleed, but includes:

- oversewing of an ulcer
- vagotomy and pyloroplasty
- partial gastrectomy
- angiographic transarterial embolization
- transjugular intrahepatic portosystemic shunt (TIPS) to treat oesophageal and gastric variceal bleeds due to portal hypertension.

Further reading

Scottish Intercollegiate Guidelines Network (SIGN). *Management of Acute Upper and Lower Gastrointestinal Bleeding.* SIGN: Edinburgh, 2008.

Gastro-oesophageal reflux disease

Gastro-oesophageal reflux disease (GORD) is a common chronic condition in which the gastric contents reflux out of the stomach and into the oesophagus. This prolongs the exposure of the oesophageal mucosa to gastric acid with a pH of less than 4. Ultimately this will damage the oesophageal mucosa, leading to oesophagitis.

Prolonged gastro-oesophageal reflux increases the risk of oesophageal adenocarcinoma by about eightfold.

Causes
- Abnormal lower oesophageal sphincter pressure.
- Hiatus hernia.
- Delayed gastric emptying.
- Medication that affects lower oesophageal sphincter pressure (e.g. calcium-channel blockers, beta blockers, theophylline, and anticholinergic drugs).

Signs and symptoms
- Heartburn, especially following meals and when lying down.
- Regurgitation of acid or bile.
- Dysphagia due to defects in peristaltic function.
- Excess salivation.

Behavioural modifications
- Reduction in fat intake, as fat delays gastric emptying.
- Weight reduction.
- Smoking cessation.
- Small regular meals.
- Try not to eat within 3 h before going to bed.
- Avoid hot drinks and alcohol prior to bedtime.
- Avoid drugs that affect oesophageal motility or damage the oesophageal mucosa.

Pharmacological therapies
- Proton pump inhibitors.
- H_2 antagonists.

Surgical interventions
- Required if pharmacological interventions fail.
- Laparoscopic anti-reflux surgery.
- The oesophageal sphincter is reinforced by wrapping the upper portion of the stomach around the lowest portion of the oesophagus.

Further reading
Van Baalen C. Managing gastro-oesphageal reflux disease the surgical way. *Gastrointestinal Nursing* 2008; 6: 24–9.

Gastric tumours

The incidence of gastric tumours in the UK has declined by 50% in the last 50 years. However, it still carries a poor prognosis due to non-specific symptoms in the early stages resulting in a late diagnosis. It rarely occurs before the age of 40 years, and the majority of cases occur after the age of 55 years and in the seventh decade.

The tumour can occur anywhere in the stomach, but the number of gastric tumours occurring at the gastro-oesophageal junction is increasing. This is thought to be due to the rising incidence of GORD. The majority of gastric tumours are adenocarcinomas which are classified as diffuse or intestinal. Diffuse adenocarcinomas are more common and have a poorer survival rate.

Risk factors
- Age over 60 years.
- Male gender.
- Low socio-economic status.
- Smoking.
- Obesity, as it increases the risk of GORD.
- Chronic infection with *H. pylori*.
- A diet that is high in salt, and low in fruit and vegetables.
- Diagnosis of oesophagitis or GORD.
- Family history of a parent or sibling being diagnosed with a gastric tumour.
- Radiation exposure.

Common early signs and symptoms
- Heartburn.
- Feeling bloated.
- Loss of appetite.
- Persistent stomach pains.

Later signs and symptoms
- Unexplained weight loss.
- Anaemia.
- Jaundice.
- Dysphagia.
- Nausea and vomiting.

Diagnosis and staging
- Gastroscopy allows both visualization of the tumour location and biopsy.
- The size, position, and extent of the tumour enable staging.
- CT scan of the thorax, abdomen, and pelvis is routine to detect metastases.

Treatment of resectable gastric tumours
- Partial or total gastrectomy.
- Lymph node resection of locoregional nodes.
- Laparoscopic resection.
- Endoscopic mucosal resection for early gastric tumours.
- Chemotherapy before or after surgery.
- Radiotherapy.

Treatment of unresectable or metastatic gastric tumours
- The aim of surgery should be to relieve symptoms.
- Gastric bypass.
- Gastroscopy and/or placement of a jejunostomy tube for enteral feeding.
- Chemotherapy.
- Radiotherapy.
- Endoscopic insertion of self-expanding stents to treat obstructions.

Further reading
Bailey K. An overview of gastric cancer and its management. *Cancer Nursing Practice* 2011 10: 31–7.
Cancer Research UK. *Stomach Cancer Incidence Statistics.* Cancer Research UK: London, 2011 www.cancerresearchuk.org/health-professional/cancer-statistics/statistics-by-cancer type/stomach-cancer/incidence

Bariatric surgery

Obesity is an increasing health problem that has associated health risks which affect the cardiovascular, respiratory, and endocrine systems. Body mass index (BMI) is a crude measure of overall nutritional status. It is calculated by dividing the person's weight in kilograms by their height in metres squared.

Bariatric surgery is an option for individuals with severe obesity, and its use has increased in recent years. This is partly due to improved surgical techniques which are less invasive, leading to reduced mortality and length of stay in hospital.

Criteria for surgery

The National Institute for Health and Care Excellence (NICE) has produced guidelines[1] which suggest that bariatric surgery should be considered for people who:

- have a BMI of ≥ 40 kg/m^2
- have a BMI of 35–40 kg/m^2 and a disease such as hypertension or type 2 diabetes, which would improve with weight loss
- with non-surgical measures have failed to achieve a clinically beneficial weight loss over at least a 6-month period
- are fit enough to undergo surgery and a general anaesthetic
- are committed to long-term follow-up.

Types of surgery

There are three types of bariatric surgery:

- gastric restriction
- malabsorptive procedures
- combined restrictive and malabsorptive surgery.

Gastric restrictive surgery

Gastric restrictive surgery is aimed at producing a small pouch, so that the patient feels 'full' after only eating small amounts. However, it may not be successful, as the patient can still drink higher-calorie drinks. The following types of procedure are undertaken:

- vertical banding, which involves stapling part of the fundus of the stomach, to produce a reservoir and a band narrowing the diameter of the outlet
- laparoscopic adjustable gastric banding, which consists of an inflated silicone band that is placed around the upper part of the stomach
- vertical sleeve gastrectomy, which involves removing 85% of the stomach while ensuring that the pylorus and nerve supply remain intact. This procedure is irreversible, whereas the other two types are reversible.

Malabsorptive procedures

These procedures aim to reduce the absorption of nutrients as a result of a large percentage of food bypassing the stomach and directly entering the small bowel. The length of the small bowel is reduced, thereby decreasing the transit time of food and reducing absorption.

Careful management and monitoring are required following these procedures, due to the risk of electrolyte imbalances and vitamin deficiencies.

- The biliopancreatic diversion involves removal of the lower part of the stomach, with a direct anastomosis to the jejunum.
- A variation of the biliopancreatic diversion involves a duodenal switch, whereby the pylorus is retained, preventing increased transit into the small intestine.

Combined malabsorptive and restrictive surgery

The Roux-en-Y bypass involves the creation of a small pouch, following the transaction of the stomach. The pouch is joined to the jejunum, bypassing the rest of the stomach and the small intestine.

Surgical complications following bariatric surgery

- Venous thromboembolism.
- Gastrointestinal leakage at the surgical site.
- Wound dehiscence and major wound infection due to obesity.
- Small bowel obstruction.
- Malnutrition leading to anaemia, vitamin B_{12} deficiency, and osteoporosis.
- 'Dumping syndrome'—a condition in which food leaves the stomach too quickly and enters the small intestine largely undigested. Symptoms include nausea, vomiting, bloating, cramping, diarrhoea, dizziness, and fatigue.
- Abdominal hernia.
- Gallstones due to rapid weight loss.
- Inflammatory hepatitis due to rapid weight loss.

Reference

1 National Institute for Health and Care Excellence (NICE). *Obesity: guidance on the prevention of overweight and obesity in adults and children.* CG43. NICE: London, 2006. www.nice.org.uk/guidance/cg43

Further reading

Scottish Intercollegiate Guidelines Network (SIGN). *Management of Obesity: a national clinical guideline.* SIGN: Edinburgh, 2010.

Gastrointestinal perforation

Gastrointestinal perforation involves intestinal contents leaking into the abdominal cavity from the stomach, small intestine, or large bowel. Perforation of the stomach can lead to leakage of gastric acid, and perforation of the intestine can result in bacterial contamination of the abdominal cavity. Whatever the cause or the location within the gastrointestinal tract, this condition is a medical emergency.

Causes
- Gastric ulcer.
- Appendicitis.
- Diverticulitis.
- Ingestion of corrosive substances or foreign bodies.
- Gastrointestinal cancer.
- Trauma, including penetrating injury or blunt trauma.
- Inflammatory bowel disease.
- Injury caused during endoscopy, endoscopic retrograde cholangiopancreatography (ERCP), or colonoscopy.

Signs and symptoms
- Severe abdominal pain.
- Rigid abdomen.
- Nausea and vomiting.
- Rebound tenderness.
- Pyrexia.
- Signs of hypovolaemic and/or septic shock.

Diagnosis
- Clinical examination.
- Abdominal X-ray showing free gas in the abdominal cavity.
- CT scan.
- Raised white blood cell count.

▶▶ Treatment
- Depends upon the cause, but generally involves surgery.
- Exploratory laparotomy and closure of perforation with peritoneal washout.
- Fluid resuscitation.
- Antibiotics.
- Nil by mouth (NBM) and nasogastric aspiration/drainage.

▶ Peritonitis
Gastrointestinal perforation can lead to peritonitis, which is inflammation of the peritoneum (the thin tissue covering the abdominal cavity, abdominal organs, and the outside of the intestines).

Causes

Peritonitis can be acute or chronic, but the following are the most common types:

- *Primary bacterial* peritonitis is an infection that occurs as a complication of ascites which is associated with chronic liver disease.
- *Secondary bacterial* peritonitis is caused by bacteria entering the peritoneum following perforation of the abdominal viscus.
- *Tertiary* peritonitis is caused by recurrent or persistent infection.
- *Continuous ambulatory peritoneal dialysis (CAPD)-associated* peritonitis is caused by bacteria or fungi entering the abdominal cavity via the dialysis catheter.

Signs and symptoms

- Abdominal pain, tenderness, and guarding.
- Rigid abdomen.
- Nausea and vomiting.
- Pyrexia.
- Signs of hypovolaemia and/or septic shock.

Diagnosis

- Clinical examination.
- Full blood count, arterial blood gas analysis, and blood cultures.
- Peritoneal fluid analysis.
- Ultrasound scan.
- CT scan.

▶▶ Treatment

- Fluid resuscitation and correction of electrolyte disturbances.
- Intravenous antibiotic or antifungal therapy.
- Surgery to repair the perforation or drain the abscess.

Oesophageal disease

Barrett's oesophagus

Barrett's oesophagus refers to a change in the appearance of the oesophageal lining due to acid and bile refluxing into the lower oesophagus, resulting in inflammation. The squamous epithelium of the lower oesophagus becomes replaced by red columnar epithelium, similar to the cells that line the stomach. These changed cells have an increased risk of developing into pre-cancerous cells, increasing the risk of a person with Barrett's oesophagus developing oesophageal adenocarcinoma.

Risk factors
- GORD.
- Male gender.
- Age 50–70 years.
- Smoking.
- Obesity.

Symptoms
- Heartburn.
- Pain in the upper abdomen and chest.
- Nausea and an acid taste in the mouth.
- Belching and bloating.

Diagnosis and treatment
- Endoscopy and biopsies if Barrett's oesophagus is suspected.
- Pharmacological treatment of acid reflux.
- Laser therapy of abnormal cells.
- Photodynamic therapy.
- Epithelial radio-frequency ablation.
- Argon plasma coagulation.
- Endoscopic mucosal resection to remove affected oesophageal cells.

Oesophageal cancer

Oesophageal cancer is rare in the UK, but its incidence has risen in the last 20 years, with about 7500 cases diagnosed each year. It has a poor prognosis due in part to the late presentation of symptoms. The two main types of oesophageal cancer are adenocarcinoma and squamous-cell carcinoma.

Adenocarcinoma occurs in the lower third of the oesophagus and at the gastro-oesophageal junction, with dysplastic changes being mainly due to reflux. Squamous-cell carcinoma mainly occurs in the middle and upper oesophagus, and is linked to alcohol, diet, and smoking.

Risk factors and causes
- GORD.
- Alcohol and smoking.
- Barrett's oesophagus.
- Male gender and age over 45 years.
- Obesity.

Symptoms
- Dysphagia.
- Acid indigestion.
- Weight loss.
- Hoarseness or chronic cough.
- Haematemesis.

Diagnosis and staging
- Endoscopic biopsy provides histology for diagnosis.
- Clinical examination and blood tests.
- CT scan of the chest and abdomen for evidence of spread to lymph nodes and major organs such as the lungs or liver.
- Endoscopic ultrasound to diagnose the extent of spread in the oesophageal wall.
- Laparoscopy to detect peritoneal spread.
- Staging of tumour based on the tumour–node–metastasis system.

Treatment
- Oesophagectomy for localized tumours provides the only chance of cure, but only 20% of patients will survive to 5 years.
- Pre-operative chemotherapy for adenocarcinoma increases the survival rate, and post-operative chemotherapy is also used to destroy micrometastases.
- For metastatic disease, single-dose brachytherapy is used to shrink the tumour and treat obstruction of the oesophagus. This involves the insertion of a radioactive material in or near the tumour.
- Palliative chemotherapy is used in selected patients.

Post-operative care following oesophagectomy
- Pain management is key to reducing cardiopulmonary complications.
- Chest physiotherapy to prevent atelectasis and pneumonia.
- Accurate fluid balance to restore circulating volume due to fluid shifts while preventing fluid overload as the patient is at risk of pulmonary oedema.
- Nasogastric tube to drain air and fluid from the stomach.
- NBM for 5–7 days until the anastomosis has healed.
- Jejunostomy for feeding.

Further reading
Stahl M et al. Esophageal cancer: Clinical Practice Guidelines for diagnosis, treatment and follow-up. *Annals of Oncology* 2010; 21 (Suppl. 5): 46–9.

Pancreatic disease

The pancreas is located close to the stomach in the abdominal cavity. Its tail lies close to the spleen, and the pancreatic head is encircled by the duodenum. It is an endocrine gland that produces the hormones somatostatin, glucagon, and insulin in the islets of Langerhans. It is also an exocrine gland that produces the pancreatic enzymes amylase, lipase, and protease in an inactive form within the pancreatic pyramidal acinar cells.

Pancreatitis

Acute pancreatitis is a rapidly developing and potentially fatal inflammation of the pancreas, involving other organ systems. Chronic pancreatitis causes progressive and irreversible damage to the pancreas, which cannot be corrected by removing the cause.

This inflammation of the pancreas occurs when pancreatic enzymes are prematurely activated before they reach the small intestine. The enzymes leak into the pancreatic tissue, initiating autodigestion of the tissue and cell membranes. Interstitial oedema develops in the pancreatic parenchyma along with necrosis of the parenchyma and pancreatic fat, and vessel damage. This damage triggers the release of inflammatory mediators such as bradykinin, histamine, and prostaglandin, resulting in systemic complications.

Causes

- Gallstones.
- Excessive alcohol consumption.
- Accidental damage during ERCP.
- Viral infection (e.g. mumps).

Signs and symptoms

- Severe abrupt onset of abdominal pain radiating to the back.
- Nausea and vomiting.
- Abdominal distension associated with small bowel ileus or pseudocyst.
- Low-grade pyrexia.
- Septic shock.

Diagnosis

- Clinical features.
- Plasma pancreatic enzyme levels are three times higher than normal.
- C-reactive protein (CRP) concentration is > 150 mg/L at 48 h.
- Ultrasound scan should be performed if gallstones are suspected.
- Contrast-enhanced CT scan should be performed if doubt exists.
- Abdominal X-ray.

Treatment

- NBM, and severe acute cases may require enteral feeding.
- Intravenous fluids.
- Oxygen therapy.
- Analgesia.
- Removal of gallstones.
- Drainage of pseudocyst.

Pancreatic cancer

Pancreatic cancer is typically diagnosed at an advanced stage, when it has spread into neighbouring organs and structures, making resection almost impossible. The late presentation is due to individuals being asymptomatic or having vague non-specific symptoms such as weight loss, abdominal pain, dyspepsia, and fatigue.

Risk factors

- Smoking.
- Diet high in processed meats and fat.
- Cirrhosis.
- Chronic pancreatitis.
- Family history of pancreatic cancer (first-degree relative).

Diagnosis

- CT scan.
- Magnetic resonance imaging (MRI) scan.
- Biopsy and brushings may be taken using ERCP.
- Ultrasound scan.

Treatment

- Surgery:
  - Whipple procedure
  - distal pancreatectomy
  - total pancreatectomy.
- Chemotherapy.
- Radiotherapy.
- Stenting of bile ducts to relieve jaundice.

Splenic injury

The spleen is a lymphoid organ in the left upper quadrant of the abdomen. It is located beneath the diaphragm, and lies between the ninth and eleventh ribs. It is a soft blood-rich organ that filters blood, clearing it of bacteria and viruses. The spleen is the most important peripheral immune organ, as it contains more lymphatic tissue than all the lymph nodes in the body. It predominantly responds to blood-borne bacteria in septicaemia, and provides a site of lymphocyte proliferation.

Other functions of the spleen include destruction of worn out red blood cells, and delivering the breakdown products of this process to the liver. It is also a blood reservoir, and during haemorrhage empties its store of blood into the circulation.

Causes of splenic injury

- Blunt trauma due to:
  - motor vehicle accident
  - injury during contact sports
  - bicycle accident
  - domestic violence.
- Glandular fever.
- Haemolytic anaemia and certain types of lymphoma.
- Malaria.

Symptoms

- Left-sided abdominal pain under the rib cage.
- Left shoulder pain.
- Confusion.
- Fainting.
- Signs of hypovolaemic shock.

Diagnosis

- CT scan is considered to be the gold standard for evaluating and grading splenic injury.
- Ultrasound scan is the method of choice, as it is quick, easy, and non-invasive.

Grading of splenic injury

The Organ Injury Scaling Committee of the American Association for the Surgery of Trauma has devised a universal grading system for individual organs.[2,3] The splenic injury scale or an adapted version is used to guide treatment options.

- Grade 1: a subcapsular haematoma that is < 10% of surface area and a capsular tear < 1 cm in depth.
- Grade 2: a subcapsular haematoma that is 10–50% of surface area or intra-parenchymal haematoma < 5 cm in diameter and a tear 1–3 cm in depth not involving trabecular vessels.
- Grade 3: subcapsular haematoma that is > 50% of surface area or ruptured with active bleeding. Intra-parenchymal haematoma > 5 cm in diameter and tear > 3 cm in depth or involving trabecular vessels.

- Grade 4: a laceration involving the segmental or hilar vessels producing devascularization of > 25% of the spleen.
- Grade 5: completely shattered spleen or hilar vascular injury that devascularizes the spleen.

Splenic repair

- Use of adhesives for grade 1 and 2 lesions, which involves the use of fibrin glue and collagen fleece. It can be combined with other techniques.
- Parenchymal suture, although this technique is complex and unsuitable for extensive ruptures.
- Coagulation techniques are used to control bleeding from superficial lacerations, and consist of techniques such as infrared and laser coagulation.
- Partial resection for grade 2 or 3 injuries which are limited to one pole or half the spleen. This is done using a stapler and adhesives.
- Mesh splenorrhaphy is used for extensive tears involving both hilar and diaphragmatic surfaces. A vicryl mesh with an absorbable thread is wrapped around the spleen and the thread pulled together on the hilar face to achieve haemostasis.
- Splenectomy is performed when the spleen is shattered or there is separation of the hilus. Following splenectomy the patient should be immunized with the pneumococcus vaccine.

Long-term care to prevent infection following splenectomy

- Pneumococcal, *Haemophilus influenzae* type b (Hib), meningococcal, and influenza vaccines.
- Lifelong antibiotic therapy for high-risk groups.
- Low-risk groups should be counselled about the risks and benefits of antibiotic prophylaxis.
- All patients should carry a supply of appropriate antibiotics for emergency use.
- All patients should carry written or electronic information to alert health professionals to the risk of overwhelming infection.

References

2 TraumaSource. *Injury Scoring Scale: a resource for trauma care professionals*. ℜ www.aast.org library/traumatools/injuryscoringscales.aspx
3 Moore EE et al. Organ injury scaling: spleen and liver (1994 revision). *Journal of Trauma* 1995 38: 323–4.

Further reading

Davies J et al. Review of guidelines for the prevention and treatment of infection in patients with an absent or dysfunctional spleen: prepared on behalf of the British Committee for Standard in Haematology by a Working Party of the Haemato-Oncology Task Force. *British Journal of Haematology* 2011: 155: 308–17.

The gall bladder and biliary tree

The gall bladder is a small pear-shaped sac that sits in a shallow fossa on the inferior surface of the liver. Its main function is to store bile, which is required to digest fats in the small intestine. Bile flows from the liver via the left and right hepatic ducts into the common hepatic duct. This then connects with the cystic duct coming from the gall bladder, to form the common bile duct. The biliary tree consists of the gall bladder and the ducts carrying bile and other digestive enzymes to the small intestine from the liver, gall bladder, and pancreas.

Gallstones

Cholelithiasis is the medical term for gallstones, which are biliary calculi. The two main types are cholesterol stones, which form when there is an excess of cholesterol in the bile, and pigment stones, which form when there is an excess of bilirubin in the bile.

Risk factors

- Age > 65 years.
- Female gender.
- Obesity.
- Family history.
- Rapid weight loss.

Signs and symptoms

- Right upper quadrant pain which may radiate to the shoulder blades.
- Pain experienced after eating fatty foods.
- Nausea and vomiting.
- Belching and indigestion.

Diagnosis and treatment

- Ultrasound scan is the method of choice.
- ERCP if it is suspected that stones are present in the ducts.
- CT scan if it is not possible to perform ERCP.
- Low-fat diet.
- Removal of stones via ERCP.
- Lithotripsy to break up gallstones.
- Laparoscopic cholecystectomy to remove the gall bladder.
- Open cholecystectomy via a laparotomy.

Primary sclerosing cholangitis

Primary sclerosing cholangitis (PSC) is an uncommon chronic liver disease in which the bile ducts inside and outside the liver become inflamed, resulting in the development of scar tissue. The bile ducts become narrowed over time, and there is a build-up of bile within the liver, which causes inflammation and scarring of the hepatic cells.

The cause of PSC is not known, but current evidence suggests that it is triggered by an unknown bacterium or virus in individuals who are genetically programmed to develop the disorder. It frequently occurs in patients with inflammatory bowel disease, especially ulcerative colitis, but is also seen in those with Crohn's disease.

Signs and symptoms

- Tiredness.
- Abdominal discomfort in the right upper quadrant.
- Itching due to build-up of bile salts.
- Jaundice due to blockage of the bile ducts.
- Malabsorption of fat and vitamins A, D, E, and K.

Diagnosis and treatment

- ERCP.
- Magnetic resonance imaging (MRI).
- Liver function tests (LFTs) and autoantibody blood tests.
- Liver biopsy may be used to stage progression of the disease.
- Medication to relieve itching, and to supplement vitamins and bile acids.
- ERCP to stent the common bile duct may be required.
- Ultimately, liver transplantation will be required.

Cholangiocarcinoma

Cholangiocarcinoma is a cancer occurring in any part of the biliary tree. The majority are adenocarcinomas, and the rest are squamous-cell tumours. The incidence in the UK has increased significantly in recent decades, and the prognosis remains poor due to the fact that in around 50% of cases there is lymph node involvement.

Risk factors

- PSC with or without ulcerative colitis.
- Increasing age.
- Chronic intraductal gallstones.
- Congenital abnormalities of the bile ducts.

Signs and symptoms

- Jaundice with hepatomegaly.
- Abdominal pain in the right upper quadrant.
- Weight loss.
- Pale-coloured stools and dark urine.
- Itching.

Diagnosis and treatment

- Bloods to check LFTs, clotting, and tumour markers.
- MRI.
- Curative surgical resection based on the site and extent of bile duct involvement.
- Palliative surgical resection.
- Chemotherapy.
- ERCP to insert bile duct stents for relief of symptoms.

Small bowel disease

The small intestine consists of the duodenum, jejunum, and ileum, and it is here where chemical digestion of food begins in earnest. The majority of food absorption takes place within the small intestine, which has a large surface area to aid the process.

Coeliac disease

Coeliac disease is an autoimmune response to gluten in the diet, which results in chronic inflammatory disease in genetically susceptible individuals. Upon exposure to gluten the immune system reacts with the small bowel tissue, leading to an inflammatory response. This results in atrophy of the villi that line the small intestine, which leads to impairment of the absorption of nutrients.

Previously coeliac disease was considered to be an uncommon disease of childhood, presenting as diarrhoea, weight loss, and failure to thrive. Now the commonest age for presentation is 40–60 years, but it remains underdiagnosed or misdiagnosed as irritable bowel syndrome.

Risk factors and associated disorders

- Female gender.
- First-degree relative with coeliac disease.
- Thyroid disease.
- Type 1 diabetes.
- Irritable bowel syndrome.

Signs and symptoms

- Chronic or intermittent diarrhoea.
- Abdominal pain, bloating, and flatulence.
- Prolonged fatigue.
- Isolated nutritional deficiency (e.g. anaemia).
- Osteoporosis not attributed to other causes.

Diagnosis and treatment[4]

- Does the patient have any of the signs, symptoms, or related conditions?
- Are they on a gluten-containing diet?
- If the answer to these questions is yes, perform serological testing for IgA tissue transglutaminase (tTGA).
- If the tTGA test result is equivocal, test for IgA endomysial antibodies (EMA).
- Refer the patient to a gastroenterologist for small bowel biopsy to confirm or exclude coeliac disease.
- Prescribe lifelong adherence to a gluten-free diet.

Crohn's disease

Crohn's disease is a chronic inflammatory bowel disease that can affect multiple areas of the gastrointestinal tract at any one time, but in the majority of patients there is involvement of the terminal ileum. The inflammatory reaction is considered to occur when a person's immune system reacts abnormally to the presence of bacteria, food, and other substances. White blood cells accumulate in the lining of the intestines causing damage to the full thickness of the bowel.

Three types of disease activity occur in Crohn's disease:

- *inflammatory* type, characterized by diarrhoea, abdominal pain, and fever
- *penetrating* type, in which abscesses and fistulae develop, extending into the peritoneum
- *stricturing* type, which leads to bowel obstruction.

Risk factors

- First-degree relative with inflammatory bowel disease.
- Age 15–30 years, although Crohn's disease can develop at any age.
- Smoking.

Signs and symptoms

- Abdominal pain, especially in the right lower quadrant.
- Diarrhoea, which may contain mucus, blood, or pus.
- Weight loss.
- General tiredness.
- Mouth ulcers.
- Arthritis.

Diagnosis

- Blood tests, including serological antibodies.
- Stool culture and microscopy.
- Colonoscopy, including biopsies.
- Barium enema.
- Wireless capsule endoscopy.

Treatment

- Anti-inflammatory drugs containing mesalazine.
- Steroids and immune system suppressors.
- Antibiotics.
- Dietary treatment (e.g. a strict liquid diet).
- Surgery to relieve symptoms or correct complications such as abscess or blockage.
- Surgery may involve resection of part of the bowel or all of the colon leading to formation of an ileostomy.

Reference

4 National Institute for Health and Care Excellence (NICE). *Coeliac Disease: recognition and assessment of coeliac disease.* CG86. NICE: London, 2009. ℜ www.nice.org.uk/guidance/cg86

Liver disease

Acute liver failure is defined as rapid hepatocellular dysfunction that leads to coagulopathy, encephalopathy, and multi-organ failure. The high mortality and morbidity associated with acute liver failure are due to the complications that develop. These include cerebral oedema, renal failure, and cardiovascular failure due to systemic inflammatory response syndrome (SIRS) and sepsis.

Chronic liver failure is a disease process that involves the progressive destruction of the liver, resulting in fibrosis and cirrhosis (see Table 18.1).

Diagnosis and treatment

- Bloods for LFTs, glucose, full blood count, renal function, coagulation, autoimmune markers, and hepatitis serology.
- Arterial blood gas analysis and lactate level.
- Toxicology screen if overdose is suspected.
- Ultrasound scan.
- Endoscopy if oesophageal varices are suspected.
- ERCP if intrahepatic or extrahepatic biliary obstruction is suspected.
- Liver biopsy and histology.
- Treatment is based on supportive care and is guided by the cause.
- Whenever possible the precipitating cause should be removed.
- If damage is severe, the patient will require liver transplantation.

Table 18.1 Acute and chronic liver failure

Causes of acute liver failure	Causes of chronic liver failure
Paracetamol overdose	Viral hepatitis B, C, and D
Medication	Excessive alcohol consumption
Viral infection (hepatitis A, B, C, D, and E; Epstein–Barr virus)	Wilson's disease
	Haemochromatosis
Autoimmune hepatitis	Primary biliary cirrhosis
Acute fatty liver of pregnancy	PSC
Toxins (magic mushrooms, organic solvents)	Budd–Chiari syndrome
	Medication
	Cryptogenic causes

Signs and symptoms of acute liver failure	Signs and symptoms of chronic liver failure
Abnormal LFTs	Abnormal LFTs
Jaundice	Jaundice
Coagulopathy	Ascites
Hepatic encephalopathy	Spontaneous bacterial peritonitis
Pain in right upper quadrant	Variceal haemorrhage
Hypoglycaemia	Hepatic encephalopathy
Multi-organ failure	Weight loss
	Renal failure
	Pulmonary oedema

Liver transplantation

Livers for transplants come from three main donor groups:
- donors following brainstem death
- donors following cardiac death
- live donors, where part of the healthy liver from a live donor is used.

Patients require a rigorous physical, psychological, and social assessment of their suitability for liver transplantation. It is important that they understand the need for lifelong medication, lifestyle changes, and the factors that may affect their recovery.

The liver must come from a donor who is approximately the same weight and body size as the recipient. It must be free from disease, infection, or injury, and be of the same blood type as or a compatible blood type with that of the recipient.

Potential complications following liver transplantation

- Haemorrhage.
- Biliary leaks.
- Primary graft non-function.
- Acute rejection.
- Infection.
- Hepatic artery thrombosis.
- Type 2 diabetes.
- Renal failure.
- Malignancy.

Further reading

National Institute for Health and Care Excellence (NICE). *Living-Donor Liver Transplantation*. IPG194. NICE: London, 2006. ℡ www.nice.org.uk/guidance/ipg194
National Institute for Health and Care Excellence (NICE). *Stent Insertion for Bleeding Oesophageal Varices*. IPG392. NICE: London, 2011. ℡ www.nice.org.uk/guidance/ipg392

Liver tumours

Primary hepatocellular carcinoma is the most common type of liver cancer. It is a cancer of the hepatocytes, and is also known as hepatoma. It is very common worldwide, but is rare in the west. Primary hepatocellular carcinoma has a poor prognosis due to the late presentation of symptoms, and only a small percentage of tumours can be completely removed by surgery.

Risk factors
- Male gender.
- Age > 60 years.
- Hepatitis B, C, or D.
- Cirrhosis.
- Asian ethnicity, due to its association with high rates of hepatitis B.
- Excessive alcohol consumption.
- Haemochromatosis.

Signs and symptoms
- Jaundice.
- Pain around the right shoulder blade.
- Abdominal pain in the right upper quadrant.
- Loss of appetite.
- Weight loss.
- Fatigue.

Diagnosis
- Serum tumour markers, such as raised levels of alpha-fetoprotein (AFP).
- LFTs.
- Abdominal CT scan with contrast medium.
- MRI scan.
- Biopsy if the diagnosis remains in question or the result will influence the treatment plan.
- Staging of tumour.

Treatment
- Cryotherapy using liquid nitrogen or liquid carbon dioxide, to freeze and destroy abnormal cells.
- Partial hepatectomy, in which the cancerous part of the liver is removed.
- Total hepatectomy and liver transplant, in which the whole of the liver is removed and replaced with a donor liver.
- Radio-frequency ablation, which uses radio waves to heat and destroy abnormal cells.
- External radiotherapy treatment.
- Internal radiotherapy treatment using radioactive implants that are placed in or near the tumour.

- Regional chemotherapy, which is administered to the blood vessels that supply the tumour.
- Chemoembolization of the hepatic artery.
- Percutaneous ethanol injection into the tumour.

Metastatic liver disease

Metastatic cancer refers to cancer that has spread from the place of origin to another part of the body. The liver is a common site of metastatic disease, as it has a rich dual blood supply, receiving blood via the hepatic artery and the portal vein. Metastatic liver cancer is 20 times more common than primary liver cancer. It generally has a poor prognosis, with a low chance of survival at 1 year.

Primary cancers that cause metastatic liver disease include:

- colorectal cancer
- breast cancer
- lung cancer
- oesophageal cancer
- pancreatic cancer
- stomach cancer
- melanoma.

Further reading

National Institute for Health and Care Excellence (NICE). *Radiofrequency Ablation of Hepatocellular Carcinoma*. IPG2. NICE: London, 2003. ℘ www.nice.org.uk/guidance/ipg2
National Institute for Health and Care Excellence (NICE). *Microwave Ablation of Hepatocellular Carcinoma*. IPG214. NICE: London, 2007. ℘ www.nice.org.uk/guidance/ipg214

Colorectal and lower gastrointestinal surgery

Inflammatory bowel disease

There are a variety of idiopathic disorders within the category of inflammatory bowel disease (IBD), the most notable being ulcerative colitis and Crohn's disease. An unknown factor or agent (or a combination of factors) triggers the body's immune system to produce an inflammatory reaction in the intestinal tract, which then continues in an uncontrolled manner. IBD is frequently seen in the younger age group, and is defined as diseases that cause inflammation along the gastrointestinal tract, diarrhoea, pain, and weight loss. Typically, ulcerative colitis affects only the large bowel, whereas Crohn's disease can affect any part of the gastrointestinal tract from the mouth to the anus. Both conditions can produce extra-intestinal manifestations, such as joint, skin, and eye complications. Both medical and surgical treatments are offered, depending on the extent and severity of the disease process.

Ulcerative colitis

The cause of ulcerative colitis is unknown, but the typical age of onset is 18–30 years, and it often presents as an acute flare-up, sometimes following a gastrointestinal infection or a period of stress. Symptoms include bloody diarrhoea, frequency and urgency of passing faeces, abdominal pain, fever, anaemia, and elevated serum inflammatory markers.

Crohn's disease

The age of onset of Crohn's disease is variable, and all age groups are affected. The symptoms are similar to those seen in ulcerative colitis, but as any part of the gastrointestinal tract can be affected, the symptoms are dependent on the location of the disease. For example, extensive small bowel disease may result in severe malnutrition and electrolyte imbalance, due to destruction of the microvilli that are essential for absorption of fluid and electrolytes.

Complications of IBD

- Perforation.
- Strictures and obstruction.
- Profuse bleeding.
- Fistulae.
- Toxic megacolon.
- Malignancy.

Assessment

Assessment needs to be thorough for an accurate diagnosis to be obtained. It should include the following:

- A *detailed history* provides clues to the diagnosis.
- *Abdominal examination* can be used to ascertain the severity of the patient's condition and the need for immediate intervention.
- *Inspection of the anal and perineal area* will show changes associated with IBD, such as a perineal abscess, fistula, skin tags, or other areas of abnormality.

- *Biochemistry*. Blood samples should be taken regularly to measure haemoglobin (Hb), white cell count, and inflammatory markers, as well as albumin (to give an indication of the nutritional status of the patient).
- *Microbiology*. A sample of faeces should always be sent to the laboratory for evaluation. Infective elements such as *Clostridium difficile* or parasites must be identified and treated before a final diagnosis is made.
- *Radiology*. Plain abdominal X-ray, CT scan, barium X-rays of the small and large bowel, and MRI scan of the perineum are all useful modalities for assessment.
- *Endoscopic examination* allows direct visualization of the gastrointestinal tract and provides an opportunity to biopsy inflamed areas.
- *Histopathology* can provide a definitive answer. However, ulcerative colitis and Crohn's disease can appear to be very similar, and it is not always possible to distinguish between them.

Medical treatments

The aim of the following treatments is to modulate the inflammatory response:

- sulfasalazine and 5-amino salicylates (e.g. olsalazine, mesalazine, and balsalazide)
- corticosteroids (e.g. hydrocortisone)
- immunosuppressive agents/immunomodulators (e.g. azathioprine, ciclosporin, methotrexate, anti-TNFα antibody, such as infliximab)
- antibiotics
- new potential drugs (e.g. probiotics, nicotine).

Surgical treatments

Surgery is used only to control symptoms in IBD. Preservation of the gut is vital to prevent problems with malnourishment and fluid absorption if extensive and repeated surgery will be required in the future. Surgical procedures fall into four categories:

1. resection of diseased bowel (e.g. subtotal colectomy)
2. drainage of sepsis (e.g. pockets of pus in the perineum are acutely painful and need to be drained before a complete assessment can be undertaken)
3. control of fistulating disease (e.g. defunctioning stoma surgery such as a loop ileostomy can 'switch off' perianal disease and bring the symptoms under control)
4. stricturoplasty allows areas of scarred and narrow gut to be widened, thus preventing the loss of further bowel which would shorten the gut even further.

Tumours of the lower large bowel and rectum

Bowel cancer is now the third commonest cancer in the UK after lung and breast cancer. It affects both men and women, and the term refers to all tumours of the colon and rectum. Around 75–95% of these tumours are caused by lifestyle factors such as obesity, diet, and smoking, as well as an increasing propensity to the disease with age. Only a minority of cases have a genetic component.

Tumours begin as polyps growing in the lining of the bowel. If left untreated, these grow larger and invade the muscle layers underneath and can perforate through the lining. A polyp such as an adenoma, which is initially benign, will become cancerous over a period of years. Spread of the tumour can occur through the lymphatic or vascular systems, leading to liver and lung metastases.

Tumours may occur anywhere in the large bowel (see Figure 19.1). The commonest site is the colon, where two-thirds of bowel tumours are found. Rectal cancer accounts for one-third of all bowel cancers each year in the UK.

Anal tumours are very rare, with only around 500 cases a year. The majority of these are treated with a combination of chemotherapy and radiotherapy, and rarely require surgical intervention unless they recur.

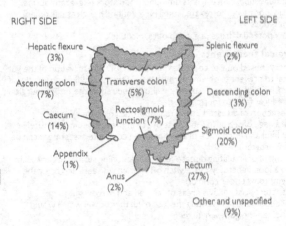

RIGHT SIDE

LEFT SIDE

Hepatic flexure (3%)

Splenic flexure (2%)

Ascending colon (7%)

Transverse colon (5%)

Descending colon (3%)

Caecum (14%)

Rectosigmoid junction (7%)

Sigmoid colon (20%)

Appendix (1%)

Rectum (27%)

Anus (2%)

Other and unspecified (9%)

Figure 19.1 Percentage of cancers that develop in the large bowel.

Symptoms

These include rectal bleeding mixed with the stool, a change in bowel habit (e.g. diarrhoea), weight loss, and rectal or abdominal pain. Symptoms in patients who are over 50 years of age warrant investigation if they have persisted for 3 weeks or more. Obstructive symptoms may be present if the tumour is large and narrowing the lumen of the bowel. These patients may present as an emergency and require urgent surgery.

Staging of the tumour

This allows the clinician to plan appropriate care based on the position and extent of the tumour.

Colonoscopy

This allows direct visualization of the whole colon. The tumour can be assessed for size and position, a biopsy can be taken, and the area can be tattooed so that it is recognizable at laparoscopy.

CT scan

This will reveal areas of further disease, such as liver or lung metastases, as well as the presence of lymph nodes involved with the tumour. If the tumour is locally advanced or perforated, treatment may need to be modified.

MRI scan

This is performed for all rectal tumours, to assess the need for pre-operative radiotherapy.

Endoanal ultrasound scan

If a rectal tumour is small it may be resectable locally, and should be assessed with an ultrasound scan.

Treatments

The gold standard treatment for both colon and rectal cancer is surgery. However, patients with rectal cancer now receive pre-operative treatment to downstage the tumour, in the form of radiotherapy delivered as either a short course over 5 days or a longer course over 5 weeks when it is combined with chemotherapy.

Surgery

This involves the resection of the affected part of the bowel, which can be performed as either a laparoscopic or an open procedure.[1] Surgical procedures are listed in Table 19.1.

Table 19.1 Surgical procedures in colorectal surgery	
Abdomino-perineal excision of rectum	Hartmann's procedure
Anterior resection	Sigmoid colectomy
Left hemicolectomy	Transverse colectomy
Right hemicolectomy	

Some tumours are unresectable. Palliative surgery may be performed to relieve symptoms, such as a bypass from one part of the bowel to another without actually removing the primary tumour, or placing of a stent.

Adjuvant chemotherapy

This is then offered to patients if histology shows features which indicate that recurrence is a possibility.

Palliative treatments

Patients with advanced disease or recurrence may no longer be suitable for surgery, but can be offered palliative chemotherapy if they are fit enough for it. Treatments may be given in combination or as part of a trial. Continuation of treatment is based on response and the patient's fitness and personal choice. Supportive care is introduced when the chemotherapy options have been exhausted or the patient declines further intervention.

Reference

1 National Institute for Health and Care Excellence (NICE). *Colorectal Cancer: the diagnosis and management of colorectal cancer.* CG131. NICE: London, 2011. ℔ www.nice.org.uk/guidance/cg131

Abdominal hernias

In general, a hernia refers to a condition that arises when an organ pushes through a weak area in the muscles or tissues that surround and contain it.

An abdominal hernia occurs when there is a tear in the inner lining of the abdominal wall (the outer layer of muscle, fat, and tissue that extends from the bottom of the ribs to the top of the thighs), causing a bulge in the abdominal wall where the organs protrude. These are generally reducible, which means that the organs can be gently palpated back when the patient is lying down, or non-reducible if this cannot be done and the bulge remains. They are caused by straining or increasing pressure on the abdominal wall, which may be due to:

- a chronic cough, such as smoker's cough
- pregnancy
- lifting heavy objects
- obesity
- persistent sneezing associated with allergies
- straining during defecation or urination.

Types of hernias
- Inguinal.
- Indirect inguinal.
- Epigastric.
- Umbilical.
- Femoral.
- Incisional.

Symptoms include a noticeable bulge when standing, pain which is worse after standing for long periods, and abdominal symptoms such as vomiting if the intestine is trapped within the hernia.

If the hernia becomes 'strangulated', this constitutes an emergency, as the bowel within the hernia sac becomes gangrenous and dies. Immediate surgery is necessary.

Treatments
These include:
- abdominal belts or supports and lifestyle changes (e.g. losing weight) to prevent recurrence
- analgesia (e.g. paracetamol) to reduce discomfort
- surgery (laparoscopic or open) to repair the hernia.

Anorectal disorders

Anorectal disorders are a group of medical disorders that occur at the junction of the anal canal and the rectum. Many are extremely painful and cause bleeding, whereas others are more complex and require more serious intervention. Examples include the following:

- An *anal fissure* is a tear in the lining of the anus, usually caused by a hard bowel movement. Fissures are painful and bleed when the tissue is stressed during bowel movements.
- An *anorectal abscess* is characterized by a pus-forming infection in the anorectal region. Painful abscesses form under the skin.
- An *anorectal fistula* is an abnormal opening or channel from the anorectal area to another surface (e.g. perineum, vagina). It can be simple or complex.
- A *rectal prolapse* is a partial or circumferential full-thickness descent of the rectum, emerging through the anus.
- *Haemorrhoids* (also known as piles) are displaced anal cushions. Anal cushions form part of the continence mechanism by sealing the anal canal. They are displaced and congested through constipation and straining.
- *Pruritus ani* is anal itching, which can be caused by haemorrhoids, a fissure, diabetes, or a skin disease. It is an intractable itch that leads to scratching of and damage to the perianal skin.

Assessment

- A comprehensive history is needed to ascertain the symptoms and relieving factors.
- Visual inspection of the perineal area will reveal skin tags, rectal prolapse, fissures or splits around the anal sphincter, an abscess, pus, or faecal material from a fistula.

Investigations

- Digital anal and rectal examination.
- Proctoscopy and flexible sigmoidoscopy.
- Examination under anaesthesia.
- MRI scan to carefully assess complex fistula tracts and anal pathology.

Treatments

The treatment depends upon the findings, but can be acute for anorectal sepsis, strangulated haemorrhoids, or thrombosed external haemorrhoids. Abscesses are drained and cavities curetted, and haemorrhoids are removed surgically.

Anal fissure

This requires conservative management with stool softeners together with advice about constipation and dietary intake. Glyceryl trinitrate (GTN) ointment is prescribed to heal the fissure initially. Anal sphincterotomy is advised for patients with persistent symptoms.

Anal fistula
- Drainage of sepsis and assessment of the fistula tract under anaesthesia with or without insertion of a seton tube.
- 'Laying open' of a fistula.
- Anorectal advancement flap.

Rectal prolapse

This requires conservative management with stool softeners together with advice about constipation and dietary intake. Surgery is offered if the problem persists and the patient is symptomatic. Techniques include:
- Delorme's procedure
- rectopexy
- rectosigmoidectomy.

Haemorrhoids

These require conservative management with stool softeners together with advice about constipation and dietary intake. Other treatments include:
- haemorrhoidectomy
- banding of haemorrhoids
- injection sclerotherapy.

Pruritus ani

This requires good perianal skin hygiene after bowel movements, advice about keeping the skin dry, and a change to the diet to avoid exacerbation of the problem.

Further reading

Keighley M and Williams N. *Surgery of the Anus, Rectum and Colon*, 3rd edn. Saunders: Philadelphia, PA, 2008.

Porrett T and Daniel N. *Essential Coloproctology for Nurses*. Whurr Publishers Ltd: London, 1999.

Acute abdomen

The term 'acute abdomen' is generally applied to conditions in which the patient presents with acute distress related to an abdominal complaint. Symptoms may include pain, vomiting, difficulty in swallowing, jaundice, distension, heartburn, or weight loss. Routine observations may reveal abnormalities in pulse rate, temperature, and blood pressure. Haemorrhage from the upper gastrointestinal tract will be obvious and can be life-threatening. It may be due to oesophageal or gastric causes, but will be accompanied by shock and collapse if severe enough, warranting immediate treatment to resuscitate the patient.

Pre-existing ill health or an underlying disease may be present, so an accurate history is vital to ensure that the appropriate treatment is initiated. Attention should be paid to:
- reproductive and menstrual history
- the possibility of pregnancy and its complications
- drug history and alcohol consumption
- previous medical history and surgical procedures.

Examination

A thorough examination of the abdomen must be performed, including the following:
- Observation to assess for shape and symmetry of the abdomen, scars, distension, visible peristalsis, colour of skin or skin lesions, swellings, and hernias.
- Palpation of the abdominal wall to elicit localized pain, pelvic organs such as the bladder and uterus, liver or spleen edge on inspiration, and kidneys and abdominal masses.
- Localized peritonitis (inflammation of the peritoneum) is evident if 'guarding' occurs even to light palpation. A 'rigid' abdomen is indicative of generalized peritonitis.
- Percussion and auscultation to distinguish between distension due to gas, fluid, or solid masses.
- Rectal examination to assess for rectal, prostatic, and pelvic pathology such as a tumour or abscess. Bleeding from the rectum could be severe, warranting fluid resuscitation and initiation of treatment.

Investigations

- Abdominal and chest X-rays, which will reveal free air beneath the diaphragm.
- Urinalysis, as this may detect kidney disease or findings such as blood or glycosuria which may be indicative of diabetes mellitus.
- Further imaging (e.g. CT scan).
- Blood tests.
- Endoscopy if appropriate.

Treatment

This is dependent upon the findings after the assessment has been made. Treatments are tailored accordingly, and may be medical or surgical. Diagnoses may include inflammatory processes such as pancreatitis, colitis, cholecystitis, and appendicitis, which are treated with antibiotics, fluid resuscitation, and possibly surgery. Obstruction may be caused by intra-abdominal or bowel tumours, and may require immediate intervention if there is a risk of perforation leading to peritonitis. Peritonitis is life-threatening and carries a 10% risk of mortality.

Further reading

Douglas G, Nicol F and Robertson C. *Macleod's Clinical Examination*, 13th edn. Churchill Livingstone: London, 2013.

Appendicitis

The appendix is a small appendage attached to the right colon. The wall of the appendix contains lymphatic tissue that is part of the immune system for making antibodies. Appendicitis is inflammation of the appendix, usually caused by a bacterial infection. However, other causes may include obstruction by parasites, faecaliths (hard stool), or lymphoid hyperplasia secondary to viral infection. After the blockage occurs, bacteria that are normally found within the appendix begin to invade (infect) the wall of the appendix. The body responds to the invasion by mounting an attack on the bacteria (i.e. inflammation).

• The most common symptoms of appendicitis are abdominal pain, loss of appetite, nausea and vomiting, fever, and abdominal tenderness.
• Appendicitis is usually suspected on the basis of the patient's history and physical examination. However, a white blood cell count, urinalysis, abdominal X-ray, barium enema, ultrasonography, CT scan, and laparoscopy may also aid the diagnosis.
• Due to the varying size and location of the appendix, and the proximity of other organs, it may be difficult to differentiate appendicitis from other abdominal and pelvic diseases.
• The treatment for appendicitis is usually antibiotic therapy and surgery to remove the appendix. This is commonly performed as a laparoscopic (keyhole) procedure, and the patient is discharged after 24–48 h.
• Complications of appendectomy include wound infection and abscess formation.
• Other conditions that can mimic appendicitis include Meckel's diverticulitis, pelvic inflammatory disease (PID), inflammatory diseases of the right upper abdomen (gall-bladder disease, liver disease, or perforated duodenal ulcer), right-sided diverticulitis, and kidney diseases.

Small bowel obstruction

Small bowel obstruction (SBO) may occur at any point along the jejunum, duodenum, or ileum which make up the small bowel. SBO is classified as mechanical or functional, partial or complete, and simple (non-strangulated) or strangulated. There are a variety of causes, including the following:
- post-surgical adhesions
- strangulated hernia
- Crohn's disease
- volvulus
- intussusception
- tumours of the small bowel (e.g. lymphoma)
- tumours of the large bowel causing extrinsic pressure on the small bowel
- gynaecological tumours causing extrinsic pressure
- peritoneal tumours.

Symptoms

In SBO, the intestine dilates above the blockage due to an accumulation of gastrointestinal secretions and swallowed air. Vomiting is typically associated with proximal SBOs. It is important to assess the type of vomit, as this will indicate the level of obstruction (i.e. bile or faecal fluid). The patient may continue to have their bowels open as bowel contents attempt to pass out below the level of obstruction. This may be very liquid, causing further fluid loss. Small bowel distension can cause lymphatic compression that leads to bowel wall lymphoedema. Increasing pressure within the lumen of the bowel can result in reduced venous and arterial blood flow and severe fluid loss, dehydration (which can lead to hypovolaemic shock and death), and electrolyte imbalance. Respiratory distress and peritonitis can occur, with mortality as high as 25%. Hiccups can occur due to irritation of the diaphragm as distension increases.

Strangulated SBOs are most commonly associated with adhesions. A loop of bowel twists, and arterial blood flow is blocked. If left untreated, intestinal ischaemia will progress to necrosis, perforation, peritonitis, and possibly death. A strangulated SBO is a surgical emergency.

Assessment

- Monitor vital signs.
- Maintain an accurate fluid balance chart.
- Abdominal and chest X-rays.
- CT scan.
- Abdominal examination.
- Biochemistry to assess renal and respiratory function.

Treatment

Simple SBO may settle spontaneously in response to resting the gut, inserting a nasogastric tube, replacing fluids intravenously, and giving adequate pain relief. Surgical resolution of the cause of the SBO is required if the patient's condition worsens. Increasing acidosis, pain, and respiratory distress are all indicators for surgical intervention.

Large bowel obstruction

Causes

The causes of large bowel obstruction (LBO) are many, and include:

- tumours
- volvulus
- constipation
- intussusception
- Crohn's disease
- adhesions
- diverticular disease
- pseudo-obstruction.

Presentation

The patient typically presents with abdominal pain and distension. They often give a history of several days of constipation which becomes absolute when no flatus is passed. Abdominal distension is present, with pain, colic, and vomiting developing as the obstruction progressively worsens.

Assessment

- Abdominal X-ray.
- CT scan.
- Contrast enema.
- Abdominal examination.
- Rectal examination to exclude rectal lesion.
- Biochemistry.

Treatment

Treatment depends on the cause and severity of the obstruction. The patient is resuscitated and rehydrated if necessary, a nasogastric tube i passed, and surgery is considered. Impending strangulation and perforation require immediate intervention. Urgent surgery may result in the formation of a stoma, as the bowel will have been unprepared for surgery and full of faeces which could compromise any join or anastomosi that is attempted.

However, it may be possible to delay surgery until the patient is nutritionally stable enough to undergo a procedure. Luminal stenting can be used as a 'bridge' to surgery. The patient's condition improves as th bowel becomes unblocked, and a safe elective procedure is performeed under optimum conditions.

It is usually possible for the surgeon to make a diagnosis at the time of surgery, and future treatments will be based upon the diagnosis. An stoma that has been formed has the potential to be reversed if the rectum remains, but this is dependent upon the diagnosis, the patient's condition, and their wishes.

Ischaemic bowel

Ischaemia occurs as a result of a compromised blood supply from the mesenteric arteries to the gut. Large sections of bowel become ischaemic and gangrene can occur as a result, a systemic inflammatory reaction occurs, and the patient presents with abdominal symptoms. There are three main types:

- acute mesenteric ischaemia
- chronic mesenteric ischaemia
- ischaemic colitis.

Causes include:

- arterial embolic disruption to the mesentery—for example, after myocardial infarction (MI) or atrial fibrillation (AF)
- venous or arterial thrombus (e.g. atherosclerosis, aortic aneurysm)
- drugs (e.g. digitalis, cocaine, antihypertensive drugs) (non-occlusive mesenteric ischaemia)
- intra-abdominal infection, tumour, portal hypertension, and venous trauma
- bacterial and viral infections caused by *Escherichia coli* and cytomegalovirus, respectively.

Clinical features

Early identification requires a high index of suspicion, but the symptoms are similar in the three main types:

- acute abdominal pain varying in severity, nature, and location occurs in 75–98% of cases
- pain is usually out of proportion to physical findings in the early stages
- rapid and forceful bowel movements
- unexplained abdominal distension or gastrointestinal bleeding may be the only features
- distension is a late feature and is often the first sign of impending bowel infarction
- stool is positive for occult blood in 75% of cases—this may precede all other features
- right-sided abdominal pain associated with the passage of maroon or bright red blood in stool, although characteristic of colonic ischaemia, also suggests the diagnosis of acute mesenteric ischaemia
- no abdominal findings early in the course of intestinal ischaemia, but as infarction develops there is increasing tenderness, rebound tenderness, and guarding as peritonitis develops
- nausea, vomiting, melaena, haematemesis, massive abdominal distension, back pain, and shock are late features and indicate compromise of bowel viability.

Investigations

- Blood tests will reveal acidosis and a raised white cell count (WCC).
- Abdominal X-ray appears normal in the early stages, but there is increased 'thumbprinting' of small bowel in the later stages, ileus, and thickened bowel wall.

- Angiography to detect embolic features (this is the gold standard investigation).
- CT can also be helpful for detecting emboli or showing gas in the bowel wall (pneumatosis intestinalis) or portal vein, bowel wall oedema, and solid organ infarction.
- Electrocardiogram (ECG) may show AF or MI.

These findings can be attributable to other conditions, including abdominal aortic aneurysm, diverticulitis, ectopic pregnancy, MI, and biliary disease, among others.

Management
Medical management may include fluid resuscitation, oxygen, and thrombolytic agents and heparin for acute ischaemia. Surgical options include angioplasty, embolectomy, and resection of gangrenous bowel.

Chronic ischaemic changes are usually due to factors that predispose an individual to atherosclerosis, such as smoking, hypertension, diabetes mellitus, and hyperlipidaemia. Management is therefore aimed at reducing these factors. Patients are often malnourished and surgical intervention is risky. Anticoagulants will be started, but surgical options would include endarterectomy of vessels, bypass to patent vessels, or angioplasty and stenting.

Ischaemic colitis
This is caused by compromise of the blood supply to the colon. The most common cause is atheroma of the mesenteric vessels, which is mainly a disease of the elderly, with the average age at diagnosis being 70. Predisposing factors can include thrombosis, shock, volvulus, drugs, recent cardiac surgery, trauma, vasculitis, and long-distance running, among others.

Presentation
The patient presents with an acute abdomen and requires investigations to confirm the diagnosis. These include blood tests which will show acidosis, colonoscopy which will reveal bluish, swollen mucosa with no contact bleeding, abdominal X-ray and CT, and stool tests to rule out infective causes.

Treatment
Treatment is aimed at resolving the cause of the hypoperfusion with bowel rest and supportive care (total parenteral nutrition). Antibiotics may be helpful.

Surgery is vital if fulminant total colitis develops, but will result in an ileostomy. Chronic segmental colitis may develop, which could require surgical intervention if stricturing occurs in the future.

Complications associated with bowel surgery

Complications following bowel surgery may occur for a variety of reasons. The patient may have comorbidities that affect their recovery, such as poor nutrition, diabetes, cardiac and circulatory problems, or chronic respiratory function problems, as well as other underlying medical conditions.

The most serious complication is an anastomotic leak, when faecal contents leak through the join made in the bowel. This can occur in the early post-operative period, or it may be a more subtle event that is not diagnosed until after the patient has been discharged from hospital. The patient normally develops pyrexia and pain, symptoms of peritonitis in severe cases, and appears unwell. The leak is confirmed with a CT scan or contrast enema. This type of complication can lead to increased mortality, wound infection, prolonged stay in hospital, and a slower recovery. It may also delay further necessary treatment, such as chemotherapy.

Minor leaks can be managed conservatively with antibiotics and/or the placement of a drain if there is a significant collection.

However, if the patient develops peritonitis, further surgery is necessary to divide the anastomosis and bring out a stoma. This is an emergency situation, and the patient may require added support such as intensive care in order to prevent further sepsis.

Other complications include:
- circulatory problems (including haemorrhage, MI, AF, etc.)
- post-operative ileus
- deep vein thrombosis or pulmonary embolism
- chest infection
- urinary tract infection
- wound dehiscence or infection
- delayed healing (typically of a perineal wound if the patient received radiotherapy pre-operatively)
- fistula formation
- hernia formation (incisional or parastomal).

Management of stomas

A stoma (derived from the Greek word for mouth) is an opening into the bowel through the abdominal wall and exteriorization of the bowel, as either a temporary or permanent measure. Both small and large bowel can be fashioned into a stoma, depending on the site of disease, and the stoma itself can be an end or a loop of bowel. An end stoma is often permanent because the rest of the bowel was removed due to disease, leaving no residual bowel for forming a join (anastomosis). A loop stoma is usually temporary and reversible, and can protect a join or rest the bowel, allowing disease to dissipate or a join to heal completely before reversal is considered. However, both types of stoma are formed in the palliative setting when there is extensive disease such as cancer which may cause an impending obstruction.

Colostomy

A large bowel stoma (called a colostomy, as it is the colon that is brought out) is normally situated on the left of the abdomen and produces formed faeces. The patient wears a closed bag and changes it on a regular basis, on average once or twice a day.

Ileostomy

When small bowel or ileum is brought out it is called an ileostomy, and the stoma is usually situated on the right side of the abdomen. The output varies from a watery fluid to thick liquid effluent depending on which region of the ileum is exteriorized.

Common conditions that result in stoma formation

Stoma formation can be indicated in a number of clinical conditions. These are listed in Table 19.2.

Table 19.2 Stoma formation

Colostomy	Ileostomy
Cancer	Ulcerative colitis
Diverticular disease	Crohn's disease
Trauma	Familial adenomatous polyposis (FAP)
Crohn's disease	Obstruction
Obstruction	Ischaemia

Stoma management

Pre-operatively, when possible, the patient is provided with both written and verbal information about their condition, the planned treatment, and stoma advice. Some patients also wish to meet an established patient with a stoma.

It is not always possible to conduct a thorough patient assessment prior to stoma surgery, particularly if the stoma is created in an emergency. However, in this case the assessment should be undertaken as soon as possible after the operation, to enable the nurse to plan individualized care and plan for discharge of the patient from hospital.

Limitations such as poor dexterity and site must be taken into consideration, as well as language barriers, ethnicity, and social factors. The patient's abdomen should also be assessed for the most appropriate site for the stoma, which will not interfere with the patient's activities of daily living, and takes into account their lifestyle and personal issues.

Patients are taught stoma management with the aim of promoting self-care and independence. This may begin before admission to hospital in the case of highly motivated patients, which not only helps to reduce the inpatient stay but also increases the patient's own confidence in their ability to handle the stoma and equipment.

The involvement of a nurse specialist who is an expert in stoma care ensures that the patient receives ongoing support, education, and information, as stoma-forming surgery can be life-changing for the patient and their family. Adequate knowledge of stoma products and problem-solving skills help to ensure that the patient is kept updated about products and the latest developments in surgery.

Stomal complications

- Stenosis.
- Prolapse.
- Herniation.
- Trauma.
- Necrosis.
- Management issues (e.g. leakage, sore skin).

Further reading

Breckman B. *Stoma Care and Rehabilitation.* Elsevier: Edinburgh, 2005.

Enhanced recovery after surgery

Enhanced recovery after surgery (ERAS) is widely practised after colorectal surgery across the UK in order to help patients to recover from their operation more quickly.

The basic principles can be summarized as follows:

- *Optimizing the patient's condition prior to surgery.* This includes improving or correcting anaemia, stabilizing diabetes, providing carbohydrate-loading drinks pre-operatively, and avoiding bowel preparation.
- *Focused management of the patient during and after surgery.* This includes admission of the patient on the day of surgery, optimization of fluid hydration, avoiding pre-operative sedatives, using minimally invasive (laparoscopic) surgery where possible, and providing individualized goal-directed fluid therapy, epidural pain management, and prevention of hypothermia.
- *Post-operative rehabilitation.* This includes early patient mobilization and oral intake, including diet, avoidance of the use of nasogastric tubes and drains, regular oral analgesia (including paracetamol and ibuprofen, while avoiding opiates), and early removal of urinary catheters.

The emphasis is on early but safe discharge from hospital (within less than 7 days), which can be achieved if the patient is not vomiting, has adequate pain relief, is able to eat and drink, is passing flatus or has had their bowels open, and is mobilizing independently. It is also important that the patient's social arrangements are adequate to support early discharge from hospital.

The importance of contacting the team if any complications (e.g. increased pain, vomiting, or fever) occur at home must be emphasized, and contact numbers provided to avoid delay if readmission is required.

Expectations with regard to the patient's participation in the ERAS process are explained in the clinic pre-operatively, and they are given information about ERAS in the form of booklets and/or a DVD. Early discharge planning to anticipate any problems is essential in order to minimize any delays to the process and address issues of concern to the patient and their family.

Further reading

Enhanced Recovery Partnership Programme, *Delivering Enhanced Recovery: helping patients get better sooner after surgery.* Department of Health: London, 2010.

Trauma and orthopaedics

Physiological response to traumatic injury

The physiological response to traumatic injury protects the individual from deterioration in their condition, conserving body fluids and providing energy to the catabolic cells (see Box 20.1). When injury has occurred, the body enters a three stage 'ebb–flow–recovery' response triggered by the sympathetic nervous system (see Box 20.2). Appropriate trauma management may attenuate the response but will not remove it, as it is essential for survival.

It is important to consider the following factors that influence the trauma response:

- Age—young males show a greater physiological response, whereas the elderly show a diminished response
- current medications (e.g. beta blockers, diuretics)
- pre-existing conditions (e.g. cardiac impairment, respiratory impairment)
- trauma history—duration and severity of traumatic injury, time to resuscitation or pain relief
- pre-existing nutritional state.

The trauma response results in protein deamination (auto-cannabilization) that is influenced by the severity of the injury. As lean body mass is used for energy there is a higher incidence of cardiac and respiratory compromise, resulting in increased mortality. Traumatic injury can result in an approximate increase in metabolic activity from 15% up to 60–70% in critical illness. Therefore it is important to closely monitor and remove any detrimental factors that may increase the trauma response further (see Box 20.3).

As a result of these factors, trauma management must include the key aspects of management listed in Box 20.4.

Box 20.1 Physiological changes during the trauma response

Increased oxygen consumption
Poor wound healing
Lean muscle depletion
Tissue oedema
Fat depletion from adipose tissue
Oliguria—'diabetes of trauma'
Hyperglycaemia
Hypernatraemia
Hypokalaemia
Increased blood osmolarity and coagulability
Increased infection risk

Box 20.2 Ebb–flow–recovery model

Ebb-phase catabolic state Starts immediately after trauma and lasts for 6–24 h	Decreased metabolic rate, reduced oxygen consumption, and reduced energy expenditure to conserve body fluids and stored fuel. Low body temperature, hypotension, and poor tissue perfusion initiate the release of stress hormone (catecholamines)
Flow-phase catabolic state Five key hormones are released to initiate the response Duration ranges from days to months depending on the severity of the condition Adaptive catabolic state at the end of the flow phase	Catecholamines—adrenaline/noradrenaline increase heart rate and respiratory rate, and peripheral vasoconstriction to divert blood to the central organs, resulting in a reduction in urinary output and gastroparesis. Adipose fat is used for cellular energy. Protein stores are 'cannibalized' for energy **Glucagon** (triggered by adrenaline) converts stored glycogen to glucose for cellular energy **Aldosterone** causes sodium and water retention to increase or maintain blood volume. However, potassium from cell damage will be excreted **Cortisol** increases blood glucose levels by antagonizing insulin production, and promotes the breakdown of fat and lean muscle mass. However, it has anti-inflammatory properties, which lead to immunosuppression and poor wound healing Metabolic rate decreases towards the norm
Recovery/ convalescent-phase anabolic state	Tissue repair and regeneration Replenishment of body stores (fat, protein, glucose)

Box 20.3 Factors that increase the trauma response further

Hypovolaemia (the most potent precipitator of the physiological response)
Hypoxia
Pain
Anxiety
Tissue injury (release of eicosanoids and leukotrienes, complement activation)
Infection and sepsis
Inadequate nutritional intake, malnutrition

Box 20.4 Important aspects of management during the trauma response

Fluid resuscitation
Tissue oxygenation
Removal of triggers
Close monitoring during the first 72 h after injury
Symptom control
Prompt surgical intervention, with good anaesthetic management
Early nutritional support

Gut barrier theory

The gut mucosal cells prevent systemic absorption of microbes from the gut lumen into the systemic circulation. Certain triggers (e.g. hypovolaemia, hypoxia) can cause failure of the gut barrier, leading to translocation of gut-derived bacteria into the systemic circulation, resulting in the release of inflammatory mediators, such as tumour necrosis factor (TNF) and interleukin-1 (IL-1), into the circulation.

This leads to sepsis, immunosuppression, and systemic inflammatory response syndrome (SIRS), resulting in multiple organ dysfunction syndrome (MODS).

The trauma response can be modified by ensuring an adequate nutritional intake to provide the essential cellular fuel during the catabolic phase. Oral/enteral nutrition must be the first choice of route to maintain the gut barrier.

Mechanisms of injury

An understanding of the circumstances and various forces involved at the time of injury may give an indication of the type, severity, and location of possible injuries. Mechanisms of injury may also be influenced by other factors, including predisposing conditions and the age and build of the injured person (e.g. a child being hit by a car may have different injuries from an adult involved in a similar incident).

Penetrating force

Caused by objects penetrating the body (e.g. stabbing, gunshot, impalement). The path and velocity of the penetrating object may also indicate the organs that may be damaged and the severity of the injury caused.

Blunt force

Caused either by a direct blow to the body with a blunt object, or by the patient striking a blunt object. Blunt forces can be localized (e.g. a baseball bat striking and fracturing the arm) or widespread (e.g. chest and abdominal trauma of a car driver striking the steering wheel of a car).

Axial/referred forces

This occurs when a load is passed along the axis of the body (e.g. a person diving into shallow water, hitting their head, and sustaining cervical spine injury).

Acceleration/deceleration forces

Sudden and often violent deceleration from speed of a moving body, which results in forward acceleration of the internal organs, leading to internal lacerations and/or contusions (e.g. coup-contrecoup injury of the brain, shearing injury of the aorta).

Blast forces

The release of a shock wave following an explosion, causing injury from:
- the shock wave itself (e.g. rapid expansion/contraction within air- and fluid-containing structures and organs, such as the lungs)
- fragments of the device and/or surrounding debris
- the casualty being thrown against surrounding objects.

Thermal injury

Exposure to extreme temperatures:
- dry heat causing burns
- wet heat causing scalds
- electrical burns
- chemical burns
- radiation burns.

Assessment of the trauma patient

Triage

A process used in emergency departments to prioritize care based on the severity of illness or injury. The most commonly used tool for hospital triage in the UK is the National Triage Scale (see Table 20.1).

Primary survey and initial management

Primary survey and initial trauma management relate to the immediate care delivered, with the appropriate treatment given for the most severe or life-threatening conditions or injuries first. To perform a primary survey, a full history is required alongside the ABCDE approach.

History

This includes assessment of the nature of the incident and mechanism of injury, the patient's name and medical history, current medication, age, gender, presenting trauma and status, current condition and conscious level using AVPU (A = alert, V = response to voice, P = response to pain, U = unresponsive/unconscious), time of last meal or fluid intake, and any allergies.

Airway with cervical spine control

Assessment of the airway may be as simple as asking the patient their name. A positive reply will confirm that they have an airway, are breathing, and have a circulation.

If the patient is unresponsive the airway may be compromised and require management, which may include:

• chin lift or modified jaw thrust if a cervical spine injury is suspected
• removal of any obstruction/suction
• use of airway adjuncts
• ensuring a definitive airway.

If a cervical spine injury is suspected, immobilization will be required, initially with an experienced and competent practitioner holding and supporting the patient's head and neck while maintaining a neutral spinal alignment. This is maintained until the patient has been immobilized with a hard cervical collar and the use of head blocks and strapping.

Table 20.1 Triage model in the UK

Category			Time to be seen
One	Immediate	Red	Immediate
Two	Very urgent	Orange	Within 10 min
Three	Urgent	Yellow	Within 1 h
Four	Standard	Green	Within 2 h
Five	Non-urgent	Blue	Within 4 h

Breathing

If the patient is not breathing, cardiopulmonary resuscitation (CPR) should be commenced with oxygen provided via a bag-and-valve mask or bag and definitive airway as per the Resuscitation Council (UK) guidelines.[1]

If the patient is breathing, a respiratory assessment is required. This should include breathing rate, depth, rhythm, breath sounds, chest expansion, and oxygen saturation. Oxygen should be administered via a non-rebreathe oxygen mask at 15 L/min. The patient should be assessed for chest trauma (see ➔ p. 470).

Circulation

- Check blood pressure, pulse, capillary refill, and cyanosis.
- Intravenous access with two cannulae (cannula size will depend on local policy and individual assessment of the patient).
- Bloods for cross-match, full blood count (FBC), urea and electrolytes (U&E), glucose, and drug screen.
- Fluid challenge (2 L of crystalloid).
- If the patient improves and then deteriorates, give colloid or O-negative blood if not cross-matched.
- Find the source and cause of bleeding and treat it.

Disability/dysfunction and Exposure

Check the patient's conscious level using the Glasgow Coma Scale (GCS). Record patient observations, findings, and symptoms. Remove all clothing from the patient and observe for signs of injury or presenting conditions. Use a top-to-toe method of assessment to perform a secondary survey. If spinal injury is suspected, both assessment of neurological status and log rolling to examine the back should be performed according to local policy.

Trauma scoring

The aim of trauma scoring is to predict the likelihood of survival following a traumatic incident. Trauma scores are used to evaluate and improve pre-hospital triage, monitor hospital care and response to treatment, and focus the priority of treatment by ranking injuries according to mortality. They can also be used as a research tool after the event, to identify preventable deaths and evaluate the effectiveness of hospital care, allowing more efficient allocation of resources.[2]

Secondary survey

This is performed following the primary survey and any subsequent emergency care, and follows a more detailed top-to-toe examination.

References

1 Resuscitation Council (UK). *Advanced Life Support: algorithm*. Resuscitation Council (UK): London, 2010. https://lms.resus.org.uk/modules/m25-v2-als-algorithm/11118/resources/chapter_6.pdf

2 Dawes M. Monitoring the trauma patient. In: RA O'Shea (ed.) *Principles and Practice of Trauma Nursing*. Elsevier Churchill Livingstone: London, 2005. pp. 289–311.

Musculoskeletal assessment and examination

Principles of orthopaedic assessment and examination

Assessment and examination of the musculoskeletal system involve the collection of information through history taking and physical examination of the patient's gait, arms, legs, and spine (GALS), followed by a regional examination of the musculoskeletal system (REMS). This should lead to the discovery of any significant musculoskeletal problem.

History

Ascertain the patient's medical history in general as well as any specific history relating to the presenting problem, including the current status of the problem, how the condition initially presented, previous injury or surgery, lifestyle choices, social and cultural background, and any associated family health problems.

Assessment

Gait

- The patient's walking pattern should be observed for symmetry, smoothness, and ability to turn.
- With the patient standing in the anatomical position, they should be observed from the anterior and posterior for bulk and symmetry of the muscles and joints, limb and spinal alignment, extension of the arms and knees, and any other obvious swellings and abnormalities.

Arms

- Assess the patient's ability to abduct and externally rotate the arm.
- Observe their hands and fingers for swelling, deformity, and muscle bulk.
- Assess the patient's grip by asking them to make a fist and then asking them to squeeze your hand so that you can assess their grip strength.
- Assess finger movement by asking the patient to bring each finger to meet their thumb (fine precision pinch).
- Gently squeeze the metacarpophalangeal joints to assess for tenderness caused by inflammatory joint disorders.

Legs

- With the patient lying down, assess flexion and extension of the knee joints.
- With the knee flexed at 90°, assess internal rotation of the hip when flexed.
- Assess for knee effusion by sliding your hand down the thigh and then pressing the patella down. If the patella taps the femur and then bounces back, this is a positive test for an effusion.

Spine

- With the patient standing, observe for scoliosis and abnormal lordosis and kyphosis.
- Assess lateral flexion of the neck by asking the patient to bring their ear towards their shoulder.
- With two fingers on the lumber vertebrae, ask the patient to bend and try to touch their toes. If your fingers move apart on flexion and back together on extension this indicates normal movement of the lumbar spine.

Regional examination of the musculoskeletal system (REMS)

- Look at the affected area, checking for symmetry, skin changes, muscle bulk alignment, swelling, and joint posture.
- Assess the skin temperature (with the back of your hand), fluctuation and movement of swelling, hard and soft swellings, and tenderness of joints.
- Test the range of movement of the joints, both actively and passively, as well as assessing for hypermobility.
- Assess function in order to ascertain how any limitation in movement affects the patient's ability to perform tasks.

Investigations

Imaging

- Plain X-rays.
- Contrast studies.
- Computed tomography (CT) scans to assess bone and some soft tissue.
- Magnetic resonance imaging (MRI) scan to assess soft tissues.
- Ultrasound scan to assess soft tissues and solid organs.
- Isotope scans to assess skeletal 'hot spots.'
- Positron emission tomography (PET) scan to assess the brain.
- Dual-energy X-ray absorptiometry (DXA) to assess bone density.

Blood tests

- FBC and U&E to check for anaemia, blood loss, renal function, and immune status.
- Immunoglobulins, erythrocyte sedimentation rate (ESR), and C-reactive protein (CRP) to assess for inflammatory disorders and infection.
- Blood cultures to assess for sepsis.
- Alkaline phosphatase to assess for disorder where there is an increase in osteoblast activity, such as Paget's disease and bone malignancy.
- Acid phosphatase and prostate-specific antigen (PSA) to assess for prostate cancer, which can metastasize to bone.
- Calcium levels to assess for parathyroid and bone disorders.

Urine tests

- Hydroxyproline—elevated levels indicate an increase in osteoclast activity, which is seen in bone destruction due to disease and/or infection.

Fracture types and classification

Definition

A fracture is commonly defined as a partial or complete break in the structural continuity of the bone,[3] which can often be displaced. If the skin over the fracture remains intact, the term *simple (closed) fracture* is used. If the skin and cavities above the fracture are breached, the term *compound (open) fracture* is used (see Box 20.5 and Figure 20.1).

Box 20.5 Classification of fractures	
Comminuted	The fracture is broken into two or more fragments, usually as a result of direct force
Transverse	The fracture occurs across the bone at 90°, usually as a result of direct force
Oblique	The fracture occurs at an oblique angle of 35–45°, as a result of either direct or indirect force
Spiral	The fracture occurs at an oblique angle and encircles the bone as a result of an indirect rotatory force
Impacted	The adjacent fracture ends of the bone are wedged together. Can be as a result of direct or indirect force
Crush/ compressed	Common in cancellous bones such as vertebrae where the bone is compacted, usually as a result of indirect forces
Avulsion	Bone is pulled apart indirectly with two opposing forces, usually a muscular/ligament or tendon pull
Depressed	Specific to the skull, where the fracture fragment is depressed below the normal surface as a result of direct force
Fatigue/stress	Undisplaced microfractures occurring as a result of repetitive stress to a bone
Physeal	Specific to patients with a growing skeleton, where a fracture occurs through or across the epiphyseal growth plate. May give rise to progressive deformity
Greenstick	Incomplete fracture, most common in children, where the bone buckles and bends as a result of direct or indirect forces
Complicated	Any fracture that causes trauma to the surrounding tissues and organs

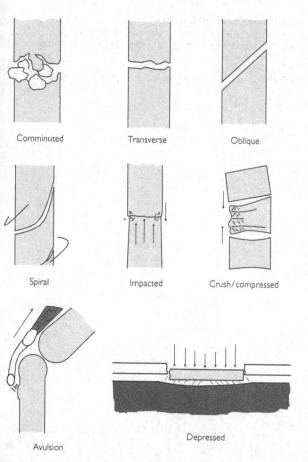

Comminuted   Transverse   Oblique

Spiral   Impacted   Crush/compressed

Avulsion   Depressed

Figure 20.1 Fracture classification. © Richard Ian Stock, reproduced with permission.

Common causes of fracture
- Direct force with fracture occurring at the point of impact.
- Indirect force where the fracture occurs at a distance from the point of force or impact.
- Repetitive stress.
- Pathological disorders (e.g. bone tumour, Paget's disease).

Reference
3 Robb J, Porter D, Keating J and Luqmani R. Clinical history and examination. In: R Luqmani et al. (eds) *Textbook of Orthopaedics, Trauma and Rheumatology*. Mosby Elsevier: Philadelphia PA, 2008. pp. 3–40.

Physiology of bone healing

Haematoma formation

Following fracture, bleeding from the bone end and possible bleeding from soft tissue damage will occur around the fracture site, forming a haematoma. During this stage the periosteum around the site is also stripped.

Cellular proliferation

Inflammation occurs at the fracture site, resulting in cellular proliferation within the periosteum. At this stage there is an ingrowth of blood vessels.

Callus formation

Initially a soft callus is formed by the production of cartilaginous tissue from chondrocytes and fibroblasts. Dead bone is resorbed at this stage, and immature woven bone begins to be laid down by osteoblasts, forming a hard callus that begins to ossify.

Callus ossification

Woven bone is replaced by lamellar bone as a result of mineralization. At this point the fracture is seen as united.

Remodelling

Once the bone is united the medullary cavity and bone shape are restored. This process can take up to 2 years.

The timing of bone fracture healing is shown in Box 20.6.

Box 20.6 Timing of bone fracture healing in a healthy adult

	Upper limb	Lower limb
Callus visible	2–3 weeks	2–3 weeks
Union	4–6 weeks	8–12 weeks
Consolidation	6–8 weeks	12–18 weeks
Adequate strength	3–6 months	3–6 months

Age-related timing of fracture healing in children: fracture at birth, united at 1 month; fracture at 8 years of age, united at 8 weeks; fracture at 3–8 years of age: rapid bone growth for 12 weeks post fracture.

Principles of fracture management

Fracture management and care can be divided into five stages, commonly known as the 5 Rs, namely resuscitation, reduction, restriction, restoration, and rehabilitation.

Resuscitation

This involves the immediate care of life-threatening injuries while ensuring care of the airway, breathing, and circulation, and providing effective analgesia.

Reduction

To ensure that the bone ends heal effectively, the fracture must be positioned into normal alignment. To prevent further soft tissue trauma and to reduce the risk of fat embolism, this needs to be performed before callus formation. Reduction can be performed either *closed*, in which case the fracture is realigned manually, or *open*, in which case the fracture is realigned surgically.

Restriction

Following reduction the fracture should be restricted. This can be achieved in a number of ways (see Box 20.7).

Restoration and rehabilitation

Restoration of function and rehabilitation involves input from the multidisciplinary team, including the medical team, nursing team, physiotherapists, occupational therapists, orthotists, dietitians, pharmacy, radiology and social services within both primary and secondary care areas.

As well as restoration and rehabilitation, it is also essential that the team works together to prevent or reduce the risks of complications resulting from the injury itself or problems associated with immobility.

Good rehabilitation also requires focus on good nutrition, ensuring effective sleep and rest, and addressing boredom, the psychological impact of trauma, possible altered body image, and the potential social impact of injury upon the person.

Box 20.7 Restriction methods in fractures

External	Internal
Splinting	Screws
Casting (e.g. plaster of Paris)	Plates
Orthoses	Intramedullary nails
Functional bracing	Wires
Traction	Nail plates
External fixators	Dynamic hip screws
	Hemi-arthroplasty
	Arthrodesis

External fixation and pin site care

External fixation is the surgical application of a metal frame to an extremity for one of the following reasons:
- stabilization and treatment of complex fractures involving soft tissue and/or skin damage
- correction of a bony deformity
- limb reconstruction
- limb lengthening (distraction).

Types of external fixation
- Monolateral—half pins are inserted into the bony cortex and attached to a bar either on one side of the limb (unilateral) or on both sides (bilateral).
- Circular—finer metal wires or pins (multiple) are inserted through the bone and attached under tension to a circular frame surrounding the limb.

Advantages of external fixation
- Rigid bone fixation allows the patient to weight bear, which will encourage faster bone healing.
- Reduction in complications resulting from reduced mobility (e.g. deep vein thrombosis).
- Easier access to traumatic wounds for wound assessment and care.
- Reduced length of hospital stay, as the patient can care for the external fixator at home.

Disadvantages of external fixation
- Pin or wire loosening, migration, or breakage.
- Pin site infection.
- Osteomyelitis.
- Joint stiffness.
- Psychological problems—body image disturbance, non-acceptance of the frame.

Pin site infection is the commonest complication that may occur, due to the invasive nature of the fixators and the length of time they may have to remain *in situ* (weeks, months, or longer).

Pin insertion sites
Following the application of an external fixator, it is normal to see a physiological response around the pin or wire insertion site. This so-called pin site reaction consists of redness, heat, tenderness, swelling, and serous discharge. This is a normal immunological response to the presence of the pin or wire (a foreign body), and it lasts up to 72 h following insertion.

However, a pin site infection must be suspected if there is a purulent discharge, increased pain and discomfort, and pin loosening.

Aspects of pin site care[4] are highlighted in Box 20.8.

Box 20.8 Pin site care

Wound dressing	Pin sites should be covered with (initially) sterile, non-shedding dressing at all times
	The dressing should have some absorptive capacity and keep exudate away from the wound
	Each pin site must be treated as an individual wound and treated separately
Frequency of dressing change	Every 7 days, but more frequently as needed if there is copious discharge or infection is suspected
Cleansing solution	Chlorhexidine in alcohol or saline if there is a skin sensitivity reaction (e.g. psoriasis, eczema)
Crust removal	Crusts are nature's own dressing, but should be gently removed when cleansing if there is evidence of increased exudate (e.g. more soft tissue involvement)
	Scabs form as part of the normal tissue healing process and should be left alone
Light compression around the pin	Recommended for 48 h post-operatively and when there is more soft tissue involvement or the pin is near a joint
	Skin tenting can occur around the pin, causing tenderness, pain, and infection. The use of compression devices can reduce this complication
	Compression can be achieved through the use of bungs, clips, or bandages
Patient hygiene	Showering is recommended prior to dressing changes. *Bathing is not recommended*
	The fixator frame should be dried after showering
Patient and carer education	The aim is for the patient to self-manage their care, so teaching sessions, information and/or leaflets should be provided on pin site care, recognition of infection, prevention of complications related to reduced mobility, and support services that are available once the patient is discharged
	A diet high in protein should be encouraged, and the importance of not smoking (if appropriate) should be emphasized
Psychological care	Body image disturbance and non-acceptance of the fixator frame may occur, which may lead to depression and poor compliance with treatment. The patient's clothing may need to be adjusted to cover the frame (e.g. tracksuit bottoms). Clothing protects the frame and reduces dust accumulation

Reference

4 Royal College of Nursing. *Guidance on Pin Site Care: report and recommendations from the 201 Consensus Project on Pin Site Care*. Royal College of Nursing: London, 2011.

Head injury

Head injury or traumatic brain injury (TBI) results from physical trauma to the head, causing major disability in all age groups, although the incidence is higher in young males (2:1). It is estimated that 1.4 million individuals attend Accident and Emergency departments annually with a head injury in the UK, and around 150 000–200 000 of these patients need hospitalization.[5] There has been a rise in more severe, complex head and cervical spine injuries since the introduction of compulsory wearing of seatbelts.

Causes of head injury

- Blunt trauma (e.g. acceleration/deceleration, coup/contrecoup, road traffic accidents, falls, assaults).
- Penetrating trauma (e.g. gunshot wounds, stab wounds).
- Blast injuries (e.g. improvised explosive device (IED) injuries).
- Shaken baby syndrome—non-accidental injury (NAI).
- Sport-related trauma.
- A combination of the above.

The different mechanisms of head injury are summarized in Box 20.9.

Box 20.9 Mechanisms of head injury	
Mechanical loading	Direct impact to the head
	High magnitude and short duration
	Causes focal lesions—skull fractures, base of skull fracture (skull bone is thinner in this region)
Impulse loading	No direct contact made with the head, but violent movement of the head and neck
	Involves inertia forces—acceleration/deceleration, coup/contrecoup
	Causes cerebral tissue to impact inside the skull on the opposite side (contralateral)
	Longer duration
	Causes diffuse injury but no skull fracture
Static loading	Compressive forces to the head—crush injury
	Longest duration
	Causes skull fractures and compression

The aim of head injury management is to prevent and/or minimize secondary brain injury resulting from cerebral hypoxia, hypercapnia, ischaemia due to haemorrhage, hypotension, and respiratory difficulties. With close observation and effective management of these events the head-injured patient can be given the best chance of recovery.

Reference

5 National Institute for Health and Care Excellence (NICE). *Head Injury: triage, assessment, investigation and early management of head injury in children, young people and adults.* CG176 NICE: London, 2014. ℘ www.nice.org.uk/guidance/cg176

Types of head injury

Head injury can be defined as damage to the scalp, bony skull, and brain tissue which may involve injury to cerebral blood vessels, and can be classified as closed (if the skull remains intact) or open (if the skull and meningeal layers are damaged).

Primary injury

This occurs at the time of the traumatic event, can cause immediate, irreversible neuronal damage or death, and can be classified as focal (localized) or diffuse (widespread).

Focal injury
- Scalp lacerations.
- Contusions.
- Skull fractures—linear, depressed, basilar.
- Coup/contrecoup (damage on opposite side of brain).
- Bleeds.

Diffuse injury
- Concussion.
- Diffuse axonal injury (DAI)—shearing and disruption of neuronal axons.

Diffuse axonal injury (DAI)
This is seen in acceleration/deceleration injuries with rotation of the brain around its axis (brainstem). Stretching of neuronal axons causes damage to or loss of neural connections. Ruptured axons form retraction balls, and petechial haemorrhages develop in the cerebral midline structures, including the corpus callosum and brainstem. There is loss of consciousness at time of the injury, and it is important to clarify this at the time of assessment and history taking. DAI is the main cause of disability in brain-injured individuals, and accounts for 35% of all brain injury-related deaths.

Secondary injury

This event occurs later, causing macro- or microscopic damage, but it can result in raised intracranial pressure (RICP), which leads to reduced cerebral perfusion and ultimately death. Early identification of RICP is vital to reduce or prevent further cerebral damage.

Macroscopic damage
- Intracranial bleeds—extradural (arterial bleeding), subdural (venous bleeding), subarachnoid, and intracerebral bleeds.
- Infection.
- Infarction (spasm of arteries resulting in cerebral ischaemia).

Microscopic damage
- Cerebral oedema following further insult (e.g. hypovolaemia, hypoxia, hypercapnia, hypocapnia, pyrexia, hypoglycaemia).
- Neuroexcitatory neurotransmitter release (glutamate, aspartate).
- Calcium influx.
- Inflammatory mediator release.

Clinical features and diagnosis of head injury

- It is important to determine the history and mechanism of injury.
- Headache, vomiting, altered motor function, dizziness, visual disturbance, seizures, tiredness, noise and light intolerance, visible head wound.
- Altered conscious state, loss of consciousness, unconsciousness, amnesia before (retrograde) or after (post-traumatic) the event.
- Irritability or altered behaviour.
- Glasgow Coma Scale (GCS) score of 13–15 (mild head injury), 9–12 (moderate head injury), or 3–8 (severe head injury).
- Skull X-ray will identify any skull fractures.
- CT scan is recommended if there has been a dangerous mechanism of injury, loss of consciousness, or amnesia.[6]
- A fall in pulse rate and rising blood pressure indicates RICP (Cushing's response).
- Pyrexia or hyperpyrexia increases the cerebral metabolic rate and oxygen consumption.
- Systolic blood pressure below 90 mmHg can compromise cerebral perfusion.
- Abnormal posturing—decerebrate (arms flexed and feet extended) or decorticate (both arms and feet extended) indicates cerebral deterioration.
- Damage to or swelling of the pituitary stalk causes diabetes insipidus (production of copious dilute urine). Nasal vasopressin (antidiuretic hormone) can be prescribed.
- Leakage of cerebrospinal fluid via the nose (rhinorrhoea) or via the ear (otorrhoea) indicates a tear in the meninges following a skull fracture, and increased risk of meningeal infection. Prophylactic antibiotics that cross the blood–brain barrier should be prescribed.
- The development of bruising behind the ear (Battle's sign) and periorbital bruising ('raccoon eyes' or 'panda eyes') is an indication of fractures to the base of the skull. These are significant diagnostic signs, as base of skull fractures are not seen on skull X-rays.

Reference

6 National Institute for Health and Care Excellence (NICE). *Head Injury: triage, assessment, investigation and early management of head injury in children, young people and adults.* CG176. NICE: London, 2014. ♫ www.nice.org.uk/guidance/cg176

Immediate management of the head-injured patient

The following factors cause a rise in intracranial pressure (ICP):
- hypoxia
- hypercapnia
- body position
- restlessness and agitation
- coughing and sneezing
- rapid eye movement (REM) sleep
- tracheal suctioning
- mechanical ventilation
- ataxic respirations
- Valsalva manoeuvre (pushing or straining on passing a stool).

The following care strategies aim to reduce ICP, maintain patient bodily functions, and promote comfort.
- Preserve life—maintain a patent airway, adequate breathing and oxygenation, and adequate circulation.
- Intubation and mechanical ventilation should be commenced if the GCS score is ≤ 8.
- Neck immobilization should be maintained until cleared by cervical X-ray.
- Commence neurological observations and GCS monitoring.
- Keep the patient in neutral alignment, with the head in the midline position and the *head end* of the bed elevated to 30°.
- Monitor the following observations every 30 min:
  - temperature, blood pressure, pulse rate, respiratory rhythm, and respiratory rate
  - record the GCS score—limb movements and motor power, best verbal response, pupil size and reaction.
- Administer oxygen via face mask or nasal cannulae to maintain arterial oxygen at 11 kPa or above.[7]
- If an ICP-measuring device is in position, monitor ICP (normal range is 10–15 mmHg).
- Maintain fluid balance to keep the patient normotensive in order to sustain adequate cerebral blood flow. If ICP is raised, osmotherapy may be prescribed (mannitol/hypertonic saline administered intravenously, loop diuretics).
- Blood glucose levels should be maintained in the range 6–8 mmol/L, as hypoglycaemia and hyperglycaemia result in a poorer outcome.[8]
- Intravenous anticonvulsant (phenytoin) may be required in the short term to prevent and control fits (common in the first 7 days after injury).
- Quiet environment with dimmed lighting to reduce stimulation.
- Avoid clustering of care activities. Deliver care in a planned, timely manner when the ICP is at normal levels.

- Analgesia should be offered, and short-acting sedation may be required before nursing interventions.
- Ensure that oxygen and suction equipment is available.
- Body alignment:
  - Maintain the head in a midline, neutral position, with elevation to 30° to facilitate cerebral venous drainage.
  - Avoid hip and knee flexion, as this increases the ICP.

References

7 Helmy A, Vizcaychipi M and Gupta AK. Traumatic brain injury: intensive care management *British Journal of Anaesthesia* 2007; **99**: 32–42.
8 Holbein M et al. Differential influence of arterial blood glucose on cerebral metabolism following severe traumatic brain injury. *Critical Care* 2009; **13**: R13.

Ongoing management of the head-injured patient

Prevention of cerebral infection

- Leakage of cerebrospinal fluid or blood from the nose or ear can indicate meningeal tears from skull fractures, which increase the risk of meningitis and cerebral abscess.
- Tetanus cover should be provided, and prophylactic antibiotics that cross the blood–brain barrier should be prescribed.

Nutritional intake and elimination needs

- There is a risk of vomiting or aspiration in a patient with a lowered conscious state.
- An orogastric tube can be passed to empty the stomach and protect the airway (avoid nasal insertion in patients with suspected base of skull fractures).
- Oral or enteral tube feeding must be established within 7 days post injury to reduce the hypercatabolic response.
- Gastrokinetic drugs may be needed (e.g. metoclopramide or low-dose erythromycin) to improve gastric motility and aid feeding.
- Dysphagia may be present in a conscious patient, so referral to the speech and language therapy (SALT) team may be necessary for assessment.
- Constipation must be avoided, as this can raise ICP. An adequate fluid intake should be maintained (if it is not contraindicated due to raised ICP). Stool softeners, mild laxatives, suppositories, or enemas may be prescribed.

Personal hygiene and prevention of complications

- Personal care must be maintained to promote comfort and regular turning of the patient to prevent the development of decubitus ulcers. During the turn, body alignment must be maintained to avoid triggering the Valsalva manoeuvre. Although interventions will cause a rise in ICP, this is only transient, and it will settle once care has been completed. Ten-minute intervals between care interventions will allow for this. Any unnecessary interventions must be avoided.
- Careful planning of care must be established to promote sufficient rest and sleep intervals.
- There is a risk of deep vein thrombosis associated with head injury.[9] Therefore prophylactic measures must be implemented, with the use of graduated compression stockings and subcutaneous low-molecular-weight heparin.
- The development of peptic ulceration (Cushing's ulcer) is linked with head injury,[10] so *prescription of H_2 antagonists is advised.*

Psychological support

- Encourage the patient's family to visit, but plan to ensure that the patient has adequate time to rest and sleep at regular intervals.
- Good communication should be established between the patient and their family, with regular information about their progress, as this may help to reduce anxiety and distress.
- An unconscious patient may still be able to hear and understand, so talk to them before starting any procedures, and be sensitive when conducting conversations around the bedside. Gentle therapeutic touch may be beneficial and can be incorporated into the care.
- The family must be made aware of the behavioural consequences that may persist following brain injury (e.g. mood swings, noise and light intolerance, headaches, irritability, anger, anxiety, impulsivity and disinhibition, poor memory). Referral to appropriate support groups or charities may be beneficial to both the patient and their family.

Surgical management

- ICP monitoring device insertion—a screw or bolt is inserted through the cranium via a burr hole and then attached to a pressure transducer to record the ICP.
- Extra-ventricular drain insertion—a catheter is placed into the lateral ventricle to allow drainage of cerebrospinal fluid to relieve the ICP.

Complications following placement of ICP monitoring devices or drains include haematoma formation, loosening or blockage of the device, and a risk of infection that becomes higher the longer the device remains *in situ*. Close monitoring of vital signs is essential in order to detect signs of infection.

- Decompressive craniotomy—a segment of the cranial bone is surgically removed and the dural layer of the meninges is opened to allow expansion of the brain tissue and reduce the ICP. Following surgery, care must be taken to protect the craniotomy site from injury.

Important points

- Close monitoring is crucial in the acute phase after injury, in order to detect further deterioration and prevent secondary brain injury and complications. Mild to severe head injuries can have devastating effects on the patient and their family.
- Lifelong adjustments will need to be made, as the head-injured person may be left with long-term symptoms and disability.

References

9 National Institute for Health and Care Excellence (NICE). *Head Injury: triage, assessment, investigation and early management of head injury in children, young people and adults.* CG176 NICE: London, 2014. ℘ www.nice.org.uk/guidance/cg176
10 Helmy A, Vizcaychipi M and Gupta AK. Traumatic brain injury: intensive care management. *British Journal of Anaesthesia* 2007; 99: 32–42.

Further reading

Brain Trauma Foundation. Guidelines for the management of severe traumatic brain injury, 3rd edition. *Journal of Neurotrauma* 2007; 24 (Suppl. 1): S1–106.

Spinal injury

Acute spinal injury (ASI) involves damage to the spinal column that may or may not involve injury to the spinal cord, and can involve the following bone damage, ligament damage, or a combination of both.
- Bone damage—fractures, dislocations, subluxations (partial dislocation), and compression, which can involve the vertebral body, transverse and spinous processes, pedicles, and lamina.
- Spinal ligaments—anterior and posterior longitudinal, supraspinatus, interspinous and capsules of facet joint ligaments.

Spinal injuries are classified as stable if further displacement is unlikely to occur, or unstable if ligament groups have been breached and progressive displacement, causing further damage, is likely to occur.

Causes of acute spinal injury
- Falls—from a height, down stairs, falling down, jumping.
- Road traffic accidents—involving four-wheeled vehicles, motorcycles, cyclists, pedestrians.
- Sport related (e.g. diving into shallow water, rugby, horse riding, altitude and water sports, gymnastics, boxing).
- Penetrating injury—criminal assault (e.g. stab wounds, gunshot injuries), self-harm.
- Blast injuries (e.g. IED, exploding pressurized canisters).

There is a high probability of other associated injuries occurring with acute spinal injuries (e.g. head, chest, abdominal, long bone, and pelvic injuries). Mechanisms and types of spinal injury are highlighted in Boxes 20.10 and 20.11.

Box 20.10 Mechanisms of spinal injury

Hyperextension	Common in the neck due to the flexibility of the spine in this region. Whiplash injury, falls down stairs, diving into shallow water, contact sports (e.g. rugby tackle)
Hyperflexion	Heavy blow across shoulders or back of neck, sudden deceleration. Causes crush/wedge fracture of vertebral body
Axial loading	Blow to the top of the head or a fall from a height onto feet
Lateral flexion	Blow to the side of the head
Flexion–rotation	Sudden deceleration with twisting of the spine. Heavy blow to one shoulder or fall onto posterior or lateral aspect of head
Distraction	Seatbelt injury with hyperflexion of the spine and vertebrae pulled out of alignment
Compression	Forces above and below the spine concurrently can cause burst fractures and high index of spinal cord damage

Box 20.11 Types of spinal cord injury

Concussion	Resulting in neurological deficits that last from minutes to hours
Contusion	Bruising and bleeding of neural tissue leading to structural damage and possible permanent disability
Laceration–transection	Causing permanent disability, with loss of sensory input and motor function; spinal shock seen
Complete	Permanent loss of all voluntary movements and sensation below the level of the injury
Incomplete	Oedema around the spinal cord may subside with some recovery of neurological function in intact nerve fibres. Classified into four main syndromes—anterior, posterior, central, and hemisection cord syndromes

Spinal cord syndromes

Anterior cord syndrome
- This is the commonest syndrome. It follows flexion–rotation forces and compression fractures of the vertebral body causing injury to the corticospinal and spinothalamic tracts.
- Compression of the anterior spinal artery occurs, resulting in spinal cord ischaemia at that level.
- There is loss of pain and temperature perception and motor power.

Posterior cord syndrome
- Posterior impact force or hyperextension of the neck injures the dorsal column, resulting in loss of proprioception (sense of position), vibration, and sense of touch.

Central cord syndrome
- This usually occurs in the elderly after hyperextension forces. There may be underlying pathology (e.g. cervical spondylosis).
- The injury results in upper limb and hand weakness or paralysis (flaccid) and lower limb spasticity.

Hemisection (Brown–Séquard) syndrome
- There is damage to the lateral half of the spinal cord, seen in stab and gunshot injuries, and lateral mass fractures.
- Loss of motor function occurs on the same side as the cord injury, but pain and temperature sensation remain intact.
- Motor function remains intact on the opposite side, but there is loss of pain and temperature sensation.

Diagnosis and complications of spinal injury

Obtain a full history in order to determine the mechanism and cause of the injury.

- *Look* for bruising and/or abrasions around the face, spine, abdomen, and pelvis, as this could indicate seatbelt injury and distraction force on the spine.
- *Move.* Ensure cervical stabilization (manual or hard collar) and neutral alignment to prevent further injury. Log roll with 'the spine in line' to examine the back for bruising and haematoma, and to remove the patient from the spinal board. An experienced team of staff should perform the turn, with the most experienced person controlling the head.
- *Feel.* Palpate the spinous processes and disc spaces along the length of the spine, observing for tenderness or pain.
- A full neurological examination must be performed, to include GCS score, motor and sensory function, deep tendon reflexes, and cranial nerve function.

Check for the six P's

The presence of any of the following signs is indicative of a cervical spine injury:

- Pain in the neck or back.
- Position of the head and trunk.
- Paralysis or weakness.
- Paraesthesia.
- Ptosis—drooping eyelid (indicating third cranial nerve involvement).
- Priapism—penile erection in an unconscious male patient.

Other cardinal signs

- Unconsciousness—treat the patient as if a spinal injury is present until it has been ruled out.
- Stuffy nose, hypotension, and bradycardia in spinal injuries at the level of the sixth thoracic vertebra or above indicate spinal shock.
- The sensation of an electric shock or water running down the back of the neck could indicate a high cervical spine injury.
- Bladder and/or bowel disturbance.

Imaging

- Plain X-ray—anterior, posterior, and lateral views, open-mouth view for the first and second cervical vertebrae, shoulder pull, and swimmer's view for visualization of the seventh cervical vertebra.
- Magnetic resonance imaging (MRI) scan—bone and soft tissue visualization, useful for ligament and spinal cord damage.
- CT scan—useful for visualizing bony damage and disc herniation.

Complications of spinal cord injury

See Box 20.12.

Box 20.12 Complications of spinal cord injury

Respiratory   Poikilothermia   Urinary
insufficiency   Hyperpyrexia   retention
Neurogenic shock   Autonomic dysreflexia   Spinal shock

Table 20.2 Respiratory insufficiency

Injury level	Muscles affected	Management
First to fourth cervical vertebrae	Paralysis of diaphragm and intercostal and abdominal muscles	Mechanical ventilation and tracheostomy are required
Fifth cervical vertebra	Weakness or paralysis of diaphragm, paralysis of intercostal and abdominal muscles	Reduced vital capacity and hypoxia may result. Short-term mechanical ventilation may be required
Fifth to eighth cervical vertebrae	Paralysis of intercostal and abdominal muscles	Reduced vital capacity and hypoxia may result. Inefficient cough mechanism and secretion clearance leading to chest infection

Respiratory insufficiency

This complication is a significant threat in cervical injuries, as hypoxia can cause further spinal cord insult and secondary cord damage. Therefore it is important that respiratory function is monitored closely (see Table 20.2).

Neurogenic shock

Loss of sympathetic autonomic outflow in high spinal injuries, at the level of T6 or above, results in a loss of vasomotor tone and 'pooling' of blood in the periphery. Hypotension and bradycardia develop and procedures such as tracheal suction stimulate vagal activity that can exacerbate the bradycardic state. The skin is warm but the core body temperature can fall until it reaches the environmental temperature (poikilothermia) causing hypothermia.

Spinal shock

There is loss of descending impulses and spinal reflex, causing flaccid paralysis, areflexia, and loss of sensation below the level of the injury. This is an acute, transient problem that occurs in the first 24–72 h after injury, and can last for up to 6 weeks. This makes injury severity assessment difficult until the shock has resolved. Neurogenic and spinal shock are different physiological states, and although they are related, they must be managed separately.

Autonomic dysreflexia (AD)

This can occur in the acute phase after spinal injury, but is more commonly seen in later stages of management and rehabilitation. It affects individuals with injuries at the level of T6 or above, and is a serious, life-threatening complication that can result in cerebral bleeds and death. It is triggered by a noxious stimulus below the level of injury (e.g. bladder distension, constipation, pain), which causes sudden excessive sympathetic overactivity. Severe hypertension, headaches, flushing or blotching of skin, cardiac arrhythmias, blurred vision, and anxiety occur as a result, and need urgent management. The patient should be positioned sitting up (with cervical spine immobilization if this is indicated), the cause should be identified and treated (e.g. unblock urinary catheter, turn patient), and analgesia and vasodilators should be prescribed.

Management of spinal injury

Spinal cord injury is a serious, life-threatening condition that must be managed by a multidisciplinary healthcare team experienced in the managing of this type of injury and the possible complications that may occur. Management should involve transfer to a specialist spinal centre once the patient has been assessed and stabilized.

The aims of management are preservation of life, prevention of secondary damage to the spinal cord, and early detection and management of complications during care and rehabilitation.

Use of a spinal bed is recommended for patients with unstable injuries, but if this is not available a firm-based bed will suffice.

Immediate management

ABCDE approach

Management is dependent on fracture stability and spinal cord involvement. Stable bony injuries may require a short period of bed rest with analgesia, followed by gradual mobilization with spinal bracing to maintain posture.

Unstable injuries can be managed conservatively until there is evidence of sufficient bone healing, or surgically stabilized with instrumentation and bone grafting.

Conservative management

Cervical spinal injury

Cervical traction can be applied with skull calipers (tongs) and weights to immobilize the region and reduce bony fractures and dislocations. The patient should be nursed supine in bed with a neck roll in place to maintain the natural cervical lordosis of the neck. Traction should be maintained for up to 6 weeks, followed by wearing of a rigid collar and mobilization as directed by the physiotherapist.

Alternatively, a halo brace and jacket can be applied for 12 weeks, giving full restriction of movement in the region and allowing for early mobilization.

Thoracic spinal injury

This tends to be a stable injury, as the ribcage naturally splints this region. Bed rest for 6–8 weeks is advised.

Thoracolumbar and lumbar spinal injury

Bed rest for 6–8 weeks is recommended, with pillows to support the natural spinal curves (neck and lumbar lordosis).

Surgical management

This is advised for unstable injuries or when there is evidence of spinal cord compression. A variety of surgical procedures are used, depending on the nature of the injury. These can involve internal fixation of fractures, vertebral segmental fusion with rods and bone grafts, bone fragment removal, and decompression of the spinal cord.

Post-operative and continuing management

- Neurological assessment, pulse, blood pressure, respiratory adequacy and vital capacity, and temperature.
- Pain assessment and management with analgesia, repositioning, and comfort measures.
- Ensure that bowel sounds are present before allowing oral diet and fluid intake.
- Oral fluids and nutrition are required—high protein content, light, and easy to digest.
- Prophylaxis for peptic ulceration—prescribe proton pump inhibitors.
- Prophylaxis for deep vein thrombosis—graduated compression stockings, subcutaneous low-molecular-weight heparin, and passive limb movement.
- Bladder care— neurogenic bladder may be spastic (resulting from lesions above T12), in which case there is reflex bladder emptying, or flaccid (resulting from lesions below T12), in which case catheterization is required.
- Bowel care—ensure adequate fluid intake; stool softeners, mild laxatives, suppositories, or enemas may be prescribed.
- Skin care—regular turning and positioning to prevent decubitus ulceration, frequent calculation of the pressure ulcer risk, use of pressure-relieving aids and pillows for positioning, use of a spinal turning bed (if this is available).
- Physiotherapy for the chest and limbs to prevent chest infection and limb contractures, respectively.
- Education of the patient and their family about the injury, prognosis, and management plan, and their involvement in care and decision making.
- Psychological care—the patient will be grieving the loss of their pre-injury life; good communication skills are therefore essential.
- Prevention of long-term complications (e.g. renal calculi, pathological fractures, limb spasticity, chronic back pain, obesity).
- Sexual dysfunction—referral to counselling services.

Further reading

North West Midlands Critical Care Network. *Spinal Care Bundle*. North West Midlands Critical Care Network: Birmingham, 2008. ℘ www.wyccn.nhs.uk/Pages/Publications.aspx

Royal College of Physicians. *Chronic Spinal Cord Injury: management of patients in acute hospital settings*. Concise Guidance to Good Practice Number 9. Royal College of Physicians: London, 2008.

Chest injuries

The chest cavity contains vital organs and structures which are protected by the bony ribcage. Trauma to the chest from blunt or penetrating trauma can result in hypovolaemic shock, hypoxia, and respiratory failure, and has been found to account for around 25% of all deaths from traumatic injury.[11]

Injuries resulting from chest trauma

Pulmonary contusion
Bruising of the lung tissue following blunt trauma, resulting in hypoxia, haemoptysis, and pain on breathing.

Pneumothorax
The presence of air in the pleural cavity following a penetrating injury, or from damaged lung tissue. There are three types—closed/simple, open/sucking, and tension pneumothorax. Tracheal deviation indicates a tension pneumothorax, which can lead to compression of the heart and cardiac arrest.

Haemothorax or haemopneumothorax
The presence of either blood or blood and air in the pleural cavity (the cavity can hold up to 3 L of blood). This compresses the lung on the affected side, leading to hypoxia and hypovolaemic shock.

Rib fractures
Ribs 4–9 are most commonly fractured. The fracture pain can cause hypoxia due to difficulty in breathing.

Sternal fracture
This occurs following severe blunt trauma to the anterior chest wall. It causes pain and hypoxia, but there may also be bruising to the lungs and heart and the development of life-threatening cardiac tamponade and rupture.

Flail chest
Three or more ribs are fractured in two or more places, resulting in one segment of the chest wall moving independently to the rest. Paradoxical breathing is present—that is, on inspiration the flail segment moves inwards, and on expiration the flail segment moves outwards. This compromises effective ventilation.

Cardiac contusion and pericardial tamponade
Bruising of the heart following blunt trauma causes chest pain and potential arrhythmias. Blood entering the pericardial sac leads to cardiac compression (tamponade) and falling cardiac output, resulting in cardiac arrest.

Ruptured oesophagus and diaphragm
Oesophageal rupture causes spillage of the oesophageal contents into the mediastinum, leading to inflammation and serious infection. Diaphragmatic rupture results in the abdominal contents moving into the chest cavity. Both conditions cause respiratory compromise and hypoxia.

Immediate management
- A—maintain a patent airway.
- B—check the respiratory rate, depth, and rhythm, oxygen saturations, skin colour, chest wall symmetry, chest expansion (bilateral equal movements), and identify any signs of respiratory compromise.
- C—observe pulse rate, rhythm, and depth, blood pressure, and central venous pressure (CVP).
- Chest auscultation and palpation. Examine the chest for bruising, grazes, seatbelt/steering wheel marks, penetrating wounds, and the presence of surgical emphysema.
- Examine for the presence of pain on palpation, breathing, and crepitus of ribs.
- High-flow oxygen should be administered through a face mask.
- Arterial blood gases, chest X-ray, and an electrocardiogram (ECG) should be performed.
- Focused assessment with sonography for trauma (FAST) is a rapid diagnostic tool, used at the bedside, which can detect pericardial fluid and solid organ injury.
- A chest drain is inserted for pneumothoraces to drain air or blood.
- Needle thoracostomy should be performed in an emergency to treat a tension pneumothorax, followed by chest drain insertion.
- Needle pericardiocentesis (needle inserted into the pericardial sac) should be performed to relieve a cardiac tamponade.

Ongoing management
- Patients should be nursed in an upright position if their condition allows (e.g. no spinal injuries, no hypotension).
- Continue with prescribed humidified, high-flow oxygen therapy.
- Frequent monitoring of vital signs and oxygen saturations.
- Assessment of pain and administration of analgesia to ease respiratory work. Consider the use of opiates, intercostal blocks, epidural infusions, and non-steroidal anti-inflammatory drugs (NSAIDs).
- Care of chest drains (see Chapter 25).
- Prevention of chest infections by encouraging coughing, and practising deep breathing exercises.
- Patients with chest wall instability and flail segments may be mechanically ventilated to stabilize the fractures.

Surgical management
Thoracotomy is indicated to explore and repair penetrating wounds, stop major bleeding, release cardiac tamponade, and repair the diaphragm and organs.

Reference
11 O'Shea RA (ed.) Principles and Practice of Trauma Nursing. Elsevier Churchill Livingstone: London, 2005.

Pelvic injuries

The pelvis consists of several bones, including the sacrum, coccyx, and two innominate bones divided into three sections (the ilium, ischium, and pubis). The pelvis has two main joints (the sacroiliac joint and symphysis pubis) which are supported by strong ligaments. The functions of the pelvis are to distribute weight from the trunk down through the lower limbs, to provide attachment points for muscles and ligaments, and to protect vital structures contained within the pelvic ring (gastrointestinal, genitourinary, and reproductive organs, major blood vessels, and nerves).

Causes of pelvic injury

High-velocity blunt trauma

Causes include motor vehicle collisions, crushing, and pedestrian accidents. Disruption to the pelvic ring requires considerable force, so these patients often have other associated injuries (e.g. head, lumbar spine, lung, and abdominal organ damage).

Low-velocity blunt trauma

These are mainly caused by falls, usually associated with the elderly, with underlying bone pathology (e.g. osteoporosis).

The different types of pelvic fractures are outlined in Box 20.13.

Lateral compression

This is most common type of fracture, caused by a side impact which results in overlapping of the pelvic wing towards the midline. Pelvic ring capacity is reduced, which means that any bleeding will be restricted. However, sharp bone fragments can cause soft tissue and organ damage (e.g. bladder, urethra).

Anterior–posterior compression

This is the second most common injury, resulting from a front impact that causes disruption of the ligaments supporting the sacroiliac and symphysis joints. There are usually multiple fractures, and the pelvic wings spring outwards in an 'open-book' position. Pelvic ring capacity is increased (from 1.5 L to 4 L in adults), and bleeding into the retroperitoneal space is associated with a high mortality rate due to hypovolaemic shock. The iliac blood vessels, abdominal organs, and soft tissues are at high risk of injury.

Box 20.13 Types of pelvic fracture

Stable pelvic injury	One fracture of the bony ring
Unstable pelvic injury	More than one fracture of the bony ring and/or disruption of the sacroiliac ligaments

---

Vertical shear

This is the least common injury, caused by a fall from a height and landing on the lower limbs. This injury can also result from lower limb impaction into the pelvis following a front impact in a motor vehicle accident (e.g. seated passenger's knees hitting the dashboard). There is a risk of renal, liver, and diaphragm damage with the upward shearing of the pelvic wing.

Combined mechanism injury

This is any combination of the injuries listed under causes of pelvic injury, leading to an unstable injury.

Immediate management

Identify and treat life-threatening problems

- A—maintain a patent airway.
- B—check respiratory rate, depth, and rhythm, oxygen saturations, and skin colour, and administer high-flow oxygen via a face mask.
- C—intravenous access, colloid/blood infusion, observe pulse rate, rhythm, and depth, blood pressure, and central venous pressure.
- Stabilize the pelvis using temporary pelvic slings/binder or sheet wrapped around the pelvis and crossed over at the front to bring the pelvic wings in, and tamponade bleeding.
- Examine the abdomen for bruising, grazes, seatbelt/steering wheel marks, pelvic asymmetry, and perineal and scrotal bruising or swelling.
- Lower limb rotation or shortening may be present.
- Abdominal X-ray and CT scan of the pelvis to determine the fracture type and associated injuries.
- FAST to detect bleeding and solid organ injury.
- Urological assessment.

Ongoing management

- Avoid log rolling. Careful handling is needed, and move the patient using a hoist or sliding board.
- Frequent monitoring of vital signs, and neurovascular assessment of limbs.
- Urinalysis to detect the presence of haematuria.

Stable injuries

Treat conservatively.

- Bed rest for 2–3 weeks.
- Analgesia.
- Gradual weight bearing.
- Deep vein thrombosis (DVT) prophylaxis, as patients with pelvic injuries are at high risk due to immobilization and venous stasis.

Unstable injuries
- Early pelvic stabilization to control bleeding.
- External compression with application of an external fixation device.
- Pin site care.
- Urinary catheter if there is no urethral damage, otherwise suprapubic catheter.
- Avoid excessive movement of the pelvis.
- Antibiotics should be prescribed if there is damage to pelvic organs.

Surgical management
- Open reduction of fractures with plates/screws and internal fixation (ORIF).

Shoulder injuries

The shoulder joint

There are several muscles associated with the movement of the shoulder. However, it is the muscles and tendons of the rotator cuff that give the shoulder its stabilization. These consist of the subscapularis, infraspinatus, supraspinatus, and teres minor, which are also involved with the rotation, abduction, and extension of the arm.

Fracture of the clavicle and scapula

These fractures can occur as a result of either direct or indirect force, and are often associated with falls onto the outstretched arm. The blade of the scapula can also be fractured by crushing forces, and clavicle fractures are nearly always displaced.

Treatment is almost always conservative, with support provided to the limb via the use of a sling, although occasionally open reduction and internal fixation may be required for clavicle fractures.

Active movement of the elbow, hand, and fingers should be commenced at an early stage. With scapula fractures, active movement of the shoulder should be encouraged as early as pain allows, whereas with clavicle fractures active movement of the shoulder may often be delayed for approximately 10–14 days, depending on severity.

Shoulder dislocation

Traumatic shoulder dislocation usually occurs as a result of indirect forces, often caused by motorcycle and sporting injuries. The shoulder most commonly dislocates anteriorly and can be complicated by damage to the rotator cuff, nerve injury, vascular injury, and damage to the glenoid labrum, leading to recurrent dislocation.

Treatment is usually non-surgical with a closed reduction, often with anaesthetic or sedation. The patient should be assessed for nerve damage and the reduction confirmed by X-ray. The arm is then usually supported with a sling as indicated by the medical team (normally for 2–4 weeks), before commencing active movement, often with physiotherapy advice.

Recurrent shoulder dislocation

Following initial shoulder dislocation, the cartilage that gives the shoulder depth (the glenoid labrum) is often torn, and this can be associated with damage to the rotator cuff, resulting in instability of the joint and an increased risk of recurrent dislocation. This is especially common in younger adults, and can affect activities that involve abduction and lateral rotation ('combing the hair' movement).

For many, care is simply a case of avoiding the movements that cause the dislocation. However, for those at high risk of recurrent dislocation, surgery to repair and tighten damaged structures within the joint may be indicated.

Rotator cuff tear

Tears within the ligaments of the rotator cuff usually occur as a result of trauma, recurrent dislocation due to glenohumeral instability, or following impingement (chronic tendonitis).

The patient commonly complains of pain, especially on abduction, which often leads to difficulty in performing activities that involve this movement (e.g. putting on a shirt or jacket). This can result in a weakness of abduction, and in chronic long-standing cases, muscle wasting can occur.

Conservative treatment consists of analgesia and steroidal injection to relieve pain and reduce inflammation, and physiotherapy to restore and/or maintain function. For complete tears or partial tears that cause persistent pain, surgery to repair the tear may be indicated.

Brachial plexus injury

The brachial plexus passes over the first rib and behind the clavicle before entering the axilla. It is formed by the spinal nerves originating from C5 to T1, which supply the upper extremities and shoulder region. Injuries usually occur as a result of direct trauma, although they are also seen following birth, as a result of traction or pressure during delivery.

Signs and symptoms include swelling and pain around the neck and shoulder region, loss of sensation, and paralysis and atrophy of the deltoid, biceps, and brachial muscles. Ptosis and unequal pupil size may indicate an incomplete injury to the lower plexus (Horner's syndrome). The arm on the affected side will hang loosely with extended elbow and pronated forearm.

Pre-ganglionic injuries have a poor prognosis for recovery, whereas post-ganglionic injuries may benefit from microsurgery, although recovery is often still limited. In some circumstances, amputation may be considered if the paralysed limb affects quality of life or chronic pain is experienced.

Fractures of the arm, wrist, and hand

Fractures of the humerus

Proximal humerus

The patient will present with the common signs and symptoms of fracture, although pain may be minimal if the fracture site is impacted. Severe bruising may be present, and it is important to assess for nerve damage to the axillary nerve and brachial plexus. Treatment will depend upon the severity and stability of the fracture.

- Simple non-displaced fractures may be treated with a sling for 4–6 weeks.
- Displaced fractures may be treated with a closed reduction and a tight body bandage for 3–4 weeks.
- More severe fractures may require open reduction with internal fixation or possible prosthetic surgery.

Humeral shaft

Fractures of the humeral shaft can occur as a result of direct or indirect forces, which can often be associated with radial nerve damage. Simple fractures may be treated with casting and traction via the weight of the arm supported within a sling. Severe fractures can be treated with open reduction and internal fixation, although comminuted fractures may require external fixation.

Distal humerus

The distal humerus consists of two bony prominences known as condyles, and fractures occur either above these prominences (supracondylar), which is more commonly seen in children, or through them (condylar), which is more frequently associated with adults. If the fracture is undisplaced, support with light cast and a sling may be indicated, whereas displaced fractures require reduction and surgical fixation. Distal fractures can be associated with vascular and nerve injury, which may lead to the development of compartment syndrome and ischaemic contracture below the level of the injury.

Fractures of the radius and ulna

Olecranon

If undisplaced, fracture of the olecranon process can be treated conservatively in a cast and/or sling. However, with this method of treatment joint stiffness is not uncommon, so physiotherapy is required following fracture healing. Displaced fractures may require surgical fixation.

Radial neck and head

Undisplaced fractures are often treated conservatively with a sling or collar and cuff bandage. In adults, displaced fractures may be treated with surgical fixation, or alternatively excision of the radial head and a prosthetic implant replacement may be considered. In children, treatment depends on the severity of the displacement, with closed manipulation considered for fractures that have an angle of less than 30°, and surgical fixation for those with an angle greater than 30°.

Ulnar and radial shaft

Displaced fractures are common, and displacement often reoccurs if treated with manipulation and casting. Therefore surgical fixation with a supportive cast post-operatively is usually indicated.

In children, greenstick fractures are often seen, and these can usually be treated with manipulation and casting. Compartment syndrome can be associated with ulnar and radial fracture, so monitoring involving neurovascular assessment and observation of the limb is required.

Distal fractures (Colles and Smith fractures)

A Colles fracture presents as a posterior displacement of the distal fracture fragment, and usually occurs following a fall onto an outstretched hand. A Smith fracture is similar in presentation, although the distal fracture fragment has an anterior displacement. If the displacement is severe, manipulation of the fracture is usually indicated, with application of a plaster cast. The initial cast often consists of a back slab until the swelling has subsided. A full cast is then usually applied later.

Fractures of the wrist and hand

Scaphoid fracture

This is a common fracture of the scaphoid carpal bone that often does not show on X-ray until a callus has formed. Therefore the fracture is often diagnosed and treated on the basis of other presenting features commonly seen with a fracture. These include stiffness around the wrist with pain within the natural depression at the base of the first metacarpal (anatomical snuffbox). For unconfirmed injuries, an X-ray should be repeated at 2 weeks after the initial injury, to detect the presence of a callus which would confirm a fracture. Most scaphoid fractures can be treated with the use of a cast, which often involves the thumb (scaphoid plaster). However, non-union and avascular necrosis are recognized as potential problems following initial treatment, when surgical fixation with possible bone grafting may be indicated.

Phalangeal fractures

Fractures to the thumb and fingers are usually treated conservatively, often by strapping the affected finger to an adjacent unaffected finger (buddy strapping), although plastic or flexible aluminium splints may often be used.

Surgery is often indicated for more severe injury, especially if there is associated ligament and/or tendon damage.

Femoral fractures

Anatomy of the femur

The femur is the longest bone of the human body, and it extends from the hip joint to the knee joint. The proximal end consists of a rounded head of femur which articulates with the acetabulum of the pelvis through a ball and socket joint, and a neck of femur which precedes two bony prominences known as the greater and lesser trochanters.

The femur extends distally along a medially curved shaft to the distal end, which articulates with the tibia and patella through a hinged joint and gliding joint, respectively. Either side of the joint at the distal end there are two bony prominences known as the medial and lateral epicondyles.

Fracture sites

- Subcapital neck of femur (across the neck below the rounded head). This can be impacted.
- Trochanteric fracture (from trochanter to trochanter).
- Upper shaft.
- Mid shaft.
- Lower shaft (sometimes called supracondylar).
- Epicondylar fractures.

Causes of fracture and predisposing factors

The healthy femur is an extremely strong bone, so usually a severe force is required to cause a fracture. Therefore most fractures in healthy bone are caused as a result of severe trauma. However, predisposing conditions and diseases can lead to weakening of the bone structure. This can result in fractures that occur through forces that would not normally cause injury in healthy bone. These conditions and diseases include:

- osteopenia and osteoporosis
- Paget's disease (osteitis deformans)
- bone malignancies
- osteogenesis imperfecta (brittle bone disease).

Presentation of signs and symptoms

- Pain associated with a fractured femur is usually severe, due to intense muscle contraction and subsequent soft tissue damage caused by the displacement of bone ends.
- Deformity, shortening, and unnatural lie. External rotation of the limb may also be seen, especially with fractures to the neck of femur.
- Swelling and severe bruising due to soft tissue damage and haematoma formation.
- Loss of power and movement.

Care management and treatment

Initial care

Due to the severity of the forces that usually cause injury, initial care involves potential resuscitation, and the assessment and treatment of other life-threatening injuries, accompanied by effective analgesia. Emergency care specific for the fracture usually involves immobilization of the limb, with traction applied if appropriate.

Traction

This is often used in the long term for patients who are high anaesthetic risks. However, this anaesthetic risk may need to be weighed against the fact that traction for long-term management requires bed rest for 10–14 weeks, which in itself carries a risk.

Intermedullary nailing

This is often the surgical treatment of choice for shaft of femur fractures, with a medullary nail inserted along the length of the femur. The nails can remain in place for a lifetime, but are often removed if indicated when the fracture is completely healed or if the nail moves.

Open reduction and internal fixation

A combination of pins, screws, and plates is used to fixate the fracture. This approach is occasionally used with fractures of shaft, but more commonly used with supracondylar fractures and trochanteric fractures to the neck of femur.

Hemiarthroplasty

This consists of a joint replacement with a stem which is inserted along the shaft of the femur, with a large artificial femoral head that articulates with a healthy acetabular cup. It is the treatment of choice for subcapital fracture of the hip due to associated vascular necrosis of the femoral head.

Total hip replacement

This is the repair of choice for a fractured neck or femur if there is any pre-existing arthritic damage to the articular surface of the acetabulum.

Knee injuries

Anatomy of the knee

The knee consists of two main types of joints:

- A hinge joint—the synovial joint consists of the distal end of the femur articulating with the proximal end of the tibia. The joint is further divided into medial and lateral compartments in relation to the condyles, and is also referred to as a condylar joint.
- A gliding joint—this consists of the femur articulating with the patella.

Within the joint capsule the surfaces of the bones are protected by hyaline cartilage, with further protection provided by two pads of fibrocartilage known as menisci. These are attached to the superior aspect of the tibia, and help to compensate for non-conformity between the femur and tibia.

The knee joint is also given extra stability on either side of the joint by the medial and lateral collateral ligaments, and anteriorly and posteriorly by the anterior and posterior cruciate ligaments.

Patella fracture

This can be caused by direct forces, often resulting in a comminuted stellate (starburst) fracture, or indirectly by muscular and/or tendon pull resulting in transverse fracture.

If the fracture is undisplaced it may be treated conservatively with bracing or a cast. Displaced fractures are usually treated with internal fixation. Early mobilization is important with both conservative and surgical interventions, with the patient usually partially weight bearing for approximately 6 weeks following injury and/or surgery.

Ligament tear

Ligament damage often occurs as a result of rotational forces associated with sport, and so is commonly (but not exclusively) seen in the young. The resulting damage causes pain and instability of the joint.

For acute injury, unless the knee is locked the treatment is usually conservative, with physiotherapy to increase and maintain movement, often using a brace to maintain stability.

For long-term instability, surgical repair and/or reconstruction is often required, usually using graft taken from the hamstring tendon or patella ligament. Following surgery there is a period of staged physiotherapy to maintain movement and strength, and a brace is often used to support the limb during this period.

Meniscal tear

Meniscal tears usually occur as a result of trauma, especially in relation to rotational forces associated with sport. However, they can also occur as a result of direct force, and in addition are seen in degenerative disorders such as osteoarthritis.

The main presenting features are sudden acute pain, immobility, and locking of the knee. Treatment depends on the severity of the tear. In acute severe cases, or if problems become persistent, arthroscopic surgery is usually performed with debridement and removal of the damaged parts of the meniscus. Post-operatively the patient is usually allowed to mobilize as soon as they are able to do so, and they are normally discharged on the day of surgery.

Fractures of the tibia and fibula

Anatomy of the tibia

The tibia is the second longest bone in the human body. It extends from the knee to the ankle, and is commonly referred to as the shin bone.

The proximal end of the bone consists of a tibial plateau and tibial spine (that articulates with the distal end of the femur to form the knee joint), a medial condyle, a lateral condyle (that articulates with the proximal end of the fibula), and a tibial tubercle (to which the distal end of the patella tendon is attached).

Distally the bone consists of an inferior articular surface that articulates with the talus bone, with a medial malleolus that forms part of a mortice for the hinge joint at the ankle.

Anatomy of the fibula

The fibula is a long bone that articulates with the proximal end of the tibia and extends distally to form the lateral malleolus, which articulates with the tibia and talus to form the ankle joint.

Fracture sites

- Tibial plateau.
- Upper, mid, and lower shaft.
- Medial malleolar (tibia) and lateral malleolar (fibula) (see ➲ p. 484).

Causes of fracture

Fractures can occur as a result of direct forces, such as a blow, or indirect forces, such as rotation of the limb.

Presentation of signs and symptoms

Tibial and fibular fractures present with pain, deformity, and shortening, loss of power and movement, and unnatural lie. Swelling and severe bruising due to soft tissue damage and haematoma formation may also occur. Compound fractures to the tibia are also common, due to limited soft tissue coverage anteriorly.

Care management and treatment

Non-surgical interventions

Undisplaced simple fractures are often treated conservatively with the use of a cast or brace to immobilize and protect the fracture, usually from the joint above the injury to the joint below.

Surgical interventions

Surgical options include open reduction and internal fixation using pins, screws, and plates to fixate the fracture, intermedullary nailing, and external fixation, especially for compound fractures.

Ankle and foot injuries

Ligament injuries to the ankle

Ligament injuries usually occur as a result of sudden twisting or rotational forces that pull the tendon to the point where it either partially or completely ruptures, causing pain, swelling, and bruising. X-rays are often required to rule out the presence of fracture.

Initial treatment relates to reduction of the swelling with rest, ice, compression bandages, and elevation, which for partial rupture may be sufficient until full movement returns. For complete rupture, immobilization in a below-knee cast may be advised for 6–10 weeks, although operative repair for severe rupture may be appropriate.

Achilles tendon rupture

The rupture occurs while pushing off from the ground, often when running or jumping, as this increases the force exerted. The patient presents with intense pain above the heel and finds it either difficult or impossible to plantar flex the foot.

The treatment can be either conservative or involve surgical repair. In both cases the foot will need to be held in plantar flexion with a cast for approximately 8 weeks. Often the patient may need to be non-weight bearing, with the use of crutches, although a walking cast with a heel may also be used, especially for patients who have difficulty using crutches.

Malleoli fracture and fracture dislocation

Ankle fractures usually occur as a result of twisting and rotational forces and are often associated with tendon ruptures, which increase the risk of dislocation. The patient normally presents with pain, swelling, and deformity, and is usually unable to weight bear through that limb.

For severe fracture dislocation, early manipulation is required due to the potential risk of neurovascular damage that may compromise the foot. Further treatment depends upon the position and stability of the fracture, and may involve either conservative treatment with a cast or surgical fixation with a cast. However, it should be noted that due to rapid and severe swelling, a full cast cannot usually be applied until this has subsided following elevation of the limb.

Calcaneal fractures

These fractures often occur following a fall from a height on to the heel of the foot. The fracture can often involve the articular surface of the talo-calcaneal joint, or can be a posterior fracture that does not affect the joint at all.

The patient usually presents with pain and swelling, so elevation and ice are often required. For undisplaced fractures, a compression bandage with a non-weight-bearing regime for up to 6 weeks may be all that is required. For displaced fractures, surgical fixation is normally required with the patient able to mobilize non-weight bearing until the fracture is healed, and then partial weight bearing for a further 4 weeks.

Tarsal and metatarsal injuries

Injuries to the tarsals and metatarsals can consist of sprain, strains, fractures, and dislocation, and usually occur as a result of rotational or blunt forces. Pain and swelling are often present, and the patient may find it difficult to stand or mobilize.

Treatment often consists of immobilization with a cast after the swelling has subsided. Manipulation, reduction, and fixation with wires may be considered for fractures and dislocations.

Phalangeal fractures

Fractures to the toes usually occur as a result of blunt trauma, and treatment usually consists of the patient being encouraged to mobilize as they are able, possibly with protective footwear, neighbourhood strapping, or splinting.

Neurovascular assessment and management

Neurovascular damage and impairment are not uncommon with injury to the arms and hands, so the patient should be monitored for the following signs and symptoms that could indicate neurovascular impairment.

- Radiating pain and paraesthesia distal to the injury, especially within the web spaces of the fingers and toes.
- Feel for the presence and strength of a pulse distal to the injury. If the pulse is difficult to feel, check the unaffected limb, as this may be normal for the patient.
- The limb may feel cold and appear pale, with a reduced capillary refill time to the limb distal to the injury.

If neurovascular impairment is suspected, any constriction must be released by the removal of bandages and the splitting and possible removal of any casts. If circulation and/or sensation are not restored, reduction of any compressing fractures and/or surgery to repair vascular injury may be required as a matter of urgency (see also compartment syndrome on ➲ p. 500).

Support and/or elevation

Following injury and/or surgery it is common to ensure that the affected limb is supported to ease pain and discomfort, and/or elevated to reduce swelling. This can often be achieved with bed pillows, although the following methods can be used.

Bradford sling

This is used to maintain elevation of the affected upper limb while the patient is lying in bed. It consists of a sling—suspended from a drip stand by the side of the bed—which supports the patient's arm.

Arm slings

This can be a simple triangular calico or cotton bandage that is used to rest and support the injured limb, or it may be a purpose-made sling designed specifically to support the limb.

Collar and cuff

This is a length of foam strap that rests around the patient's neck and wrist to allow the arm to be supported in a flexed position. As the arm is free at the elbow, a certain amount of traction to the upper arm can also be achieved.

Braun frame

A metal frame is used to elevate the lower limbs following injury and/or surgery.

Traumatic amputation

Mechanism of injury

Traumatic amputation involves the partial or complete severing of a limb, often as a result of a road traffic incident, industrial incident, or blast injury, but it also includes degloving injury of the hand or foot.

Management and care

For severe amputation, emergency assessment and management of ABC and treatment of severe bleeding are essential. Initial care involves control of bleeding with direct pressure and limb elevation. Within the hospital setting, surgery may be required to stem and control bleeding.

Tourniquet

In the case of catastrophic haemorrhage, the use of a tourniquet may be considered if direct pressure and limb elevation fail to stem the bleeding.

However, tourniquets can cause complications, including nerve paralysis, ischaemia, rapid muscle breakdown, compartment syndrome, increased intravascular coagulation, and reperfusion injury leading to rhabdomyolysis.[12]

Although traumatic amputations may be replanted, the success of surgery often depends on the severity of the injury and any subsequent damage to the amputated limb and exposed stump. In circumstances where the limb has been destroyed or severely damaged, and replantation is not an option, care of the stump and rehabilitation with prosthetics should be the focus.

To improve the likelihood of successful replantation, the injured limb should be wrapped in a damp non-adhesive non-fluffing cloth/dressing and placed within a plastic bag that is then put in ice/ice water (do not place the limb directly in contact with ice).

Post-operative care

Due to the nature of trauma, there is an increased risk of infection developing in the replanted limb or remaining stump, so good wound care is essential, and the use of prophylactic antibiotics may be considered. The neurovascular status of the limb also needs to be monitored due to poor revascularization following surgery.

For further information about post-operative care, see Chapter 21.

Reference

12 Niven M and Castle N. Use of tourniquets in combat and civilian trauma situations. *Emergency Nurse* 2010; **18**: 32–6.

Acute respiratory distress syndrome

Acute respiratory distress syndrome (ARDS) presents as acute lung injury (ALI) with hypoxic respiratory failure caused by severe pulmonary inflammation that follows a severe physiological insult. There is no evidence of a cardiogenic cause for the pulmonary oedema. Although ARDS develops as a complication of major traumatic injury, there are other causes of this syndrome.

Traumatic causes of ARDS are listed in Box 20.14.

Clinical features of ARDS

- Insidious onset of symptoms occurring 12–48 h after the insult or traumatic injury.
- Tachypnoea, acute dyspnoea, cyanosis, and severe hypoxia.
- Respiratory crepitations, atelectasis (alveolar collapse), and pulmonary fibrosis.
- Agitation and restlessness.
- Pyrexia, hypotension, tachycardia, and peripheral vasoconstriction in the presence of sepsis.
- Multisystem organ dysfunction.

Investigations

Diagnosis is based on clinical presentation and chest radiography changes.

- *Chest X-ray* shows a patchy, peripheral distribution of infiltrates but can progress to diffuse, bilateral involvement of the lungs within 72 h
- *Arterial blood gases* will demonstrate severe hypoxia.

Box 20.14 Traumatic causes of ARDS

Direct lung injury (pulmonary)

Chest contusion following trauma

Smoke inhalation

Fat embolism

Radiation injury

Indirect lung injury (extra-pulmonary)

Sepsis

Systemic causes following traumatic injury (e.g. systemic inflammatory response syndrome (SIRS), shock, disseminated intravascular coagulopathy (DIC), large blood transfusions)

Burn injury

Multiple long bone fractures, pelvic fractures, neurotrauma

- *Haematological studies* will demonstrate an immune and cytokine response, but it is important to monitor for the development of organ dysfunction (renal and hepatic) and early development of DIC (see ➔ p. 490).
- *Chest CT scan* is performed in severe cases to identify pulmonary causes and complications (e.g. pleural effusions).
- *ECG* is performed to determine whether there is a pulmonary or cardiogenic cause of pulmonary oedema.
- *Fibre-optic bronchoscopy with lavage* is used to exclude infection in patients who are not improving.

Management of ARDS

There is no specific treatment for ARDS, so it is important to identify and aggressively treat the underlying injury that has activated the syndrome, and to implement the following general supportive strategies.

- Commence high-flow oxygen via face mask. However, if hypoxaemia persists, continuous positive airway pressure (CPAP) or non-invasive positive pressure ventilation (NIPPV) via face mask will be needed to improve gaseous exchange. If these strategies are unsuccessful or the patient is non-compliant, transfer them to a critical care unit, where mechanical ventilation (IPPV) possibly with positive end-expiratory pressure (PEEP) will be required.
- Lung protection. It is important that low tidal volumes are used during IPPV to prevent ventilator-induced lung injury and worsening of ARDS.
- Recruitment therapy. Prone positioning of the patient for 12 h or longer may improve oxygenation by recruiting redundant alveoli.
- Fluid resuscitation should be given to reverse shock and optimize organ perfusion, and then reduced to conservative amounts to minimize pulmonary capillary leak syndrome. Invasive monitoring via a central venous line (CVP) can guide an accurate fluid intake.
- Antibiotic therapy should be commenced to reduce and treat pulmonary infection.
- Diuretics may be useful for managing and maintaining a conservative fluid balance.
- Heparinization may be indicated, as ARDS can trigger DIC.
- Commence early enteral feeding with a diet low in carbohydrates and high in antioxidants and omega-3 polyunsaturated fatty acids (PUFAs), as this has anti-inflammatory properties.
- Position the patient with a 45° head-up tilt to prevent aspiration of gastric contents.

Disseminated intravascular coagulopathy

This syndrome may develop following severe trauma, causing the activation of the intrinsic and extrinsic pathways of the coagulation cascade, resulting in a consumptive coagulopathy and disturbance of coagulation homeostasis. Disseminated intravascular coagulopathy (DIC) occurs in both acute and chronic forms.

- Acute—sudden exposure to pro-coagulants (tissue thromboplastin) following trauma which triggers intravascular coagulation and can lead to organ failure.
- Chronic—continuous or intermittent exposure to *small amounts* of pro-coagulants which trigger intravascular coagulation (as seen in malignancies).

Causes of DIC are outlined in Box 20.15.

Following traumatic injury there is damage to red blood cells, platelets, and the vascular endothelium (blood vessel lining). This activates the coagulation cascade, resulting in the production of pro-coagulants (e.g. tissue thromboplastin) and deposition of fibrin in the microvasculture. This produces a vast number of microclots in the capillaries *(intravascular coagulation)*, which are widespread and diffuse *(disseminated coagulation)*—hence the name of this syndrome.

Fibrin clots are broken down by plasmin, resulting in the release of fibrin degradation products (FDPs) and D-dimers which are both anticoagulants.

Depletion of clotting factors and platelets combined with the high levels of circulating FDP and D-dimer products (anticoagulants) leads to bleeding and bruising.

Box 20.15 Causes of DIC

Trauma-related causes	Non-traumatic causes
Traumatic injury	Infection
Road traffic accidents	Sepsis
Polytrauma	Severe toxaemia/inflammation
Traumatic brain injury	Rheumatoid arthritis
Burn injury	Lupus
Snake envenomation	Malignant tumours and blood cancers
Massive blood transfusions	Obstetric emergencies
Fat embolism syndrome	Vascular disorders, aortic aneurysms
	Transfusion reactions
	Organ dysfunction, hepatic failure
	Heat stroke and hyperthermia
	Recreational drugs

Clinical presentation

- Skin petechiae/ecchymosis (bruising).
- Spontaneous bleeding (e.g. gums, mucous membranes, cannulation, venepuncture, and injection sites, incisional wounds, drain sites).
- Epistaxis, haemoptysis, and haematemesis.
- Dyspnoea and cough.
- Altered conscious states and disorientation.
- Jaundice.
- Haematuria and oliguria.

Bleeding from at least three unrelated sites is highly suggestive of DIC and should be investigated further.

Investigations

Diagnosis is based on clinical presentation and the following laboratory investigations:

- platelet count
- fibrinogen levels
- APPT and PT—clotting times
- antithrombin
- FDPs and D-dimers.

Management

Treat the underlying cause that has activated the coagulation pathways, and then give supportive treatment. Any invasive procedures should be carefully followed up by administration of clotting factors and platelets.

- Monitor vital signs—blood pressure, pulse, body temperature, respiratory rate, pulse oximetry, neurological observations, and urine output.
- Correct hypovolaemia, hypotension, and acid–base balance.
- Administer haemostatic products (e.g. platelet replacement, packed red blood cells, fresh frozen plasma).
- Administer anticoagulants—heparin, vitamin K, activated protein C (APC).
- Administer antifibrinolytic agents—tranexamic acid.

Nursing care should be provided carefully to prevent further tissue trauma.

- Avoid using manual or automatic blood pressure cuffs, as they can cause bruising. Monitor blood pressure invasively.
- Avoid unnecessary needlestick procedures. Draw blood from arterial or venous lines that are already in situ.
- Perform regular skin inspection for petechial haemorrhages.

It is important to avoid or reverse hypovolaemic shock (systolic blood pressure < 90 mmHg), acidosis (pH < 7.1), and hypothermia (body temperature < 34°C), as all of these can lead to the development of DIC.

Management will involve members of the haematological and transfusion services, and if organ failure is present then critical care management should be instigated.

Rhabdomyolysis

Rhabdomyolysis occurs when crush or pressure forces cause muscle damage that leads to the breakdown of muscle tissue, with leakage of muscle proteins and toxic cellular products into the systemic circulation. It can develop following traumatic injury, but can also have non-trauma related causes.

Pathophysiology

Muscle damage results from the movement of extracellular water, sodium, and calcium into the muscle cell. Calcium activates enzyme activity that breaks down the cell membrane, causing leakage of potassium, phosphate, urate, creatinine kinase (CK), myoglobin (muscle protein), and inflammatory mediators into the systemic circulation. Cardiac arrhythmias can occur due to the hyperkalaemic state, and nephron obstruction and inflammation results from the release of myoglobin and inflammatory mediators, leading to acute kidney injury. There is a large influx of extracellular fluid into the damaged muscle (as much as 12 L over 48 h[13,14]), leading to a hypovolaemic state, which affects renal function and causes acute compartment syndrome. A combination of hypovolaemia and acidosis causes the myoglobin to precipitate in the renal tubules, resulting in obstruction and nephron damage.

Presenting features and complications

- Pain, swelling, tenderness, and bruising of muscle.
- Muscle weakness and reduced deep tendon reflex.
- Soft 'doughy' muscle on palpation.
- Pyrexia and tachycardia.
- Malaise and lethargy.
- Altered conscious state, agitation, and confusion.
- Nausea and vomiting.
- Oliguria or anuria.
- Reddish-brown urine ('Cola' colour).

Investigations and diagnosis

Rhabdomyolysis must be suspected in any patient who has suffered traumatic injury with soft tissue involvement, crush injury, or sustained prolonged periods of immobilization.

- Obtain a trauma history, including the duration of muscle pressure or compression if possible.
- Positive clinical features evident.
- ECG—peaked T waves, prolonged PR and QRS interval.
- Imaging—MRI scan will show the extent of muscle damage only.
- Urinalysis—positive for blood in the absence of red blood cells.

Biochemical tests

- CK levels are three to five times normal values.
- U&E—high potassium levels are seen.
- Lactate dehydrogenase (LDH) levels are raised.
- Serum glutamic oxaloacetic transaminase (SGOT) levels are raised.
- PT may be prolonged and platelet count may be low.

Management and care

- Treat the underlying cause or condition.
- Maintain high-flow oxygen therapy unless this is contraindicated.
- Maintain frequent monitoring of vital signs—temperature, pulse, respiratory rate and rhythm, blood pressure, oxygen saturations, and cardiac monitoring.
- Instigate early aggressive fluid resuscitation—intravenous access, and IV isotonic crystalloids to maintain urinary output at 300 mL/h (in adults).
- Commence central venous pressure monitoring, and maintain an accurate fluid intake and output record (care must be taken in patients with cardiovascular compromise).
- Maintain good urinary output. A urinary catheter should be inserted, and hourly urine volumes recorded. Intravenous mannitol or a loop diuretic can be prescribed if urinary output falls. If renal failure develops, haemofiltration or dialysis should be commenced.
- Measure urinary pH and monitor the colour. The pH must be maintained above 6.5 to prevent myoglobin precipitation. Intravenous sodium bicarbonate 8.4% can be prescribed to achieve this.
- Treat hyperkalaemia. Intravenous glucose and an insulin regime or dialysis can be prescribed.
- Observe for and treat DIC.
- Treat compartment syndrome. Monitor neurovascular signs on the affected limb. Initial treatment is with IV mannitol. If this is not successful, surgical fasciotomy is required (see ➲ p. 501).
- Pain management should consist of frequent pain assessment and administration of opiate analgesics.

It is important that high-risk patients are identified, closely monitored, and aggressively managed in the acute phase of illness in order to reduce the mortality rate and improve patient outcome.

References

13 Greaves I, Porter K and Smith J. Consensus statement on the early management of crush injury and prevention of crush syndrome. *Journal of the Royal Army Medical Corps* 2003; 149: 255–9.

14 Childs S. Rhabdomyolysis. *Orthopaedic Nursing* 2005; 24: 443–7.

Psychological impact of trauma

Trauma can end the life as the person knew it and signal the beginning of a journey of uncertainty and physical and psychological distress over which they have no control. It is important that psychological problems following trauma are identified early, and that care interventions are commenced to reduce psychological distress and physiological complications and allow the person to commence the rehabilitation journey and a return to normal life.

Trauma can affect an individual in various ways:

- Physical impact—pain, disability, wounds/scars, limb loss, and the stress response initiated by secretion of catabolic hormones.
- Psychological impact—numb or dazed feeling, anger, anxiety, fear, helplessness, sadness, loss of control and independence, grief, denial, loss of identity, vulnerability, threat to body image, low self-esteem, and loss of confidence.
- Social impact—separation from family and friends and normal life, isolation, role change, loss of employment, loss of income, loss of social life, dependency.

Certain factors will further increase psychological distress after trauma, such as being involved in or witnessing overwhelming events that pose a threat to life and personal safety. Severe injury and an anxiety-prone personality type, along with poor personal coping mechanisms, increase the risk, especially if there has been previous traumatic experience.

Body image disturbance

Traumatic injury can temporarily or permanently disrupt a person's bodily appearance, and is classified as temporary or permanent (see Box 20.16).

Box 20.16 Body image disturbance

Temporary changes	Permanent changes
Intravenous lines, urinary catheters, nasogastric tubes, wound drains, dressings, bandages, plaster of Paris, splints, external fixators, use of walking aids, wheelchairs, traction	Scars, surgical wounds, pin site scars, burns, traumatic limb loss or surgical amputations, stomas, phantom limb sensation/pain
Medication—steroids	Tetraplegia or paraplegia following spinal injury
Phantom limb sensation/pain	Fasciotomy scars following compartment syndrome
Hospital clothing	Traumatic brain injury

Post-traumatic stress disorder (PTSD)

This is a condition of psychological distress that continues for more than 1 month after a traumatic event and can persist for 1 year or more. The diagnostic criteria for PTSD are listed in Box 20.17. PTSD can be divided into three types:
- acute—sudden onset, duration of at least 6 weeks but no longer than 6 months
- chronic—gradual onset, duration of more than 6 months
- delayed—onset more than 6 months after the traumatic event.

Psychological management of the trauma patient
- Provide a safe and secure caring environment.
- Develop a trusting relationship with the patient and their family.
- Offer and implement interventions, services, and support to help the patient to psychologically process the traumatic event.
- Good communication skills are essential—be open, honest, and genuine, and listen.
- Use expressive touch and complementary therapies.
- Give information (the right amount at the right time) to ensure that the patient and their family are fully informed and can make decisions.

Box 20.17 Diagnostic criteria for PTSD

Core diagnostic criteria for PTSD[15]

Life-threatening event outside normal human experience

Re-experiencing the trauma—intrusive memories, nightmares, flashbacks to the event, distress when faced with events that resemble the trauma

Avoidance of stimuli associated with the trauma

Evidence of heightened arousal—sleep disturbance, irritability, hypervigilance, exaggerated startle response

Duration > 1 month

Other common indications of psychological distress

Poor concentration and attention span, poor memory and retention of information

Mood changes—anger, withdrawal, sadness, anxiety state, denial, numbness

Poor appetite, nausea, poor sleep patterns, loss of libido

Physiological changes—tachycardia, increased blood pressure (if not losing fluid volume), increased respirations, clammy skin, immunocompromised

- Give the patient control with regard to decision making and participation in care planning and realistic goal planning. This will empower the patient.
- Provide positive role models, especially other patients who have been through a similar experience.
- Arrange referral to a clinical psychologist, counselling services, or follow-up clinics if required.
- Allow the patient to wear their own clothing in hospital—patient identity, use of mirrors.
- Talk about and look at the injury, to help to promote acceptance of the event.

For PTSD, consider trauma-focused cognitive behavioural therapy (CBT) and eye movement desensitization and reprocessing (EMDR) therapy. Drugs (e.g. antidepressants, hypnotics) should not be used until CBT has been tried.[16]

References

15 American Psychiatric Association. *Diagnostic and Statistical Manual of Mental Disorder*. Fourth Edition, Text Revision. American Psychiatric Association: Washington, DC, 2000.
16 National Institute for Health and Care Excellence (NICE). *Post-Traumatic Stress Disorder (PTSD): the management of PTSD in adults and children in primary and secondary care*. CG26. NICE: London, 2005. ₰ www.nice.org.uk/guidance/cg26/resource guidance-posttraumatic-stress-disorder-ptsd-pdf

Fat embolism syndrome

This syndrome is characterized by the clinical triad of dyspnoea, petechial skin rash, and altered conscious state. Fat embolism syndrome (FES) is a complication associated with long bone fractures and following orthopaedic surgical procedures on long bones, although it has been associated with non-traumatic and non-orthopaedic conditions (e.g. pancreatitis, fatty liver, bone marrow transplants, steroid use).

High-risk patients

- Long bone fractures—proximal/middle shaft.
- Multiple fractures.
- Pelvic fractures.
- Fracture re-manipulation.
- Arthroplasty procedures.
- Intramedullary nailing.
- Young patients (< 35 years old) who have suffered trauma (it is rarely seen in children, as their bone marrow has more haematopoietic tissue).

Pathophysiology

The presence of fat globules in the lung and peripheral circulation causes hypoxia and altered conscious state due to decreased alveolar diffusion of oxygen.

The physiological theories of FES are summarized in Box 20.18.

Box 20.18 Psychological theories of FES	
Theory	Clinical presentation
Mechanical infiltration	Increase in bone intramedullary pressure following injury or surgery
	Bone marrow is forced into venous sinusoids in bone and systemic circulation
	Enters the pulmonary circulation and occludes pulmonary capillaries
	Smaller fat globules continue through the pulmonary circulation and out into the systemic arterial circulation, and lodge in cerebral and renal vessels and skin capillaries
Coagulation disturbance	Release of fat and tissue thromboplastin following bone fracture or surgery
	Increase in blood viscosity and coagulation
	Sludging of cells in pulmonary and cerebral capillaries
Biochemical	Release of catecholamines following injury or surgery
	Mobilization of lipids from adipose tissue
	Circulating lipids become trapped in pulmonary capillaries, causing inflammation and endothelial damage

The general consensus is that there is a biphasic course of events involving a combination of the theories outlined in Box 20.18, such that initial mechanical obstruction is followed by coagulation disturbance and fat toxicity in the lungs.

Clinical presentation
- Around 46% of cases present within 24 h following injury or surgery.
- Around 91% present within 72 h following injury or surgery.
- The average time span is 12–24 h after injury or surgery.

The clinical changes associated with FES are listed in Box 20.19.

Box 20.19 Clinical changes associated with FES	
Respiratory changes	Dyspnoea, tachypnoea, hyperventilation, cyanosis
	Chest rattles, haemoptysis
	Severe hypoxia—PaO_2 < 7.9 kPa (60 mmHg)
	Hypocapnia initially leading to hypercapnia; as the condition worsens, pulmonary oedema
	Chest X-ray—diffuse, bilateral infiltrates, 'snowstorm' appearance of acute respiratory distress syndrome (ARDS)
Cerebral changes	Fluctuating conscious state—restlessness, confusion, agitation, disorientation, stupor, coma
	Fits, limb rigidity, cerebral oedema
	Rapid spike in body temperature (38–40°C) due to cerebral emboli
Skin changes	Around 50–60% of patients have petechial haemorrhages* where skin capillaries have been occluded and rupture
	Found in the upper chest, axilla, back of neck, and conjunctiva of the eyes
Cardiovascular changes	Tachycardia, hypotension, fall in cardiac output, raised cerebral venous pressure (CVP)
	Right-sided cardiac failure, raised pulmonary artery pressure
	Chest pain in some cases, ECG changes (depressed ST segment, right bundle branch block (RBBB), inverted T wave)
Ocular changes	Around 50–60% of patients have intravascular emboli in retinal capillaries
	Complaints of having blurred vision like 'cotton wool before the eyes'
Renal changes	Reduced urinary output
	Lipuria in very severe cases; all patients with bone fractures have fat in their urine, but most do not present with FES

* This is a late sign which disappears within hours and may be missed.

Management of fat embolism syndrome

There is no treatment for FES. Therefore management is purely supportive.

The main aim is to prevent or detect the condition early by identifying the 'at-risk' patient and closely monitoring them through the critical period of time, which is up to 72 h post injury or surgery.[17,18]

Important points to remember

- Identify high-risk patients.
- Closely monitor them for 72 h post injury or surgery.
- Use appropriate assessment tools.
- Provide early definitive fracture treatment (within 10 h).
- Provide optimal fluid management and organ support.
- Always consider patient safety.
- Education of the healthcare team is important.

References

7 Powers K and Talbot L. Fat embolism syndrome after femur fracture with intramedullary nailing: case report. *American Journal of Critical Care* 2011; **20**: 264–7.
8 Kirkland L. Fat embolism. *Medscape* 2009. ℘ http://emedicine.medscape.com/article/460524-overview

Further reading

atif A et al. Fat embolism and fat embolism syndrome. *Professional Medical Journal* 2008; **15**: 407–13.
Vhite T, Petrisor B and Bhandari M. Prevention of fat embolism syndrome. *Injury* 2006; **37** (Suppl. 4): S59–67.

Acute compartment syndrome

Muscle groups and compartments

Muscle compartments are enveloped and divided into their muscle groups by fascia, which is an inelastic connective tissue that ensures muscle compartments and their respective vessels and nerves are maintained.

Causes of compartment syndrome

Compartment syndrome occurs as a result of swelling within the fascia, usually due to traumatic haemorrhage and/or oedema. A cycle of events then occur as follows:

- The fascia is unable to expand to accommodate the swelling, and therefore compresses nerves and blood vessels, compromising blood flow to the muscles and other tissues within the compartment.
- Muscle ischaemia occurs as a result of this compression and reduced blood flow, which will lead to an inflammatory response.
- As part of the inflammatory response, chemical mediators (including histamine, prostaglandins, and cytokines) are released.
- These mediators increase the vascular permeability, resulting in further oedema and swelling within the area, and thus causing further compression.
- This continues until necrosis of the nerves, blood vessels, and subsequently the muscles occurs within the affected compartments.

Although the swelling usually occurs as a result of direct trauma, it can also be associated with severe infection within the compartment. A similar cycle of events can also occur as a result of swelling of a limb within a plaster cast.

Presentation of signs and symptoms

Pain

Increasing pain that is not relieved by analgesia or immobilization is an early sign and should not be ignored when it is present with an associated injury. Increased pain and discomfort of passive flexion or hyperextension of the limbs below the affected area is also commonly seen.

Paraesthesia, pallor, paralysis, and pulseless limb

These are also commonly seen, but are later signs, due to the fact that the arterial supply is under greater pressure than the other blood vessels and is therefore affected later in the cycle. Within compartment syndrome the nerves are also less sensitive to ischaemia than the muscle itself.

Compartment pressures

Compartment pressures can be measured by means of various devices (e.g. Stryker needle). Normal compartment pressure is less than 10 mmHg, and pressure values higher than this may suggest cause for concern. However, treatment is often indicated by clinical presentation

Treatment

If compartment syndrome is suspected, urgent decompression is required. Any casts, bandages, or constrictive dressings must be removed, and the limb is positioned flat, as elevation reduces end capillary pressure, which results in increased ischaemia. If compartment pressures or sign and symptoms are at a level that is causing concern, a surgical incision into the fascia (fasciotomy) is indicated to relieve the increasing pressure.

Infection

Causative factors

All traumatic and orthopaedic surgical wounds are at risk of developing infection, which usually occurs:

- directly at the time of surgery
- directly as a result of trauma
- from a haematogenous focus of infection elsewhere within the body
- from a localized infection such as an infected wound associated with a fracture
- due to poor wound care following injury or surgery.

Localized wound infection

Localized wound infection often involves staphylococcal or streptococcal bacteria, and usually resolves following antibiotic therapy and appropriate aseptic wound care.

Cellulitis

Localized infection, especially if not treated appropriately, can develop further into the dermis and subcutaneous layer of the skin, causing cellulitis. Treatment in this situation normally involves the use of IV antibiotics as well as rest and elevation of the affected limb. The patient will often show systemic symptoms of infection (e.g. pain, heat, swelling, inflammation, pyrexia, tachycardia, malaise), which will also need to be monitored and managed.

Necrotizing fasciitis

This can be caused by many types of bacteria, and can initially present with similar signs and symptoms to those of cellulitis. Toxins released by the bacteria cause rapid necrosis of the deeper subcutaneous tissue, fascia, and muscle. The deeper infection may present with:

- severe pain
- blistering, hardening, discoloration, and necrosis of the skin and deeper tissues
- life-threatening sepsis.

Treatment consists of urgent excision and debridement of the affected area, followed by IV antibiotics. However, amputation may also be indicated. Patients who are severely compromised often require intensive care support.

Gas gangrene

Infection can be caused by various bacteria belonging to the genus *Clostridium* that release toxins which generate gas and cause necrosis of the surrounding soft tissue. The patient may present with similar signs and symptoms to those of necrotizing fasciitis, although in addition there will be subcutaneous emphysema and an odorous discharge. Care and management are similar to that of necrotizing fasciitis, although hyperbaric oxygen may also be administered.

Tetanus

This is caused by toxins from *Clostridium tetani*, which cause muscle spasm, often around the face, although in severe established cases all muscles can become affected. Treatment of tetanus infection may consist of IV or IM antibiotics and muscle-relaxing drugs for mild cases. However, severe cases usually require intensive care with tetanus immunoglobulin. Prophylactic immunization programmes have reduced the risk of tetanus infection.

Septic arthritis

This infection presents with pain, tenderness, and swelling, and inflammation within a joint which is associated with systemic symptoms of infection and sepsis. Later pustulant abscesses and sinuses can form, and eventually joint destruction will occur if the infection is left untreated. Children and older adults are often at risk, as well as those who:

• are immunosuppressed
• have trauma to a particular joint
• have a prosthetic joint implant
• have diabetes mellitus
• have rheumatoid arthritis.

Care and management usually consist of IV antibiotics, rest, splinting, drainage, and aspiration. Patients with a prosthetic implant may require removal of the prosthesis and insertion of an antibiotic block or beads, with later revision when the infection has resolved.

Osteomyelitis

This is a bacterial, fungal, or parasitic infection of the bone structure that can lead to a chronic infective condition which, if left untreated, results in ischaemic bone tissue and necrosis. This infected bone can separate to form loose bone (known as sequestra) encased within its own periosteum of live bone (involucrum). The formation of sequestra is often associated with sinus development, which occurs if the involucrum cracks (cloacae), allowing the pustulant contents of the sequestra to escape. Infection is also associated with septic arthritis, especially if the infection is located close to a large synovial joint.

Presentation of signs and symptoms

In the early acute stages the patient will usually present with common signs and symptoms of infection, including pain around the area of infection, increased body temperature, and general malaise. The affected area may often be red and hot to touch, and this can be associated with localized swelling and possible joint effusion.

X-rays may show abnormalities, such as bone destruction, pathological fracture, and sequestra formation, but in the early stages they may not show any abnormality at all. CT scans can also highlight bone abnormalities, and MRI scans can detect any involvement of bone marrow and other tissue. Blood cultures, wound swabs, and biopsy can also be used to confirm culture and sensitivity, and normal infective indicators such as an increase in WCC, ESR, and CRP may also be seen.

Treatment

Early treatment for a patient with an acute onset includes:
- analgesia
- IV antibiotics
- rest and splintage of the affected area
- aseptic care of any wounds and drainage.

Treatment for chronic osteomyelitis includes:
- wound irrigation
- insertion of antibiotic beads
- surgical debridement of the bone, with reconstruction using a bone graft
- amputation of the affected limb.

Osteoarthritis and rheumatoid arthritis

Osteoarthritis

Osteoarthritis is a degenerative condition of the joint, the initial cause of which is non-inflammatory, although the aetiology is uncertain. The condition is often idiopathic. However, secondary factors are also known to have a causative effect, including previous trauma, extreme stresses to the joint, obesity, smoking, hormonal changes, congenital and anatomical abnormalities, previous infection, and chronic alcohol intake. The condition develops in five stages, starting with the breakdown of the articular surface, followed by synovial irritation, eburnation of the bone, attempted remodelling, and finally disorganization of the joint. The presenting features and non-surgical interventions are listed in Box 20.20.

Rheumatoid arthritis

Rheumatoid arthritis is an inflammatory disorder that primarily affects the synovium of the joint, leading to degenerative changes. The condition is usually symmetrical and bilateral, and generally affects multiple joints. As with osteoarthritis, the aetiology is uncertain, as it appears to be multifactoral, with links having been made to immune system dysfunction as well as to genetic, hormonal, and dietary factors.

Box 20.20 Presenting features of and non-surgical interventions for osteoarthritis

Presenting features	
Pain	X-ray changes
Stiffness	Narrowing of joint space
Crepitus	Subchondral sclerosis
Deformity	Osteophytes at joint margins
Joint instability	Subchondral cysts
Heberden's/Bouchard's nodes on hands	Muscle wasting

Non-surgical interventions	
Pain relief using analgesic and/or non-steroidal anti-inflammatory drugs	Modification of activities and lifestyle. Avoiding causes of the pain
Physiotherapy to maintain movement and function of the joint	Reducing the load on any affected weight-bearing joints, with the use of mobility aids and weight loss
Periods of rest	

The disorder usually progresses through three stages, starting with cellular changes that cause thickening of the synovial membrane and oedema within the affected soft tissue. This leads to an inflammatory response that increases swelling and results in synovitis and development of pannus (a fibrovascular tissue). Finally the joint will enter a phase that results in cartilage and bone destruction with muscle atrophy and joint deformity. The presenting features and non-surgical interventions are listed in Box 20.21.

Juvenile chronic idiopathic arthritis

This disorder presents in children in a variety of forms, including pauci-articular (affecting four or fewer joints), polyarticular (affecting four or more joints), and systemic arthritis (affecting other internal organs as well as joints).

For most children, recovery is good, with often minimal deformity and limitation of movement. However, some children can be left with severe deformity and other associated problems, including joint stiffness, retarded growth, and reduced sight due to chronic iridocyclitis.

Box 20.21 Presenting features of and non-surgical interventions for rheumatoid arthritis

Presenting features

Stiffness of the affected joints, especially in the morning	Rheumatoid factor may be present
Reduced mobility of the affected joints	Enzyme-linked immunosorbent assay (ELISA), latex test may be positive
Pain	Antinuclear antibodies (ANA) may be present
Swollen warm joints	Nodules
Joint deformity	Tenosynovitis
Tenderness	Bursitis
Muscle atrophy	Synovial cysts
Rheumatoid nodules	Ligament laxity

Non-surgical interventions

Analgesia	Physiotherapy
Steroidal joint injections	Change of lifestyle
Steroidal medication	Diet
Non-steroidal anti-inflammatory drugs	Alternative medicine
Rheumatic disease suppressants	Splintage
	Weight loss

Developmental disorders

Osteochondritis and osteonecrosis

Bone damage and death can occur following repetitive stress, trauma, and interruption of the blood supply to bone. These factors result in bone compression, fragmentation, and bone separation from the growth plates, causing pain, swelling, and limited movement. The carpal and tarsal bones of the hands and feet, and the patella, elbow, tibial tuberosity, femoral head, and condyles are the sites affected in the skeleton.

Osteochondritis dissecans and Osgood–Schlatter disease

The signs and symptoms that are seen in osteochondritis dissecans and Osgood–Schlatter disease are pain, swelling, joint effusion, and locking of the knee joint. The aim of management is to rest the joint. This may include restriction of movement in the affected area, temporary cessation of sporting activities, and providing pain relief. In the case of osteochondritis dissecans, if the necrotic bone fragment is displaced then minor surgical intervention is recommended to fixate or remove the fragment. It can take up to 2 years for the lesion to heal.

Perthes disease (also known as Legg–Calvé–Perthes disease)

This is a disorder that occurs in children aged 4–10 years, and it is four times more common in boys. There is necrosis of the femoral head caused by an interruption in the blood supply, followed by bone fragmentation, resolution, and then remodelling. This process can take 2 years. Perthes disease is a major cause of hip pain in children.

Presenting features

- Pain in the hip and groin, which may be referred to the inner thigh and knee. There is also pain on internal rotation of the leg.
- Limp—may be painless and intermittent.
- Movement—limited abduction of the leg.
- Positive Catterall's sign—passive hip flexion causes external rotation of the leg.

Investigations

- Plain X-rays—anterior/posterior, lateral frog views (full abduction).
- MRI scan—detects infarction in femoral head blood vessels.
- Bone scan—highly sensitive (97%), shows void in the femoral head.

Management

This is dependent on the severity of the disease and age of the child.

Conservative management

Outpatient follow-up with further X-rays to observe the disease progression. Short-term rest (non-weight-bearing) for several weeks during acute pain episodes (skin traction may be used), with the use of non-steroidal anti-inflammatory drugs for pain relief. Abduction braces or splints may be used to obtain full containment of the femoral head while the bone is regenerating and remodelling.

Surgical management

Realignment osteotomies are performed through the pelvis or femur to achieve femoral head containment which will protect the shape of the head until bone re-ossification has occurred. Post-operatively the child will need to be non-weight bearing in the short term, and this is assisted by the application of traction or a hip spica.

Slipped upper femoral epiphysis (SUFE)

This is a condition seen in older children, in which the head of the femur slips off the growth plate (physis). It occurs mainly in boys aged 9–16 years, and less commonly in girls aged 8–15 years. It can be bilateral in 25% of cases, which means that both hips should be investigated.

Predisposition to SUFE

Many cases of SUFE are idiopathic, but obesity and delayed puberty are factors commonly seen in these children. It seems that there may be an imbalance between growth and sex hormone production, leading to delayed fusion of the growth plates.

Presenting features

- Pain in the hip, groin, and anterior thigh, which may be referred to the knee.
- Limp on mobilizing.
- Shortening of the limb by 1–2 cm.
- External rotation of the leg.
- Limited abduction and internal rotation.

Investigations

- Plain X-rays—anterior/posterior, lateral frog views (full abduction).
- MRI and CT scan for pre-surgical assessment.
- Bone scan—may detect a pre-slip and avascular necrosis of the bone.

Management

Surgical intervention is needed to secure the slip and prevent it from worsening, but the procedure chosen will depend on the severity of the slip.

Minor slips will be pinned under imaging. Major slips will be pinned and a compensatory osteotomy will be performed to realign the hip.

Bone malignancy

A variety of benign and malignant tumours affect the musculoskeletal system, involving bone (osteo-), cartilage (chondro-), smooth muscle (leio-), skeletal muscle (rhabdo-), and bone marrow, where the prefixes in parentheses indicate the tumour type.

Bone malignancy accounts for less than 1% of all new cancer cases diagnosed in the UK each year, and in 2008 a total of 600 bone tumour cases and 1630 soft tissue tumour cases were recorded in the UK.[19] These malignancies present a major challenge to the healthcare team, as they are rare and difficult to diagnose early, which means that there may be metastatic spread (usually to the lungs) by the time of diagnosis. Management of bone malignancies can involve treatments that cause long-term side effects and disfigurement, and because of all these issues patients should be managed in a specialist bone tumour centre where the necessary expertise, resources, and support systems are available.

The most common bone malignancies are listed in Box 20.22.

Certain factors can predispose to musculoskeletal tumour development. These include Paget's disease of bone, previous trauma, radiation injury, chronic bone infection, osteogenesis imperfecta (brittle bone disease), and some genetic conditions (e.g. Ollier's disease, retinoblastoma).

Presenting features

These vary depending on the tumour type and location.
- Pain—non-mechanical, night-time, ranging from deep aching to acute, may radiate if nerves are involved.
- Palpable lump or swelling—hard or soft depending on the site, may be warm and tender.
- Unexplained limp, and limited mobility if the tumour involves or is near a joint.
- Non-specific aches and pains that will delay diagnosis.
- Low-grade pyrexia.
- Fatigue and recent weight loss—these are late signs.

Box 20.22 The most common bone malignancies

Tumour	Age group affected (years)	Common sites of tumour
Osteosarcoma	10–20 > 40 (in Paget-related osteosarcoma)	Distal femur, proximal tibia
Chondrosarcoma	40–60	Central skeleton—pelvis, ribs, proximal bone ends
Ewing's sarcoma	5–20	Diaphysis (shaft) of long bones—femur, pelvis

Diagnosis and investigations

Following the history taking and clinical examination it will be necessary to determine the presence, type, and extent of malignancy by performing the investigations outlined in Box 20.23.

Management of bone malignancy

Treatment of the malignancy is dependent on the tumour type, histological staging and grading, extent of spread, age of the patient, prognosis, quality of life, and lifestyle issues. Most benign tumours are treated by surgical excision, and further recurrence is unlikely. Malignant tumour treatment may involve chemotherapy to shrink the tumour before surgery, with further post-operative doses to kill micrometastases. This is dependent on tumour sensitivity, as some malignancies are resistant to chemotherapy. Radiotherapy can be used in some cases to prevent recurrence, or for palliative management to relieve pain.

Surgical interventions
Benign tumours
- Simple excision of the tumour, or curettage and insertion of bone grafting or bone cement to stabilize the remaining cavity to prevent pathological fractures.
- Percutaneous ablation (destruction) by heat or laser via a minimally invasive procedure under imaging guidance.

Malignant tumours
- Bone excision with a cuff of healthy bone to reduce recurrence of the tumour.
- Limb amputation is considered in patients in whom major vessels or nerves are involved, or in the very young if the affected limb is not going to develop properly.

Box 20.23 Investigations for bone malignancy

Plain X-ray—anterior, posterior, and lateral views

CT scan—bone, soft tissue, and neural structures involved. Used to check metastatic spread to the lungs

MRI scan—more sensitive than CT scan for soft tissue tumours, to view tumour extent and spread

Bone scan—will detect asymmetrical 'hot spots' in the skeleton

Biopsy.* Excision biopsy (for benign malignancies, to remove the tumour). Open biopsy (under a general anaesthetic a section of the tumour is removed for analysis). Needle/core biopsy (under imaging guidance, a needle or drill is used to remove a core of the tumour; this is the least invasive method)

* Biopsies should be performed in a specialist bone tumour centre, as it is essential that the procedure does not seed tumour cells or contaminate the surrounding healthy tissue, as this would cause spread of the malignancy.

Limb-sparing surgery

This consists of the following procedures to retain the limb:

- Allograft—the tumour and bone are removed, and the bone is replaced by donated human bone. This procedure is infrequently performed due to the increased risk of infection post surgery.
- Autograft—the tumour and bone are removed and the bone is replaced by the patient's own bone from another body area (e.g. fibula implanted into tibia or pelvis).
- Endoprosthetic replacement (EPR)—removal of malignant bone (e.g. femur, tibia, humerus) with margins of healthy bone to prevent tumour recurrence. An extendable custom-made metal prosthesis is implanted, which may incorporate a joint.
- Rotationplasty—a type of autograft in which the diseased portion of the limb is removed and the remaining lower limb below the tumour is rotated and reattached to the stump, forming a joint (e.g. the ankle becomes a knee joint).

Nursing considerations

A key worker should be allocated who has the necessary expertise and knowledge to coordinate the patient's care journey, liaise with the healthcare team, and advise and give information to the patient and their family.

Physical considerations

Ensure that the patient is infection-free prior to surgery—dental and oral check, nasal screening, urine screening.

Psychological considerations

- Psychological care—at the time of diagnosis, breaking bad news, side effects of chemotherapy and/or radiotherapy (e.g. hair loss, infertility), body image disturbance after surgery.
- Children—education/schooling needs.

Reference

19 National Institute for Health and Care Excellence (NICE). *Improving Outcomes for People with Sarcoma*. CSGSARCOMA. NICE: London, 2006. ℬ www.nice.org.uk/guidance/csgsarcoma

Further reading

Gibson F and Soanes L (eds). *Cancer in Children and Young People: acute nursing care*. John Wiley & Sons Ltd: Chichester, 2008.

National Institute for Health and Care Excellence (NICE). *Improving Outcomes in Children and Young People with Cancer*. CSGCYP. NICE: London, 2005. ℬ www.nice.org.uk/guidance/csgcyp

Common surgical orthopaedic interventions

Arthroscopy
Arthroscopy is a surgical procedure in which a rigid scope is inserted into a joint. It is most commonly used to view the knee and shoulder joint. The procedure can be used for diagnostic and therapeutic surgical interventions, such as biopsy debridement, meniscectomy, ligament repair and microfracture.

Arthrotomy
Arthrotomy involves the surgical opening of the joint space and, like arthroscopy, is used for diagnostic and therapeutic surgical interventions.

Osteotomy
An osteotomy is a procedure whereby the bone is shortened, lengthened (distraction), or realigned, either to correct deformity or to alter the weight-bearing angle of a joint.

Arthrodesis
Arthrodesis is the surgical fusion of a joint. It is indicated for painful or unstable joints when the resulting stiffness will not greatly affect the function of the joint.

Arthroplasty
Arthroplasty is the creation of an artificial joint for the correction of degenerative arthritis. This is achieved by the insertion of an implanted prosthetic joint or the surgical excision of the articular surfaces without implanting a prosthetic replacement (excision arthroplasty). The aim of the procedure is usually to relieve pain and/or improve the movement and function of the joint.

Arthroplasty surgery

Shoulder resurfacing

This involves the insertion of a resurfacing prosthesis onto the humeral head with another prosthesis covering the surface of the glenoid cavity. The surgery is usually less invasive than a total shoulder replacement.

Total shoulder replacement

This involves the removal of the head of the humerus and the insertion of a stemmed prosthesis that articulates with the prosthetic covering of the glenoid cavity.

Specific post-operative care for shoulder arthroplasty

- The shoulder is rested either in abduction or in a sling, with physiotherapy commenced to exercise and strengthen the shoulder muscles.
- Return to work should be assessed on an individual basis, but is anywhere between 6 to 16 weeks, depending on the nature of the patient's occupation. Driving is usually allowed after about 6 weeks.

Total hip replacement

This involves the removal of the femoral head and insertion of a stemmed prosthesis, which can either be cemented into position or may be cementless. The femoral prosthesis has a rounded head that articulates with an acetabular cup prosthesis, which may also be cemented or cementless. The prosthetic implants often have a stainless steel femoral component that articulates with a polyethylene cup, although many designs are now made from titanium, ceramic materials, and other metal alloys.

Hip resurfacing

This involves the insertion of a resurfacing prosthesis onto the femoral head, which articulates with a prosthetic acetabular cup. Due to having a larger femoral head it is less prone to post-operative dislocation. Most implants are usually metal on metal. The surgery is generally performed in younger patients, as bone is preserved. Older patients also tend to have contraindications that would prevent resurfacing, such as poor bone stock, osteoporosis, and bone cysts.

Specific post-operative care for hip arthroplasty

- Abduction wedge or trough will be in place.
- An epidural, patient-controlled analgesia (PCA), or femoral nerve block may be used for immediate post-operative pain. Thereafter the use of oral analgesia is encouraged.
- Physiotherapy usually commences 1 day post-operatively, initially with a walking frame, and then progressing to sticks or crutches.

- The patient can be discharged home when it is considered safe to do so.
- Due to the risk of dislocation, the patient is educated not to flex their hip past 90° or adduct their hip for approximately 12 weeks post surgery. Occupational therapy is required to ensure that any adaptations and aids are in place to prevent these movements (e.g. raised toilet seats, raised armchairs).

Total knee replacement

This involves the insertion of a metal resurfacing prosthesis onto the distal end of the femur, which then articulates with a polyethylene on metal prosthesis that is inserted into the proximal end of the tibial plateau. A polyethylene patella button may also be inserted to articulate with the femoral component. The prosthesis can be either cemented or cementless. The procedure is usually performed in older patients (over the age of 65 years), although it can be used for younger patients with severe joint disease and destruction.

Unicompartmental knee replacement

This involves the insertion of a metal resurfacing prosthesis onto the medial femoral condyle, which then articulates with either a polyethylene or polyethylene-on-metal prosthesis that replaces the medial tibial condyle. The polyethylene-on-metal component may slide or rock. The prosthesis is suitable for patients with arthritis within the medial compartment of the knee, especially younger patients, as the joint is preserved for future knee replacement.

Specific post-operative care for knee arthroplasty

- An epidural, PCA, or femoral nerve block may be used for immediate post-operative pain. The use of oral analgesia is then encouraged.
- Knee flexion, knee extension, and straight leg exercises are used to strengthen the quadriceps.
- A continuous passive motion (CPM) machine may be used to assist flexion, depending on the surgeon's preference and local policy, protocol, or instruction.
- Cold therapy is applied to the knee (e.g. using the CryoCuff).
- Physiotherapy usually commences 1 day post-operatively, initially with a walking frame, and then progressing to sticks or crutches.
- The patient is discharged home when it is considered safe to do so.
- Outpatient physiotherapy will be necessary in order to maintain extension and increase flexion.

General post-operative care for all arthroplasty procedures

- The patient may have a drain in place. This is normally removed 24–48 h after surgery, when the dressing is also reduced.
- The use of analgesia is encouraged.
- Neurovascular observations are performed as indicated by the patient's condition and local policy.
- Precautions should be taken to prevent DVT.

Spinal surgery

Spinal conditions and low back pain

Low back pain is a symptom associated with the following spinal conditions:
- degenerative disc disease
- facet joint arthritis
- spondylolysis (stress fracture)
- spondylolisthesis or instability
- spinal fracture due to trauma
- spinal deformity
- lumbar disc herniation
- spinal stenosis
- tumours
- inflammatory conditions (e.g. ankylosing spondylitis, rheumatoid arthritis)
- neuropsychiatric conditions.

Before surgery for spinal cord impingement is considered, conservative treatments will usually have been exhausted. These may include:
- physiotherapy
- health advice and lifestyle changes, including smoking cessation, weight loss, exercise, and advice on good posture (especially when moving, handling, and lifting objects)
- analgesics
- heat or cold therapy
- supportive corsetry
- non-steroidal anti-inflammatory drugs
- epidural steroidal injections.

Spinal decompression

This is a general term that refers to the process of surgically relieving the pressure impingement on the spinal cord and spinal nerves. The following are classed as spinal decompression procedures:
- *Laminectomy* is performed when there is a narrowing of the spinal canal (spinal stenosis). It involves the partial or complete removal of the lamina of the affected vertebrae.
- *Discectomy* or *microdiscectomy* is performed in order to relieve the pressure caused by a prolapsed or herniated intervertebral disc. The affected part of the disc is removed, and this procedure may be performed in combination with a laminectomy. For disc lesions of the lumbar spine a posterior approach is used, whereas an anterior approach may be used for disc lesions of the cervical spine.

Spinal fusion

This procedure may be considered for severe degenerative disorders, injuries, and deformities of the spine, especially in the lumbar region. During surgery the disc is removed and a bone graft (usually an autograft from the iliac crest) is inserted to fuse the bone together. Surgical metalwork may also be inserted to support the fusion, especially if more than one bone is involved.

As with discectomy, a posterior approach is normally used for the lumbar region, whereas an anterior approach may be considered for the cervical region.

Scoliosis

This is a lateral C or S-shaped spinal deformity, with rotation of the vertebrae. It can result from bad posture or be caused by a structural abnormality of the spine.

It can affect all parts of the spine, but is most commonly seen in the thoracic and lumbar area. If untreated, scoliosis leads to problems with body image, balance problems, cardiopulmonary compromise, and pain caused by degenerative changes in the spinal joints.

Types of structural scoliosis

There are six types of structural scoliosis—congenital, infantile, juvenile, neuromuscular, adolescent, and adult. The most commonly seen type is adolescent scoliosis (also known as idiopathic scoliosis, as there is no apparent cause).

Management of scoliosis

See Box 20.24.

Post-operative care for all spinal surgery patients

- The patient usually stays in hospital for 2–4 days, but hospitalization may be longer, especially after spinal fusion and scoliosis surgery.
- IV or IM opioid analgesia is given post-operatively, progressing to oral pain relief following discharge.
- Chest drains will be *in situ* after scoliosis surgery.
- Close observation of vital signs, cardiac and respiratory function monitoring, and neurovascular observations are required following scoliosis surgery.
- Restricted fluids and diet may be required until bowel sounds are heard.
- Catheterization may be required until the patient is mobilizing.
- Log rolling and sitting up in alignment.
- Perching to wash and eat.
- Possible bracing or support corset may be needed for up to 6 months.
- The patient should be instructed to avoid bending and lifting heavy weights for 3–6 weeks after decompression and for 3–6 months after spinal fusion.

Box 20.24 Management of scoliosis	
Conservative	Physiotherapy, spinal bracing to slow spinal curve progression
Surgical	Spinal segmental rodding and spinal fusion. Anterior discectomy and costoplasty may be performed to loosen the curve and aid instrumentation

Hand and foot conditions

Common conditions that affect the hand and wrist

Rheumatoid arthritis

This is usually treated non-surgically, especially in the early stages (see ➲ Box 20.21, p. 506). Surgical procedures such as synovectomy for severe synovitis, stabilization surgery for deformity, and arthrodesis or arthoplasty for joint destruction may be considered.

Osteoarthritis

As with rheumatoid arthritis, a non-surgical approach is usually the first line of treatment, although arthrodesis or arthroplasty is also considered if there is severe joint destruction.

Dupuytren's contracture

This involves the thickening and contracture of the palmar fascia, which can progress to the index and ring fingers, producing flexion deformities.

A Z-shaped surgical dissection of the palmar fascia (Z-plasty) is usually considered, and skin grafting may also be required following dissection. Occasionally amputation may be the best option in severe cases.

Trigger finger

This occurs as a result of a thickening of the tendon sheath within which the flexor tendon becomes trapped until the finger is forced into extension (although occasionally the finger cannot be extended). Many cases resolve without any intervention, although steroidal injections can often be effective. Occasionally an incision of the tendon sheath is indicated if the condition is recurring and/or persistent.

Carpal tunnel syndrome

This presents as pain and paraesthesia along the median nerve into the hand, as well as the thumb, index finger, middle finger, and lateral side of the ring finger. It is common in middle-aged women, and is often seen during pregnancy, but usually resolves after the pregnancy.

The condition results from any swelling in and around the carpal tunnel of the wrist, through which the median nerve passes.

Splinting and steroidal injections may be used, although in persistent cases surgery to decompress the carpal tunnel may be indicated.

Common conditions that affect the foot and ankle

Rheumatoid arthritis and osteoarthritis

As with the hand, a non-surgical approach is the first line of treatment, with similar surgical options considered for synovitis, deformity, and joint destruction.

Pes planus (flat feet)

This condition can be congenital, as a result of fusion of the tarsal bone from birth, or acquired, as a result of ligament laxity that is often caused by inflammatory arthritis. Non-surgical treatment is generally considered to be the best option, usually with the use of orthotics. Surgical treatment, when considered, may involve tendon surgery and/or fusion to increase the medial arch.

Hallux valgus with bunions or corns

This condition usually develops as a result of wearing narrow shoes that force the first metatarsal phalangeal joint laterally, exposing a hard bony prominence over which a bursa may develop. The skin over this prominence becomes hardened and/or inflamed, and pressure from footwear can also cause pressure sores to develop.

Orthotics and the use of anti-inflammatory drugs may be considered as a first-line treatment, although surgical straightening (osteotomy) of the toe is often considered, with removal of the bunion.

Congenital talipes equinovarus (clubfoot)

This is a congenital deformity in which either one or both feet internally rotate at the ankle. Treatment is usually conservative, with the foot being gently manipulated into position and supported with a cast. This procedure is repeated several times over a period of 4–5 weeks until the deformity has been corrected (the Ponseti method). Following correction, supportive orthotics are often required, and occasionally corrective surgery to adjust the ligaments may also be needed.

Morton's neuroma

This is a benign growth within the intermetatarsal plantar nerves that results in pain and/or paraesthesia in the sole of the foot, especially when weight bearing. Treatment may involve the use of orthotic footwear, steroidal injections, or surgical removal of the neuroma.

Post-operative care

See the section on hand and wrist injuries on p. 478 and the section on foot and ankle injuries on p. 484.

Chapter 21

Vascular surgery

Symptoms of vascular disease

Of the population with peripheral artery disease (PAD), 20–50% are asymptomatic.

Patients who lead a sedentary lifestyle will not walk far enough to develop the symptoms of claudication. Therefore population screening for PAD, using the resting Ankle Brachial Pressure Index (ABPI), will always detect cases in individuals without any symptoms.

Intermittent claudication is present in 10–35% of the population with PAD, and most commonly affects the calf muscle (3–5% of the adult population), although it can also affect the thigh and buttocks in rare cases. Patients describe a cramping aching discomfort on walking a specific distance, which is relieved by resting for less than 10 min. The pain is always reproducible on walking, and is worse when walking uphill, carrying a heavy object, or when walking at a faster pace. The pain is not evident at rest or when standing.

Critical limb ischaemia is present in 1–3% of the PAD population, and symptoms include the following:
• Night pain—toe pain on elevation of the limb, which is relieved with dependency. Patients typically report these symptoms at night when lying in bed, but can develop them on elevation at any time of the day and the patient usually stops sleeping in bed but favours a chair, as their legs are dependent when they are seated in a chair.
• Rest pain—as well as having night pain, patients can also develop true rest pain, which is pain in the toes and/or foot that is experienced continually, not just on elevation.
• Tissue loss—ulcers and gangrene.

The classification of peripheral arterial disease according to Fontaine's stages is shown in Table 21.1.

Table 21.1 Fontaine's stages

Stage	Clinical presentation
I	Asymptomatic
IIa	Mild claudication
IIb	Moderate to severe claudication
III	Ischaemic rest pain
IV	Ulceration and gangrene

Assessment of the vascular patient

Intermittent claudication

- Objective assessment of symptoms:
  - How long have the symptoms been present?
  - How far can the patient walk on the flat before developing symptoms?
  - Do the symptoms feel like cramp, and do they resolve with a rest of less than 10 min?
  - Do they only occur on exertion (e.g. walking on the street)?
  - Do they occur in the muscle groups of the legs?
  - Does the patient have pain at rest or when the limb is elevated?
- Foot assessment:
  - Assessment of skin condition, including any wounds or ulcers.
  - Temperature of limbs, assessing both together to assess for any difference in temperature.
  - Is hair and nail growth normal and equal on both limbs?
- Palpation of pulses:
  - Palpation of peripheral pulses, including femoral, popliteal, dorsalis pedis, and posterior tibial.
  - Remember that diabetic patients can have bounding pulses but have significant arterial disease.

Ankle Brachial Pressure Index (ABPI) measurement

- Values of less than 0.9 indicate arterial insufficiency.
- Values higher than 1.2 suggest calcification of arteries and render the test inconclusive.
- Resting or exercise ABPIs can be completed. Exercise ABPIs detect a drop in pressure following exercise, and provide information on functional walking distance as well as pressure readings.
- Patients with an isolated iliac stenosis may have no pressure decrease across the stenosis at rest, and will therefore have a normal resting ABPI. However, on exercise the increased blood flow down the leg will make such lesions significant.

Duplex imaging

This ultrasound-guided technique allows the arterial flow to be assessed throughout the arterial tree, from the aorta through to the pedal arteries. It provides detailed images of the location and size of arterial stenosis, and aids clinical decisions on treatment options.

Factors that influence vascular disease

Smoking

Smokers are three times more likely to develop symptomatic PAD than non-smokers. The association between smoking and PAD may be even stronger than that between smoking and coronary heart disease. Heavier smokers have more severe disease than less heavy smokers (see Table 21.2).

Hypertension

Hypertension is associated with arterial disease in any arterial bed, but the relative risk of developing PAD is less for hypertension than it is for diabetes or smoking.

Diabetes mellitus

- Symptomatic PAD is twice as common in diabetic patients compared with non-diabetic patients.
- Patients with confirmed diabetes have a 26% increased risk of PAD with every 1% increase in glycated haemoglobin (HbA1C) levels.
- Diabetic patients develop more aggressive PAD, with earlier large vessel disease, than non-diabetic patients.
- The need for major amputation is 5 to 10 times higher in diabetic patients than in non-diabetic patients.
- Insulin resistance can occur pre-diabetes, and includes a myriad of risk factors, including hyperglycaemia, dyslipidaemia, hypertension, and central obesity, and raises the risk of symptomatic PAD by 40–50%.

Dyslipidaemia

A fasting cholesterol level higher than 7 mmol/L has been associated with a doubling of the incidence of symptomatic PAD. Treatment of hyperlipidaemia reduces both the progression of arterial disease and the incidence of symptomatic disease.

Age

The prevalence of symptomatic PAD increases with age, and ranges from a prevalence of 3% in patients aged 40 years, to 6% in patients aged 60 years.

Gender

Symptomatic PAD is more common in men from the relatively younger age groups, but at older ages there is little difference between men and women.

Genetics

It is recognized that arterial disease can be genetically linked, and it may be due to the genetic links for hyperlipidaemia and type 2 diabetes.

Hyperhomocysteine

An increased homocysteine level is high in the PAD population. Hyperhomocysteinaemia is detected in 1% of the general population and in 30% of young patients with symptomatic PAD.

Table 21.2 Intermittent claudication: risk factors and associations of vascular disease. Reproduced with permission from Greg McLatchie, Neil Borley and Joanna Chikwe, *Oxford Handbook of Clinical Surgery*, 3rd edition, 2007, p. 576, with permission from Oxford University Press.

Risk factor	Association
Hypertension	Obesity
Hyperlipidaemia	Diet
Diabetes mellitus	Sedentary lifestyle
Tobacco smoking	Gender
Positive family history	Occupation

Chronic ischaemia of the limbs

Chronic ischaemia is treated conservatively with best medical therapy and lifestyle modifications.

Best medical therapy (BMT)

- Complete smoking cessation.
- Commence antiplatelet therapy. Clopidogrel 75 mg should be prescribed daily to prevent occlusive vascular events.[1]
- Commence statin therapy. All patients who have been diagnosed with peripheral arterial disease should be commenced on statin therapy, as they are at high risk of future arterial events, including myocardial infarction (MI) and cerebrovascular accident.[1] Aim for total cholesterol 4 mmol/L and LDL-cholesterol 2 mmol/L.
- Control blood pressure: ≤ 135/85 mmHg. Blood pressure of 140/90 mmHg warrants ambulatory blood pressure monitoring.[2]
- Control diabetes. Aim for HbA1C levels to be less than 7% or as close to 6% as possible.[3]

Lifestyle modifications

- Check diabetic status yearly, even if the patient is not known to have any metabolic syndrome or confirmed diabetes.[3]
- Low-fat diet.
- Weight reduction, aiming for a healthy BMI of 18–25 kg/m^2.
- Purposeful daily walking; exercise has been shown to build a collateral blood supply that can compensate for the diseased artery. The collaterals grow in response to the pain that develops during walking. Therefore a purposeful daily walk to cause the pain can help to relieve the symptoms in the long term.

Surgical interventions

Surgical intervention is considered if the patient's walking distance has not improved or if it has deteriorated. Treatment options include angioplasty and stent and bypass graft surgery.

Angiography

- This allows progression to therapeutic angioplasty, stent, or thrombolysis.
- Stop warfarin prior to the procedure. Metformin may be stopped post procedure for 48 h.
- Can be performed as a day-case procedure or an inpatient procedure.
- Usual post-operative observations for 4 h, assessing for haemorrhage.
- Assessment of puncture site for haematoma and evident bleeding.
- Closure devices seal the artery and allow early mobilization, but if not used the patient should lie supported for 4 h before sitting up and then eventually mobilizing.
- Foot observation and pain assessment are important to assess for embolic events. Increasing foot pain should be assessed by the medical team.

Bypass graft surgery

- Prior to the procedure a venous duplex of the legs and/or arms is undertaken to assess whether a suitable vein can be used for the procedure.
- The preferred choice is a vein graft, as they have better patency rates, but prosthetic grafts can be used.
- Veins can be either harvested, reversed, and then used as a bypass graft, or can be *in situ* and replumbed into arterial vessels.
- The diseased artery is bypassed with either the vein or prosthetic graft, so that blood flows around the diseased or occluded section and rejoins the native vessel below the level of disease.
- The usual post-operative care is required.
- Foot checks are needed after the procedure, to ensure that the foot is well perfused.
- Length of stay is variable, depending upon the type of graft, site of graft, patient's condition before the procedure, and comorbidities.
- Post-procedure infra-inguinal vein grafts are surveyed, using duplex scans, checking for graft stenoses and inflow or outflow problems. This is to try to prevent graft failure.

References

1 National Institute for Health and Care Excellence (NICE). *Clopidogrel and Modified-Release Dipyridamole for the Prevention of Occlusive Vascular Events*. TA210. NICE: London, 2010. www.nice.org.uk/guidance/ta210
2 National Institute for Health and Care Excellence (NICE). *Hypertension*. QS28. NICE: London, 2013. www.nice.org.uk/guidance/qs28
3 Norgren L et al. Inter-society consensus for the management of peripheral arterial disease (TASC II). *Journal of Vascular Surgery* 2007; **45 (Suppl. S):** S5–67.

Acute ischaemia of the limbs

Acute limb ischaemia is defined as any sudden decrease in limb perfusion that causes a potential threat to limb viability in patients who present within 2 weeks of the acute event.[4]

Causes
- Embolism.
- Trauma.
- Peripheral aneurysms with emboli.
- Native thrombosis.
- Reconstruction (graft) occlusions.

Physical examination and the 5 P's
- Pain: time of onset, location and intensity, change over time.
- Pulselessness: absent pedal pulses. The accuracy of pulse detection is highly variable, so ABPI measurements should be recorded immediately. Usually very low pressure is obtained or the Doppler signals may be absent.
- Pallor: change of colour and temperature is common, especially if there is a marked difference from the contralateral limb. Venous filling may be slow or absent.
- Paraesthesia: numbness occurs in more than 50% of patients.
- Paralysis: this is a poor prognostic sign.

Limb viability
Following physical examination the severity of the acute limb ischaemia and the viability of the limb must be assessed. Table 21.3 shows the three categories of limb viability.[4]

Table 21.3 Three categories of limb viability

Category	Description and prognosis	Sensory loss	Muscle weakness
1. Viable	Not immediately threatened	None	None
2a. Threatened marginal	Salvageable if promptly treated	Minimal (toes) or none	None
2b. Threatened immediate	Salvageable with immediate revascularization	More than toes, associated with rest pain	Mild, moderate
3. Irreversible	Major tissue loss or permanent nerve damage inevitable	Profound, anaesthetic	Profound paralysis (rigor)

Three findings which help to separate 'threatened' from 'viable' extremities are:
- presence of rest pain
- sensory loss
- muscle weakness.

Investigations

The following investigations are performed in order to establish a cause for the acute ischaemia.
- A 12-lead electrocardiogram (ECG) to look for atrial fibrillation, myocardial infarction (MI), and ventricular aneurysm.
- Standard biochemistry to see whether dehydration is the cause.
- Full blood count to check for polycythaemia.
- Clotting times—inherited prothrombotic states.
- Imaging of arterial flow—aneurysm, intermittent claudication.

Imaging in the form of angiography or duplex images will assist the planning of treatment options.

Treatment

- All patients with suspected acute limb ischaemia should be reviewed immediately by a vascular specialist, who will decide what treatment should be implemented and when.[4]
- Pharmacological thrombolysis is the initial treatment of choice in patients in whom the degree of severity allows time (category 1 and 2). A lytic agent is administered via a catheter for 22–48 h. Repeat angiography is usually undertaken after 24 h to assess progress.
- Other endovascular techniques include percutaneous aspiration thrombectomy suction using a 50-mL syringe to remove an embolus or thrombus from native arteries, bypass grafts, and run-off vessels. It can be used independently or as a joint treatment plan with thrombolysis.
- Surgical embolectomy.
- Graft thrombosis involves removing the clot and correcting the underlying lesion that caused the thrombosis. This is usually completed with angioplasty, stent or bypass grafting, or surgical revision of previous graft.
- Thrombosed popliteal aneurysm is treated with either surgical bypass grafting to tibial vessels or regional thrombolysis.
- Amputation, with the ratio of above-knee to below-knee amputations being 4:1 in acute limb ischaemia, compared with 1:1 for critical limb ischaemia. The incidence of major amputation is 25%. Around 10–15% of patients are thought to be salvageable, undergo therapy, and ultimately require major amputation.

Reference

4 Norgren L et al. Inter-society consensus for the management of peripheral arterial disease (TASC II). *Journal of Vascular Surgery* 2007; **45** (Suppl. S): S5–67.

Carotid disease

Pathophysiology

Hardening of the arteries (atherosclerosis) causes most cases of carotid artery disease. Atheromatous plaques form at the bifurcation of the common carotid artery, and advance into the external and internal carotid arteries. A cerebrovascular accident (CVA) or stroke can be caused by atheroma of the carotid arteries, when the plaque in a carotid artery cracks or ruptures. Occlusion of the vessels in carotid disease is from plaque stenosis or thromboembolism. A CVA can also be caused by an intracerebral haemorrhage. Due to the anatomical structure of the circle of Willis, blood flow may be sufficient to support brain tissue during the acute phase and prevent severe damage.

Clinical features

Signs and symptoms are of sudden onset over hours or even days.
- Amaurosis fugax (a dulling of vision described by the patient as being like a blind being pulled down).
- Weakness.
- Slurred speech.
- Paralysis (hemiparesis).
- Ataxia or aphasia.

A CVA if the patient's symptoms last for ≥ 24 h.
  Transient ischaemic attacks (TIAs) have the same symptoms as CVA but last for ≤ 24 hours.
  Crescendo TIAs are ≥ 2 in a week.

Diagnosis

The carotid plaque is assessed by a carotid duplex scan, and two forms of measurement are used:
- The North American Symptomatic Carotid Endarterectomy Trial (NASCET). Patients who require carotid artery revascularization need to have carotid stenosis of 50–99% according to NASCET.
- The European Carotid Surgery Trials (ECST). Carotid stenosis needs to be 70–99% before revascularization is performed.

Patients may also require a magnetic resonance angiograph (MRA) or CT angiography.

Treatment

Patients who clinically present with symptoms of a TIA and are at high risk for stroke should receive the following immediate treatment:
- aspirin started immediately at 300 mg daily
- assessment and investigations within 24 h
- introduction of measures for secondary prevention
- assessment for carotid endarterectomy or stenting within 7 days of symptoms
- surgery or intervention to be performed within 2 weeks
- best medical treatment.

Carotid endarterectomy is the treatment of choice for patients with symptomatic carotid stenosis who are suitable for surgery. Carotid artery stenting should be considered as an option for patients who require carotid artery revascularization to prevent stroke, and who are at increased risk of developing surgical complications.

Complications associated with carotid stenting

- Hypertension.
- Allergy to contrast.
- Poor renal function.
- Calcified carotid artery.
- Difficult anatomy and irregular plaque within carotid arteries.

Carotid endarterectomy

Carotid endarterectomy removes the plaque that is blocking the carotid artery, and can be performed using a local or general anaesthetic.

Pre-operative care for carotid endarterectomy

- Patients are assessed in a vascular pre-admission clinic.
- Pre-operative blood tests should include full blood count, clotting, and renal and liver function.
- 12-lead ECG.
- Diabetic patients will require a recent HbA1C.
- Chest X-ray.

Surgical procedure

- An incision is made near the sternomastoid muscle in the neck, and the carotid artery is opened.
- The internal, common, and external carotid arteries are clamped, the lumen of the internal carotid artery is opened, and the atheromatous plaque substance is removed.
- The artery is closed, homeostasis is achieved, and the overlying layers are closed.
- Many surgeons lay a temporary shunt to ensure a blood supply to the brain during the procedure.
- A Dacron patch may be used in closure if required.
- Transcranial Doppler is used peri-operatively and post-operatively in patients who are having a general anaesthetic, and only post-operatively in patients who are having a local anaesthetic.

Post-operative care following a carotid endarterectomy

- The patient is nursed in a post-anaesthetic care unit or an enhanced care unit immediately post-operatively for 1–24 h depending on patient needs. They are returned to a surgical ward once they are stable.
- Continual monitoring of vital signs, intravenous fluids until oral fluids are tolerated, and analgesics as needed.

- Observe for:
  - bradycardia
  - change in level of consciousness and/or loss of motor control
  - dysphasia
  - visual disturbances
  - ipsilateral headache
  - bleeding or swelling at the wound site
  - cranial nerve damage.

Complications

Complications can arise during or following surgery, as well as underlying conditions that led to the blockage of the patient's arteries in the first place. Stroke is the most serious intra-operative and post-operative risk. If it occurs within 12–24 h after surgery, the cause is usually an embolism. Other major complications that can occur are:

- myocardial infarction
- death
- respiratory difficulties
- hypertension
- nerve injury, which can cause problems with vocal cords, saliva management, and tongue movement
- cerebral haemorrhage
- restenosis, the continuing build-up of plaque, which can occur from 5 months to 13 years after surgery.

Discharge

- 1–3 days following surgery.
- Removal of clips or sutures (if not dissolvable) at 7–10 days.
- Outpatient appointment 4–6 weeks post-operatively.
- The patient cannot drive until they have been seen in outpatients post-operatively.

Abdominal aortic aneurysm (AAA) disease

An aneurysm is a balloon-like swelling in the wall of an artery, which may be due to degenerative disease or infection that damages the muscular section of the vessel. It can also be due to a congenital deficiency in the muscular wall.

Common sites for aneurysms
- Thoracic aorta.
- Abdominal aorta.
- Iliac artery.
- Popliteal artery.
- Carotid artery.
- Cerebral arteries.

Risk factors
- Family history.
- Hypertension.
- Peripheral arterial disease.
- Smoking.
- Marfan syndrome (a genetic disorder of connective tissue).
- Untreated syphilis.

Clinical features
- Asymptomatic, usually found incidentally.
- Strong abdominal pulsation or a pulsatile mass felt on clinical examination.
- Occurs in the older population unless there is a strong family history (there is a 1 in 4 chance of siblings having AAA).
- Can develop trash foot or distal gangrene from emboli.

Medical management and treatment
- Anteroposterior (AP) diameter 3.0–5.5 cm: regular ultrasound scans and best medical therapy.
- AP diameter ≥ 5.5 cm: surgical repair if the patient is fit for surgery.

Best medical therapy
- Control of hypertension.
- Smoking cessation.
- Antiplatelet therapy.
- Statin therapy.
- Healthy lifestyle advice, including diet and exercise.

Clinical features of rupture
- Back pain radiating round to the groin.
- Unconsciousness.
- Raised blood pressure and low pulse.
- Pallor.
- Distended abdomen.
- *This is a medical emergency.* There is only a 10% chance of survival.

Types of surgery

Open repair

- Hospitalization for 7–10 days.
- For the first 48–72 h the patient is nursed on a high-dependency unit or critical care unit.
- Bowel obstruction care.
- Epidural care.
- Recovery period is 3–6 months.
- Standard follow-up in clinic.

Endovascular aneurysm repair (EVAR)

- A stent is inserted under sterile X-ray fluoroscopic guidance.
- In some centres this is performed as day-case surgery, but it generally involves a stay of 1–3 days in hospital.
- Spiral CT assessment of graft position at 1 month, 3 months, and then yearly for 5 years.

Amputation

Amputation is the severing of a limb, or part of a limb, from the rest of the body. A minor amputation involves partial removal of a foot, such as toe amputations or forefoot resections. A major amputation involves removal of the leg above or below the knee (see Figure 21.1).

The aim of surgical amputation is to increase the quality of life for the patient by alleviating pain, infection, and reduced mobility, while producing a soundly healed stump that the patient can mobilize on and that will allow early rehabilitation with a prosthesis.

Epidemiology

- The population of amputees is thought to be around 52 000.
- There is significant geographical variation in amputation rates.
- The incidence is higher in smokers, rises steeply with age (most amputees are over 60 years old), and is higher in men.
- Diabetes is a significant factor, accounting for 50% of the total amputee population. Diabetic patients are 12.5–31.6 times more likely to have an amputation than non-diabetics.

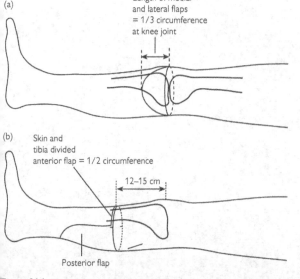

Figure 21.1 Common levels of lower limb amputation. (a) Through-knee amputation. (b) Below-knee amputation. Reproduced with permission from Hands L, Murphy M, Sharp M et al. *Oxford Specialist Handbook of Vascular Surgery*, 2007. Oxford: Oxford University Press, p. 341, Figures 15.3 and 15.4.

Aetiology

- Approximately 85–90% of amputations in the developed world are caused by peripheral vascular disease, with the remaining 10–15% caused by infection secondary to diabetic foot ulceration (see Table 21.4).
- In the UK, 72% of amputations are due to peripheral vascular disease.

Table 21.4 Causes of amputation

Cause of amputation	Percentage
Dysvascularity	72%
Trauma	7%
Infection	8%
Neurological disorder	1%
Neoplasia	3%
Other	5%
No cause provided	4%

Rehabilitation of the amputee

There are three important aims of rehabilitation:
- The production of a soundly healed stump and a patient who can walk. The level of amputation is crucial. Above-knee amputations heal readily, but many patients do not master walking on a prosthesis. The opposite is true of below-knee amputations.
- Early rehabilitation with a prosthesis.
- Cost-effectiveness.

Process of rehabilitation

Before the stump has healed

The patient should be mobilized using the pneumatic post-amputation mobility (PPAM) aid under the supervision of an experienced physiotherapist. Initially, parallel bars are used for support, slowly graduating to elbow crutches. The patient will then be referred to the local disablement service centre to be assessed and measured for a prosthesis. If it is unlikely that they will be able to walk, a wheelchair will be provided.

Once the stump has healed

The patient will receive their first prosthesis with a temporary socket. Occasionally a temporary limb may be used if the patient is frail, requires a light prosthesis, or if there is doubt whether they will use a prosthesis. The length of time spent standing is slowly increased, at first on the flat and later on slopes and uneven surfaces. The patient is taught how to pick up objects on the floor, climb stairs, and get up again after falling. Close supervision by occupational therapists and physiotherapists is therefore essential. A home visit will be completed to assess for structural changes or re-accommodation requirements.

Stump care

- Examine the stump regularly in the early stages for oedema and infection.
- Swelling is controlled with stump compression socks (only to be used after the stump has healed).
- Infection is treated with antibiotics and rest.
- Stump socks are provided and worn with the prosthesis to avoid chafing by the fit of the limb.
- Problems with weight-bearing areas of the stump and the interface of the prosthesis will arise as the stump shrinks and the socket becomes loose.

Causes of stump pain

- Neuromas.
- Osteomyelitis—growth of a bony spur.
- Ischaemia.
- Phantom limb pain.

The psychological impact of amputation

- This is often described in the same emotional terms as a bereavement. The patient passes through the stages of bereavement while coming to terms with the amputation.
- Feelings can be intensified by phantom limb pain.
- The psychological impact is generally more pronounced in the elderly population.
- The patient should have time to decide upon amputation, and will need time with the medical team to ensure that they make the right decision.
- Referral to either a counsellor or a psychiatric team for support may be required.

Work

- Amputees should be encouraged to return to work.
- People who can no longer work within their usual role should get support from their workplace occupational health or social care.

Driving

- Amputees must inform the Driver and Vehicle Licensing Centre (DVLC) and their insurance company about their disability.
- An amputation should not debar the patient from driving, as a car can be modified.
- The DVLC will recommend an automatic transmission car. If the driver is a bilateral amputee, hand controls are required.
- All amputees should be advised to contact the British School of Motoring or a local agency for a trial assessment, and they should join the Disabled Drivers Association.

Varicose veins

Varicose veins are superficial veins that have become widened and tortuous. They are often visible in leg tissues.

Pathophysiology

Valves in the superficial system become incompetent, leaking and causing back flow into the veins, putting pressure on the veins and nearby valves and creating venous hypertension and varicosities. Saphenofemoral junction incompetence is the most common cause of reflux from the deep to superficial vein systems. Other causes may include:

- genetics
- venous outflow obstruction due to deep vein thrombosis (DVT) or trauma
- external compression by surrounding tissue (e.g. tumour)
- pregnancy.

Prevalence

In the UK, around 40% of varicose veins occur in men and 32% in women. However, more women present for treatment. Influencing factors include:

- pregnancy
- age
- obesity.

Presentation

- Cosmetic, due to unsightly tortuous veins, reticular veins, or telangiectasia (thread veins). Asymptomatic.
- Symptomatic, with discomfort and heaviness in the legs, particularly after standing for long periods and by the end of the day. Itching and aching may also occur.
- Symptoms are often more severe in the early and later stages of the condition.

Complications

- Thrombophlebitis.
- Skin changes: haemosiderin to lipodermatosclerosis, eczema.
- Bleeding.
- Ulcers.
- Associated with incompetent valves and venous hypertension.

History

- Family history.
- Previous venous disease, including DVT.
- Coexisting cardiovascular disease.
- Complications, including healed ulcers.
- Quality-of-life issues relating to varicose veins.

Physical examination

- With the patient standing, note the area of varicosity and distribution
- Varicosities relating to the short saphenous vein normally present below the knee and posteriolaterally.
- Varicosities relating to the long saphenous vein normally present the length of the leg and medially.
- Oedema.
- Skin changes.
- Location of saphenofemoral junction to assess thrill.
- Abdominal examination to observe for causes of external venous compression.

Investigations

- Duplex ultrasound is the gold standard, and colour flow imaging may be added.
- Doppler (hand-held).

Treatment options

Support hosiery
- Used to provide relief from aching.
- Absence of arterial disease should be confirmed prior to prescribing.
- The patient should be measured as per the manufacturer's guidelines
- Compliance issues.

Intervention
- Surgery: saphenofemoral ligation, stripping of the long saphenous vein, and avulsion.
- Radiofrequency/laser ablation: insertion of a probe into the long saphenous vein using ultrasound guidance. Ablation using radiofrequency or laser.
- Sclerotherapy: sclerosant is injected into the veins, causing them to spasm, and sections of vein are destroyed. May be mixed with air or gas to produce foam and then injected.
- After all interventions, bandaging and compression hosiery are required.

Possible complications of intervention include:
- bruising
- haemorrhage
- wound infection
- skin staining (foam sclerotherapy)
- paraesthesia
- reoccurrence
- DVT
- skin burns (radiofrequency/laser ablation).

Lymphoedema

Causes of primary lymphoedema

Inherited primary lymphoedema is caused by poorly developed or missing lymph nodes or vessels in the body. It may be present at birth, develop at the onset of puberty (praecox), or become apparent many years into adulthood (tarda).

Causes of secondary lymphoedema

- Injury to lymphatic vessels, most commonly after lymph node dissection, surgery, radiation therapy (for breast cancer or head and neck cancer), or DVT.
- Cancer patients can develop symptoms months or years after treatment has been completed.
- Accidents.
- Parasitic infections (filariasis).

Pathophysiology

The flow of lymph from the legs to the heart is the result of the calf muscle pump (soleus muscle). As a person walks, this muscle contracts, squeezing lymph out of the leg via the lymphatic system. When the muscle relaxes, the valves in the vessels close, preventing the fluid from returning to the extremities. Lymph from the leg is filtered through the inguinal lymph nodes (groin) to the thoracic duct and then into the venous circulation through the left subclavian vein.

Stages of development

Grade 1 (mild oedema)
Lymphoedema involves the distal body parts, such as the forearm and hand, or lower leg and foot. The difference in circumference is less than 4 cm, and other tissue changes are not yet present.

Grade 2 (moderate oedema)
Lymphoedema involves an entire limb or corresponding quadrant of the trunk. The difference in circumference is more than 4 cm but less than 6 cm, and tissue changes such as pitting are apparent. The patient may develop infection of the skin (erysipelas).

Grade 3a (severe oedema)
Lymphoedema is present in one limb and its associated trunk quadrant. The difference in circumference is more than 6 cm. Significant skin altera-tions, such as cornification or keratosis, cysts and/or fistulae are present. In addition, the patient may experience repeated attacks of erysipelas.

Grade 3b (massive oedema)
The same symptoms are present as in grade 3a, except that two or more extremities are affected.

Grade 4 (gigantic oedema)

Also known as elephantiasis, in this stage of lymphoedema the affected extremities are huge, due to almost complete blockage of the lymph channels. Elephantiasis may also affect the head and face.

Diagnosis

- Physical examination of the leg.
- Determine whether elevation relieves the swelling.
- Measure the circumference of the affected limb with a tape measure. There should be a 4 cm difference in size between the affected limb and the contralateral limb. This measurement can be used in future assessments to determine whether the symptoms are improving.
- Check for pulses (femoral, popliteal, posterior tibial, and dorsalis pedis).
- Assess the degree of swelling with fingertip pressure.
- Check whether the groin lymph nodes are enlarged, which would suggest that infection is present.

Treatment

- Manual compression lymphatic massage performed by a trained specialist.
- Compression bandaging (wrapping) utilizing several layers of padding and short-stretch bandaging to reduce swelling.
- Sequential gradient pump therapy (multi-chambered pneumatic sleeve with cells that overlap to promote fluid movement). This can help to soften fibrotic tissue and therefore enable more efficient lymphatic drainage.
- Compression with garments (either specifically measured or over-the-counter products).
- Exercise therapy.
- Usually a combination of all of the above is used to treat the affected limb.

Aetiology of venous leg ulcers

Venous leg ulcers account for approximately 70% of leg ulcers, and venous hypertension is the largest contributory factor in leg ulceration.

Chronic venous hypertension

- Valvular damage allows the reflux of blood, resulting in high pressures in the capillaries damaging the microcirculation, leading to leakage of red blood cells causing pigmentation. Thinning of the dermis occurs, leaving the skin susceptible to trauma.
- The condition may be exacerbated by calf or foot pump failure, with peripheral oedema leading to tissue ischaemia.

The progression from chronic venous hypertension to ulceration is unclear and much debated. The main theories can be summarized as follows:

- White cell entrapment—trapped leucocytes release inflammatory mediators that alter the permeability of capillary vessels, allowing tissue breakdown.
- Fibrin cuffs are found around capillaries in areas of lipodermatosclerosis. These may act as a barrier to oxygen, causing localized ischaemia.
- Mechanical theory—ulceration occurs as a result of mechanical stress on the leg from oedema.
- Trap growth factor theory—tissue repair is prevented by growth factors being trapped in fibrin cuffs.

Alone or in combination, these are thought to cause venous ulcers. Ulcers may be insidious or they may be exacerbated by trauma to tissues.

Further reading

Moffatt C, Martin R and Smithdale R. *Leg Ulcer Management*. Blackwell Publishing Ltd: Oxford, 2007.

Assessment of venous leg ulcers

History
- Family history of venous disease.
- Medical history of:
  - trauma
  - soft tissue injuries
  - DVT
  - phlebitis
  - fixed or limited ankle joint function
  - varicose veins
  - symptoms of venous insufficiency.
- Ulcer:
  - duration
  - pain
  - site.

Appearance
The ulcer is shallow, and occurs in the gaiter area, most commonly to the medial aspect with the presence of granulating tissue to wound bed and an irregular border.

Skin changes to the lower leg include the following:
- haemosiderin—brown staining caused by leakage of blood into the interstitial space
- lipodermatosclerosis—hard wood-like skin caused by fibrous tissue being laid down. This creates a change in leg shape (inverted champagne bottle)
- ankle flare—tiny varicose-type veins around the ankle which are usually due to incompetent perforators
- atrophie blanche—layers of white avascular tissue surrounded by hyperpigmentation
- varicose eczema—due to irritation from leaking capillaries.

Lifestyle factors
- Intravenous drug abuse.
- Obesity.

Investigations
- Foot pulses.
- ABPI > 0.8. Remember that diabetic patients may have increased pressures due to calcification.
- Duplex scan if there is a history of DVT or varicose veins.
- Blood tests, including full blood count, erythrocyte sedimentation rate, renal function, and glucose to check for diabetes.
- Wound swab if infection is suspected.
- Wound biopsy for non-healing or irregular ulcers.

Differential diagnosis
Arterial ulcer, mixed aetiology ulcer, vasculitic ulcer, or malignancy.

Wound assessment
- Site.
- Size—width, length, and depth.
- Wound bed appearance.
- Exudate.
- Wound margins.
- Surrounding skin condition.
- Pain.
- Photograph and wound map.

Management of venous ulcers

Compression therapy
- This is the mainstay of management of venous ulcers.
- External graduated pressure is applied to reduce oedema, reverse venous hypertension, and promote venous return.
- A pressure of 40 mmHg at the ankle is calculated to reverse venous hypertension (decreasing to 17 mmHg at the knee).
- Laplace's law:

$$\text{bandage pressure} = \frac{\text{bandage tension} \times \text{number of layers} \times 4620}{\text{circumference of limb} \times \text{bandage width}}$$

All of the factors in this equation affect the level of compression.

Methods
- Bandaging: multi-layer, short-stretch, vari-stretch.
- Hosiery used as both treatment and prevention when ulcer has healed.
- Intermittent pneumatic compression.

Factors to consider
- Leg shape.
- Pressure sites.
- Foot deformity.
- Exudate.
- Skin condition.
- Infection.
- Concordance.
- Mobility and dexterity.
- Pain.
- Lifestyle.
- Patient choice.
- Allergy.

Wound management
Dressings
A simple dressing should be used underneath compression bandaging. Consider:
- cost
- infection
- possible debridement
- patient preference and comfort.

Medication
- Pentoxifylline may be used alongside compression therapy or alone. Compression therapy remains the mainstay of treatment.
- Antibiotics should *not* be routinely given.
- Emollient to protect the surrounding skin.
- Analgesia if needed.

Surgery

This may be indicated on conformation of superficial venous incompetence.

Medical management

Management of underlying comorbidities (e.g. arthritis, diabetes).

Education and health promotion

- Understanding of the causation and treatment promotes concordance.
- Lifestyle advice.
- Leg elevation.
- Exercise, including leg and foot exercises.
- Skin care—regular washing and use of emollient.
- Healthy diet, and weight loss if obese.
- Smoking cessation.
- Hosiery care.

Urology and renal surgery

Anatomy of the male urinary tract

The anatomy of the male reproductive and urinary tract is divided into internal and external organs.

External organs

The penis

The male sexual reproductive organ is defined by its three main parts— the root (which is attached to the perineal membrane), the body (or shaft), and the glans. The body of the penis is cylindrical in shape and consists of three internal chambers—the corpus spongiosum and two corpora cavernosa. These chambers consist of special, sponge-like erectile tissue. The urethra emerges from the perineal membrane after passing through the prostate, and traverses the whole length of the corpus spongiosum to open on the glans.

The scrotum

This is the sac-like structure containing the testes. The scrotum has a protective role, and also optimizes conditions (temperature lower than core body temperature) for sperm production and survival.

The testes

These are the two small ovoid structures that are responsible for producing testosterone and generating sperm.

The epididymis is a coiled tube on the posterior aspect of each testicle. It transports and stores sperm cells. It also brings the sperm to maturity.

Internal organs

The vas deferens is a long muscular tube that connects the epididymis to ejaculatory ducts that then open into the prostatic urethra (also known as the seminalis colliculus).

The urethra is the tube that carries urine from the bladder to the outside of the body, as well as sperm during sexual intercourse.

The seminal vesicles are sac-like pouches that attach to the vas deferens near the base of the bladder. They produce a fluid rich in fructose to ensure sperm survival after ejaculation.

The prostate gland is a structure located at the base of the bladder, anterior to the rectum. The prostate gland adds fluid to the ejaculate.

Bulbourethral glands (also known as Cowper's glands) are small round structures located on the sides of the urethra just below the prostate gland. They produce fluid to lubricate the urethra.

The ureter is a tubular structure arising at the renal pelvis. It inserts into the trigone (base) of the bladder, and provides urinary drainage from the kidney to the bladder.

The kidney is an organ located in the retroperitoneum, with blood flow supplied via the renal arteries. Its functions include:

• urine production and excretion
• haemostatic functions (e.g. maintaining acid–base balance, blood pressure control)
• hormone and enzyme production (e.g. calcitriol, erythropoietin, renin).

Anatomy of the female urinary tract

The female reproductive system is usually divided into internal and external organs, which are described in Chapter 28.

Internal organs

- Two ovaries.
- Two Fallopian tubes.
- Uterus (womb).
- Vagina.

The internal organs of the urinary system are the same in both sexes, with the kidneys draining into the bladder via the ureters.

In the female, urine is also excreted via the urethra, the opening of which lies anterior to the vaginal orifice.

History taking, and signs and symptoms of urological problems in the male patient

General considerations

Taking a thorough genito-urinary history is a critical part of understanding urological conditions. The patient must be assessed in terms of their age, gender, and past medical and surgical history. Privacy and comfort for both the history and examination are essential. It is important to be confident in your approach and also to establish a good rapport. Due to the presenting condition it may be appropriate and necessary to include details about the patient's sexual and psychosexual history.

Male genito-urinary history

History taking follows the same format as described in Chapter 4, and includes the following main features:

- presenting complaints
- history of presenting complaints
- past medical and surgical history
- medications and allergies
- social history
- systems review.

Systems review is a more specific assessment of urological problems, and it is important to understand the patient's description of urinary symptoms, including:

- dysuria
- frequency of micturition, and the presence of any nocturia
- post-void dribbling
- hesitancy
- the fullness of the urinary stream
- sudden or gradual onset of symptoms
- any incontinence or urgency of micturition
- pain, haematuria, and discharge.

Urethral discharge is also a relatively common presenting symptom i men. Further questions about the following are needed to understan the cause:

- dysuria
- where a sexually transmitted disease is suspected or likely, given the patient's history:
  - past and present sexual partners, sexual orientation, and previou sexually transmitted diseases
  - any symptoms in the partner
- any other more generalized symptoms, including:
  - joint pains
  - eye inflammation, pain, or grittiness
  - gastrointestinal symptoms
  - fever.

Testicular pain is common in men, and it is crucial to understand the nature of this in order to exclude the possibility of torsion. It is important to ascertain whether the pain is associated with:

- trauma
- speed of onset (sudden or slow)
- other conditions (e.g. mumps)
- other urinary symptoms (e.g. dysuria, urethral discharge).

Possible causes include trauma, infection, torsion, and epididymitis.

Impotence

Impotence covers a number of different conditions and causes. Consider:
- emotional and psychological factors
- drugs and alcohol
- any association with other relevant diseases (diabetes mellitus, neurological disease, cardiovascular disease).

It is important to establish whether there is:
- loss of libido
- erectile failure.

Other symptoms

- When faced with a history of loin to groin pain, consider calculus, which can cause ureteric obstruction.
- The sudden onset of pain in renal colic or acute urinary retention can be differentiated from the gradual onset seen in outflow obstruction such as benign prostatic hyperplasia.
- Systemic symptoms of acute kidney injury or chronic renal failure (e.g. anorexia, vomiting, fatigue, pruritus, peripheral oedema).
- Consider in an elderly male patient the possibility of bone metastases secondary to prostate cancer.
- Some patients have no symptoms, but abnormalities are discovered on measuring blood pressure or during routine urinalysis, renal function testing, or serum biochemistry.

History taking, and signs and signs and symptoms of urological problems in the female patient

History taking and assessment should take into consideration the privacy and comfort of the patient. It is crucial that a good rapport is established and maintained. Intimate questions should be handled with sensitivity.

Menstrual history

- Age at menarche:
  - average age in the UK is 12 years 11 months
  - there are variations based on ethnicity
  - body weight is a factor (average weight at onset is 48 kg)
  - onset of secondary sexual characteristics if puberty is delayed or early.
- The pattern of the menstrual cycle. Record the following:
  - first day of last normal menstrual period (LNMP)
  - number of days of blood loss
  - length of cycle
  - whether blood loss is heavy (number of tampons and/or pads used, presence of clots).
- Ascertain whether any contraception is being used.

Abnormal patterns of bleeding

- *Polymenorrhoea*: unusually frequent periods.
- *Oligomenorrhoea*: unusually infrequent periods.
- *Menorrhagia*: unusually heavy periods.
- *Polymenorrhagia*: unusually heavy and frequent periods.
- *Intermenstrual bleeding* (bleeding between periods) may be due to:
  - breakthrough bleeding on the pill
  - diseases of the uterus and cervix
  - mucosal disorders.
- *Dyspareunia*.
- Postmenopausal bleeding: bleeding that occurs over 12 months after the onset of the menopause.
- Dysfunctional uterine bleeding:
  - abnormal bleeding that cannot be ascribed to pelvic pathology
  - a regular pattern suggests that ovulation is occurring
  - an irregular pattern suggests anovulatory cycles.

Vaginal discharge

Ask the patient about the following:

- when the discharge started, its frequency, and whether or not it is related to the menstrual cycle
- whether it is scanty or profuse
- colour and consistency
- odour
- any bloodstaining
- associated symptoms (pain, fever, itching, burning).

Physiological discharge is:
• scanty, mucoid, and odourless
• not associated with pruritus
• exacerbated by cyclical changes, pregnancy, and sex.

Pain

See Table 22.1.

Table 22.1 Conditions to consider by region of origin of pain

Region of origin	Conditions to consider
Suprapubic region	Ovarian cysts, ovarian torsion, bladder infections
Umbilical region	Ectopic, renal pathology, or other abdominal pathology (e.g. appendicitis, pancreatitis, ulcer, heartburn)
Iliac fossa	Ovulatory (other abdominal pathology, e.g. appendicitis)
Low abdominal region	Pelvic infection, bladder infection, haemorrhagic cyst, ovarian torsion, endometriosis (cycle related)
Abdominal region	Pelvic infection, ovarian pathology, ectopic

Physical examination of the male patient

Abdominal examination

Bedside examination should take note of general signs, such as weight loss. Then check specifically for:
- shape and symmetry of the abdominal wall
- abdominal distension
- scars and striae
- prominent veins
- hernia.

Note that visual fullness of the upper abdomen is an extremely rare and non-specific finding of hydronephrosis or a kidney or abdominal mass.

Bladder palpation and percussion can be used to confirm distension and urinary retention. Percussion of the lower abdomen may elicit a dullness that may suggest bladder distension, as a full bladder cannot be percussed above the symphysis pubis.

Rectum

A digital rectal examination can detect prostate problems. This may include a prostate that is:
- enlarged—symmetrical or asymmetrical
- hard, soft, or nodular
- tender.

Prostatitis is often felt as a boggy, tender prostate. Focal nodules are less discrete hard areas, and can be indicative of growths or possible prostate cancer. The prostate may also be symmetrically enlarged, rubbery, and non-tender, with benign prostatic hyperplasia.

Groin and genitals

Inguinal and genital examination should initially be performed with the patient standing.

Inguinal hernia or adenopathy may explain scrotal or groin pain. Gross asymmetry, swelling, erythema, or discoloration of the testes may indicate infection, torsion, tumour, or other pathology (e.g. hydrocoele). Horizontal testicular lie (bell-clapper deformity) indicates an increased risk of testicular torsion. Elevation of one testis (normally the left testis is lower) may be a sign of testicular torsion. The penis should be examined with and without retracting the foreskin. Inspection of the penis can detect:
- hypospadias or epispadias in young boys
- Peyronie's disease in men
- priapism, ulcers, and discharge in both groups.

Palpation may reveal an inguinal hernia. Cremasteric reflex may be absent with testicular torsion. Location of masses in relation to the testis and the degree and location of tenderness may help to differentiate the various types of testicular masses (e.g. spermatocoeles, epididymitis, hydrocoeles, tumours). If swelling is present, the area should be transilluminated to help to determine whether the swelling is cystic or solid. Fibrous plaques on the penile shaft are signs of Peyronie's disease.

Physical examination of the female patient

General examination

This should detect conditions which may either be present in or complicate genito-urinary disease. Examples include:

- hirsutism and/or acne, reflecting possible endocrine disorders
- anaemia, which commonly accompanies menstrual disorders
- conditions that are associated with menstrual symptoms:
  - thyroid disease
  - Cushing's syndrome
  - anorexia nervosa
  - other chronic diseases
- breast disease: examination is required
- lymphadenopathy, especially inguinal nodes
- assessment of secondary sexual characteristics.

Abdominal examination

The uterus, vagina, and adnexa lie within the pelvis, but findings relevant to the genito-urinary system may be visible, palpable, and percussible in the abdomen. Careful abdominal examination may detect the following.

Abdominal masses arising from the pelvis

- Large ovarian cysts, which can be detected by abdominal percussion revealing central dullness.
- Pregnancy (often used to equate the size of other pelvic tumours):
  - 12 weeks—palpable above the pubic bone
  - 16 weeks—palpable midway between the pubic bone and umbilicus
  - 20 weeks—just below the umbilicus
  - 28 weeks—just midway between the umbilicus and xiphisternum
  - 34 weeks—just below the xiphisternum

Ascites

Percussion reveals lateral dullness and a tympanic central abdomen.

Examination of the external genitalia

Prepare for the examination.

- With the help of a chaperone, position the patient on the couch (supine, with flexed hips and knees and the heels together, and thighs abducted).
- Cover the patient's abdomen with a sheet.
- Position the lighting to give a clear view of the external genitalia.
- Put on disposable gloves.

Examination of the vulva
- Explain the procedure to the patient.
- Systematically examine the labia majora, labia minora, introitus, urethra, and clitoris.
- Bartholin's glands are not normally palpable.
- Assess atrophic changes in the menopause, and in pubertal development in teenagers.

Examination of the vagina
- At this point it is appropriate to assess whether further examination (both digital and speculum) is appropriate or possible. If the patient has an intact hymen and is not using tampons, further internal examination would be inappropriate.
- The practice of rectal examination to assess the genitalia indirectly (although technically possible) is rarely necessary or appropriate. It should not be performed in children. The advent of ultrasound make such an intrusive procedure unnecessary.
- Separation of the labia and asking the patient to 'bear down' allows the examiner to visualize the vestibule and to identify:
  - cystocoele
  - rectocoele
  - uterine descent or prolapse.

Urological imaging and investigations

Ultrasound scans

- *Renal and bladder scans* assess bladder and renal cancer, hydronephrosis, acute and chronic renal failure, and infection (to assess the bladder it needs to be full, so if the patient is catheterized the catheter should be clamped).
- *Transrectal ultrasound scan* measures the prostate accurately and allows systematic biopsy for detection of cancer.
- *Scrotal ultrasound scan* evaluates acute scrotum from a suspected testicular cancer, infection, or varicocoele.

Intravenous urogram (IVU)

- This provides more functional information than ultrasound.
- It provides superior imaging of the ureter.
- It has been replaced by greater use of the CT urogram.

Computed tomography (CT) scans

The CT modality has become increasingly used for urological imaging and diagnostics. Pre- and post-contrast scans provide functional information about arterial and venous blood flow and the excretory function of the kidneys. Different CT approaches can be used for urological pathologies, including:

- CT KUB (non-contrast) for renal calculi
- CT urogram for transitional-cell carcinoma
- CT renal for cysts, renal lesions, and renal mass staging.

Magnetic resonance imaging (MRI) scans

- These provide a higher level of accuracy than CT in assessment of the prostate capsule and seminal vesicles.
- They offer a sensitive test for the presence of bone metastases.

Flexible cystoscopy

- This examines the urethra and bladder.
- It is performed using local anaesthetic gel.
- There is limited potential for intervention.

Rigid cystoscopy

Under general anaesthetic this permits biopsy, and the use of a resectoscope allows resection of tissue.

Ureteroscopy

- Rigid and flexible ureteroscopes provide access to the ureter and pelvicalyceal system.
- Allows the passage of instruments and laser fibres for the treatment of stones, stenting, and for biopsy.

Prostate disease

The prostate gland is a small gland located between the penis and bladder, and it surrounds the urethra. The prostate gland produces a liquefied protein called prostate-specific antigen (PSA).

Conditions that affect the prostate include:
- prostate enlargement
- prostatitis (inflammation of the prostate gland)
- prostate cancer.

Benign prostatic hyperplasia

Prostate enlargement is a common condition associated with ageing. About one-third of all men over 50 years of age display symptoms. The anatomical position of the urethra running through the prostate result in a number of symptoms associated with micturition, including:
- hesitancy
- reduced urine flow
- straining to pass urine
- increased frequency
- nocturia.

Treatment options include:
- dietary and behavioural advice on drinking prior to sleep, and reducing the consumption of urinary irritants such as caffeine and alcohol
- the use of alpha blockers to help to relax the prostate gland muscles, making it easier to urinate
- in severe cases, a transurethral resection of the prostate (TURP) or interventional embolization.

Prostatitis

Prostatitis is a poorly understood condition in which the prostate gland becomes inflamed and swollen. In most cases infection is not detected. Prostatitis affects 15% of males during their lifetime. It is most common in the 30–50 years age range.

Symptoms of prostatitis include:
- pelvic pain
- testicular pain
- pain when urinating (although this can be associated with urinary tract infection)
- pain when ejaculating
- pain in the perineum that is often worse when sitting.

Prostatitis can be treated using a combination of painkillers and other medication, such as alpha blockers, which can help to relieve the symptoms.

Prostate cancer

In the UK, prostate cancer is the most common type of cancer in men, with over 40 000 new cases diagnosed every year. Cases occur in men who are 50 years of age or older, and the incidence increases with age. Cancer of the prostate has a higher incidence in African and Afro-Caribbean men, and is less common in Asian men.

Symptoms
- Frequency and nocturia.
- Urgency (needing to rush to the toilet).
- Hesitancy.
- Straining or taking a long time while urinating.
- Weak flow or reduced flow.
- Bladder not feeling empty.

Treatment
- Prostatectomy (removal of the prostate gland).
- Radiotherapy and brachytherapy.
- Hormone therapy, using medication to block the effects of testosterone.

Urinary tract stones

Urinary tract stones may be found anywhere within the collecting system, but mainly occur within the renal pelvis or bladder. They vary considerably in size, from small 'gravel-like' stones to large staghorn calculi. The calculi may remain in the position where they are formed, or migrate, producing symptoms as they do so.

Presenting features
- Severe 'ureteric colic' or 'renal colic'—an intermittent, stabbing pain that radiates from the loin to the groin.
- Microscopic haematuria (rarely frank).
- Nausea and vomiting.
- Pyrexia.
- Loin or renal angle tenderness.
- Urinary retention secondary to obstruction proximal to the position of the calculus, resulting in hydroureter and hydronephrosis.

Investigations
- Stick testing of urine for the following:
  - red cells
  - white cells and nitrites (which suggest infection)
  - pH (values above 7 suggest urea-splitting organisms such as *Proteus* species. whereas values below 5 suggest uric acid stones).
- Midstream specimen of urine for microscopy (pyuria suggests infection), culture, and sensitivities. Any concurrent antibiotic therapy should be noted.
- Blood for FBC, CRP, renal function, electrolytes, calcium, phosphate, urate, and creatinine.
- Haemoglobin (Hb), platelet count, prothrombin time, and international normalized ratio (INR) if intervention is planned.

Other more detailed tests include:
- CT urogram and/or CT KUB
- renal ultrasound scan for hydronephrosis.

Treatment and management
Initial management in an emergency
- Analgesia (e.g. diclofenac 100 mg per rectum), anti-emetic (e.g. metoclopramide 10 mg IV).
- IV fluids and oral rehydration.
- Conservative management can take 1–3 weeks with small stones being passed.
- Emergency surgical treatment with percutaneous nephrostomy and/or ureteric stent insertion is necessary if the patient is obstructed with resultant deterioration of renal function.

Elective presentations and management
- Extracorporeal shock wave lithotripsy (ESWL).
- Percutaneous nephrolithotomy (PCNL).
- Endoscopic treatment.

Urinary tract infections (UTIs)

UTIs are defined as a significant bacteriuria in the presence of symptoms. They are classified on the basis of clinical symptoms, laboratory data, and microbiological findings. They are divided into uncomplicated UTIs, complicated UTIs, and sepsis.[1] An uncomplicated UTI is one in which the urinary tract is structurally and functionally normal. The majority of patients with this type of UTI are female (women and girls are at increased risk of developing UTIs because they have a short urethra), who respond quickly to a short course of antibiotics for 3 days.

In complicated UTI the patient has an underlying anatomical or functional abnormality, such as a neurological condition, bladder outlet obstruction, detrusor–sphincter dyssynergia in spinal cord injury, bladder fistula (between bladder and bowel, or between bladder and vagina), renal or bladder stones, diabetes mellitus, an indwelling urinary catheter, immunosuppression, or a history of recent urinary tract intervention. Pregnancy is another factor to consider in this group. Most UTIs in men are associated with a structural or functional abnormality, and are therefore considered to be complicated.

Bacteriuria is the presence of bacteria in the urine. This may be symptomatic or asymptomatic.

Negative urinalysis dipstick results should be followed up by a urine culture if the patient has symptoms of UTI, as the probability of a positive culture is 81%.

Bacteriuria without pyuria indicates bacterial colonization of the urine rather than active infection.

Pyuria is the presence of white blood cells in the urine. In the absence of bacteriuria, other pathology should be considered (i.e. bladder stones, TB infection, carcinoma in situ, or other inflammatory conditions).[3]

Recurrent UTI is defined as more than two infections within 6 months or three infections within 12 months. Recurrent UTI may be caused by a chronic bacterial prostatitis, urethral diverticulum, bladder diverticulum, bladder fistula, bacteria within calculi, or an obstructed or atrophic infected kidney (as well as the causes of complicated UTI listed earlier).

Unresolved infection can be the cause of inadequate treatment, reinfection, or infection by a different organism.

The bacteria most often seen in UTIs are of faecal origin. Most acute UTIs in patients with normal anatomical structure and function are caused by certain strains of Escherichia coli.

Other pathogens that can cause UTIs include Staphylococcus aureus, Staphylococcus saprophyticus, coagulase-negative Staphylococcus, Klebsiella pneumoniae, Proteus mirabilis, Enterococcus species, and Pseudomonas aeruginosa, although this list is not exhaustive. In rare cases, Candida albicans can cause UTI (e.g. in diabetic patients).[2]

Complicated UTIs often recur, and can take longer to respond to treatment—hence the need for a longer course of antibiotics.[3]

It is good practice to repeat a urinalysis 7–14 days after completion of antibiotics to ensure clearance of infection, especially in pregnant women with asymptomatic bacteriuria, because this is associated with pyelonephritis and premature delivery.[4–6]

Manifestations

Urethritis

Most of the cases of purulent urethritis without cystitis are sexually transmitted. The inflammation and infection are limited to the urethra. Pathogens such as *Chlamydia trachomatis*, *Neisseria gonorrhoeae*, *Ureaplasma urealyticum*, and *Trichomonas vaginalis* are the most common causes of urethritis. The disease occurs in men and women. Complaints include discomfort during voiding, but there are usually no symptoms of post-void suprapubic pain or urinary frequency.

Cystitis

This results from irritation of the lower urinary tract mucosa. Pyuria i present. Common signs and symptoms of acute uncomplicated lower UTI/cystitis include dysuria, frequent and urgent urination, suprapubic pain or tenderness, and possibly haematuria, but with the absence of vaginal discharge. The presence of vaginal symptoms should prompt alternative diagnoses. Differential diagnoses in women include vaginitis, acute urethritis, interstitial cystitis, and pelvic inflammatory disease. Other organisms that mimic acute cystitis include *Chlamydia*, *Neisseria gonorrhoeae*, *Candida*, and herpes simplex virus.[7]

Pyelonephritis

This usually results from the ascension of bacteria to the kidney from the lower urinary tract, but also can arise by haematogenous spread (e.g. from the lungs in patients with pneumonia). Unlike cystitis, pyelonephritis is an invasive disease. Symptoms include many of those associated with cystitis, but may also include fever, loin and/or flank pain and tenderness, nausea and vomiting, and peripheral leukocytosis. Urinary urgency and frequency may be present or absent. Pyuria is present. Complications of pyelonephritis can include sepsis, septic shock and death.

Septicaemia

Bacteraemia is the presence of pathogenic organisms in the blood stream, leading to septicaemia or sepsis. The diagnosis is confirmed by positive blood cultures of specific organisms, accompanied by a systemic response including two of the following symptoms: fever $> 38°C$ or hypothermia $< 36°C$, tachycardia of > 90 beats/min in patients not taking beta blockers, raised respiratory rate of > 20 breaths/min, white cell count $> 12\,000$ cells/mm^3, < 4000 cells/mm^3, or 10% immature (band) forms. Severe sepsis is a state of altered organ perfusion or evidence of dysfunction of one or more organs, including one or more of the following symptoms: oliguria, altered mental state, hypoxaemia, or lactic acidosis. Septic shock is severe sepsis with hypotension, organ dysfunction, and hypoperfusion.

Gram-negative aerobic bacteria

These are common causes of urosepsis (e.g. *E. coli*, *Proteus* species, and *Klebsiella* species). In urinary tract operations involving the bowel, anaerobic bacteria may be the cause of urosepsis.

Investigations

- Urine dipstick and/or midstream urine culture and sensitivity. Analysis for pH, blood, protein, glucose, leucocytes, and nitrites. Cloudy urine that is positive for nitrites and leucocytes is very likely to be infected.
- The pH varies between 4.5 and 8, with an average value in the range 5.5–6.5.
- Proteinuria suggests the presence of renal disease or multiple myeloma, but it can also occur following strenuous exercise.
- White blood cells—leucocyte esterase, which is produced by neutrophils, detects the presence of white blood cells in urine. Not all patients with bacteriuria have significant pyuria. Causes of false-negative results include concentrated urine, glycosuria, consumption of large amounts of ascorbic acid, and the presence of urobilinogen. False-positive results are usually caused by contamination.
- The presence of nitrites suggests bacteriuria. Nitrites are not normally found in urine, and a positive nitrite dipstick test has more than 90% specificity for bacteriuria. False-positive results for nitrites are usually caused by contamination.[3]
- Depending on the severity of the symptoms, a renal ultrasound scan or intravenous (IV) pyelogram or renal CT scan may be required.

Microbiological findings

The number of bacteria present is considered relevant for a diagnosis of UTI. The following are considered to be 'clinically relevant results':

- ≥ 103 cfu/mL of uropathogens in a midstream specimen of urine (MSU) in acute uncomplicated cystitis in women
- ≥ 104 cfu/mL of uropathogens in an MSU in acute uncomplicated pyelonephritis in women
- ≥ 105 cfu/mL of uropathogens in an MSU in women, or ≥ 104 cfu/mL of uropathogens in an MSU in men, or in 'straight-catheter' urine in women, in a complicated UTI
- asymptomatic bacteriuria is diagnosed if two cultures of the same bacterial strain taken 24 h apart show bacteriuria of ≥ 105 cfu/mL of uropathogens
- in a suprapubic bladder puncture specimen, any count of bacteria is relevant.[1]

Treatment

- A course of empirical antibiotics for 3–5 days is usually sufficient for uncomplicated UTIs (e.g. trimethoprim 200 mg twice a day or nitrofurantoin 50 mg four times a day as first-line therapy).[8]
- Complicated cystitis may require co-amoxiclav 625 mg orally three times a day, or if there is an allergy to penicillin, ciprofloxacin 500 mg orally twice a day, and review at 5 days.

- Pyelonephritis and urinary sepsis may require co-amoxiclav 1.2 g IV three times a day alongside a daily dose of IV gentamicin 5 mg/kg lean body mass, or if there is an allergy to penicillin, ertapenem 1 g IV daily alongside a daily dose of IV gentamicin 5 mg/kg lean body mass daily. Alternatively, discuss the case with a microbiologist if the patient has an allergy to ertapenem and/or meropenem. Review the treatment at 48 h.
- Known ESBL 'coliform' colonization requires advice from a microbiologist to check sensitivity to gentamicin, or for an alternative if resistant.
- If the likely source is UTI, treat with a daily dose of IV gentamicin 5 mg/kg lean body mass whether or not the patient is allergic to penicillin.
- If the source is not UTI or the patient is septic, consider giving ertapenem 1 g IV daily alongside IV gentamicin 5 mg/kg lean body mass daily, and review at 5 days.[9]

References

1 Grabe M et al. Guidelines on Urological Infections. European Association of Urology: Arnhem 2015. http://uroweb.org/wp-content/uploads/19-Urological-infections_LR2.pdf

2 Chamberlain NR. Urinary Tract Infections (Urethritis, Cystitis, Pyelonephritis). A.T. St University (ATSU): Kirksville, MO, 2009. www.atsu.edu/faculty/chamberlain/website/lectures/lecture/uti.htm

3 Reynard J, Brewster S and Biers S. Oxford Handbook of Urology: a quick reference guide urological diagnosis and management, 2nd edn. Oxford University Press: Oxford, 2009.

4 Carr J. Urinary tract infections in women: diagnosis and management in primary care. British Medical Journal 2006; 332: 94–7.

5 Health Protection Agency. Diagnosis of UTI: quick reference guide for primary care. www. gov.uk/government/uploads/system/uploads/attachment_data/file/345784/UTI_quick_ref_guidelines.pdf

6 Scottish Intercollegiate Guidelines Network (SIGN). Management of Suspected Bacterial Urinary Tract Infection in Adults. SIGN: Edinburgh, 2006. www.sign.ac.uk/guidelines/full-text/88/index.html

7 Pattman R et al. (eds) Oxford Handbook of Genitourinary Medicine, HIV, and Sexual Health, 2nd edn. Oxford University Press: Oxford, 2010.

8 www.medicinescomplete.com

9 University Hospitals Coventry and Warwickshire NHS Trust. Antibiotic Policy. University Hospitals Coventry and Warwickshire NHS Trust: Coventry, 2015.

Further reading

Agency for Healthcare Research and Quality (AHRQ). Treatment for acute uncomplicated lower UTI. In: Diagnosis and Management of Lower Urinary Tract Infection. AHRQ: London 2012. www.guideline.gov/syntheses/synthesis.aspx?id=35626

Urinary retention

Acute urinary retention (AUR) is an urgent urological condition. It is characterized by sudden inability to pass urine and by the painful distension of the bladder. It can be relieved almost instantly by urinary catheterization. It is a common condition. More than 1 in 10 men in their 70's will experience AUR, and the risk for men in their eighties is nearly 1 in 3.[10] The main cause of AUR is usually benign prostatic hyperplasia (BPH). It can be precipitated by surgery (especially lower abdominal surgery) or over-distension of the bladder (as a result of either a large fluid intake or prescription of diuretics) (as can constipation).[11]

Most acute hospitals admit patients who present with AUR. In one UK survey, 65% of responding hospitals stated that they admitted these patients, with 20% admitting them only if renal function was deranged.[12] However, there is evidence that it is safe to send AUR patients home after they have been catheterized, provided that they are not uraemic, septic, ill, or dehydrated. A trial without a catheter could be arranged at a later date.[13]

Chronic urinary retention (CUR) is painless. If the bladder wall becomes weaker, an increasing amount of urine (residual) remains after voiding. When this residual becomes larger than the normal bladder capacity (300–500 mL) it can be defined as CUR.[11] Chronic retention with low pressure may reach 2–3 L. It may be relatively asymptomatic or present with urinary frequency, or overflow incontinence. Chronic retention with overflow is a probable cause of incontinence in the elderly.[11] CUR is not always an indication for immediate catheterization. In elderly men, who seem to be relatively asymptomatic, usually no harm is caused by such retention, and it may well be best not to perform any major intervention.

High-pressure CUR is less common, but is important, as it can be complicated by hydronephrosis and renal failure. Urinary catheterization would be indicated in this case, and is usually associated with diuresis. Although this is partly due to the correction of the fluid retention, covering the patient with an intravenous infusion during the initial recovery period would be indicated.[11]

References

10 Willis S and McNeil A. New trends in acute urinary retention: developing a management protocol. *Urology News* 2004; 8: 5.6–10.

11 Kirk D. *Managing Prostate Disease.* Altman Publishing: St Albans, 2007.

12 Manikandan R et al. Management of acute urinary retention secondary to benign prostatic hyperplasia in the UK: a national survey. *BJU International* 2004; 93: 84–8.

13 Pickard R, Emberton M and Neal DE. The management of men with acute urinary retention. *British Journal of Urology* 1998; 81: 712–20.

Penile disease

Peyronie's disease

This is a disorder of the penile connective tissue, identifed by François Gigot de la Peyronie in 1743. Fibrous plaque formation occurs in the corpus cavernosum's tunica albuginea. There is inflammatory thickening with fibrin deposition, increased collagen production, decreased quantity of elastic fibres, and subsequent fibrosis with or without calcification. This process results in penile angulation or an hourglass-like deformity.

Treatment

Medical treatment

This is indicated for those able to tolerate intercourse in the early stage of the disease.

- Oral treatment options: colchicine, vitamin E, or potassium aminobenzoate.
- Intralesional injections: verapamil or collagenase.
- Treatment of associated erectile dysfunction.

Surgical treatment

This is indicated for those with stable lesions but a more severe deformity.

- Plication techniques—plication of the tunica opposite the deforming plaque.
- Grafting techniques—the plaque is excised and the defect grafted.
- Prosthesis insertion within the corpora cavernosa—generally reserved for patients with severe erectile dysfunction refractory to medical therapy.

Priapism

Priapism is an abnormally sustained erection unrelated to sexual stimulation. It is classified as either high flow (arterial) or low flow (veno-occlusive).

Low-flow priapism

Causes include:

- drugs—intracavernosal prostaglandin and papaverine, psychotropic drugs (e.g. trazodone, chlorpromazine)
- abnormal blood viscosity—sickle cell, myeloma, leukaemia, thalassaemia, total parenteral nutrition
- neurological disease (e.g. spinal or cerebrovascular disease).

Treatment includes:

- ice packs to reduce swelling
- correction of underlying abnormalities—sickle cell (rehydration, oxygen, transfusion), myeloma (plasmapheresis)
- oral B-agonists
- intracavernosal phenylephrine
- corpora cavernosa aspiration (up to 50 mL) plus manual pressure
- surgical techniques augment venous drainage of the corpora cavernosa.

High-flow priapism

High-flow priapism is rarer than the low-flow type, and usually less painful. It is the result of a ruptured artery from an injury to the penis or the perineum (the area between the scrotum and the anus), which prevents blood in the penis from circulating normally.

Treatment consists of selective pudendal arteriography and embolization.

Foreskin conditions

Common foreskin conditions include phimosis and paraphimosis, as well as dermatological conditions such as balanitis (inflammation of the glans).

Phimosis

This condition occurs when the foreskin cannot be retracted over the glans of the penis. At birth, a physiological phimosis is present due to adhesions between the glans penis and foreskin. Gradual separation then occurs as the penis develops. The deposition of epithelial debris (smegma) under the foreskin leads to division of the adhesions and the ability to retract the foreskin. Around 90% of boys can retract their foreskin by 3 years of age, and only 1% are non-retractile by 16 years of age.

However, phimosis can also be acquired and develop in a previously retractile foreskin. This typically occurs after balanitis or foreskin trauma.

Paraphimosis

Paraphimosis occurs when a tight foreskin retracted over the glans penis becomes oedematous and cannot be returned to its normal anatomical position (see Figure 22.1).

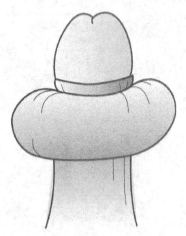

Figure 22.1 Paraphimosis. Reproduced from Mark Davenport and Agostino Pierro, *Paediatric Surgery*, 2009, with permission from Oxford University Press.

Causes

It typically occurs in young men who do not pull back their foreskin after washing, sexual intercourse, or masturbation, and in elderly men who do not have their foreskin replaced after urethral catheterization.

Symptomology

Paraphimosis is typically painful. The retracted foreskin is swollen and oedematous, and may develop an area of ulceration. The swelling lies behind a tight band (constriction ring) of foreskin immediately behind the glans penis, which also swells.

Treatment

Paraphimosis may initially be treated non-operatively, and then, if required, operative techniques may be used.

Non-operative management

Initial management is aimed at reducing the swelling and oedema, so that the foreskin can be replaced over the glans. The glans and distal penis should be compressed slowly for several minutes. Pain may be reduced by applying lidocaine gel or administering a dorsal penile nerve block (typically using 0.5% plain bupivacaine), although children and adolescents may require a general anaesthetic. Once the swelling has reduced, the retracted foreskin may be drawn over the glans.

To aid reduction of the swelling and oedema, the following modifications of this procedure have been described.
- The 'iced-glove' technique: prior to compression, but after administration of anaesthesia, the penis is invaginated into the thumb of a rubber glove containing ice, and left for several minutes before compression and subsequent reduction are attempted.
- The 'Dundee' technique:[14] prior to compression, but after administration of a dorsal penile nerve block and broad-spectrum antibiotics, the foreskin and glans penis are cleaned with skin preparation. A fine needle is then used to puncture the oedematous foreskin at multiple sites. The oedema fluid is then squeezed out of the foreskin before reduction is attempted.

As paraphimosis has a tendency to recur, a circumcision is then usually undertaken. However, this is normally performed electively after the swelling has resolved.

Operative management

If non-operative techniques fail, surgical intervention is required. The two operative techniques most commonly used are:
- The dorsal slit procedure: after administration of a dorsal penile nerve block and antibiotics, a longitudinal incision is made in the constriction ring of the foreskin and the foreskin is reduced. The incision should then be closed transversely to increase the circumference of the foreskin and decrease the chance of recurrence. However, the patient should be followed up, as phimosis may subsequently develop.

- Circumcision: if the patient is taken to theatre for treatment after failed manual reduction, the definitive treatment is a circumcision. Due to the oedematous and swollen nature of the foreskin, the patient should be counselled about the higher risk of complications compared with an elective circumcision. Particular attention should be paid to the risks of subsequent infection and wound cosmesis.

Reference

14 Reynard JM and Barua JM. Reduction of paraphimosis the simple way – the Dundee technique. *BJU International* 1999; 83: 859–60.

Scrotal problems

The anatomy of the male scrotum is outlined in the section on male anatomy (see ➲ p. 548). Problems with the scrotum can lead to serious illnesses, including hormonal imbalances, sexual problems, and infertility. Some of the more common conditions that affect the testes include testicular lesions, trauma, inflammatory conditions, testicular torsion, and benign and malignant lesions.

Testicular lesions

Intratesticular lesions
- Malignant testicular tumours.
- Benign intratesticular lesions.
- Simple intratesticular cysts or epidermoid cysts and benign teratoma (especially in the prepubertal testis).

Extratesticular lesions
- Scrotal pearls.
- Testicular/epididymal appendages.
- Inguinoscrotal hernias.

Inflammatory lesions
- Acute epididymo-orchitis or viral orchitis.
- Chronic tuberculous epididymo-orchitis, schistosomal epididymitis, and sperm granuloma.

Traumatic lesions
- Scrotal haematoma.
- Haematocoele (haematoma within tunica vaginalis).
- Testicular haematoma (haematoma within tunica albuginea testis).

Investigations
- Urinalysis for microbial culture and sensitivity.
- Blood tests.
  - Consider tumour markers (AFP, β-HCG) and inflammatory markers (CRP, WCC).
- Ultrasound scanning of the scrotum.
- Examination of the abdomen to identify masses.
- Colour flow Doppler ultrasound is useful in cases of torsion or infection.

Treatment

Testicular cancers
- Orchidectomy (surgical removal of the testis).
- Follow-up chemotherapy depending upon spread will involve several cycles.
- Can cause infertility, and patients are counselled about sperm banking.
- Epididymal cysts/spermatocoele may be aspirated, but recurrence is common. Can be surgically excised, but can return with an associated possible effect on fertility.

- Hydrocoeles should be treated if symptomatic. This can involve aspiration and drainage, or surgical incision.
- Varicocoele should be treated if symptomatic, and is commonly associated with infertility. Venous embolization and retroperitoneal ligation (laparoscopic or open) of the testicular vein have similar results. Minimally invasive treatments are preferable.

Cancer of the kidney

Renal-cell carcinoma (RCC) is the most common tumour of the kidney in adults, accounting for 86% of neoplasms arising from this organ. Renal cancer occurs in hereditary and non-hereditary forms. RCC can be further subdivided into:

- conventional (80–90%)
- papillary (10–15%)
- chromophobe (4–5%)
- collecting duct carcinoma (1%).

Clinical features

- Symptoms include haematuria, groin pain, and awareness of a mass arising from the flank.
- Chest symptoms and bone pain may be present with metastases to these sites.
- Positive family history.
- Renal carcinomas are often small and may be multiple.

Diagnosis and investigations

- Blood tests: FBC and U&E.
- IV contrast-enhanced CT scan of chest and abdomen.
- Isotope bone scan if there are concerns about bony metastases.

Treatment

Surgical options
- Radical nephrectomy is recommended for large tumours.
- Partial nephrectomy may be suitable for peripheral tumours less than 4 cm in diameter.

Medical therapy
Medical approaches are often used for metastatic disease.
- Biological therapy can involve the use of immune modulators such as interferons and interleukins.
- Chemotherapy is rarely used.
- Hormonal therapy (androgens and tamoxifen) may be of some benefit.
- Radiotherapy is useful for palliating painful bony metastases.

Prognosis

- The outcome following nephrectomy is unpredictable.
- Tumours that are pathologically confined to the kidney have a good prognosis. Poor prognostic indicators include extracapsular spread, invasion of the renal vein, and lymph node involvement.
- Cure is likely if the tumour is less than 4 cm in diameter and if there is no local or distant spread or invasion—for example, stage 1 is associated with 90% survival, compared with 50% for stage 2.
- Periodic radiological follow-up is recommended in most cases, so that locally recurrent or metastatic disease can be detected at an early stage.

Cancer of the bladder

Bladder cancer is the fourth most common cancer in men in the UK. It is the most frequently occurring tumour of the urinary system, and accounts for around 1 in 30 new cases of cancer each year in the UK. Bladder cancer is the eleventh most common cancer in women.

Risk factors

- About 50% of bladder cancers are caused by smoking.
- Industrial exposure to aromatic amines in dyes, paints, solvents, leather dust, inks, combustion products, rubber, and textiles.
- Environmental pollution.
- Genetic predisposition.[15]
- Radiation to the pelvis.
- Cyclophosphamide.
- Coffee may increase the risk of bladder cancer, but there is no established dose-related risk.[16]
- There is a small amount of evidence that chronic infection is associated with bladder cancer (e.g. HIV, herpes simplex, TB, schistosomiasis).

Clinical features

- The majority of cases present with painless haematuria.
- Other features include painful micturition, renal colic due to blood clot, disturbance of the urinary stream, and retention of urine.

Diagnosis and investigation

- Urine cytology to identify cancer cells.
- Cystoscopy to biopsy the bladder, or ultrasound scan of the full bladder for imaging.
- Transurethral resection to perform resection and larger biopsies.
- Ultrasound imaging to assess the bladder wall (with the bladder full).

Treatment

Treatment is dependent upon the tumour type, site, and spread.

Superficial transitional-cell tumours

- Surgical removal by endoscopic resection.
- Recurrence is common, and regular endoscopic surveillance with check cystoscopy should be performed.
- Intravesical chemotherapy can be given to reduce tumour recurrence.

Carcinoma *in situ*

- Requires thorough therapy to prevent invasive transitional-cell carcinoma.
- Immunotherapy with intravesical BCG is effective in around 60% of cases.
- Close endoscopic surveillance with regular bladder biopsy is required.

Invasive transitional-cell carcinomas

- Muscle-invasive tumours are of high grade and have a poor prognosis (dependent upon spread).
- Curative therapy can be offered with radical cystectomy or radical radiotherapy.

Squamous cell and adenocarcinoma

Radical cystectomy can be performed if the patient's general condition allows this. These tumours do not respond well to radiotherapy and chemotherapy.

Radical surgery

Cystectomy with urinary diversion offers the best chance of cure if the cancer is localized to the bladder. The usual operation is either cystectomy and formation of an ileal conduit, or bladder reconstruction (neo-bladder).

Radical radiotherapy

- This is useful if the patient cannot tolerate surgery. It offers bladder conservation, although the results are poor in multifocal disease.
- Frail patients who are unfit for radical surgery or radiotherapy may benefit from palliative radiotherapy to the bladder.

Neoadjuvant chemotherapy

- Cisplatin-based chemotherapy given before cystectomy or radiotherapy offers a modest survival benefit of around 5% improvement at 5 years.
- For patients with good performance status, concomitant chemotherapy and radiotherapy may offer improved response rates over radiotherapy alone.

References

5 Bellmunt J et al. Bladder cancer: ESMO Practice Guidelines for diagnosis, treatment and follow-up. *Annals of Oncology* 2014; 25 (Suppl. 3): iii40–48.
6 National Institute for Health and Care Excellence (NICE). *Bladder Cancer: diagnosis and management*. NG2. NICE: London, 2015. ℘ www.nice.org.uk/guidance/ng2

Erectile dysfunction

Erectile dysfunction (ED) or impotence is defined as the inability to achieve and maintain a penile erection sufficient for sexual intercourse. It is a common condition, affecting around one-third of men aged 40–70 years. Its prevalence increases with age, and it is more likely to occur in men who smoke or who have hypertension, hyperlipidemia, diabetes mellitus, or heart disease.[17]

ED is commonly categorized according to two main causes, psychogenic and organic, although in fact it is often multifactorial.

Psychogenic causes

These may account for the majority of ED. Psychogenic ED typically has a sudden onset.

Many psychological conditions may either cause or aggravate ED. These include:

- performance anxiety
- relationship difficulties
- lack of sexual attraction
- depression
- stress.

Organic causes

ED of more insidious onset is more likely to have an organic origin. However, notable exceptions to this are ED caused by trauma, surgery, and drugs, in which the onset is usually acute.

Organic ED occurs as a result of changes in the vascular, nervous, and endocrine pathways that are responsible for erectile function. Numerous clinical conditions can cause ED. These include:

- trauma to the penis or perineum
- scleroderma
- renal failure
- liver cirrhosis
- haemochromatosis
- cancer and associated treatment
- epilepsy
- stroke
- multiple sclerosis
- Alzheimer's disease
- Parkinson's disease
- endocrine conditions (hyper- and hypothyroidism)
- malnutrition
- zinc deficiency
- sickle-cell anaemia
- leukaemias.

Medications may also cause ED. These include:

- antidepressants
- antipsychotic drugs
- antihypertensive agents (for treatment of high blood pressure)

- anti-ulcer drugs (e.g. cimetidine)
- hormonal medications
- alcohol
- marijuana and cocaine.

Surgical conditions that can cause ED include:
- procedures performed on the brain and spinal cord
- retroperitoneal or pelvic lymph node dissection
- aorto-iliac or aorto-femoral bypass
- abdominal perineal resection
- proctocolectomy
- radical prostatectomy
- transurethral resection of the prostate
- cryosurgery performed on the prostate
- cystectomy.

Psychological impact

Sexual activity and ability can have a profound effect on emotional and psychological well-being.

Treatment

A range of treatment options are available.
- Vacuum devices—these create effective erections and are relatively reliable for most men, although they can cause bruising, pain, loss of sensation, and discomfort.
- Medication—sildenafil citrate is the most commonly used medication. It requires initial normal stimulation to occur, and improves the overall erection. Side effects include headache, and it is contraindicated in patients who are taking nitrate cardiac medication.
- Testosterone is sometimes used in men with low libido, but not for ED per se. The synergistic effect of this with other agents is effective.
- Injection therapy—intracavernosal injection of medication (e.g. alprostadil) into the penis. This method remains an effective alternative to oral agents.

Reference

7 Eardley I. The incidence, prevalence, and natural history of erectile dysfunction. *Sexual Medicine Reviews* 2013; 1: 3–16.

Renal transplantation

There are two main sources of kidney for transplantation—living donors and cadaveric and beating heart donors.

Living donors

In the UK, live donation accounts for 33% of all renal transplants. Living donors are often related (siblings, parents, or children), and are authorized by the Human Tissue Authority. Non-related 'altruistic' transplants are rare, with only four recorded cases in the UK. Living donor transplants provide the opportunity to assess the donor and recipient for tissue compatibility, and allow time to optimize them prior to surgery. Living donors are admitted to the same hospital, and often the same ward, prior to the operation. Operatively, the removal of the donor kidney and transplantation occur in adjoining operating theatres in order to reduce the ischaemic time from removal to re-instituting blood flow, and thus improve the outcome. Typically, the donor spends 7–10 days in hospital, compared with 3–5 days for the recipient.

Cadaveric and beating heart donors

In the case of patients who have suffered a serious brain injury, which has resulted in certified brain death, organs may be harvested for use with the patient's prior consent (i.e. if they are an organ donation card holder or after discussion with the family about the patient's wishes prior to the event. Brain death is established using the following criteria:

- identifiable cause of brain death (head injury, cerebral bleed), confirmed through expertise and investigations such as CT scan
- exclusion of other causes of brainstem suppression (i.e. pharmacological therapy, hypothermia, biochemical disturbances)
- no spontaneous respiration, with a confirmed $PaCO_2$ of > 6.7 kPa
- the following brainstem tests, conducted by two independent doctors:
  - fixed, dilated, and unresponsive pupils
  - absent corneal reflex
  - absence of vestibular–ocular reflex
  - absence of motor response to peripheral painful stimuli
  - absence of respiratory effort when disconnected from ventilator
  - absence of cough and gag reflex.

Therapeutic management of the patient must continue to preserve the organs up until the donation procedure. This requires continuous monitoring of ECG changes, arterial pressure, CVP, urine output, and temperature. Inotropic support is avoided where possible, due to the vasoconstrictive effects on the donor kidney.

Once the organs have been removed, they require preparation before rapid transport to the recipient. Minimizing the ischaemic time will significantly improve the graft survival. However, modern techniques mean that this can be extended to 6 h. Typically, the kidney is infused with preserving solution and stored at a temperature of 4–10°C.

Complications of renal transplantation

There are a number of common complications that occur in the recipient of a renal transplant. These include wound complications, graft dysfunction due to renal artery and vein problems, lymphocoeles, urological problems, infections, and rejection.

Wound complications

Wound complications are the most frequent cause of post-operative complications in the transplant patient. However, post-operative infections are often more serious in the transplant patient, due to the need for immunosuppressive drug regimes. Wound complications can be noted as:

- surgical site wound infection
- wound dehiscence
- hernia.

Wound infections will occur, although their incidence will be reduced by strict adherence to sterile practices during the procedure and the administration of prophylactic antibiotics during surgery. It should be noted that organisms from the bladder (which is opened to allow the ureter to be implanted) can be present, and bladder irrigation prior to surgery can be used to reduce this effect.

Graft dysfunction

The kidney, once transplanted, may not work optimally, and this is best detected by observing the production of urine. Urine output may not be reliable in the immediate post-operative period, due to the significant amounts of intra-operative diuretics that are given. However, during the first 24 h close attention should be given to an absence or trending reduction in urine output and rising serial creatinine levels. If blood pressures remain consistent during this period, urgent investigation, diagnosis, and treatment are required. The patient may need a short period of dialysis to provide additional support and clearance as the transplant function improves.

Renal artery and vein problems

Renal artery stenosis (RAS) is a frequent complication, and is characterized by reduced blood flow to the kidney. Although stenosis can occur at any stage after the transplant, it typically occurs 3–12 months after surgery. Immediate stenosis is often related to kinking of the artery or an anastomotic problem as a result of surgery, and is treated as an urgent surgical problem. However, RAS has three main forms, namely anastomotic, diffuse, and discrete narrowing of the renal artery. The anastomotic form is often related to the suture line, which can create a purse-string effect with increased arterial pressure narrowing the lumen. It can also be caused by arterial trauma during the procedure, either from the clamp or from kinking in the artery after the procedure. Diffuse stenosis occurs along the renal artery, whereas discrete stenosis occurs only in the distal portion of the vessel. After investigation, several options are available to improve blood flow, including angioplasty, stenting, and surgical reconstruction of the vessel.

Although uncommon, renal vein problems such as thrombosis are potentially severe for the graft and the patient. Thrombus can form for a variety of reasons, including haematoma compression of the vein, lymphocoele, hypotension, and technical difficulties during surgery. This results in blocking of the renal vein, resulting in a poor prognosis for graft survival.

Lymphocoeles

Intra-abdominal lymphatic fluid is found in most post-transplant patients, as a result of lymphatic disruption caused during preparation of the kidney and arterial site for transplant. The lymphatic fluid drains into the intra-abdominal space. In most cases this fluid is reabsorbed over time and causes few problems. However, larger collections can form between the kidney and the bladder, causing increased pressure on vessels such as the renal artery, renal vein, and ureter. If larger collections cause symptoms, percutaneous drainage can be performed or, less frequently, laparotomy for direct access.

Urological problems

Post transplant, the patient can develop urological problems from the ureteral connection to the bladder, resulting in urine leakage into the abdominal cavity. In addition, lymphocoeles can cause ureteral obstruction, leading to more complicated hydronephrosis. They will often require surgical intervention to manage the primary source of the problem, or in the case of late-developing ureteral strictures, dilatation may be used.

Neurological and spinal surgery

Neurological assessment and examination

Neurological examination

This is performed:
- as a routine part of medical examination on admission for surgery
- to diagnose whether symptoms of illness in the patient are caused by a neurological condition, and if so, where in the nervous system any pathological lesion(s) are located.

Disease or abnormality of neurological functions may involve:
- the nervous system itself
- body systems that have an effect on the function of the nervous system; there is usually disturbance of cardiovascular, respiratory, renal, or metabolic function
- general symptoms (e.g. headache) that have neurological implications

Neurological examination is an important part of the pre-operative examination of patients before surgery. This may reveal previously unsuspected neurological problems. Also, some elderly patients have memory problems which may affect their ability to understand procedures, or give informed consent. Medical staff frequently seek specialist neurology advice.

Diagnosis of neurological illness (e.g. epilepsy, brain and spinal tumours) can have serious consequences, and must be very carefully communicated to patients and their families. This is supported by multidisciplinary teams (MDTs), and sometimes by specialist nurses.

Signs and symptoms of neurological illness
- Abnormality or loss of sensory function—tingling, burning, or numbness.
- Abnormality or loss of motor function—paralysis of head, trunk, or limbs.
- Abnormality or loss of function in the cranial nerves that arise from the brain and brainstem.
- Abnormality or loss of autonomic function (e.g. blood pressure, pulse, bladder or bowel function).
- Higher mental functioning—cognitive and behavioural aspects, including memory and language.

The neurological examination is performed by medical staff, but certain aspects pertaining to the patient's neurological and/or musculoskeletal status and their capacity to carry out activities of daily living may be assessed by other members of the MDT (e.g. assessment of sensorimotor function by physiotherapists, assessment of speech and swallowing by speech and language therapists).

Neurological assessment

This is a term applied to the short appraisal of key aspects of a patient's neurological status by nursing staff using a recognized neurological observations chart (in the form of a hand-held computer record system). This includes:

- the Glasgow Coma Scale (GCS) (see ⊃ p. 458), which allocates a numerical score to eye opening, verbal response, and limb movements; an adapted paediatric coma score is used in children
- shape, size, and equality of pupils
- strength and control of limbs to given instructions
- pulse, blood pressure, respiration rate, and temperature.

If the patient is unable to respond to commands, a painful stimulus is used to arouse them to maximum wakefulness. This stimulus, which has to be repeated frequently, must not cause damage to the patient's tissues, and local policy should be followed about approved methods of applying a painful stimulus to a central body location (e.g. trapezius muscle). *Do not use nailbed pressure or sternal rub.*

Special points

It is very important that patients with impaired consciousness and/or at risk of deterioration are assessed at appropriate intervals by suitably trained and experienced staff.

Nurses who are performing neurological observations must be trained and supervised to ensure that their observations are consistent, accurate, and reliable. A joint assessment by both nurses at handover maintains continuity of patient assessment and ensures that any changes are not missed.

Assessments should be continued through the night, and the patient woken fully at scheduled times until they are stable and observations can be reduced in frequency. This is essential for all age groups, but is particularly significant in children and the elderly, in whom deterioration may follow an injury that initially appears to be trivial.

For any patient who has a reduced GCS score, the observations should be repeated after a short interval, and medical attention sought immediately. Slight changes in patient behaviour can signal imminent deterioration. Confused, irritable, or noisy behaviour in an at-risk patient should not be attributed to alcohol, drug ingestion, or poor conduct. It may be an early sign of brain injury.

Further reading

Hickey JV. *The Clinical Practice of Neurological and Neurosurgical Nursing*, 7th edn. Wolters Kluwer Health: Philadelphia, PA, 2013.

Posner JB, Saper CB, Schiff N and Plum F. *Plum and Posner's Diagnosis of Stupor and Coma*, 4th edn. Oxford University Press: Oxford, 2007.

Woodward S and Mestecky C (eds). *Neuroscience Nursing: evidence-based theory and practice*. Blackwell Publishing Ltd: Oxford, 2011.

Recent advances in neurosurgical techniques

During the last 20 years there have been significant advances in all areas of neurosurgery, which have revolutionized the treatment of patients. Surgical techniques have been developed that would not have been possible without advances in brain imaging, advanced computerized operating systems, and neuroanaesthesia.

Surgical techniques

Surgical openings to access intracranial structures include the following:

- Burr hole/twist drill—a hole is made in the skull using a neurosurgical drill. This can be used to insert an intracranial pressure monitoring device, external ventricular drain, neurosurgical endoscope, or biopsy device.
- Craniotomy—removal of a section of cranium (a bone flap), which at the end of surgery is put back in place; it then heals like any bony fracture.
- Craniectomy—an enlarged burr hole is made, involving more extensive removal of bone. It is most commonly used to gain access to the base of the brain, and occasionally used for extensive removal of a bone flap to allow swelling of the brain after head injury (i.e. bilateral decompressive craniectomy).
- Trans-sphenoidal access through the nasal passages to the pituitary gland.

Sterotaxis

Stereotactic procedures use both MRI and CT imaging, with an external frame attached to the patient's head. This imaging produces accurate three-dimensional targets that define the precise location of specific brain structures for surgery. As the frame is placed prior to surgery, the patient will need physical and psychological support.

Neuronavigation

This refers to advanced operating systems in which the use of advanced mathematical modelling combined with real-time computer-guided imaging creates a three-dimensional model of the brain and allows the surgeon to map the brain, guide the tip of a surgical instrument to precise location, and avoid vital structures (e.g. optic nerve or arteries). Sophisticated neuroimaging technologies can thus be related to the patient during surgery.

Neuroimaging
- CT scan—this two-dimensional image of the brain is particularly useful for the demonstration and differentiation of haemorrhage. CT angiography is used for the imaging of aneurysms.
- MRI scan—this uses powerful magnetic fields to construct images, and is particularly effective for soft tissues (e.g. for differentiating brain tumour from normal brain tissue). It avoids the use of ionizing radiation. Advances in MRI techniques include diffusion MRI (also known as diffusion tensor imaging), MRI angiography, MR spectrometry, and functional MRI.

Neurovascular procedures
Neurovascular abnormalities include aneurysms, arteriovenous malformation, and vascular narrowing.

Improved intravascular devices allow access to vascular abnormalities within the cranium via an artery, thus avoiding the need for open cranial surgery. Recent advances in the surgical treatment of acute stroke include the use of intra-arterial devices to remove thrombus from intracranial arteries (mechanical embolectomy).

Radiosurgery
This involves the use of non-invasive methods of delivering precise targeted ionizing radiation to patients with benign and malignant tumours, particularly those that are difficult to access.

Examples include:
- cyberknife—a frameless robotic radiosurgery system
- gamma knife— does not involve the use of a 'surgical knife', but the surgically precise delivery of gamma radiation to target the tumour.

Nursing neurosurgical patients
It is important to note that even with the possibilities that have now been opened up by advanced surgery, the recovery of all neurosurgical patients depends on the following key nursing skills:
- clinical observation of the patient's neurological status
- prevention of neurosurgical complications, particularly the recognition and treatment of raised intracranial pressure, and prevention of post-operative complications such as infection
- prevention and management of respiratory complications
- prevention of the complications of coma and immobility
- rehabilitation.

Further reading
Woodward S and Mestecky C (eds). *Neuroscience Nursing: evidence-based theory and practice.* Blackwell Publishing Ltd: Oxford, 2011.

Hydrocephalus

Cerebrospinal fluid (CSF) is a clear fluid produced by the intraventricular choroid plexus. It flows through the cerebral ventricles, over the surface of the brain and spinal cord, and is reabsorbed into the cerebral venous sinuses. The total volume of CSF is 120–150 mL, but around 500 mL are secreted and reabsorbed over a period of 24 h. The normal pressure of CSF within the ventricles is the same as intracranial pressure (below 10 mmHg in adults).

Hydrocephalus can be either acute or chronic, and occurs when CSF pressure rises and produces symptoms of raised intracranial pressure. The ventricles appear enlarged on CT scan. Many adults with hydrocephalus first developed the condition as babies or children, and require lifelong management.

Causes
- Obstruction to normal flow (obstructive or non-communicating hydrocephalus). This can be:
  - congenital—due to malformation of the ventricular pathway; often there are other coexisting CNS abnormalities (e.g. hindbrain herniation syndromes, spina bifida)
  - acquired—resulting from space-occupying lesions (e.g. brain tumour obstructing the ventricular pathway, traumatic brain injury).
- Blockage of the site of reabsorption in the venous sinuses (communicating hydrocephalus), usually due to:
  - meningitis, particularly bacterial (septic) meningitis
  - traumatic or spontaneous subarachnoid haemorrhage.
- Overproduction of CSF—this is rare.

Normal-pressure hydrocephalus is a condition of older adults caused by cortical atrophy. The characteristic symptom pattern (triad) of dementia, incontinence, and gait disturbance is caused by enlargement of the ventricles without elevation of CSF pressure. This is occasionally treated surgically.

Signs and symptoms of hydrocephalus
- Infants develop enlarged head circumference, full appearance of the fontanelle, downward deviation of the eyes, irritability, and poor feeding.
- Older children and adults develop the following signs of raised intracranial pressure:
  - headaches
  - blurred vision
  - vomiting
  - drowsiness or coma.

Investigations

- CT scan shows enlarged ventricles and the underlying cause.
- MRI scan.
- Lumbar puncture—*this must not be performed in patients with signs of acute raised intracranial pressure*, due to the risk of sudden deterioration. Seek neurosurgical advice.

Treatment

- External ventricular drainage (EVD). An intraventricular catheter is placed via a burr hole into the lateral ventricle on the non-dominant side. CSF flow is diverted as a temporary measure to reduce the pressure. Complications of this medical device include under- and over-drainage, infection, and displacement. *This requires specialist nursing observations and care* (see Further reading list at the end of this section).
- Ventriculo-peritoneal (VP) shunt. An intraventricular proximal catheter is inserted into a lateral ventricle. A long distal catheter is tunnelled through the soft tissues into the peritoneal cavity. A specialized unidirectional flow valve under the skin at the back of the head connects the proximal and distal catheters, allowing CSF to flow through the valve into the peritoneal cavity to be reabsorbed into the venous circulation.
- Endoscopic third ventriculostomy. Using a neurosurgical endoscope via a burr hole, an internal diversion is made between the third ventricle and the subarachnoid space on the undersurface of the brain. This procedure is complex due to the proximity of vital structures and major blood vessels.

Special points of care

- Post-operative management is as for neurosurgical patients.
- Maintain neurological observations for continuing signs of raised intracranial pressure, and report them.
- Observe, monitor, and report signs of infection.

Complications of surgery

Cranial and abdominal complications can occur, including:
- blockage of VP shunt catheters or failure of valve
- infection of the ventricular catheter
- infection or displacement of the abdominal catheter
- long-term effects on cerebral functioning (usually affecting cognition) may occur due to complex changes in the brain
- some children have multiple complex disabilities (e.g. spina bifida) that require life-long specialist management. The management of potential complications related to the shunt is only one aspect of their medical needs.

Further reading

Hickey JV. *The Clinical Practice of Neurological and Neurosurgical Nursing*, 7th edn. Wolters Kluwer Health: Philadelphia, PA, 2013.

Woodward S and Mestecky C (eds). *Neuroscience Nursing: evidence-based theory and practice*. Blackwell Publishing Ltd: Oxford, 2011.

►► Management of raised intracranial pressure

The most important aspect of nursing is the close observation of the at-risk patient by staff trained and experienced in assessment using a neurological observation chart that incorporates the Glasgow Coma Scale (GCS), pupil reactions, limb responses, and vital signs.

The motto 'time is brain' is a reminder of the life-threatening consequences of delay in recognizing and reporting deterioration. Raised intracranial pressure is treated by removing the cause of the rise, and managing the patient—usually in the intensive care unit—during the period of maximum risk.

Pathophysiology

The cranium essentially forms a rigid box containing the following three components, maintained in equilibrium by physiological mechanisms (e.g. autoregulation of cerebral blood flow):
- brain tissue (80%)
- CSF in the ventricles and subarachnoid space
- blood in the intracranial vasculature.

The Monro–Kellie hypothesis states that an increase in one component (e.g. brain mass) results in a corresponding decrease in the other two. This results in compromise of the cerebral blood supply, obstruction to CSF flow, and compression of vital structures.

Compensatory adjustments in CSF flow and blood flow permit small, slow increases in volume to be tolerated in the early stages (e.g. slow-growing brain tumour). The patient may experience some weeks of nausea and headaches before seeking medical help.

A sudden increase in intracranial volume (e.g. haemorrhage due to head injury) results in rapidly rising intracranial pressure, and is a *life threatening medical emergency*. The patient may deteriorate rapidly, with little warning, to coma and respiratory arrest due to cerebral herniation.

Main causes
- Traumatic brain injury.
- An intracranial mass or space-occupying lesion (e.g. brain tumour, cerebral haematoma, cerebral abscess, or other abnormality).
- Cerebral or subarachnoid haemorrhage.
- Cerebral infection—meningitis or encephalitis.
- Diffuse swelling of the brain—caused by severe hypoxia, sepsis, or a wide range of other systemic metabolic disorders (e.g. liver failure, hypertensive encephalopathy).
- Hydrocephalus—as a complication of head injury, cerebral infection, or brain tumour. It may also be due to a blocked ventriculo-peritoneal shunt in children or adults.

▶▶Signs of raised intracranial pressure

Avoid any delay. Report changes immediately and increase the frequency of neurological observations. In unstable patients these should take place at least every 30 min.

Signs of raised intracranial pressure include:

- headache
- nausea and vomiting
- confusion, drowsiness, and coma
- change in respiratory rate, rhythm, depth, and sound—noisy breathing and irregular rhythms are danger signs
- papilloedema (swelling of the head of the optic nerve at the back of the eye) and blurred vision
- bradycardia and hypertension—this is usually a late sign
- increasing pupil size with sluggish or absent reaction to light; unequal pupils or bilateral abnormal pupils
- weak or paralysed limbs with abnormal posture in response to noxious stimuli.

▶Investigation

Urgent CT scan of the head.

Management

- Maintain close observation and do not leave the patient unattended, as they may deteriorate rapidly.
- Maintain patient safety. The patient may be restless and confused.
- If the patient is unconscious, maintain airway and safe position.
- The patient may be at risk of seizures, so observe closely for this.
- Ensure that there is an intravenous cannula for venous access.
- Measure oxygen saturations and administer oxygen if prescribed.
- Maintain 30° head-of-bed elevation (on medical instruction), and prevent neck flexion or constriction to ensure unobstructed venous return from the head.
- Maintain normothermia (core temperature of or below 37°C).

Transfer to critical care unit or a specialist neurosciences unit

- Sedation, intubation, and ventilation are needed if the GCS score is < 8.
- Osmotherapy (mannitol, furosemide, or hypertonic saline) may be given to reduce cerebral oedema and facilitate transfer.

Principles of management in critical care

- Transfer to the operating theatre for neurosurgical treatment of the underlying cause (e.g. haematomas).
- Monitoring of intracranial pressure using an intracranial pressure monitoring device.
- Insertion of an external ventricular drain into lateral ventricle, and diversion of CSF into a specialized drain.
- In severe cases, craniectomy (removal of a bone flap) to allow swelling of the brain.

Neurosurgical aspects of cranio-cerebral trauma

The commonest causes of head injury are falls, assaults, and sports and road traffic accidents.

Head injury is a significant cause of death and serious disability in young people. Children and older adults are at increased risk due to impaired environmental awareness, sight, hearing, and balance. Children with a history of previous head injury are at increased risk.

The most important public health aspect is prevention and education in relation to driver and pedestrian safety, including alcohol awareness.

Trauma to the head can include combined injury to:
- soft tissues of the scalp and face—bleeding can be profuse
- the skull vault or base—this can be accompanied by facial or orbital fractures, and it can involve penetrating injuries and entry of air or bone fragments into the brain. There is a high risk of intracranial infection
- the brain, through direct injury and haematoma formation, or through secondary brain injury which appears in the hours and days after the initial insult:
  - hypoxic/ischaemic injury
  - cerebral oedema
  - raised intracranial pressure
  - hypotension
  - pyrexia
  - seizures.

Grading of injury

It is important to obtain as much information as possible from the patient or witnesses at the scene. This includes:
- history of injury (e.g. speed of vehicle, distance of fall)
- duration of loss of consciousness—the patient may appear normal immediately after the event, but deteriorate suddenly (lucid interval) with coma and signs of brain herniation
- recollection of the event or accident—the patient's recall of events before the injury (retrograde amnesia) and after it (anterograde amnesia)
- GCS score
- pupil size and reaction to light—this is an important indicator
- focal neurological signs—note motor deficit
- severe headache
- vomiting
- vital signs—record, and report any change
- any history of seizures before or after the event
- bleeding from the nose or ear, bruising around the orbit or behind the ear, leakage of clear fluid from the nose or ear.

Investigation and management of head injury

Follow the guidelines produced by the National Institute for Health and Care Excellence (NICE) for the investigation, management, and transfer of head-injured patients.[1] Patients who require neurosurgery should be transferred urgently to a neurosciences unit.

Neurosurgical management

This is required in any of the following situations.

Open head injury

Compound skull fracture and penetrating brain injury (e.g. knife injury, gunshot injury, road traffic accident).

- Debridement and removal of skull fragments. Replacement of bone flap may later be required.
- Development of seizures is a significant complication and requires prophylactic anti-epileptic medication.

Closed head injury

A combination of acceleration and rotational forces applied to the head cause the following:

- Intracranial haematomas, which are usually but not always associated with skull fracture. Haematomas are classified as follows:
  - Extradural—tearing of arteries between the outer meningeal layer (dura) and the brain, often due to tearing of the middle meningeal artery in the temporal/parietal region. Formation of haematoma leads to a rapid rise in intracranial pressure, and requires urgent neurosurgery to evacuate the haematoma and monitor brain swelling.
  - Subdural—bleeding over the surface of the brain, which may be acute or chronic. This also requires urgent neurosurgery and monitoring.
  - Intracerebral—bleeding within the substance of the brain (the most common type of haematoma). It may be improved by neurosurgery, but can be associated with other significant brain injury, with a poor prognosis.
- Diffuse axonal injury—tearing and disruption of axons throughout the brain substance.

Principles of management

- Frequent assessment of the patient's neurological status using the GCS score.
- Monitoring of intracranial pressure using an intracranial pressure-monitoring device (intracranial pressure bolt).
- Alleviation of cerebral swelling by the use of an extraventricular drain and temporary diversion of CSF.
- Prevention and management of secondary brain injury.

Reference

National Institute for Health and Care Excellence (NICE). *Head Injury: triage, assessment, investigation and early management of head injury in infants, children and adults.* CG56. NICE: London, 2007. www.nice.org.uk/guidance/cg56

Management of brain tumours

Management of brain tumours involves both neurosurgery and oncology management by an MDT.[2] Clinical nurse specialists support patients and their families during complex treatments. Primary brain tumours are rare. Although there are improved treatments, the prognosis for high-grade primary brain tumours remains poor.

Types of brain tumour

Intracranial tumours can be classified as follows:

- intrinsic—developing from glial cells in the brain substance (parenchyma), such as astrocytes. They include glioblastomas and astrocytomas
- extrinsic—developing from other structures inside the cranium (e.g. meninges, nerve sheaths, pituitary gland).

The commonest types in adults are primary brain tumours, meningiomas, and metastatic tumours. In children the commonest types are medulloblastomas and cerebellar astrocytomas.

Metastases in the central nervous system occur in up to 25% of patients with a primary tumour elsewhere (e.g. breast or lung). Central nervous system lymphomas can affect immunocompromised patients.[2]

Classification of tumours

- A complex system based on histological grading and tumour.
- Tumour grades 1 and 2 are considered low grade.
- Tumour grades 3 and 4 are considered high grade, and may be termed malignant. They are more aggressive, with rapid growth.

Clinical presentation

- Raised intracranial pressure—headaches, vomiting, papilloedema, and drowsiness which may progress to coma.
- Seizures—partial seizures (with or without loss of consciousness) or generalized seizures.
- Impaired function of a cerebral hemisphere or lobe—this may include cognitive, memory, or behavioural changes, dysphasia, or hemiplegia
- Endocrine abnormalities occur with tumours of the pituitary gland.
- Symptoms depend on the hormone involved. The condition often presents as Cushing's syndrome. Abnormal growth and menstrual problems also occur.

Investigation

- CT scan—shows the location, size, and number of tumours.
- MRI scan—used for demonstration of tumours in the posterior fossa and for differentiation of tumour and surrounding oedema, small or multiple lesions.

Medication

- Steroid therapy (dexamethasone) to reduce cerebral oedema around the tumour.
- Anticonvulsant medication for seizure control.

Surgery

The surgical approach will be dependent on tumour location:

- craniotomy—access to supratentorial structures via a bone flap, which can be aided by a stereotactic frame or image-guided operating system
- craniectomy—enlarged burr hole in the occipital region to gain access to the posterior fossa
- trans-sphenoidal approach—access via the nose through the sphenoidal sinus to the pituitary fossa.

Surgical excision may involve:

- biopsy only—tumour histology
- partial removal (decompression or debulking)—surgical removal of the tumour mass without unacceptable neurological impairment due to loss of tissue in 'eloquent' areas (e.g. loss of speech and language). Surgery is occasionally performed with the patient awake for part of this procedure ('awake craniotomy')
- complete removal—most likely to be used for benign tumours (e.g. meningioma, acoustic neuroma). It is rarely possible for primary brain tumours, as they are by nature infiltrative.

Radiotherapy

This is given on an outpatient basis over a period of 2–6 weeks. It may be used with benign or malignant tumours, but must be carefully planned to avoid damage to adjacent normal brain. Patients in poor health may have a shorter treatment period. A variety of methods are available, including:

- conventional fractionated radiotherapy
- stereotactic radiosurgery—used for small well-defined tumours that are unsuitable for surgery or conventional radiotherapy.

Side effects can include:

- increased cerebral oedema during treatment
- cognitive impairment in a small percentage of patients
- radionecrosis, with onset a few months after treatment.

Chemotherapy

The current 'gold standard' treatment of aggressive grade 4 tumours combines oral chemotherapy (temozolomide) with radiotherapy. This regime is given on a daily basis for 42 days.

An alternative is implanted chemotherapy, which is a localized treatment using carmustine implants.

Palliative care

Patients and their families benefit from specialized advice and support from a specialist neuro-oncology nurse.

Reference

2 National Institute for Health and Care Excellence (NICE). *Improving Outcomes for People with Brain and Other CNS Tumours: the manual*, NICE: London, 2006. ℜ www. nice.org.uk/guidance/csgbraincns/evidence/improving-outcomes-for-people-with brain-and-other-cns-tumours-the-manual2

Further reading

Louis DN et al. (eds). *WHO Classification of Tumours of the Central Nervous System*, 4th ed. World Health Organization: Geneva, 2007.

Management of subarachnoid haemorrhage, cerebral aneurysms, and arteriovenous malformations

Subarachnoid haemorrhage (SAH), a type of haemorrhagic stroke, is a *medical emergency*. The peak incidence is in the age range 40–60 years, and the cause is usually a ruptured cerebral artery aneurysm. Outcome is predicted by the World Federation of Neurological Surgeons (WFNS) clinical grading[3] and other indicators, such as the amount of blood in the subarachnoid space, and the GCS score on admission. Morbidity and mortality rates tend to be high.

Clinical presentation

- Sudden onset of very severe headache. The patient may collapse without warning, and the condition may be fatal at onset.
- Nausea and vomiting.
- Altered conscious level, ranging from mild drowsiness through to coma.
- Meningism—neck stiffness, photophobia, and irritability.
- Seizures.
- Focal neurological signs (e.g. unequal dilated pupils).
- Signs of raised intracranial pressure—headache, vomiting, impaired consciousness, papilloedema.

Pathology

There is bleeding into the subarachnoid space between the skull and brain. Blood circulates over the surface of the brain and spinal cord in the CSF, and tends to pool in the basal cisterns.

- Aneurysms develop on the circle of Willis at the base of the brain; around 50% affect the anterior cerebral arteries or the anterior communicating artery. This is associated with familial factors and other cardiovascular risk factors (e.g. hypertension, smoking).
- Arteriovenous malformations (AVM)—uncommon abnormalities of cerebral blood vessels.

Immediate care

- The patient must be transferred to a specialist neurosciences facility for management unless this is contraindicated by their clinical condition. They are assigned a grade from 0 (unruptured aneurysm) to V (deep coma) on the WFNS scale.
- Start frequent neurological observations immediately and continue them at least every 30 min until the patient's condition has stabilized.
- Report any deterioration in GCS score immediately.
- Patients who are admitted to a ward area are nursed on bed rest in a quiet environment to help to reduce headache and photophobia, but must be under close supervision.
- Position patients with impaired consciousness so as to protect their airway, and observe respiration and oxygen saturation.

- Provide analgesia and anti-emetic for severe headache and vomiting.
- Prevent straining during toileting, or other causes of elevated blood pressure (e.g. control the number of visitors).

Investigation
- Urgent CT scan shows haemorrhage around the brain.
- Lumbar puncture—this should only be performed in CT-negative patients without signs of raised intracranial pressure. It detects blood in the CSF, and may reveal non-aneurysmal bleeding.
- CT angiography (CTA) shows the size and location of aneurysms or AVMs. These may be single or multiple.

Treatment
Patients are at high risk of a further bleed within hours or days of the first event. The aim of neurosurgery is prevention of further bleeding by closure of the origin of haemorrhage. This is undertaken as soon as the patient is medically stable and fit for surgery.

Types of surgery
- Endovascular coiling. This has replaced craniotomy as the procedure of choice in recent years. The aneurysm is approached indirectly via a guided arterial catheter. Tiny platinum coils are inserted into the sac, causing embolization and obliteration of the aneurysm.
- Craniotomy. This involves a direct approach by craniotomy, and placement of a surgical clip across the neck of the aneurysm. Aftercare is the same as for cranial surgery.
- Microsurgical resection of cranial arteriovenous malformations.

Complications of SAH
- Re-bleeding.
- Raised intracranial pressure—extravasation of blood into the intracranial cavity leads to a sudden rise in intracranial pressure; vomiting, coma, and respiratory arrest may follow.
- Meningeal inflammation, which causes severe headache, nausea, and vomiting (meningism).
- Delayed cerebral ischaemia (DCI) associated with vasospasm—this is a complex response of the cerebral circulation, with constriction of the arterial blood supply and ischaemic or infarctive changes similar to stroke. It requires specialist prevention and management, including nimodipine 60 mg 4-hourly, which is prescribed to prevent vasospasm. Observe the blood pressure 4-hourly and report changes.
- Hydrocephalus.

Medical treatment

Patients with a GCS score of < 8 are transferred to the critical care unit for advanced airway management.

Aftercare

- Close post-procedure observation of the arterial puncture site for patients who have undergone endovascular coiling.
- Neurological observations using the GCS score, blood pressure, respiration, and temperature are also recorded.
- It is essential to maintain a fluid intake/output chart. Monitor urinary output.

Reference

Teasdale GM et al. A universal subarachnoid hemorrhage scale: report of a committee of the World Federation of Neurosurgical Societies. *Journal of Neurology, Neurosurgery and Psychiatry* 1988; **51**: 1457.

Further reading

Woodward S and Waterhouse C (eds). *Oxford Handbook of Neuroscience Nursing*. Oxford University Press: Oxford, 2009.

Deep brain stimulation for neurological conditions

Functional neurosurgery refers to the surgical treatment of condition such as:
- movement disorders (e.g. Parkinson's disease, dystonias)
- severe neuropathic pain syndromes
- psychiatric conditions (e.g. Tourette syndrome, obsessive-compulsive disorder), although this is uncommon in UK practice
- refractory epilepsy.

The most common type of functional neurosurgery is deep brain stimulation (DBS) for patients with Parkinson's disease. Ablative neurosurgery in which a small area of brain is permanently destroyed (e.g. pallidotomy thalamotomy), is less usual. Neurosurgery is not suitable for all patients due to age, infirmity, or their disease progression. Some patients d not want neurosurgery because of the potential risks. Neurosurger requires very careful pre-operative patient evaluation and counselling.

Parkinson's disease

This chronic progressive neurological condition affects about 100 00 people in the UK, with about 8000 new cases diagnosed every year.[4] is mainly a disease of older people, but a significant group of individua diagnosed with young-onset Parkinson's disease may live with unpleasan symptoms of either the disease or medication side effects for many year

Clinical presentation

The diagnosis is based almost entirely on clinical presentation. There ar a number of other differential diagnoses, including essential tremor an multi-infarct dementia. The symptoms include:
- tremor—initially unilateral, but progressing to the limbs, head, and trunk
- rigidity—experienced as stiffness in movement
- bradykinesia and hypokinesia—slowness in movement affecting man motor activities (e.g. speaking, writing, chewing, smiling)
- dysphagia
- postural instability, leading to falls
- autonomic dysfunction, with a tendency to postural hypotension an bowel and bladder problems
- sleep disorder (e.g. restless leg syndrome, nightmares)
- depression and dementia.

Treatment

The cause is depletion of the neurotransmitter dopamine in the bas ganglia of the brain, due to death of dopaminergic cells in the substant nigra of the midbrain. The cause of this is not yet known, but is like to be multifactorial. The mainstay of management of Parkinson's d ease is drug treatment through replacement of cerebral dopamine wi oral levodopa. After a few years of successful treatment the patie may develop dyskinesias (uncoordinated and distressing limb or fac movements) or other unpleasant side effects. This seems to be more severe in younger patients. Treatment may also cease to be effective.

Deep brain stimulator surgery

It is extremely important that prescribed medications are given exactly on time both before and after surgery, and that neurosurgical instructions about medication regimes on the day of surgery are followed.

A stereotactic frame and sophisticated brain imaging are used during the operation. A neurosurgical burr hole or twist-drill hole is made to allow insertion of the stimulator device. This part of the operation may be conducted under general anaesthetic, and the patient may be woken during part of the operation so that the precise target area of the basal ganglia can be identified. This is possible because the brain itself is insensitive to pain. Special care is taken by the operating department team to ensure the patient's comfort during this part of the procedure.

Electrodes are advanced into the chosen target area, which will depend on the condition. In Parkinson's disease, electrodes are inserted in the basal ganglia (e.g. subthalamic nucleus) and connected to a stimulus generator under the skin of the upper chest. A continuous stream of impulses is transmitted to the brain in order to block the neuronal activity that is causing the abnormal movements.

Potential specific post-operative complications include:
- raised intracranial pressure as a result of intracranial bleeding or swelling—observe carefully using the GCS, and report headache, nausea or vomiting, drowsiness, or visual disturbance
- superficial infection around the wound
- serious infection of the inserted device
- displacement of the device.

It is important to consider general post-operative needs:
- The patient may be older, with multiple health needs.
- It is a long operation, and strict measures are needed to prevent deep vein thrombosis, tissue breakdown, and respiratory infection.

After full recovery at home, the stimulator is programmed and the level of stimulus is increased until the patient experiences improvement. The patient uses a hand-held magnet across the skin of the upper chest to switch the device on or off. Most patients experience improvement in all of the symptoms of their illness, and medication regimes can usually be reduced. Some patients have a bilateral procedure, with the second operation being performed later.

Reference

4 Parkinson's UK. *What is Parkinson's?* ℘ www.parkinsons.org.uk/content/what-parkinsons

Further reading

Bain P, Aziz T, Liu X and Nandi D (eds). *Deep Brain Surgery*. Oxford University Press: New York, 2009.
Clarke C. *Parkinson's Disease in Practice*, 2nd edn. Royal Society of Medicine Press: London, 2007.
Parkinson's UK. ℘ www.parkinsons.org.uk

Surgical options for epilepsy

Seizures are episodic events in which there is a sudden onset of neurological symptoms, with or without loss of consciousness, caused by abnormal discharge of neuronal electrical activity. There may be sensory, motor, or psychogenic types of seizure, or a complex mixture of features. Nurses who are observing seizures should take careful note of the type, time, and duration, as this can be very helpful in establishing a diagnosis.

Epilepsy is a condition in which a person is liable to recurrent seizures. It is not usually diagnosed unless one or more seizures have occurred over a 2-year period, and there were no obvious provoking factors (e.g. stroke, head injury, alcohol withdrawal). Epilepsy is relatively common in the wider population. Most people with epilepsy have no underlying neurological disease or abnormality, their seizures are controlled with anti-epileptic medication, and their quality of life is good, although their choice of career and sports activities may be affected.

A smaller number of patients require multiple anti-epileptic medication regimes to achieve seizure control, some drugs have significant side effects, and some patients find adherence to their medications difficult. Patients can develop drug resistance.

Classification of seizures and epilepsy

Epilepsy is classified by seizure type and/or by epilepsy syndrome. Diagnosis and classification can be complex, but in general epilepsy is classified as either:

- partial or focal epilepsy, with or without loss of consciousness
- generalized epilepsy, in which awareness is lost.

Status epilepticus is a medical emergency in which seizure activity is continuous or intermittent over 30 min without recovery. There are multiple causes. It must be reported to medical staff immediately and treatment implemented to prevent life-threatening complications.

Patients who have had a head injury or cranial neurosurgery are at risk of developing seizures, and prophylactic anticonvulsant medication prescribed. Patient and family education is essential to maintain compliance with medication, which may be difficult if the patient has short-term memory loss or a problematic lifestyle (e.g. excessive alcohol intake).

Epilepsy surgery

A small number of adults and children with epilepsy are significantly helped by surgery. Epilepsy is sometimes associated with learning difficulties or severe complex neurological disease. Recurrent seizure activity disrupts nutrition, mobility, family life, and schooling, and surgical intervention may improve quality of life.

Investigations

Patients are admitted for:
- CT or MRI scan to visualize the suspected lesion or area
- electroencephalography (EEG) studies, with simultaneous EEG monitoring and video recording (video telemetry)
- patients may also have intra-operative and post-operative EEG studies to monitor their progress.

Types of surgery

- Craniotomy and removal of the epileptogenic area of brain. The dissection must be performed extremely carefully to avoid any 'eloquent' area of brain (e.g. speech area). It often involves the hippocampal area of the temporal lobe (hippocampal sclerosis), which causes temporal lobe epilepsy. In severe cases, where there is significant damage to or abnormality of a lobe or hemisphere, this may be removed, but this is more frequently seen in children than in adults.
- Craniotomy and division of white matter tracts to prevent seizure activity spreading over large areas of the cortex (e.g. corpus callosotomy).
- Electrical stimulation using a vagal nerve stimulator (VNS) device. The mechanism of action is not well understood, but it appears to reduce the frequency and severity of seizures. Electrodes are attached to the vagus nerve (tenth cranial nerve) in the left side of the neck, and a battery-powered pulse generator is implanted under the skin of the left chest. The patient is taught how to recognize and avert seizure activity by triggering the stimulator with a hand-held device.
- Deep brain stimulation.

Side effects of VNS device

- Sleep apnoea and daytime drowsiness.
- Laryngeal symptoms (e.g. vocal hoarseness, cough).
- Cardiac problems (e.g. bradycardia).

Patient care

- Patients require careful management of their medication regimes before and after surgery.
- Neurological observations and seizure chart.
- Patients frequently continue to experience seizures in the post-operative period, and require careful observations and support.
- Other care is the same as for craniotomy.
- Aftercare for the VNS device is organized by the epilepsy specialist nurse working with the medical team and MDT.

Further reading

Epilepsy Society. ℘ www.epilepsysociety.org.uk
Shorvon S. Handbook of Epilepsy Treatment, 3rd edn. Wiley-Blackwell: Chichester, 2010.

Disc prolapse and degenerative disease of the spine

The function of the intervertebral discs is to act as shock absorbers and facilitate movement of the spinal column. The discs need to be strong and compressible in order to withstand the body weight, and consist of two layers:

- annulus fibrosus—a strong outer fibrocartilage ring (tyre-like)
- nucleus pulposus—inner hydrophilic gel that attracts water to maintain the disc pressure, giving it a 'spongy' property.

Discs have a poor blood supply, relying on nutrients and oxygen from nearby tissues and vertebral bone. Therefore when injury or degenerative changes occur, repair and regeneration are very poor. Degenerative disease commonly starts in the late twenties or early thirties, and is a major cause of back pain later in life.

The main cause of degenerative disc disease is ageing, but other factors can increase progression of the degenerative changes, such as obesity, tall stature, smoking, occupation (driving, manual work, frequent lifting, twisting, or vibration movements), and a genetic predisposition (see Table 23.1). The most commonly affected regions of the spine are cervical C5–6, C6–7 (more flexible), and lumbar L5–S1 joint, followed by L4–L5 (these areas bear the axial load of the body).

Table 23.1 Degenerative cascade and resulting problems

Ageing process causes reduced water content of the nucleus pulposus	Flattening and bulging of disc (protrusion)
	Appearance of tears in the annular ring
	Herniation of disc material through the tears (disc prolapse)
Extruded disc material compresses and irritates spinal nerve roots	Back pain, discogenic pain
	Referred pain—radicular/sciatic distribution through buttocks, back of leg, and foot
Reduced disc space Spinal stenosis—narrowing of spinal canal and cord compression Cauda equina syndrome	Abnormal movement of vertebrae causing osteoarthritis of facet joints and osteophyte development (bony spurs)
	Mechanical back pain
	Neurological deficit—sensory (pain, numbness, tingling), motor (muscle weakness, wasting, paralysis, abnormal reflexes)
	Bladder and bowel disturbance, perianal anaesthesia, sexual dysfunction

Diagnosis

- Plain X-ray and CT scan—bony changes, arthritis, osteophyte formation.
- MRI scan—soft tissue damage, disc herniation, nerve compression.
- Radiculogram—will show disc herniation impinging on the nerves and spinal cord.
- Discogram—to assess the physical integrity of the disc; tears seen.
- EMG and nerve conduction—nerve damage, muscle weakness.

Conservative management

The majority of cases will respond to short-term rest (several days), with a return to full activity aided by the use of the following:

- analgesia, non-steroidal anti-inflammatory drugs, muscle relaxants, and epidural steroid injections
- back exercise programmes under the direction of a physiotherapist
- patient education about weight reduction, smoking cessation, and lifestyle adaptation
- short-term use of back orthoses (corsets)
- acupuncture.

Surgical management

This is recommended if there has been no improvement following conservative measures, or if there is neurological involvement, bladder and/or bowel disturbance, or intractable pain. Cauda equina syndrome requires urgent surgical decompression to minimize permanent neurological damage.

- Minimally invasive surgery—microdiscectomy by instrumentation or laser.
- Open surgery—partial or full laminectomy, decompression, and spinal fusion with pedicle screws, rods, cages, or bone grafts; disc arthroplasty, in which an artificial disc is inserted in the disc space.

Benefits of minimally invasive surgery

It is a day-case procedure that results in minimal tissue damage, reduced blood loss and infection risk, reduced post-operative pain, improved osmesis, and shorter recovery time and hospitalization.

Complications of surgery

These include recurrence of disc prolapse, arthritic changes above or below fusion points, instrumentation failure or breakage, dural tear and CSF leakage. There is more tissue damage, increased blood loss, a higher risk of infection and nerve damage, and a larger scar. All of these factors will result in a longer hospitalization.

Nursing considerations
- Neurological observations to detect any sensory or motor loss affecting the limbs.
- Observe bladder and bowel function for urinary retention and sphincter paralysis.
- Observe the wound site for bleeding, haematoma formation, signs of infection, and CSF leakage. Wound drains are removed 24 h post-operatively.
- Pain relief allows early mobilization which will prevent complications of decubitus ulcers, chest infection, and deep vein thrombosis.
- The patient should be advised not to sit or stand for long periods, and to use a back corset if this has been recommended. They should roll on to their side, lowering their legs over the side to get out of bed.
- Psychological care is needed to support the patient, and discussion of realistic long-term outcomes, as there may be a need for future revision surgery.

Spinal cord tumours

Spinal tumours are rare, but potentially cause rapid onset of spinal cord compression and paralysis, which is a medical emergency.

Patients with spinal cord compression require urgent referral to a specialist spinal or oncology team. Nurses caring for cancer patients must be particularly vigilant for new-onset pain and neurological symptoms in the neck, back, or legs.

It is important to remember that back pain is a very common problem in the general population, and most causes of back pain are due to musculoskeletal problems.

General practitioners use so-called 'red flag' indicators that prompt urgent referral. Ideally treatment needs to start within 24 h of onset in order to prevent permanent loss of function.

Types of spinal tumour

- Extradural tumour. This is the most common type. Around 70% occur at spinal thoracic level. They are mostly metastatic lesions of bone, but also include myeloma, neurofibroma, and lymphoma. Primary tumour may be breast, lung, prostate, or kidney. About 4000 patients develop metastatic spinal cord compression each year in the UK, and although many have a diagnosed primary malignancy, about 25% of patients have no previous cancer diagnosis, and the onset of spinal symptoms may be the first presentation.[5]
- Intramedullary tumour. Rare—usually meningioma or schwannoma. These tumours can be treated by neurosurgery in some cases.
- Intrinsic (intramedullary) tumour. Rare—usually astrocytoma or ependymoma. They are often slow growing, and may not present with pain.

Patient symptoms

- Pain in the neck or back is usually the first symptom. It may also occur in or around the chest, as many tumours affect the thoracic spine. Pain tends to get more severe over time, and is worse at night or on moving. It may radiate along the path of a spinal nerve in the arm or leg.
- Severe localized tenderness over the spine.
- Abnormal sensation in the limbs or trunk—numbness or tingling or burning feelings.
- Weak arms or legs—difficulty in walking, or sudden loss of ability to stand or walk.
- Bladder or bowel dysfunction.
- Sexual dysfunction (e.g. new erectile difficulty).

Pathophysiology

The spinal cord lies in the spinal canal of the vertebrae, extending from the lower border of the skull to the first lumbar vertebra. The meningeal layers and blood and lymphatic vessels lie between the spinal cord and the bone of the vertebral column. Spinal cord neurons are vulnerable to injury (e.g. compression) and ischaemia, and do not regenerate, so removal of compression is urgent.

There is little room for the expansion of a mass (e.g. tumour) or an abscess. Although the tumour may be slow growing, eventually compression of the spinal cord (myelopathy) or spinal nerve roots (radiculopathy) causes pain and loss of function. The higher the position of the tumour in the spinal cord, the more neurological function is lost. For example, a cervical cord lesion could cause paralysis of all four limbs (tetraplegia) and loss of autonomic function. Typically the patient has signs of upper motor neuron lesion damage, namely paralysis with abnormally brisk reflexes, and stiff or spastic muscles.

Below the end of the spinal cord, between the lower border of the first lumbar vertebra and the termination of the spinal canal in the lower sacrum, an expanding tumour can compress multiple spinal nerve roots (cauda equine syndrome) inside the spinal canal, causing severe pain, weakness or paralysis of the legs with absent or reduced reflexes, flaccid muscles, and bladder and bowel problems. This is termed cauda equine compression.

Investigation
- Urgent MRI scan of the spine.
- Investigation of the source of unknown primary.

Treatment
Depending on the patient's clinical status, prognosis, tumour histology type, and the patient's preference, a combination of the following treatments is used.

Drug treatment
- Corticosteroids (dexamethasone) to improve neurological functioning.

Surgery
- Decompressive spinal surgery and removal of tumour.
- Anterior or posterior approach and spinal stabilization depending on the size and location of the tumour.

Radiotherapy
- Many patients receive urgent external beam radiotherapy.

Palliation
Around 5–10% of cancer patients are thought to develop spinal metastases. A significant number who develop paralysis will not regain the ability to walk, despite treatment, and management of pain is essential.

Specific nursing needs
- Bladder catheterization and a strict care protocol are required.
- Tissue protection is essential.

Reference
5 National Institute for Health and Care Excellence (NICE). *Metastatic Spinal Cord Compression: diagnosis and management of adults at risk of and with metastatic spinal cord compression*. CG75. NICE: London, 2008. ℰ www.nice.org.uk/guidance/cg75

Medical stimulators in surgery

Medical stimulators are used for conditions in which the usual medical management for pain or other unpleasant symptoms is ineffective. They are not considered until other modes of treatment have been fully tri-alled. Patients usually have complex conditions, and require skilled care and rehabilitation in addition to detailed pre-operative assessment in relation to the device.

Medical electrical devices alter the functioning of the nervous system (this is referred to as neuromodulation). Spinal cord stimulators are likely to be the most commonly encountered device, but there are many potential targets for treatment as these devices are constantly being technically improved.

Examples of use

- Failed back surgery syndrome.
- Complex regional pain syndromes.
- Intractable angina.
- Refractory abdominal, thoracic, or pelvic pain.
- Peripheral vascular disease.
- Painful peripheral neuropathy (e.g. diabetes).
- Phantom limb pain.
- Severe neck or head pain.

There is also an increasing focus on the development of functional devices for the stimulation of movement (e.g. after spinal cord injury or nerve injury, or to assist prosthetic devices after limb loss).

Devices usually consist of electrodes which deliver pulsed electrical signals, and a battery-powered electrical pulse generator. An alternative method uses non-invasive external magnetic stimulation.

Note that people with implanted devices must not have MRI imaging.

External non-invasive devices (transcutaneous)

These are applied as pads to the skin surface. The well-known com-mercially available transcutaneous electrical nerve stimulation (TENS) machine is used to relieve pain. These devices are thought to work by inhibiting the propagation of nociceptive impulses from the periphery to the brain, based on the gate control theory of pain proposed by Melzack and Wall.[6] They are most commonly used in the home to relieve back pain.

Percutaneous devices

These involve the introduction of a fine needle under ultrasound guid-ance into a localized area. They may be used to provide a course of treat-ment on an outpatient basis, or as a trial before permanent placement of electrodes.

Examples include the following:

strengthening muscle contraction, improving motor control, and reducing spasticity

electrical stimulation of the pelvic floor muscle as part of the treatment and rehabilitation of people with some types of urinary incontinence

- percutaneous tibial nerve stimulation (PTNS) to treat urinary or faecal incontinence[7]
- occipital nerve stimulation to treat severe headache.

Permanently implanted devices

Spinal cord stimulators (SCS)

Fine electrodes are inserted into the epidural space, which contains spinal nerve roots, blood vessels, and lymphatic vessels, and lies between the outermost layer of the spinal meninges (dura) and the bone of the vertebral column. These electrodes are connected to an impulse generator implanted in a suitable superficial anatomical site (e.g. the abdominal wall).

Implanted peripheral nerve stimulators

These are used for a number of painful syndromes (e.g. complex regional pain syndromes). They are occasionally used for severe intractable pain syndromes affecting the head (e.g. occipital neuralgia, severe cluster headache, migraine).

Functional electrical stimulation

This is the stimulation of muscles to initiate standing, locomotion, or cycling movements, as an adjunct to rehabilitation for spinal cord injury or brachial plexus injury.

Patient education

Patients need help and advice to understand and respond to the sensations produced by the device (usually warm or 'buzzing' feelings). The response is individual, but in carefully selected patients this treatment is effective. Patients may experience pain which 'breaks through' the sensations produced by the stimulator, and sometimes pain relief becomes less effective over time, due to habituation.

Complications

Any patient with an implanted device needs help in understanding the use of the stimulator and assistance with other strategies (e.g. other analgesic treatments), and rehabilitation. Careful observation of the patient is required for the following:

- infection around the wound site (redness and localized pain). The most common organism is *Staphylococcus*. Pre-operative screening for MRSA is extremely important
- leakage of CSF due to incidental dural tear
- headache or other complaints of new pain or discomfort
- failure or breakage of the device or leads.

References

1 Melzack R and Wall PD. Pain mechanisms: a new theory. *Science* 1965; 150: 971–9.
2 National Institute for Health and Care Excellence (NICE). *Percutaneous Posterior Tibial Nerve Stimulation for Overactive Bladder Syndrome.* IPG362. NICE: London, 2010. ℵ www.nice.org.uk/guidance/ipg362

Further reading

British Pain Society. *Spinal Cord Stimulation for the Management of Pain: recommendations for best clinical practice.* British Pain Society: London, 2009.
National Institute for Health and Care Excellence (NICE). *Spinal Cord Stimulation for Chronic Pain of Neuropathic or Ischaemic Origin.* TA159. NICE: London, 2008. ℵ www.nice.org.uk/guidance/ta159
National Institute for Health and Care Excellence (NICE). *Percutaneous Tibial Nerve Stimulation for Faecal Incontinence.* IPG395. NICE: London, 2011. ℵ www.nice.org.uk/guidance/ipg395

Peripheral nerve injury

Peripheral nerve injury is complex. The capacity for recovery varies according to the extent and location of the injury. Recovery tends to be better in younger people.

The mechanism of injury may involve lacerations (e.g. caused by glass or knives), penetrating injuries (e.g. gunshot wound), or trauma to the limbs (e.g. fractures, sports injury). A small number are iatrogenic (i.e. associated with medical treatments or medical devices).

Peripheral nerve injury is classified according to the criteria described initially by Seddon in 1943[8] and Sunderland in 1951,[9] ranging from mild (first degree) to severe (fifth degree). This may include:

- temporary disruption of neuronal impulses due to compression of the nerve or its blood supply—this usually improves slowly over a period of a few weeks
- serious injury with crushing or stretching of the nerve—recovery can potentially occur, but it takes months to years
- complete transection.

Pathophysiology

Peripheral nerves consist of bundles of neurons sheathed by three protective layers of connective tissue (endoneurium, perineurium, and epineurium). These permit sliding and stretching of nerves during movement. Nerves contain:

- afferent fibres, which convey sensory information from the periphery to the spinal cord, and thence to the brain for processing and integration of peripheral stimuli
- efferent fibres, which convey motor impulses to target voluntary muscle groups
- autonomic fibres, which stimulate target glands and organs.

Injury damages not only individual nerve fibres, but also myelin sheath, connective tissue, and small blood vessels supplying the nerves. Surgery thus involves careful alignment of fibres, nerve sheaths, and blood vessels. When peripheral nerves are severed (e.g. by a cut), the distal part of the damaged neuron is separated from its cell body, and consequently degenerates. The surviving proximal part of the neuron undergoes complex changes that promote repair, aided by Schwann cell activity.

Symptoms

- Damage to motor nerves—weakness or complete paralysis, muscle cramping and twitching, muscle wasting, weakening of the skin and bones in affected limbs.
- Damage to sensory nerves—usually numbness, but the patient may have neuropathic pain, which is a severe burning pain that is not relieved by usual measures. Pain may be triggered by minor irritation (e.g. clothing, cold breezes).

Important clinical note

Patients are particularly vulnerable to nerve injury when they are unconscious or anaesthetized, and operating department procedures regarding padding and positioning of limbs must be followed meticulously. New complaints of numbness, tingling, or weakness of limbs must be reported promptly.

Location of injury

- Upper and lower extremities—these are particularly common locations. They may involve digits or a limb. Hand injuries with damage to the nerves and tendons that control the fingers have a serious impact on function (i.e. grasp and manipulation of objects).
- Shoulders and pelvic girdle, including injury to brachial and lumbar plexuses. Brachial plexus injuries may result in a permanently paralysed and insensitive arm, with profound disability.
- Face and neck—affecting movement and sensation of facial muscles, including eye opening and closure, chewing, speaking, and swallowing.

Diagnosis

- Electromyelography and nerve conduction studies.
- MRI scanning to visualize soft tissues.
- CT myelogram to diagnose brachial plexus injury.

Surgical treatment

If planned, this will consist of one of two options:
- immediate repair, particularly for cutting or severing injuries
- delayed surgery (i.e. delay of a few weeks), which may be preferred if there is extensive injury.

Rehabilitation

This is an important part of the patient's recovery, but due to the slow pace of repair of peripheral nerves, patients require encouragement to persist with long-term rehabilitation plans. Treatment of neuropathic pain associated with the injury is required.

While a limb is paralysed or numb, joints can develop other problems such as arthritis or stiffening as a result of disuse. The physiotherapy team will prescribe measures to protect the affected joints, and exercises to ensure full range of movement.

References

Seddon HJ. Three types of nerve injury. *Brain* 1943; 66: 237–88.

Sunderland S. A classification of peripheral nerve injuries producing loss of function. *Brain* 1951; 74: 491–516.

Further reading

ster R, Santy J and Rogers J. *Oxford Handbook of Orthopaedic and Trauma Nursing.* Oxford University Press: Oxford, 2011.

Burns and plastic surgery

Burns physiology

A burn is a thermal insult to the skin and underlying tissue (see Box 24.1).

It is imperative to have a sound grasp of burns physiology in order to effectively manage the care required to optimize recovery from this potentially life-threatening injury.

All burns will have a local response at the site of the injury, but burns that involve more than 30% of total body surface area (TBSA) will also elicit a systemic response.

Local response

At a local tissue level, a burn can be divided into three zones, identified by Jackson in 1947[1] (see Figure 24.1).

Zone of coagulation

This is the area in a burn that was nearest the heat source, and that has suffered the most damage as evidenced by clotted blood and thrombosed blood vessels. The damage in this zone is irreversible.

Zone of stasis

This is the area surrounding the zone of coagulation, which is characterized by decreased blood flow. Any resuscitation and cooling is targeted at increasing perfusion to this area, to prevent the tissue degradation in this area from becoming irreversible.

Box 24.1 Types of thermal injury

Types of burns
- Flame
- Scalds
- Contact
- Electrical
- Chemical
- Radiation

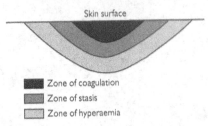

Skin surface

■ Zone of coagulation
■ Zone of stasis
□ Zone of hyperaemia

Figure 24.1 Jackson's burn wound model.

Zone of hyperaemia

This is the peripheral area around the burn, which has an increased blood flow.

These zones are three-dimensional through the affected tissue. Therefore as the zone of stasis increases, the wound will expand in depth and width.

Systemic response

The release of inflammatory mediators from the wound has a systemic effect in burns that involve more than 30% TBSA. This will have the following effects:

- Circulatory effects: capillary permeability is increased, leading to a large shift of proteins and plasma from the intravascular to interstitial space. This will lead to a significant hypovolaemia and oedema that will begin gradually post injury, with a peak at 8–12 h, and continue for 24–48 h post injury.
- Respiratory effects: inflammatory mediators will cause bronchoconstriction, and in large burns this can develop into adult respiratory distress syndrome.
- Metabolic effects: the inflammatory mediators will trigger an up to threefold increase in the basal metabolic rate, which can also be complicated by under-perfusion to the gut due to the hypovolaemia.

All of these effects mean that the major burn presents significant challenges. These major insults respond best to goal-driven therapy managed by a multidisciplinary team (MDT), as outlined in the section on the management of major burns (see ➲ p. 621).

Reference

Jackson D. The diagnosis of the depth of burning. *British Journal of Surgery* 1953; **40**: 588–96.

First aid and referral guidance

First aid

- Check for and remove or make safe any immediate danger to the patient and yourself (e.g. ensure that the electricity is turned off).
- Stop the burning process, either by smothering the flames with a fire blanket or similar device, or if the burn has been caused by hot fluids remove the affected clothing.
- Cool the burned area with cool water for 10–20 min, or for longer if this is having a therapeutic analgesic effect. The use of ice and iced water should be avoided, as this can cause the burn to become deeper. Care should be taken to prevent or avoid hypothermia, especially in children and the elderly. Cooling of the burn can be effective up to 2 h post burn.
- Cover the burn with cling film and refer the patient to the appropriate service. For chemical burns, copious amounts of water should be used, and contact with the effluent avoided to prevent further chemical burns. Specialist locations may have alternative neutralizing agents, such as Diphoterine®. The chemical involved should be documented.
- For electrical burns, ensure that the electricity supply has been turned off and the patient is not still in contact with the electricity.
- For burns to the face and/or flame burns that occurred in an enclosed space (e.g. house fire), check for signs of inhalation injury and observe the airway closely.

Referral guidance

- National thresholds for referral have been published by the National Network for Burn Care (NNBC).[2]
- As a general principle, referral to a specialist burn service should be considered for any burn of more than 2% TBSA in a child, more than 3% TBSA in an adult, full-thickness burns, chemical and electrical burns, burns to the face, hands, feet, and perineum, inhalation injuries, or burns with other complications.
- England and Wales Burn Care Services are divided into four Burn Care Networks, which consist of:
  - burn centres
  - burn units
  - burn facilities.
- These burn services will advise on treatment and investigations recommended prior to transfer.

Reference

2 National Network for Burn Care (NNBC). *National Burn Care Referral Guidance.* NNBC: London, 2012. ℘ www.britishburnassociation.org/downloads/National_Burn_Care_Referral_Guidance_-_5.2.12.pdf

Burns assessment

It is important to obtain a comprehensive history, including the mechanism of injury, the time that has elapsed since the burn, and any treatment that has already been initiated. The assessment should be performed using an ABCDE approach, bearing in mind the specific potential effects of a burn injury.

- *Airway*: the impact of the inflammatory mediators leads to bronchoconstriction. Assess for the likelihood of an inhalational injury:
  - history of burns in an enclosed space
  - burns to the face, neck, or upper chest
  - singed nasal hair
  - carbonaceous sputum
  - hoarse voice
  - stridor.
- *Breathing*: full-thickness circumferential burns of the chest may restrict chest expansion. In cases of smoke inhalation, products of combustion (e.g. soot) will act as an irritant to the bronchioles, leading to further inflammation and bronchospasm. History of fire in an enclosed space should raise the suspicion of carbon monoxide poisoning, which will not be detected by pulse oximetry, so if it is suspected the patient will require an arterial blood gas and venous sample for carboxyhaemoglobin levels.
- *Circulation*: the increased capillary permeability will lead to a significant fluid shift and resultant hypovolaemia commencing approximately 3 h post injury and continuing for 24–48 h. The rate of fluid loss is influenced by the size of the burn and the time that has elapsed since injury, rather than the depth of the burn—hence the need for an accurate history. The peripheral circulation should be checked, especially if there are any circumferential deep or full-thickness burns present, as these may require escharotomies.
- *Disability*: hypoxia or hypovolaemic shock may lead to alteration in the patient's conscious level. At this stage other injuries should be identified and managed.
- *Exposure*: at this stage, assessment of the burn size and depth should be completed. All jewellery should be removed. The patient should be kept warm to prevent hypothermia.

Assessment of burn area

This is calculated as a percentage of TBSA. In the case of a relatively small burn, the patient's palm is roughly equivalent to 1% of their TBSA, and can therefore be used to calculate the extent of a small burn.

The Wallace rule of nines (see Figure 24.2) is a reasonable way of estimating larger burns in adults, where the body is divided into areas of 9%. Accuracy can be increased further when assessing adults, and especially children, by using a Lund and Browder chart (see Figure 24.2), which takes into account the differences in body proportion with age.

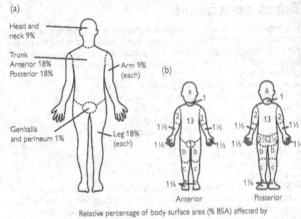

Relative percentage of body surface area (% BSA) affected by growth

Body Part	0 year	1 year	5 year	10 years	15 years
a = ½ of head	9½	8½	6½	5½	4½
b = ½ of 1 thigh	2¾	3¼	4	4¼	2½
c = ½ of 1 lower leg	2½	2½	2¾	3	3½

Figure 24.2 (a) Wallace rule of nines. (b) Lund and Browder chart. Reproduced from Robert Crouch OBE, Alan Charters, Mary Dawood, and Paula Bennett, *Oxford Handbook of Emergency Nursing*, 2009, with permission from Oxford University Press.

Assessment of burn depth

Burns can be divided into three categories—superficial, partial thickness, and full thickness—depending on the layers of the skin that are penetrated by the heat source (see Figure 24.3).

- Superficial/epidermal (sunburn)—the burn affects the epidermis but not the dermis. This appears as a reddened painful wound with brisk capillary refill. These burns usually heal without intervention over a period of 7 days, with no residual scarring.
- Partial thickness/dermal—the heat penetrates through the epidermis into the upper layers of the dermis, resulting in fluid escaping to form blisters or a moist raw surface. In most cases, burns at this depth will be painful.

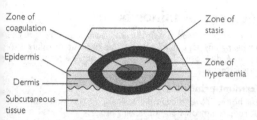

Figure 24.3 The skin and depth of burn. Reproduced from Jason Smith, Ian Greaves, and Keith Porter, *Oxford Desk Reference Major Trauma*, 2010, with permission from Oxford University Press.

- Deep dermal/full thickness—the burn involves all of the dermal layer, and may extend into underlying structures, such as muscle. A deep dermal burn will be red in colour, but will not blanch. A full-thickness burn will appear leathery or waxy, and sensation will be dulled or absent because the burn has extended past the nerve endings. If the full thickness extends circumferentially, this will need to be released surgically.

It should be borne in mind that most burns involve a mixture of depths, and may extend in depth for up to 48 h post burn, depending on the quality of first aid and fluid resuscitation.

Management of minor burns

A minor burn can be classed as a small burn, usually less than 10% TBSA
and not involving any special area that would necessitate referral to a
specialist unit. A diagnosis of a minor burn can only be made after the
full initial assessment.

Key treatment principles

- Analgesia both to cover the initial dressing and to provide continued
  cover as required throughout the healing process.
- The burn wound should be thoroughly cleansed and any dead skin
  from large blisters removed.
- A non-adherent absorbent dressing should be applied and the wound
  initially reviewed within 48 h, or sooner if:
  - exudate has seeped through the dressing
  - there is excessive pain
  - there are signs and symptoms of infection.
- If there is a high risk of infection occurring or the wound is infected,
  an antimicrobial dressing should be considered.
- Advice regarding care of the dressing should be given. The patient
  will also require additional information about nutritional intake and
  avoiding exposure of the healed tissue to the sun.
- At subsequent wound reviews, if there is any index of suspicion of
  complications or psychosocial issues, advice should be sought from
  the local burns service.

Management of major burns

A major burn is a significant life-threatening insult that requires a coordinated approach from a large MDT over a substantial period of time, in order to restore the patient to full function. In this section the emphasis will be on the initial 48 h after the burn has occurred.

The treatment of a major burn will commence following the initial assessment and calculation of the burn area and depth. In order to accurately tailor the management of these critically ill patients, it is essential that the team is aware of the time and type of burn, and any treatment that has already been initiated.

Analgesia
- This is essential in order to carry out the assessment and treatment.
- Give IV morphine diluted to 1 mg/mL titrated to the pain score.
- The pain-related needs of a burn patient will be complex, and specialist advice should be sought in addition to the above.

Fluid management
- Fluid resuscitation is usually started when the burn is greater than 15% TBSA in adults and 10% TBSA in children.
- There are many fluid replacement formulae for burns, but the most widely used is the Parkland formula (see Box 24.2).
- The patient should be catheterized and their urine output measured hourly.
- Fluid resuscitation should aim for a urine output of 1–2 mL/kg/h.
- The hourly fluid rate should be adjusted to maintain this target.
- The full clinical picture, including type of burn, laboratory results, and invasive monitoring parameters, will also contribute to the adjustment of fluid resuscitation.

Environment
- The patient should be nursed in a cubicle because of their increased susceptibility to infection.
- In patients with a major burn it is common for the hypothalamus to 'reset' itself approximately 1°C above normal. Therefore the ambient temperature needs to be closely regulated, usually between 28°C and 33°C. This is especially important during dressing changes and at any time when the patient's body is exposed.
- Ideally patients with major burns should be nursed in a high-dependency type of environment.

Box 24.2 The Parkland formula
Parkland formula
4 mL of Hartmann's solution × patient's weight × %TBSA

Half is given in the first 8 h and the remainder in the following 16 h.

This is calculated from the time of the burn.

Surgical management

At the time of assessment a decision will be made as to which areas can be managed by dressings, and which deeper areas may require surgical excision and skin grafting. This will be carried out as early as possible within the first 24 h. Depending on the size of the burn and the patient's physiological status, the excision and grafting may be undertaken in a series of procedures.

Wound management

It is important to remember that during dressings a significant proportion of the patient's body surface area is exposed, rendering them highly susceptible to infection, fluid loss, increased pain levels, and a dramatic fall in temperature.

- Accurate assessment and management of pain is vital. Initially this may involve the use of intravenous sedation and opioid analgesia.
- A heated room is required, and prior preparation of dressing materials to ensure that the patient is exposed for the minimum amount of time necessary.
- The burn wound should be cleansed by showering. This is also helpful for removing the dressing if it has adhered to the wound.
- Any blisters should be deroofed, and devitalized skin should be removed to prevent it from becoming a focus of infection.
- The wound should then be assessed and documented at each exposure in order to ensure that the appropriate dressing is selected.
- There are a range of suitable dressings available, including biological dressings (e.g. Biobrane™). Any dressing should have the following properties:
  - antimicrobial properties if there is a risk or presence of infection
  - a non-adherent surface
  - a bulky layer that can absorb substantial amounts of exudate.

The dressing should be secured to prevent slippage and the risk of shearing, usually with crepe bandage or tubular net bandage.

Therapy

Burn wounds, particularly those over moving surfaces, are at risk of contractures as the wound heals. The physiotherapist and occupational therapist are important members of the MDT, and regular physiotherapy will be required to reduce contractures and maintain range of movement and function.

Nutrition

- Enteral feeding should commence as soon as possible after admission, because of the risk of Curling's ulcer and bacterial translocation due to under-perfusion of the gut.
- A patient with increased metabolic rate and significant tissue loss requires a high-protein, high-calorie feed.
- Referral to a dietitian is essential.

Psychological care of the burns patient

Burn wounds are perhaps the most highly visible trauma injury, which will have a significant psychological impact on the patient, their family, and the care team. It is important to remember that the patient will be very conscious of any reaction conveyed by the facial expressions of those approaching them. Management issues include:

- assisting the patient in working through issues of altered body image and loss
- supporting the family
- reintegration of the patient into society after discharge
- assessment for safeguarding issues.

These issues will require referral to relevant members of a psychosocial team.

Scar management

A scar is formed in the final stage of the wound healing process, as the body lays down collagen fibres to repair the damaged tissue. Initially the scar is red, thickened, firm, and tender. Over a period of months it matures and becomes paler, softer, and less sensitive. This is due to the remodelling of the collagen fibres, which are initially laid down in disordered manner. Skin normally makes collagen and breaks it down at the same rate. If an injury occurs, collagen is then formed at an increased rate. This can continue after the wound has healed.

If only the epithelial layer is repaired, there may be little scarring because healing has occurred via regeneration as opposed to repair. Hypertrophic and keloid scars are unique to humans.

Factors that affect scar healing

- The length of time that it takes to heal—if the wound takes more than 2 weeks to heal, the resultant scar will usually be hypertrophic.
- Race—darker skin is more susceptible than Caucasian skin.
- Age—younger people scar more than older people because they have a higher skin tension and increased rate of collagen synthesis.
- Location—the sternum, upper back, shoulders, buttocks, and dorsum of the feet are more likely to develop hypertrophic scars.
- Tension—increased tension leads to increased inflammation, causing the fibroblasts to secrete more collagen.
- Infection.
- Movement or loss of graft.

Scar assessment

There are various scar assessment tools that can be used. The Vancouver Scar Scale and the Patient and Observer Scar Assessment Scale are commonly used, and assess pigmentation, vascularity, pliability, and height of the scar.

Treatment of scars

- The scar should be massaged with a non-perfumed moisturizing cream. This promotes collagen remodelling by applying pressure to the scar and providing moisture and pliability to the area. It can also help to reduce itching.
- Silicone sheets or gel—the mechanism of action is not really understood, but it is thought to mimic the stratum corneum and reduce water vapour transmission, which decreases collagen deposit. They should not be used over open wounds, and the patient should be monitored for allergic reactions.
- Pressure garments—these apply pressure to the scar, causing it to blanch. Pressure is thought to remould the collagen and push the blood away. If there is less blood the amount of oxygen and nutrients is reduced, and less collagen is made. Pressure is also thought to aid realignment of the collagen fibres so that they lie parallel to the epidermis again. The pressure garments are usually worn for between 4 months and 1 year, until the scar matures. They need

to be replaced as their elasticity decreases, and they are worn for approximately 23 h a day, with breaks for hygiene, massage, and moisturizing the skin. If a burn heals over a period of > 10 days a pressure garment should be used. It is most effective if used within 2 weeks of healing. After 6 months, pressure is less effective. It should not be applied if there is a risk of damage by shearing.

• Adhesive contact media (e.g. permeable non-woven adhesive tape).
• Steroid injections—given every 4–6 weeks for 6–10 months. There is potential for local side effects, such as dermal thinning and atrophy, and pigment changes. Systemic side effects are rare. They can be painful. Initially the scar is hard and inflexible, but it gradually softens as inhibition of blood flow leads to reduced protein synthesis and eventually a flattened scar.
• Cosmetic camouflage —there are special make-up products available which can be matched to skin tone and help to camouflage the scar.
• Dermabrasion—this can be used in conjunction with sprayed skin cells cultured from a biopsy of the patient's own skin to improve the appearance of the scar.
• Surgery—this may also exacerbate the problem, especially if there is keloid scarring.
• Laser therapy—the use of carbon dioxide and argon laser is associated with a recurrence rate similar to that for surgery. The pulsed-dye laser can be effective in reducing redness and itching.
• Radiotherapy—this is used post-operatively, and it is thought to inhibit fibroblast proliferation.
• Cryotherapy.
• Collagen injection.

Further reading

osworth-Bousfield C. *Burn Trauma: management and nursing care*, 2nd edn. Whurr Publishers: London, 2002.

earmonti R, Bond J, Erdmann D and Levinson H. A review of scar scales and scar measuring devices. *ePlasty* 2010; 10. ℘ www.eplasty.com/index.php?option=com_content&view=article&id=457&catid=171:volume-10-eplasty-2010&Itemid=121

ettiaratchy S, Papini R and Dziewulski P (eds). *ABC of Burns*. Blackwell Publishing Ltd: Oxford, 2005.

car Information Service. ℘ www.scarinfo.org/scar_facts.html

Skin grafts

A skin graft involves taking skin from one area of a body (animal or human) and applying it to another area on the same or a different body.

Classification of skin grafts

- By species:
  - autograft—taken from the patient's own body
  - allograft—taken from another person's body
  - homograft—taken from a human
  - isograft—taken from an identical twin
  - heterograft—taken from another species
  - xenograft—taken from an animal.
- By depth or type:
  - split-thickness or partial-thickness graft—only a partial thickness of the skin is harvested, which means that the donor site will still have epithelial islands, so healing can occur. The thicker the graft that is taken, the longer the healing process will be
  - full-thickness graft—the full thickness of the skin is taken, and the wound needs to be directly closed
  - sheet graft—the harvested skin is applied in one sheet. It may be fenestrated to allow exudate to escape
  - meshed—the harvested skin is put though a machine that makes cuts in the skin so that it can be stretched and thus can cover a larger area. The resulting appearance is rather like a string vest or fishnet stockings
  - pinch graft—this is one of the first types of graft, in which the skin is pinched and cut.

The differences between full-thickness and split-thickness grafts are summarized in Table 24.1.

Harvesting of skin grafts

Split-thickness skin grafts can be harvested from anywhere on the body, but are most commonly taken from the thighs and buttocks using a dermatome. Full-thickness skin grafts are usually taken from areas that can be directly closed, such as the post-auricular region and groin.

Table 24.1 Differences between full-thickness and split-thickness skin grafts

Full-thickness skin graft (FTSG)	Split-thickness skin graft (STSG)
Takes less readily	Revascularizes readily
Contracts initially but re-expands	Constricts
Better skin colour and texture	Can be expanded (e.g. meshed)
Regains sensation	Acquires ingrowth of nerves from the edge, but sensation can be reduced
Donor site requires suturing or an STSG	
Contains hairs and sweat glands	Donor site heals
	Breaks down and ulcerates if subjected to repeated trauma

Skin graft take

This occurs in three phases.

- The first phase, *serum imbibition*, occurs during the first 24–48 h. The graft is attached to the recipient bed by a fibrin layer, and nutrients are then diffused from the recipient bed to the graft.
- In the second phase, *inosculation*, a vascular network of capillaries is established between the graft and the recipient bed.
- In the third phase, *organization*, new vessels grow and fill, and the graft is usually fully adhered to the recipient bed by 5–7 days. After about 4 weeks, nerve fibres grow in from the recipient bed and surrounding area.

Key treatment principles

Donor site

- Keep the site clean and dressed. A range of dressings can be used.
- Observe for any excess bleeding.
- Analgesia should be given (the donor site is often more painful at the start of mobilizing).
- The dressing is usually left intact for 7–10 days unless this is contraindicated.
- When the site has healed, apply moisturizer twice a day until the redness disappears.
- For at least 1 year afterwards the patient should be advised to avoid direct exposure of the donor site to sunlight.

Graft site

- Use a protective dressing to prevent shearing, formation of haematomas, and infection.
- Topical negative pressure therapy can also be used for more complex grafts.
- The dressing is usually left intact initially for 2–7 days. Care needs to be taken when removing the dressing, to avoid damaging the fragile graft.
- The amount of movement permitted initially will depend on the location of the graft and local protocols.
- For at least 1 year afterwards the patient should be advised to avoid direct exposure of the graft site to sunlight.

Reasons for skin graft failure

Movement of the graft.

Infection.

An inadequately vascularized bed.

Accumulation of fluid beneath the graft.

Graft placed on bare bone, tendon, cartilage, or nerves.

Flaps

A flap involves the movement of tissue, with its blood supply, from one part of the body to another.

Indications for a skin flap

- The defect does not contain an adequate blood supply for the survival of a skin graft.
- A large hollow defect.
- An area of wear and tear.
- An area where other tissue is required.
- An area that requires reconstruction.
- Congenital defect.

Classification of flaps

By anatomical content

- Cutaneous flap—contains skin.
- Muscle flap—contains muscle.
- Myocutaneous flap—contains skin and muscle.
- Fasciocutaneous flap—contains skin and fascia.
- Fascial flap—contains fascia.
- Osseous flap—contains bone.
- Osseomyocutaneous flap—contains skin, muscle, and bone.

By blood supply

- Random pattern flaps—these flaps have a random vascular pattern, and consequently their length:breadth ratio is important. The breadth must exceed the length if the flap is to have a good chance of survival.
- Axial pattern flaps—these flaps follow an artery and vein, so they can be longer and narrower than random pattern flaps.
- Free flaps—the blood supply is disconnected from the area from which the flap is raised, and then reconnected at the recipient site.

By area

- Local flaps:
  - Z-plasty
  - advancement flap
  - rotational flap
  - transposition flap.
- Distant flaps:
  - groin flap
  - pedicle flap
  - cross-limb flap.

Key treatment principles

- Pre-operative explanation of the procedure, and education about what will be required following surgery.
- The aim of post-operative care is to ensure optimal vascularization of the flap and to detect any problems early on. If the flap fails the procedure cannot be performed again, as the tissue is no longer available. Therefore patient compliance is essential.

- Flap observations (often performed every 30–60 min for the first 24 h):
  - colour
  - temperature (skin/touch)
  - capillary refill
  - sensation
  - pulse
  - position
  - oedema and blistering
  - bleeding and drainage.
- It is vital to detect any deterioration in the flap's blood supply early on, to enable any rescue actions to be undertaken.
- Positioning—to prevent pressure and tension on the flap.
- Environmental temperature—the flap needs to be kept warm to prevent vasoconstriction.
- Fluids—sufficient fluid intake is essential to maintain adequate perfusion.
- Nutrition.
- Caffeine and nicotine must be avoided, as these can cause vasoconstriction and impair the blood supply.
- Psychological support.

Causes of flap necrosis

- Tension and kinking.
- Haematoma.
- Pressure.
- Venous congestion.
- Infection.
- Gravity.
- Arteriosclerosis.

Reconstructive surgery following trauma

Reconstructive surgery following trauma is predominantly performed to restore function and form (appearance), with the main emphasis or restoring function. Depending on the severity of the trauma, this will be a lengthy process that requires multiple operations, and it will need the skills of a wide-ranging MDT. Reconstruction and treatment will be based on restoring function utilizing the least invasive rung within the 'Reconstructive Ladder' outlined in Box 24.3.

Key pre-operative treatment principles

- Assess—all patients will require an appropriate trauma evaluation and initial management following the ABCDE principles.
- Stabilize—any fracture dislocations or interruption in circulation will need urgent manipulation and splinting to restore or maintain the circulation.
- Optimize—provide fluid resuscitation and haemodynamic monitoring.
- Analgesia.
- Psychological preparation:
  - The sudden nature of the injury and the potential for permanent disfiguration will cause anxiety, and can lead to post-traumatic stress disorder (PTSD) in a proportion of patients.
  - Early assessment and ongoing support by a mental health professional should be considered.

Depending on the mechanism of injury, multiple areas of the body may be involved.

Facial injuries

- Any lacerations will be sutured if direct closure is possible, otherwise skin grafts or flaps may be required.
- Fractures of the face may include some of the following structures:
  - orbital floor
  - zygomatic bone (cheekbone)
  - maxillary fractures, Le Fort I, II, and III fractures
  - mandibular fracture (open or closed).

Box 24.3 The 'Reconstructive Ladder'

- Free flap (top rung)
- Pedicle flap
- Random pattern flap
- Tissue expansion
- Full-thickness graft
- Split-thickness graft
- Delayed primary closure
- Primary closure
- Healing by secondary intention (bottom rung)

Key treatment principles

Assessment

- Assess the airway.
- Observe for CSF leakage via the nose or ears—this is indicative of basal skull fracture.
- Assess the eyes for acuity and normal range of movement.
- Radiographic investigations are needed to confirm the location of the fractures and the degree of displacement.

Treatment

- If there is not a life-threatening need for immediate surgery, surgical treatment may be delayed to allow a reduction in swelling.
- Any displaced fractures will require surgery in the form of open reduction and internal fixation (ORIF) using small plates.
- Some mandibular fractures may require a combination of plates and wires to keep the jaw shut.
- The approach is usually underneath the hairline or via the mouth where possible, in order to minimize scarring.
- Structures are realigned and pre-injury mandibular occlusion (bite) is restored.

Specific post-operative care

- The patient should be nursed in a semi-recumbent position in order to minimize swelling.
- If wiring has been used to stabilize the jaw, wire cutters and suction should be available at the bedside. Regular anti-emetics may be advisable.
- The patient should have a soft or liquid diet for up to 6 weeks, and will require referral to a dietitian.
- In the case of maxillary and zygomatic fractures, the patient should be advised not to blow their nose for up to 4 weeks post-operatively.
- If the surgical approach was via the mouth or the patient has their jaw wired, regular mouth care using a soft brush and mouthwash will be required.

Complications

Transient or residual paraesthesia.
Infection.
Haematoma.
Malunion of fractures.

Reconstructive surgery following limb trauma

Hand injuries

Hand injuries that require reconstruction usually involve:

- lacerations
- fractures
- neurovascular damage
- severing of the extensor or flexor tendons.

Key treatment principles

Assessment

- The mechanism of injury is important. Tendon or nerve damage as a result of crush injury has a much poorer prognosis than severing due to laceration.
- If the history indicates the possible presence of foreign bodies, X-ray should be taken to exclude this.
- The location of any lacerations is important.
  - Dorsal lacerations most commonly indicate extensor tendon injury.
  - Palmar lacerations are more commonly associated with flexor tendon injury.
- The full range of movement should be assessed in order to confirm the affected tendons.
- Viability and suitability for repair may be confirmed by ultrasound or MRI.
- Assessment of the nerve distribution is required in order to identify deficits.

Treatment

- Severed or partially severed tendons will require surgical repair, usually under a general anaesthetic. The ends of the tendon are located and sutured together. The limb and forearm are then immobilized in a back slab.
- Severed digital nerves also require surgical repair. The limb and forearm are then immobilized in a back slab.

Specific care

- The limb should be elevated in a Bradford sling.
- Regular observations of colour, temperature, and sensation should be performed in order to detect early signs of complications.
- A hand therapist will replace the back slab with a bespoke splint approximately 48 h post-operatively.
- The patient will need to attend for an intensive course of essential physiotherapy for 3–6 weeks post repair. *The importance of this for optimizing the final outcome should be emphasized to the patient pre-operatively.*
- Sutures should be removed 10 days post-operatively.

Complications
- Haematoma.
- Infection.
- Reduced function.
- Surgical adhesions, which can impair tendon movement.

Lower limb injuries
Lower limb injuries in this category generally result in a combination of soft tissue loss and an open fracture. The treatment is usually completed collaboratively by the orthopaedic and plastic surgical teams.

Key treatment principles
- Assessment.
- The limb should be assessed for viability to ensure that adequate perfusion remains.
- Radiological assessment involving X-ray, CT scan, and MRI.
- Treatment.
- Initially the wound will be debrided, and all devitalized tissue removed.
- Any fractures will then be fixated. This is commonly undertaken via external fixation (see section on external fixation and pin site care on ➲ p. 453 in Chapter 20).
- Tissue coverage will then be achieved with the use of flaps, ideally utilizing a local flap, or if necessary a free flap.
- Specific care.
- Regular observations of colour, sensation, and movement in the limbs distal to the procedure.
- Specific care of the fixation (see section on external fixation and pin site care on ➲ p. 453 in Chapter 20).
- Care of skin flaps.
- Analgesia—patients with this type of injury benefit from review by the acute pain service if this is available.

Complications
- Malunion of fractures.
- Flap necrosis.
- Circulatory insufficiency to the distal limb.

Breast surgery

Breast surgery may be performed for a number of reasons:
- to treat congenital abnormalities (e.g. hypoplasia of the breasts) or chest wall abnormalities (e.g. in Poland's syndrome)
- following mastectomy
- to treat gynaecomastia
- to correct breast asymmetry
- for aesthetic reasons
- during gender reassignment
- to relieve back and shoulder pain and psychological distress in women with large breasts.

Breast implants
- These are available in different shapes and sizes, and are filled with silicone or saline.
- Potential complications include:
  - infection
  - haematomas or seromas
  - capsule formation
  - implant rupture
  - asymmetry
  - shape distortion
  - scarring
  - alteration of nipple sensation
  - silicone granuloma.
- Breastfeeding following a breast implant is possible, but can be affected by the surgical incision or procedure used.
- The incidence of breast cancer in women with a breast implant does not appear to be any higher than that in the general population.

Breast reduction
- The aim is to reduce the size of the breast while maintaining the aesthetics and function and preserving the nipple.
- Potential complications include:
  - infection
  - haematomas and seromas
  - dehiscence
  - nipple numbness
  - nipple necrosis
  - shape distortion
  - scarring
  - fat necrosis.
- Post-operatively it is important to monitor nipple circulation and observe for haematomas.
- Drains may be used.
- The suture lines may be taped as a dressing and to help to improve scarring. The tape is usually left in place for at least 1 week.
- Support bras are worn for 4–8 weeks.
- Lactation is usually still possible after breast reduction.

Autologous breast reconstruction

There are several techniques that can be used, and the choice of technique will depend on various factors, including the amount of tissue removed, whether there has been radiotherapy treatment of the breast area, the patient's general health status and body build, the patient's preference, and the surgeon's skills.

The following techniques can be used:

- latissimus dorsi flap
- transverse rectus abdominis myocutaneous (TRAM) flap
- deep inferior epigastric perforator (DIEP) flap
- gluteal artery perforator (GAP) flap
- transverse upper gracilis (TUG) flap
- nipple reconstruction.

Key treatment principles

Pre-operative

- Education about the patient's options and their post-operative care and expectations.
- Photographs.
- Avoidance of nicotine and aspirin.
- Examination and surgical marking of the breasts while the patient is sitting up.
- Psychological considerations.

Post-operative

- Adequate analgesia.
- Flap observations and general principles of caring for a patient with a flap.
- Wound care:
  - observation
  - drains
  - dressings.
- Correct positioning—usually in a semi-recumbent position to reduce swelling and avoid pressure on the reconstructed breast and donor area. For abdominal flaps, a pillow may be required under the knees to reduce the tension on the abdomen.
- Physiotherapy:
  - chest
  - range of motion.
- Gentle mobilization is usually encouraged the next day.
- A correctly fitting non-wired support bra will be required.

Potential complications

- Numbness or a tingling sensation in the arm on the affected side.
- Breast asymmetry.
- Tissue necrosis.
- Infection.
- Abdominal hernias if abdominal muscle has been used.
- Chronic seroma.
- Limited shoulder movement if the latissimus dorsi muscle has been used.
- Scarring.

Cutaneous lesions

These involve the abnormal and uncontrolled growth of skin cells which can metastasize to other parts of the body. Skin cancer is the most common of all cancers, and its incidence is increasing. It can develop in all age groups, but it is rare in children

Risk factors

- UV light.
- Age usually > 50 years.
- Skin colour.
- It is more common in men.
- Previous skin cancers.
- Immunosuppression.
- Radiation exposure.
- Chemical exposure.
- Long-term skin damage.
- Solar keratosis.
- Family skin disorders.
- Bowen's disease.

Basal-cell carcinoma (BCC)

- Affects the cells in the basal layer (bottom) of the epidermis, and occurs on sun-exposed areas or on burnt or scarred skin.
- Is slow growing, and rarely spreads to other parts of the body.
- Also known as a 'rodent ulcer.'
- The most common skin cancer (six to eight times more common than malignant melanoma). Rare in people with dark skin, and more common in men than in women.
- Usually curable with surgery. If left untreated it will grow slowly, ulcerate, and damage nearby structures.

Signs and symptoms

- Small lump on skin.
- Usually smooth and pearly or waxy.
- May bleed or crust.
- May simply be a flat scaly red spot.
- May be a firm red lump.
- Usually painless.

Key treatment principles

- Biopsy is taken to confirm the diagnosis.
- Surgery is performed to remove the lesion. Mohs surgery is commonly used, in which the lesion is excised one layer at a time, and each layer is examined peri-operatively under a microscope until all of the margins are clear of cancerous cells.

- Other treatments:
  - cryotherapy
  - photodynamic therapy
  - curettage or cautery
  - radiotherapy
  - laser surgery
  - topical creams.

Squamous-cell carcinoma (SCC)

- An overgrowth of squamous cells that affects the outermost cells of the skin.
- Less common than BCC. Although usually slow growing, it grows faster than BCC.
- Occasionally spreads to other parts of the body. If left untreated it will penetrate the underlying tissue and may metastasize.
- Bowen's disease is an early, non-invasive stage of SCC.

Signs and symptoms
- Scaly in appearance.
- Often has a hard horny cap.
- Can feel tender.
- Usually occurs on sun-exposed skin.

Key treatment principles
- These are similar to those for BCC.

Melanoma

- A malignant lesion arising from the melanocytes in the epidermis.
- Commonly develops from a mole, but can occur on previously normal skin.
- There are four basic types:
  - superficial spreading melanoma
  - lentigo maligna
  - acral lentiginous melanoma
  - nodular melanoma.
- The most frequent locations are the trunk, legs, and arms, and the scalp in men.
- The incidence of melanoma is four times higher than it was 30 years ago.[3]

Signs and symptoms
- Increase in size.
- Change in shape, or asymmetrical.
- Change in colour, or multiple colours.
- Irregular edge.
- The elevation of a mole or lesion may suggest that the lesion is malignant.
- Itching.
- Bleeding.

Key treatment principles
- Surgical excision of the lesion with a 1–3 cm margin.
- Further investigations may be required to detect any metastases.
- For lesions over 1 mm thick, a block dissection of affected lymph nodes may be indicated.
- There is no proven adjuvant treatment, but trials of new treatments are being conducted.
- Regular follow-up by the surgeon and GP.
- Self-examination for signs of recurrence and metastases.

Reference

3 Cancer Research UK. *Melanoma Skin Cancer.* ℰℎ http://cancerhelp.cancerresearchuk.org/type/melanoma

Further reading

Chiu T and Kong T. *Key Clinical Topics in Plastic and Reconstructive Surgery.* JP Medic Ltd: London, 2015.
National Institute for Health and Care Excellence (NICE). *Skin Cancer Prevention: informatic resources and environmental changes.* PH32. NICE: London, 2011. ℰℎ www.nice.org.uk/guidance/ph32

Useful websites

Cancer Research UK. *Skin Cancer (Non Melanoma).* ℰℎ http://cancerhelp.cancerresearchu.org/type/skin-cancer/
Skin Cancer Foundation. ℰℎ www.skincancer.org/

Pre-operative evaluation and assessment for cosmetic surgery

Patients may have many motives for seeking cosmetic surgery, but ultimately their goal will be to improve the aesthetics of an area of their body. It is important that these motives are fully explored in a comprehensive assessment to ensure that surgery is the appropriate route for the patient. This will require the expertise of a wide-ranging MDT, including:
* consultant plastic surgeon
* nurse with plastic surgery expertise
* counsellor
* dietitian
* medical photographer.

Goals of effective pre-operative assessment
* Ensure that the patient has realistic expectations of the outcome and the length of time to final maturation. The use of photographs of the surgeon's previous work during the recovery phases may be helpful.
* Exclude body dysmorphic disorder, in which the person becomes fixated about a part of their body which they perceive to have a defect. It has been demonstrated that surgery is unlikely to cure this perception.
* For some procedures, such as breast reduction and abdominoplasty, a target weight may need to be set in order to minimize the risk of wound dehiscence post-operatively.
* Ensure that the patient realizes the significant risks that caffeine and nicotine pose to revascularization of any reconstructive work, such as skin grafts or flaps.
* Pre-operative photographs should be taken.
* A full explanation should be given of any aftercare that will be required, such as the use of pressure garments after liposuction or rhytidectomy, and the implications of poor compliance.

Facial surgery

Rhinoplasty

This involves manipulation of the cartilage or bone structure of the nose in order to refine its form, or in the case of a deviated septum or previous misaligned fracture, to improve its function. If minor changes to the cartilage or septum are required, the incision is usually made inside the nostrils. The cartilage is then resected, the wound is directly closed, and a bolster is applied. An external splint will be applied to preserve the revised contour. If the procedure requires the bridge of the nose to be refined, or the nose to be re-fractured, the incision line is usually on the undersurface of the nose. The wound will still be directly closed, and the nostrils may require packs. An external splint will be applied to preserve the revised contour.

Key treatment principles

- The patient should be nursed in a semi-recumbent position to minimize swelling.
- Respiratory function must be closely monitored due to nasal occlusion.
- A nasal bolster is worn for 12 h.
- Nasal packs, if present, are removed 24–48 h post-operatively.
- External nasal splints should remain in place for at least 7 days post-operatively.
- The patient should be instructed not to blow their nose for 7–10 days post-operatively.

Complications

- Altered sense of smell.
- Post-operative haemorrhage.
- Impaired nasal breathing.

Rhytidectomy (facelift)

This is used to decrease the signs of ageing by reducing skin wrinkling and gravitational changes. It can also be performed in conjunction with liposuction. Incisions are made behind the ears and beneath the temporal hair line. The skin is then undermined and the muscles and supporting soft tissues repositioned and tightened. The incision lines are then sutured, and pressure bandages are applied.

Key treatment principles

- Pre-operative surgical marking with the patient sitting, prior to administration of a general anaesthetic.
- Post-operatively the patient should remain elevated at 30° for at least 24–48 h.
- Analgesia.
- Follow-up and bandage removal 3–5 days post-operatively, usually as an outpatient.

Complications
- Haematoma.
- Infection.
- Paraesthesia.
- Decreased range of emotive expression.

Blepharoplasty

This is the surgical removal of excess skin from the upper and/or lower eyelids. It can be performed as a cosmetic procedure, but can also be used to restore function when loose skin in the upper eyelid interferes with function. In an upper blepharoplasty, an incision is made in the fold of the upper eyelid, excess skin and fat are removed, and the wound is directly closed. In a lower blepharoplasty, an incision is made directly below the eyelash line, and the excess skin is removed before direct closure.

Key treatment principles
- Surgical marking of incision lines should be performed pre-operatively with the patient upright.
- The patient should sleep sitting up for 24–48 h post-operatively.
- Antibiotic ointment should be applied to the suture line.
- Removal of sutures takes place 3–5 days post-operatively.
- Contact lens use should be avoided for up to 4 weeks after the procedure.

Complications
- Injury to the lacrimal duct.
- Haematoma.
- Infection.
- Eyelid paraesthesia.

Non-surgical facial treatments

Botulinum toxin

Clostridium botulinum produces a poisonous toxin that can cause paralysis. Despite its dangerous potential, botulinum toxin is used to treat various conditions, such as strabismus, spasticity, blepharospasm, and hyperhidrosis. Several commercial preparations of botulinum toxin A are used to treat wrinkles and facial creases, of which Botox® is possibly one of the most well known. Botulinum toxin inhibits acetylcholine release at neuromuscular junctions, thereby blocking nerve signals to the muscles, so that the injected muscle can no longer contract. This results in relaxation of the wrinkles.

Key treatment principles

- Alcohol and non-steroidal anti-inflammatory drugs (NSAIDs) should be avoided prior to the treatment.
- The toxin is injected into the relevant muscles.
- The patient should not lie down for several hours and should not massage the area for at least 12 h after the procedure, to prevent the toxin from travelling to other areas and causing undesired paralysis.
- Application of ice to the injection site may reduce pain, swelling, and bruising.
- It may take 1–3 days for the clinical effect to be achieved, reaching a peak at 1–2 weeks.
- The benefit lasts for 2–6 months.

Contraindications

- Infection or inflammation of the area.
- Previous allergic reactions.
- Pregnancy and breastfeeding.
- Pre-existing neuromuscular conditions.

Complications

- Bruising.
- Headaches.
- Hypoaesthesia.
- Paralysis.
- Decreased range of emotive expression.
- Immunity to the toxin.

Chemical peels

A chemical peel is the controlled use of chemicals to remove layers of skin in order to improve the appearance of the skin. This can range from superficial peeling that only penetrates as far as the papillary dermis, to deep peeling that penetrates to the mid-reticular dermis. The damage caused by the chemical allows the regeneration of new, remodelled dermal tissue that is increased in volume, so wrinkles and defects of the skin are reduced.

Key treatment principles

- After thorough cleansing of the skin, the peeling agent is applied to the areas to be treated. After the appropriate period of time the chemical is neutralized, and the face is then washed with water. The strength of the chemical peel and the length of time for which it remains *in situ* will determine the depth of the peel.
- Care needs to be taken to prevent the chemical solution from entering the eyes and ears.
- An ointment such as petroleum jelly should be applied to the affected area, or biosynthetic occlusive dressing to reduce pain and prevent scab formation.
- A burning sensation and oedema occur for 24–48 h after the procedure, so regular analgesia is required.
- Following a chemical peel the patient should stay out of the sun for at least 6 months.
- Following the procedure the skin will exfoliate and look unattractive for a period of time.
- The use of make-up and sunscreen should be avoided until the skin is completely healed.

Contraindications

- Hypersensitivity to the peeling agent.
- Facial cancers, although this procedure can be used for some skin cancers.
- Irradiated or severely sun-damaged skin.
- Dark skin tones.
- Oily skin.

Complications

- Pigment changes.
- Pruritus.
- Scarring.
- Infection.
- Acne and milia.

Injection augmentation

Collagen or autologous fat can be injected under the surface of the skin in order to plump up the area, reduce contour defects, and produce a more youthful appearance.

- Injection augmentation with collagen or fat cells is not permanent, as the body reabsorbs the material over a period of 4–12 months, depending on the material used.
- A topical anaesthetic is applied to the area in order to reduce pain from the injection.
- Some patients may be allergic to the collagen preparation, so a pre-test should be undertaken. Allergic reactions are not a problem with fat injections, as the fat is harvested from the patient.
- Exposure to the sun should be avoided until the skin is fully healed and all bruising has disappeared.

Complications
- Infection.
- Abscess.
- Itching and sensitivity.
- Uneven contour.
- Patient dissatisfaction.

Skin treatments

Laser treatment

The word 'laser' is an acronym for Light Amplification by Stimulated Emission of Radiation. Laser treatment in cosmetic surgery can be used for tattoo removal, bleaching of skin lesions (e.g. port-wine naevi), hair removal, as an alternative to chemical peels and dermabrasion, or as an adjunct to facelift procedures. The laser transmits a high-energy beam that generates heat in targeted areas, causing either charring or cauterization, or penetrating into the tissues, vaporizing the water in the cells and causing them to rupture.

The different types of lasers are named after the medium in which the light is generated—for example, carbon dioxide, erbium YAG (yttrium aluminium garnet). Each has a different wavelength and energy density characteristics which need to be matched to the tissue and effect required in order to optimize the treatment.

Laser safety protocols should be in place to reduce any hazards that can be associated with the use of lasers. Every organization that uses lasers should have a Laser Safety Officer who can provide more detailed information about laser safety and local protocols. Further information and advice has been provided by the Medicines and Healthcare products Regulatory Agency (MHRA).[4]

The treatment principles and complications are similar to those described for chemical peels and dermabrasion.

Dermabrasion

Dermabrasion is the surgical abrasion of the surface layers of the skin, which leads to remodelling of the dermal tissue in an organized manner, resulting in the production of firmer smoother skin on healing. Dermabrasion is used to treat scars, tattoos, wrinkles, and actinic keratosis. Microdermabrasion exfoliates only the dermis, and is only suitable for superficial skin conditions.

Key treatment principles

- Often a test patch is undertaken to estimate healing and pigmentation outcomes.
- The aim is for moist wound healing, either by a closed wound dressing method using non-adherent hydrogel dressings for 3–5 days, or by an open method with the use of topical emollients.
- Other treatment principles are similar to those for chemical peels. Re-epithelialization will take 10–14 days.

Complications
- These are similar to those following a chemical peel.

Contraindications
- Recent facial surgery (e.g. rhytidectomy).
- Radiation therapy.
- Disorders that may delay healing (e.g. diabetes mellitus, immunosuppression).
- Freckled skin, as the freckles in the treated area may disappear.
- Herpetic lesions.
- Patients who are prone to keloid scarring.

Reference

4 Medicines and Healthcare products Regulatory Agency (MHRA). *Lasers, Intense Light Sou[...]
  Systems and LEDs: guidance for safe use in medical, surgical, dental and aesthetic practic[...]
  MHRA: London, 2015. www.gov.uk/government/uploads/system/uploads/atta[...]
  ment_data/file/458799/Guidance_on_the_safe_use_of_lasers__intense_light_sour[...]
  systems_and_LEDs.pdf

Body contouring

Liposuction

This is the use of suction to remove adipose tissue through small cannulae that are inserted into the skin through small incisions. It is commonly used to improve cosmetic appearance when diet and exercise have been unsuccessful. However, it is also used for lipomas, and as an adjunct to other surgery, such as abdominoplasty, gynaecomastia, and lymphoedema.

In addition, it can be used to sculpt the body to improve its shape and/or contour and increase muscle definition (liposculpture). Normally the fat cells removed by liposuction are not replaced. However, the remaining fat cells can hypertrophy.

There are several liposuction techniques.

• Dry technique—a vacuum is created using a syringe or vacuum pump, and fat is removed by suction. A general anaesthetic is required and there may be significant blood loss, so this technique is now rarely used.
• Tumescent (wet) technique—a solution of anaesthetic and adrenaline is injected locally to reduce pain and bleeding, and to aid fat aspiration. It can be used in conjunction with the ultrasound- and laser-assisted techniques.
• Ultrasound-assisted technique—ultrasonic vibrations are used to liquidize the fat before it is removed by suction.
• Laser-assisted technique—lasers are used to melt the fat before it is removed by suction.
• Water jet-assisted technique—the fat cells are separated by a fine high-pressure water jet, making them easier to remove by suction.

Liposuction is not a treatment for obesity, and careful patient evaluation for suitability, as well as patient education, are required prior to the procedure. A review of the patient's medications should be undertaken, as some medications (e.g. non-steroidal anti-inflammatory drugs) may need to be stopped prior to surgery.

Key treatment principles

• Elasticated support bandages or garments are usually required for several weeks. These help to reduce swelling and bruising.
• Care of the small insertion sites is required. These may be sutured or left to heal by secondary intention, and therefore need a dressing. Regular observation for infection is required.
• There is likely to be bruising and swelling, which can last for several months. If there is bruising, aspirin and other anti-inflammatory medications should be avoided.
• There may be some numbness in the area, which should disappear within 2 months.
• Ambulation and light activity should be encouraged, but strenuous activity should be avoided for several weeks.

Potential complications
- Asymmetries and contour deformities.
- Lumpy uneven results.
- Significant blood loss.
- Fluid overload.
- Thrombophlebitis.
- Thrombosis.
- Haematomas.
- Infection.
- Fat embolism.
- Pulmonary oedema.
- Internal damage.
- Skin burns.

Abdominoplasty

Abdominoplasty is the surgical excision of surplus abdominal fat layers. Any excess skin is also removed, the muscle wall is repaired, and the umbilicus is repositioned. Panniculectomy is the removal of the abdominal apron of fat in obese patients. Abdominoplasty is not a minor procedure, and can carry the risk of serious complications, particularly in obese patients. However, with careful patient selection, planning, and patient education, these complications can be minimized.

Key treatment principles
- Flap observation and care are critically important.
- Analgesia—patient-controlled analgesia or an epidural may be indicated.
- The patient is usually nursed in semi-Fowler's position with pillows under the knees to minimize stress on the abdomen.
- Mobility is initially restricted, and will depend on the extent of the surgery.
- Deep vein thrombosis prevention measures are needed (e.g. anti-embolic stockings).
- Pressure ulcer prevention measures are needed.
- Drains and a urinary catheter may be *in situ*.
- Physiotherapy.
- An abdominal support garment may be used.
- Strenuous activity should be avoided for at least 6 weeks, or as advised by the surgeon.

Complications
- Wound infection.
- Wound dehiscence.
- Fat necrosis.
- Haematoma and seroma formation.
- Thromboembolism.
- Fat embolism.
- Poor scarring.
- Altered sensation in the area.

Contraindications
- Smoking.
- Diabetes.
- Cardiovascular and thromboembolic disease.
- Previous abdominal surgery.
- Future planned pregnancies.
- Unrealistic patient expectations.

Body contouring after excessive weight loss

Massive weight loss can lead to redundant folds of skin that can be painful, debilitating, and result in a negative body image. This excess skin can affect the abdomen, thighs, back, face, and neck. In addition to abdominoplasty, liposuction, and face lifts, several other procedures have now been developed to remove this excess skin.
- Brachioplasty—removal of excess skin from the upper arm.
- Upper body lift—consists of mastopexy in women, or mastectomy in men, and removal of excess skin from the upper back.
- Thigh lift—removal of excess fat and skin from the thigh.
- Lower body lift—consists of abdominoplasty and removal of excess skin from the lower back.

Often a combination of procedures may be required once stable weight loss is maintained. Multiple operations may be necessary, so a multidisciplinary approach and a detailed treatment plan will be required. The potential complications and risks are similar to those for abdominoplasty. However, in addition, blood loss during surgery can be considerable, and there is a risk of asymmetry and relapsing skin laxity due to poor skin tone.

Further reading

Chiu T and Kong T. *Key Clinical Topics in Plastic and Reconstructive Surgery*. JP Medical Ltd: London, 2015.
Grey J and Harding K. *ABC of Wound Healing*. Blackwell Publishing Ltd: Oxford, 2006.
Storch J and Rice J. *Reconstructive Plastic Surgical Nursing: clinical management and wound care*. Blackwell Publishing Ltd: Oxford: 2005.

Useful website

British Association of Plastic Reconstructive and Aesthetic Surgeons (BAPRAS). ℳ www.bapras.org.uk

Thoracic surgery

Introduction

The thorax consists of 12 thoracic vertebrae, 12 pairs of ribs, and th
sternum, which are separated from the abdomen by the diaphragm. Th
main organs found within the thoracic cavity are the heart and lungs (se
Figure 25.1).

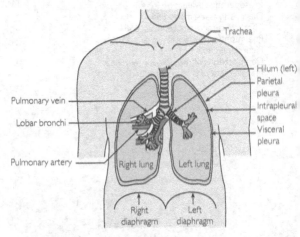

Figure 25.1 Thoracic cavity. Reproduced from Peter Wagner, Airways and
alveoli, in DA Warrell, TM Cox, and JD Firth, *Oxford Textbook of Medicine*, 5th
edition, 2010, with permission from Oxford University Press.

Indications for thoracic surgery

- Cancer.
- Interstitial lung disease.
- Emphysema.
- Tuberculosis (TB).
- Infection.
- Spontaneous pneumothorax.
- Fibrosing alveolitis.
- Sarcoidosis.
- Trauma.

Pre-operative evaluation

Lung cancer is common in the UK, with around 39 000 new cases pe[r] year and over 35 000 deaths.[1] It is therefore a priority that early diagnos[is] and staging are performed, to determine the most appropriate manage[-] ment interventions. Patients will undergo a comprehensive assessmen[t] in terms of fitness for surgery and operability, which will consider th[e] following factors.

Age

Peri-operative morbidity increases with age, and elderly patients unde[r-] going lung resections are more likely to require intensive peri-operati[ve] support. Nurses should be aware that lung resection is associated wi[th] a higher mortality risk.

Cardiovascular morbidity

Patients with existing cardiac disease are at increased risk of myocardi[al] infarction (MI) or death within 30 days of non-cardiac surgery. Thes[e] patients should have:
- a pre-operative ECG
- an echocardiogram if an audible murmur is heard
- a cardiac referral prior to thoracic surgery if they have had an MI within the previous 6 months
- optimization of cardiac treatment and commencement of secondary prophylaxis for coronary disease.

Exercise testing

Numerous studies have demonstrated an inverse relationship betwee[n] exercise capacity and post-operative complications. Exercise testi[ng] is recommended in order to determine the patient's surgical risk. T[he] British Thoracic Society has suggested that desaturation during testing more than 4% SaO_2 indicates that the patient is a high risk for surger[y.] For patients with a moderate to high risk of post-operative dyspnoe[a] the following tests should be considered:
- a shuttle walk test (400 m cut-off for good lung function)
- cardiopulmonary exercise testing.

Pulmonary function

Poor respiratory function is a concern because of the risks of pe[ri-] operative morbidity and mortality. Lung function tests will inclu[de] spirometry and peak expiratory flow rate. Forced expired volume in t[he] first second (FEV1) is regarded as the best predictor of complications [for] lung resection.[2] If the post-bronchodilator FEV1 is > 1.5 L for a lobe[ct-] omy and > 2.0 L for a pneumonectomy, with no evidence of inters[ti-] tial lung disease or shortness of breath, no further respiratory functi[on] tests are required. In addition, the patient may undergo a physiothera[py] assessment and a segment count to predict post-operative lung functi[on.]

Patients who are not clearly operable should have:
- extensive pulmonary function tests, which should include an estimation of the transfer factor for carbon monoxide (T_{LCO})
- oxygen saturations in air and at rest
- a quantitative isotope perfusion scan if a pneumonectomy is being considered.

Weight loss and nutrition

A history of weight loss, poor nutritional status, and poor performance status has been associated with poor outcomes in patients with lung cancer. A pre-operative assessment may consider:
- body mass index
- serum albumin measurements.

Further pre-operative assessments may include:
- chest X-ray
- bloods for clotting, cross-matching, and haemoglobin (Hb) levels
- sputum examination
- arterial blood gas analysis
- educational advice regarding smoking cessation, and the offer of nicotine replacement therapy
- psychological status.

References

National Institute for Health and Care Excellence (NICE). *Lung Cancer: the diagnosis and treatment of lung cancer*. CG121. NICE: London, 2011. ℗ www.nice.org.uk/guidance/cg121
British Thoracic Society and the Society for Cardiothoracic Surgery in Great Britain and Ireland. Guidelines on the radical management of patients with lung cancer. *Thorax* 2010; 65 (Suppl. 3): iii1–27.

Diagnostic assessment

Bronchoscopy

This is used to diagnose and stage many patients with lung cancer. A bron choscope is advanced into the trachea to visualize the upper airways an the airways distal to the main bronchial tree, where it can be used t assess central tumours and tumours in relation to the main bronchus.

Complications

- Pneumothorax.
- Bleeding.
- Cardiac arrhythmias.
- Hypoxia.

Video-assisted thoracoscopic surgery (VATS)

This is a minimally invasive approach to the pleural space via 1–4 por or incisions. It is used for:

- taking biopsies from the lung and the lung lining
- removal of lymph nodes
- treatment of pleural effusions.

Transthoracic needle biopsy

This involves taking diagnostic samples from lesions that are not acce sible through the bronchial tree, and where there is no lymph involve ment. A biopsy needle is inserted into the lungs to obtain aspirate f cytology or tissue samples for histology.

Mediastinoscopy

This is the gold standard for staging the mediastinum prior to thoraco omy and nodal dissection, and it establishes the histology of enlarge mediastinal lymph nodes. An incision is made midway between the bo tom of the sternal notch and the cricoid cartilage, which allows examin tion of the mediastinum and enables all of the lymph nodes around th central airway to be identified and biopsied.

Complications

- Hoarseness due to damage to the laryngeal nerve.
- Pneumothorax.
- Haemorrhage.

Computed tomography (CT) scan

This is recommended as a staging procedure for patients with non-sma cell lung cancer. It is undertaken:

- to identify enlarged mediastinal lymph nodes which will determine the best approach for biopsy or aspiration cytology
- to determine the T stage to ensure that resection is a realistic optio
- to identify metastases in the chest, liver, and adrenal glands
- to provide information on coexisting disease (emphysema, pulmona emboli, and cardiac and vascular disease).

Multidetector computed tomography (MDCT) with the administration of contrast medium

This provides rapid coverage of the chest and upper abdomen. CT coverage should also include the lower neck, for the detection of supraclavicular nodal metastases.

Positron emission tomography with computed tomography (PET-CT)

This is the most accurate imaging investigation for confirming or excluding intrathoracic lymph node metastases from lung cancer. It is best used alongside CT scanning for accurate localization and interpretation.

Magnetic resonance imaging (MRI)

This is a non-invasive procedure in which hydrogen atoms in the patient's body are aligned by a magnetic field. Radio waves passed through the body are absorbed by the hydrogen, and their subsequent movement causes a detectable change in the magnetic field. MRI provides high-resolution cross-sectional images of lung structures, and will trace blood flow. Different tissue types have different concentrations of hydrogen, which is how an image can be constructed. MRI clarifies the degree of invasion of the mediastinum, the root of the neck, the chest wall, and the diaphragm.

Ventilation perfusion scan

This is performed in order to evaluate ventilation/perfusion (V/Q) mismatch, detect pulmonary emboli, and evaluate pulmonary function.

Nuclear medicine scanning

This involves the use of a gamma camera to detect energy from a radioactive substance that has been injected, usually via the arm, into the patient. The scan can be used to visualize structures and diagnose many conditions, including cancers, injuries, and infections.

Thoracic surgery procedures

Thoracotomy

This is a surgical incision into the thoracic cavity in order to locate an examine abnormalities such as tumours, bleeding sites, and thoracic injuries, perform a biopsy, or remove diseased lung tissue. In an exploratory thoracotomy (open and closed) the thorax is opened and the lung tissu is examined. If a tumour has spread too far to be operable, a biopsy w be taken and the thorax closed. The national average for this procedur is approximately 5%, with reasons for inoperability including invasio of the heart or pericardium, trachea, or chest wall, or paralysis of th phrenic nerve.

Procedure

A common approach is to use a posteriolateral incision through th fourth, fifth, sixth, or seventh intercostal space, with the chest muscle being incised in layers. The incision is approximately 20–22 cm long. commences in the submammary fold of the anterior chest and is draw below the scapula tip and along the ribs, and then curved posterior towards the spine of the scapula. This incision allows optimal access t all parts of the hemithorax. Following incision the surgeon may take biopsy, locate and tie off bleeding, locate and repair injuries within th thoracic cavity, or spread the ribs and expose the lung area for excisio

Wedge resection

This is the removal of a small portion of the lung without regard to se ments. A thoracotomy or video-assisted thoracic surgery (VATS) performed, and a wedge-shaped section of the lung is removed. The inc sion is closed and a chest drain is inserted to allow drainage of fluid th may build up. Indications for this procedure include benign or maligna lesions, which are localized and discrete.

Lobectomy

This is the removal of one or two of the five lung lobes when the patho ogy is limited to one area of the lung. A thoracotomy incision is mac and the location is dependent on the lobe to be resected. On enteri the pleural space, the lung involved is collapsed, and lobar vessels a bronchus are ligated and divided. Following lobectomy, two tubes a left in the chest, one at the apex to evacuate air and allow the remaini lobe to expand and fill the space, and the other at the base of the thor to evacuate any blood drainage. Indications for this procedure inclu bronchogenic carcinoma, TB, lung abscess, emphysematous blebs or b lae, and benign tumours, localized fungal infections, and bronchiectasi

Segmentectomy

Bronchopulmonary segments are subdivisions of the lung that function as individual units and are held together by delicate connective tissue. Disease processes may be limited to a single segment, and therefore it is essential to preserve functional lung tissue. This procedure involves blunt dissection and resection of the bronchopulmonary segment, and chest drains are inserted post procedure, to assist with lung re-inflation and drainage of fluid. Patients with limited pulmonary reserve are usually considered for this procedure.

Pleurectomy

This involves stripping off the parietal pleura, away from the apex and posterolateral surface of the lung, by a thoracotomy incision or using VATS. This induces an inflammatory response that causes adhesion of the visceral pleura to the chest wall.

Video-assisted thoracoscopic assessment

This is used as a diagnostic and staging modality where:
- biopsies can be taken from the tumour mass
- tumour invasion in central mediastinal structures can be directly assessed
- it can be assessed whether complete resection of tumour is possible prior to a thoracotomy.

Pleurodesis

This procedure involves the stimulation of an inflammatory response to enable the formation of pleural adhesions either by the instillation of iodized talc or by mechanical abrasion of the pleural surfaces. The procedure can be undertaken via either a thoracotomy or a VATS procedure, and is usually performed to prevent recurring pleural effusions.

Pneumonectomy

This procedure has a mortality rate of 6–8%, and is performed whe
tumours affect the hilum of the lung. The surgeon will ligate and seve
the pulmonary arteries, clamp the main stem bronchus leading to th
affected lung, divide it, remove the lung, and staple the bronchial stump
A pneumonectomy is performed when a less radical approach canno
remove all of the diseased tissue.

Indications
- Bronchogenic carcinoma.
- Infection (e.g. TB).
- Bronchiectasis.
- Lung abscess.

The pneumonectomy space
Following resection, changes occur in the pneumonectomy space, whic
is reduced by the elevation of the diaphragm. Post-operatively the spac
first fills with air and then bleeding occurs, which produces a visible flui
level on chest X-ray. This fluid level may be regulated by clamping of th
chest drain for the first 24 h. The volume of gas within the space fu
ther decreases as carbon dioxide and oxygen are reabsorbed, and th
fluid then changes to a solid substance. The final stages consist of reab
sorption of nitrogen and the development of negative pressure, whic
promotes the formation of low-protein fluid to fill the remainder of th
space, and results in a slight shift in the centrality of the mediastinum.

Specific nursing care of the pneumonectomy patient
- Nurse the patient upright or on the affected side to prevent bleeding
  into the remaining lung.
- If a chest drain has been inserted, keep it clamped and release it for
  30–60 s every hour (or as indicated by the consultant or ward policy)
  to allow fluid to accumulate slowly in the pneumonectomy space.
- Never attach the drain to suction.
- Removal of a chest drain usually takes place after 24 h (or in
  accordance with the surgeon's instructions or ward policy).
- Antibiotic prophylaxis.
- Antithrombolytic stockings.
- Encourage gentle, early mobilization from day 1 post-operatively.
- Posture at least four times a day on the same side as the operation.
- Routine chest X-ray to assess the level of air–fluid rise in the
  post-pneumonectomy space.

Complications
- Mediastinal shift.
- Atrial fibrillation as the fluid level within the lung cavity rises and
  presses on the atrium (approximately day 3–5).
- Bronchial stump breakdown (bronchopleural fistula) may occur
  if infection is present (day 5–7 onwards). This is where there is a
  communication between the airways and the pleura following surgery.
- Dyspnoea.

Pleural infection

This is a frequent clinical problem, with an incidence of up to 80 000 reported cases in the UK and the USA combined.[3] The associated mortality and morbidity are high. In the UK, 20% of patients with empyema die and 20% require surgery. Studies have shown that prompt recognition and intervention reduces mortality and morbidity. Causes of pleural infection include bacterial pneumonia, lung abscess, prolonged use of chest drains, penetrating chest trauma, non-bacterial infections, and iatrogenic causes (after thoracic or oesophageal surgery).

Empyema

Most pleural infections change from a simple self-resolving parapneumonic pleural effusion into a complicated multiloculated fibrinopurulent collection associated with the features of sepsis. Empyema is an accumulation of thick purulent fluid within the pleural space, often with fibrin development and a walled off area where infection is located. There are three stages of empyema.

Simple exudative stage (simple parapneumonic effusion)

During this first stage there is extensive free-flowing fluid movement into the pleural space due to capillary vascular permeability and the production of pro-inflammatory cytokines. This exudate has a low white cell count, a lactate dehydrogenase level less than 50% of that in serum, normal pH and glucose levels, and no bacterial organisms.

Fibrinopurulent stage (complicated parapneumonic effusion)

During the second stage the effusion becomes loculated, and is soft, friable, and completely fibrinous. This is due to increasing fluid and bacterial invasion of the damaged endothelium, which fuels the immune response, promotes the recruitment of neutrophils to the site of injury, and activates the clotting cascade, resulting in an increased procoagulant state but a depression in fibrinolytic activity. This results in an increase in lactic acid and carbon dioxide production, a fall in pleural pH, an increase in glucose metabolism, and an increase in lactate dehydrogenase levels due to leucocyte death.

Organizing stage, with scar tissue (pleural peel) formation

During this third stage, fibroblasts proliferate and a solid fibrous peel encloses the lung, which prevents re-expansion, impairs lung function, and creates a persistent pleural space.

Management

The pleural effusion is identified by either a lateral X-ray or pleural ultrasonography. The latter is the preferred investigation, as it confirms the location of any fluid collection and enables guided diagnostic aspiration to be performed if necessary. Patients with a pleural effusion over 10 mm in depth that is associated with sepsis, pneumonia, recent chest trauma, or surgery should have diagnostic fluid sampling.

Indications for pleural fluid drainage
- Frank purulent cloudy fluid on sampling.
- The presence of organisms identified by Gram stain and/or culture.
- Pleural fluid pH < 7.2.
- Poor clinical progress during treatment with antibiotics.

Chest tube drainage
Chest tube insertion should be performed under imaging guidance wher ever possible, as infected effusions will be loculated. Insertion should be performed according to the British Thoracic Society's pleural disease guidelines.[3] A small-bore 10–14F tube is recommended for most case of pleural infection, but this requires regular flushing to avoid catheter blockage.

Antibiotics
Patients should receive antibiotics based on the results of pleural flui blood cultures and sensitivities, but in the absence of results, empirical antibiotics must cover the likely pathogenic organisms.

Surgical intervention
Patients should be considered for surgery if they have persistent seps and pleural collection despite chest tube drainage and antibiotic treat ment. Failure of sepsis to resolve within 5–7 days is suggested to indicat the need for immediate review by a thoracic surgeon. The procedure that are performed are dependent on factors such as age, comorbidit and the surgeon's preferences, and may include any of the following:
- a VATS procedure to remove all infected fibrinous material from within the chest
- open thoracic drainage, which requires a rib resection to enable the insertion of a large-bore chest drain. This drain is cut short and inserted into a drainage bag, but does not require an underwater seal, as the empyema cavity is sealed by the fibrous coating with no connection to the pleural space
- decortication involves removal of the thick fibrous crust from the lun surface and chest wall via a thoracotomy.

Reference
3 Davies H, Davies R and Davies C. Management of pleural infection in adults: British Thora Society pleural disease guideline 2010. *Thorax* 2010; 65 (Suppl. 2): ii41–53.

Complications of thoracic surgery

- Atelectasis.
- Respiratory insufficiency.
- Sputum retention.
- Acute respiratory distress.
- Chest infection.
- Cardiac arrhythmias related to the effects of hypoxia or the surgical procedure.
- Pulmonary oedema caused by over-infusion of fluids.
- Pneumothorax.
- Haemorrhage.
- Post-operative pain due to surgical incision and chest drain.
- Nausea and vomiting.
- Post-operative chest infection.
- Wound infection.
- Frozen shoulder on the incision side, due to reduced movement in the post-operative period.
- Increased risk of deep vein thrombosis or pulmonary emboli.
- Surgical emphysema.
- Bronchopleural fistula.

Nursing interventions

The following nursing interventions need to be considered.

Maintaining gas exchange and breathing

- Measure the respiratory rate every 15 min until the patient's condition stabilizes.
- Check the rate, depth, and rhythm of respiration.
- Continuously monitor oxygen saturations and undertake arterial blood gas measurements in order to assess the adequacy of ventilation and oxygenation.
- Administer prescribed humidified oxygen and/or nebulizers.
- Encourage breathing exercises (diaphragmatic and purse-lip breathing) to expand the alveoli and prevent atelectasis and post-operative pneumonia.
- Elevate the head of the bed to 30–40° to facilitate ventilation and chest drainage, if the patient's condition is stable.
- Assess and monitor chest drainage.
- Observe for symptoms of pulmonary oedema, including dyspnoea, crackles, bubbling sounds in the chest, tachycardia, and pink frothy sputum.
- Auscultate the lungs in order to evaluate the rate, quality, and depth of the patient's respiration.
- Assess the patency of drainage from the chest drain.

Maintaining an airway
- Ensure that the patient has a patent airway.
- Encourage an effective cough and ensure that the patient has adequate analgesia.
- Encourage the patient with regard to their breathing programme and posture at least four times a day.
- Minimize incisional pain during coughing by supporting the incision, o encouraging the patient to do so.
- Monitor the amount and viscosity of sputum.
- Liaise with the physiotherapist.

Maintaining cardiovascular stability
- Administer fluids cautiously in order to prevent pulmonary oedema.
- Assess the patient for signs of bleeding and shock by monitoring temperature, pulse, and blood pressure every 30 min, and reduce th frequency when the patient stabilizes.
- Monitor central venous pressure (follow local policy).

Optimizing the patient's pain relief and comfort
- Regularly review the patient's pain, using a pain assessment tool.
- Liaise with the pain control team and use an analgesic ladder for pain control recommendations.
- Commence arm and shoulder exercises to restore movement and prevent painful stiffening of the affected arm and shoulder.
- Adhere to local policy on the use of patient-controlled analgesia, epidurals, and nerve blocks.

A thoracotomy without lung resection reduces forced vital capacity b 25% due to diaphragmatic dysfunction. It is therefore important to mob lize the patient in order to promote lung expansion and improve ventil tion/perfusion matching.

Prevention of complications of immobilization
- Observe pressure areas for signs of deterioration.
- Complete the Waterlow score daily, and action as necessary.
- Ensure that thromboembolism-deterrent stockings are worn.
- Ensure that deep vein thrombosis prophylaxis is commenced.

Prevention of wound infection
- Observe theatre dressings and observe for bleeding of the incisional site.
- Leave surgical dressings intact (or follow ward protocol).
- Observe the wound site for exudate and infection.

Management of chest drains

The National Patient Safety Agency (NPSA) has issued recommendations for safer practice in relation to chest drain insertion.[4] Chest drains are inserted into the pleural space to drain air, fluid, or pus from the pleural cavity and thus enable re-expansion of the underlying lung.

Insertion sites

Chest drains are inserted aseptically and through the triangle of safety. Using the safe triangle minimizes the risk to the internal mammary artery and avoids damage to muscle and breast tissue. Chest drain insertion is a painful procedure, and the patient should receive analgesia prior to insertion.

Two sutures (stay and closing sutures) are used to assist closure of the wound after the drain has been removed, and to secure the drain.

Drainage systems

Chest drains are attached to a one-way underwater seal drainage device, which allows one-directional flow out of the pleural space. The tube is placed under water to a depth of 3 cm, with a side vent to allow the escape of air. The water in the system prevents air from entering the pleural space when the patient breathes in and restores negative pressure to the pleural space.

Management of a chest drain

Visual observations

- If the patient has a pneumothorax, air bubbles will be visible in the closed drainage system as air is drained from the pleural space and the lung re-expands.
- Bubbling occurs intermittently as the patient breathes out or coughs, but this will decrease once the pneumothorax has resolved.
- Respiratory swing will be observed as fluid in the chest drain tubing oscillates as the patient breathes, which confirms the correct position in the pleural space and tube patency.
- Monitor and document the chest drain for swinging and bubbling.
- Ensure that the air and suction port is not occluded while the bottle is attached to the patient, as this seals the bottle and could result in a tension pneumothorax.

The chest drain will stop swinging and bubbling as the lung re-expands. However, a sudden stoppage may indicate that the chest tube has become blocked or displaced, and results in respiratory distress.

Suction

If suction is required, a high-volume, low-pressure system should be used (10–20 cmH$_2$O).

Drainage
- The drainage system should be below the level of the patient's chest. If it is above this level, siphoning into the pleural space will occur.
- If the drainage fluid becomes cloudy and the patient becomes pyrexial, a sample should be sent for culture.
- The drainage bottle should be changed as per trust policy.
- The drainage bottle should not be overfilled, as excessive submersion of the water seal level increases the hydrostatic level that the intrapleural air must exceed before it can escape from the chest, making it difficult for air to escape from the pleural space.

Clamping
- Never clamp a bubbling chest tube,[5] as this may result in a tension pneumothorax. Situations in which chest drain tubes are clamped include accidental disconnection, damage to the drainage system, or when bottles or tubing are changed.
- If a chest tube for pneumothorax is clamped, this must be under supervision, and the patient should be managed in a specialist ward.
- Non-traumatic clamps must be used to prevent air entry while new tubing and/or an underwater seal drain are being attached, and clamps should always be kept at the patient's bedside.

Chest drain removal
The chest drain should be removed either while the patient performs Valsalva manoeuvre or during expiration, with a brisk firm movement. Two people are needed to perform this procedure. As one person removes the drain the other person ties the placed closure suture.

References
4 National Patient Safety Agency (NPSA). *Risks of Chest Drain Insertion*. Rapid Response Report NPSA/2008/RRR003. NPSA: London, 2008.
5 Davies H, Davies R and Davies C. Management of pleural infection in adults: British Thoracic Society pleural disease guideline 2010. *Thorax* 2010; 65 (Suppl. 2): ii41–53.

Further reading
Laws D, Neville E and Duffy J. BTS guidelines for the insertion of a chest drain. *Thorax* 2003; (Suppl. 2): ii53–9.
National Institute for Health and Care Excellence (NICE). *Lung Cancer: the diagnosis and treatment of lung cancer*. CG121. NICE: London, 2011. ♒ www.nice.org.uk/guidance/cg121

Useful website
National Patient Safety Agency (NPSA). ♒ www.npsa.nhs.uk

Cardiac surgery

Cardiac anatomy

The heart is the size of a human fist, and sits between the lungs in the inferior mediastinum. It is enclosed within a double-walled sac called the pericardium. The outer fibrous pericardium protects the heart and anchors it to surrounding structures such as the sternum and diaphragm. The inner serous pericardium produces a serous fluid, enabling the heart to beat in a relatively frictionless environment.

Starting with the outermost layer, the heart wall consists of the following:

- epicardium
- myocardium
- endocardium.

Internal structure of the heart

There are four chambers within the heart—two thin-walled atria at the top which receive blood, and two thick-walled ventricles at the bottom which are the actual pumps of the heart.

The right atrium receives deoxygenated blood from the venous system via the superior and inferior vena cavae, which then passes through the tricuspid valve into the right ventricle. The right ventricle pumps the deoxygenated blood through the pulmonary valve into the pulmonary artery. In the lungs, gas exchange takes place, with the unloading of carbon dioxide and loading of oxygen into the pulmonary bloodstream. Four pulmonary veins carry the oxygenated blood to the left atrium, and then it passes through the mitral valve into the left ventricle, which has significantly thicker walls than the right ventricle. The left ventricle pumps blood through the aortic valve into the aorta. The aorta supplies the body with blood rich in oxygen and nutrients.

Heart valves

The atrioventricular valves (mitral and tricuspid valves), which are located between the atria and the ventricles, prevent blood from flowing back from the ventricles into the atria. The valves are attached to the ventricles by chordae tendineae, and are pushed upwards into the closed position when the ventricles are closed. When the heart is relaxed and blood is passively filling its chambers, the atrioventricular valves hang limply in the ventricles.

The semilunar valves (pulmonary and aortic valves) have three leaflets which fit together when the valve is closed. The ventricles contract, forcing blood out of the heart, opening these leaflets and flattening them against the walls of the arteries. When the ventricles relax, blood flows backwards towards the heart, causing the leaflets to fill with blood and close the valves.

Cardiac circulation

The left and right coronary arteries branch off from the ascending aorta and supply the heart muscle with oxygen and nutrients (see Figure 26.1). The coronary arteries are compressed when the ventricles contract, and fill when the heart is relaxed. The cardiac veins drain the myocardium and empty into the coronary sinus, which empties into the right atrium.

- The left coronary artery branches into the anterior interventricular artery and the circumflex artery.
- The right coronary artery branches into the posterior interventricular artery and the marginal artery.

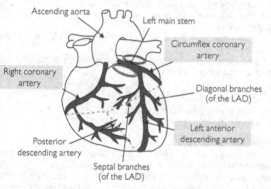

Figure 26.1 Coronary artery anatomy. LAD, left anterior descending artery. Reproduced from SG Myerson, RP Choudhury and ARJ Mitchell, *Emergencies in Cardiology*, 2nd edition, 2009, with permission from Oxford University Press.

Acute coronary syndrome

Acute coronary syndrome (ACS) is a spectrum of conditions caused by the same disease process. Atherosclerotic plaques build up over time in the lumen of the coronary arteries, and their development is influenced by the following risk factors:

- smoking
- hypertension
- hyperlipidaemia
- diabetes
- familial factors.

ACS occurs when an atherosclerotic plaque fissures, causing:

- a haemorrhage within the plaque, which restricts the lumen of the artery due to swelling
- the smooth muscle in the vessel wall to contract and also restrict the lumen of the artery
- a thrombus to form on the plaque, which completely or partially obstructs the lumen of the artery.

ACS consists of:

- unstable angina
- non-ST-segment-elevation myocardial infarction (NSTEMI)
- ST-segment-elevation myocardial infarction (STEMI).

Unstable angina

Angina pectoris is the term used to describe the pain caused by myocardial ischaemia. This occurs due to reduced blood supply to the heart muscle, caused by either obstruction or spasm of the coronary arteries. It is usually felt across the centre of the chest as tightness or indigestion like aching, and can radiate to the throat, arms, and back. Unstable angina is defined as being:

- angina on exertion which is provoked by progressively less exertion
- episodes of angina increasing in frequency, which are not predictable and not related to exercise
- an unprovoked and prolonged episode of chest pain, without ECG or laboratory evidence of myocardial infarction.

Non-ST-segment-elevation myocardial infarction (NSTEMI)

Myocardial infarction is commonly referred to as a heart attack, and occurs when there is an interruption to the blood supply to the heart muscle, resulting in the death of cardiac myocytes (muscle cells).

The patient with NSTEMI presents with acute chest pain suggestive of myocardial infarction, but on the 12-lead ECG there are non-specific abnormalities (e.g. ST-segment depression, T-wave inversion). Troponin levels are raised, indicating that myocardial damage has occurred. Complete occlusion of the coronary artery is less likely to occur in NSTEMI. However, there is a risk of progression to complete occlusion

ST-segment-elevation myocardial infarction (STEMI)

The patient with STEMI has acute chest pain, and on a 12-lead ECG they have acute ST-segment elevation, due to acute complete occlusion of a coronary artery.

Early management of acute coronary syndrome

Guidance from the National Institute for Health and Care Excellence (NICE)[1] recommends the following early management of acute coronary syndrome:

- loading dose of aspirin 300 mg orally, to be continued at a dose of 75mg
- loading dose of clopidogrel 300 mg, to be continued at a dose of 75mg
- low-molecular-weight heparin if angiography is likely to occur within 24 h
- a full clinical history, including cardiac history
- 12-lead ECG
- blood tests, including troponin, renal function, full blood count, and glucose levels
- coronary angioplasty should be offered within 96 h of admission, if the patient is classed as being at intermediate or higher risk of an adverse cardiovascular event.

Reference

National Institute for Health and Care Excellence (NICE). *Unstable Angina and NSTEMI: the early management of unstable angina and non-ST-segment-elevation myocardial infarction.* CG94. NICE: London, 2010. ℘ www.nice.org.uk/guidance/cg94

Further reading

Marshall K. Acute coronary syndrome: diagnosis, risk assessment and management. *Nursing Standard* 2011; 25: 47–57.

Overview of cardiac medication

Angiotensin-converting-enzyme (ACE) inhibitors

ACE inhibitors work by inhibiting the conversion of angiotensin to angiotensin 2 by the angiotensin-converting enzyme in the lung. Angiotensin 2 is a very potent vasoconstrictor.

Indications
- Hypertension.
- Heart failure.
- Post myocardial infarction.

Examples
- Ramipril.
- Lisinopril.
- Perindopril.

Aldosterone antagonists

Aldosterone antagonists are diuretic drugs that block the actions of aldosterone. Aldosterone is a hormone produced by the adrenal cortex which acts on the distal tubules and collecting ducts of the nephron. Sodium is reabsorbed and potassium is excreted, resulting in reduced urine production, as sodium has a strong osmotic pull.

Indications
- Resistant hypertension.
- Moderate to severe heart failure.
- Oedema and ascites in liver cirrhosis.

Examples
- Spironolactone.
- Eplerenone.

Beta blockers

Beta blockers block the beta-adrenoreceptors in the heart, peripheral circulation, bronchi, pancreas, and liver. They slow the heart rate and depress the myocardium by reducing the effects of adrenaline and noradrenaline.

Indications
- Angina.
- Cardiac arrhythmias.
- Heart failure.
- Cardiac protection following myocardial infarction.

Examples
- Sotalol.
- Propranolol.
- Esmolol hydrochloride.

Calcium-channel blockers

Calcium-channel blockers work by reducing the movement of calcium ions into cardiac muscle cells, blood vessels, and smooth muscle. This delays cardiac conduction, slows the heart rate, and relaxes the arterioles.

Indications
- Angina.
- Hypertension.
- Arrhythmias.

Examples
- Verapamil.
- Amlodipine.

Nitrates

Nitrates dilate the coronary arteries and reduce the preload by dilating the veins, which increases the oxygen supply to the myocardium and reduces the myocardial workload.

Indications
- Angina.
- Myocardial infarction.
- Severe hypertension.

Examples
- Glyceryl trinitrate (GTN).
- Isosorbide mononitrate.

Heart failure

Heart failure has been defined by NICE as 'a complex clinical syndrome that suggests impairment of the heart as a pump supporting physiological circulation. It is caused by structural or functional abnormalities of the heart.'[2]

Acute heart failure develops rapidly over a period of minutes to hours, whereas chronic heart failure develops more slowly. Patients with chronic heart failure can have episodes of acute or subacute decompensation.

Causes
- Ischaemic heart disease.
- Acute coronary syndrome.
- Hypertension.
- Valve disease.
- Arrhythmias.
- Cardiomyopathies.
- Alcohol.
- Infections of the heart wall (e.g. endocarditis).
- Thyroid dysfunction.

Signs and symptoms
- Shortness of breath due to pulmonary congestion.
- Dry cough due to bronchial hyperactivity.
- Fatigue.
- Oedema of the ankles and legs due to fluid retention.
- Tachycardia and haemodynamic instability.
- Nausea and loss of appetite.

Treatment
The Scottish Intercollegiate Guidelines Network (SIGN) recommends that treatment is based on the following:[3]
- behavioural modifications
- pharmacological therapies
- interventional procedures.

Behavioural modifications
- Reduction of alcohol consumption.
- Smoking cessation.
- Regular low-intensity physical activity.
- Salt and fluid restriction.

Pharmacological therapies
- ACE inhibitors to reduce preload.
- Beta blockers to slow heart rate.
- Aldosterone antagonists (e.g. spironolactone).
- Diuretics to treat fluid retention.
- Digoxin to treat arrhythmias.
- Anticoagulants if there is a history of thromboembolism.
- Inotropes for acute decompensation.

Interventional procedures
- Implantable cardiac defibrillator.
- Coronary artery bypass grafting.
- Intra-aortic balloon pump counterpulsation.
- Corrective surgery for valve disease.
- Cardiac transplantation.

References

National Institute for Health and Care Excellence (NICE). *Chronic Heart Failure: management of chronic heart failure in adults in primary and secondary care.* CG108. NICE: London, 2010. ℗ www.nice.org.uk/guidance/cg108

Scottish Intercollegiate Guidelines Network (SIGN). *Management of Chronic Heart Failure.* SIGN Guideline No. 95. SIGN: Edinburgh, 2007. ℗ http://sign.ac.uk/guidelines/fulltext/95/contents.html

Further reading

Whitlock A and MacInnes J. Acute heart failure: patient assessment and management. *British Journal of Cardiac Nursing* 2010; **5**: 516–25.

Cardiomyopathies

Cardiomyopathy is a chronic heart muscle disease that is not caused by ischaemia, hypertension, valvular disease, or a congenital condition. It can be acquired or inherited. There are four main types of cardiomyopathy:
- dilated
- hypertrophic
- arrhythmogenic right ventricular
- restrictive.

Dilated cardiomyopathy

This is the most common type, and it is characterized by dilation and impaired contraction of either the left or both ventricles. It is a biochemical abnormality of the cardiac muscle.

Hypertrophic cardiomyopathy

This is a congenital disease of the myocardium that leads to thickening of the myocardium. It is frequently asymptomatic and results in sudden cardiac death.

Arrhythmogenic right ventricular cardiomyopathy

This is characterized by the progressive replacement of normal right ventricular muscle cells with fibrous tissue and fat. The patient is at high risk of ventricular tachyarrhythmias and sudden death.

Restrictive cardiomyopathy

This causes restricted filling and reduced diastolic volume in both or only one of the ventricles. The heart's rhythm and pumping ability remain normal, but the restricted filling reduces blood flow, which leads to heart failure.

Causes
- Viral infections.
- Chronic alcohol abuse.
- Chemotherapy.
- Pregnancy.
- Familial.
- Neuromuscular (i.e. muscular dystrophy).
- Idiopathic.

Signs and symptoms
- Shortness of breath.
- Chest pain.
- Tachycardia and arrhythmias.
- Reduced exercise tolerance.
- Thromboembolism.
- Fatigue.

Pharmacological therapies

- ACE inhibitors to reduce preload.
- Beta blockers to slow heart rate and treat angina.
- For patients of Afro-Caribbean origin or those who cannot tolerate ACE inhibitors or angiotensin-receptor blockers, treat with a combination of hydralazine and isosorbide dinitrate.
- Calcium-channel blockers for comorbid hypertension and/or angina.
- Diuretics to alleviate oedema and dyspnoea.
- Amiodarone to suppress arrhythmias.
- Anticoagulants for patients with atrial fibrillation or a history of thromboembolism.

Interventional procedures

- Implantable cardioverter defibrillators.
- Biventricular pacemaker.
- Left ventricular assist devices.
- Cardiac transplantation.

Further reading

Griffin B (ed.). *Manual of Cardiovascular Medicine*, 4th edn. Lippincott, Williams & Wilkins: Philadelphia, PA, 2012.

Walker R. An introduction to dilated cardiomyopathy. *British Journal of Cardiac Nursing* 2008; 3: 506–10.

Percutaneous coronary intervention (PCI) and stenting

Percutaneous coronary intervention (PCI), which in clinical practice is often called coronary angioplasty, is a surgical intervention that is used in the treatment of ischaemic heart disease (IHD). It involves passing catheter through the arterial tree in a retrograde fashion, until it reaches the root of the aorta, where the coronary arteries originate.

In IHD it is often the case that the coronary arteries (the blood vessels that supply the heart muscle with oxygenated blood) are narrowed and eventually become blocked as a result of atherosclerosis. This narrowing impairs the flow of blood to the myocardium, and therefore reduces the supply of oxygen.

As the degree of coronary artery stenosis increases, delivery of oxygen to the myocardium decreases, and the mismatch between myocardial supply and myocardial demand increases, resulting in the clinical features of angina pectoris (chest pain, nausea, dizziness, and breathlessness). If a coronary artery narrows to such an extent that it becomes completely occluded, a myocardial infarction may ensue, requiring more immediate emergency treatment.

Benefits of PCI

- Reduction in the symptoms of angina (often alongside pharmacological agents).
- Reduction in the damage caused by a myocardial infarction and reduced mortality rates compared with best medical therapy.

This is achieved by inflating a balloon within the narrowed coronary artery to reduce the stenosis. This may be augmented by the use of a stent.

Stents

A stent is a wire mesh tube that is widened within the lumen of the artery in order to keep it patent (see Figure 26.2).

Stents come in two forms:
- metal (uncoated) stents
- drug-eluting stents, which are coated with medication to help to reduce the rate of re-narrowing.

How PCI is performed

1. Access to the arterial tree is obtained by cannulating an artery (commonly the femoral artery, although the brachial artery is an appropriate alternative).
2. The hole in the artery is dilated in order to allow passage of the catheter.
3. The catheter is inserted and guided to the root of the aorta. This is done under X-ray guidance.
4. The coronary arteries are visualized by injecting contrast into each coronary artery in turn. This procedure is known as coronary angiography, and is the definitive diagnostic test for coronary artery disease.

5. Once the narrowing has been located, the affected coronary artery is entered by another catheter which has a balloon at its tip. This balloon may or may not be surrounded by a stent.
6. This catheter is passed through the affected coronary artery to the point of narrowing.
7. The balloon is inflated several times in order to widen the artery, and if a stent is used this is left in the vessel.

Complications of PCI
- Myocardial infarction.
- Anaphylaxis.
- Arrhythmias.
- Contrast-induced nephropathy.
- Stroke.
- Bleeding.
- Death.
- Conversion to an emergency coronary artery bypass graft (CABG).

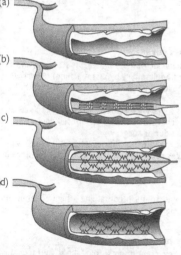

Figure 26.2 Angioplasty and coronary stenting. A guide wire is introduced across the static segment of artery (a) and is used to position the stent (b). The stent is deployed by inflating the balloon (c). The balloon and guide wire are removed, leaving the stent in place (d). Reproduced from P Ramrakha and J Hill, Oxford Handbook of Cardiology, 2nd edition, 2012, with permission from Oxford University Press.

Coronary artery bypass surgery

Coronary artery bypass surgery is performed in order to bypass blocked coronary artery to restore normal blood flow to the myocardium. Arteries or veins from elsewhere in the patient's body are grafted to the coronary arteries to bypass the vessel narrowing and improve the blood supply.

Choice of graft

The surgeon decides which graft(s) to use, based on the location and size of the coronary artery blockage. Grafts are usually taken from three primary sites:
- saphenous veins (from the leg)
- internal thoracic artery (ITA), also known as the internal mammary artery (IMA)
- radial artery (the arm).

Number of bypass grafts

- Single bypass (one).
- Double bypass (two).
- Triple bypass (three).
- Quadruple bypass (four).
- Quintuple bypass (five).

Types of cardiac bypass surgery

- In *open heart surgery (traditional bypass)* the heart is stopped, and a heart–lung machine (cardiopulmonary bypass machine) takes over the work of the heart and lungs while the surgeon performs the bypass procedure.
- *Off-pump coronary bypass surgery* is only used on carefully selected patients. The patient's heart is still beating, but special devices are used to stabilize the heart during surgery.
- *Minimally invasive direct coronary artery bypass (MIDCAB)* can only be performed if the blockages can be treated through small incisions in the chest.

Stopping the heart

Cardioplegic solution (cooled solution containing a high concentration of potassium) is infused at high pressure into the aortic root, and causes immediate asystole.

The cardiopulmonary bypass machine

This consists of several key components that allow extracorporeal circulation.
- Venous drainage cannulae are either placed directly into the right atrium, or both the superior vena cava and the inferior vena cava are cannulated.
- A venous reservoir helps the surgeons to clear any blood from the operating field, and prevents the formation of gas emboli.
- A pump drives the blood forward.

- An oxygenator takes over the role of the lungs, not only oxygenating the deoxygenated blood, but also removing the carbon dioxide.
- A heat exchanger.
- A filter to trap macro- and microemboli.
- An arterial cannula is often inserted into the aorta to take filtered oxygenated and temperature-regulated blood back to the patient.

Complications of bypass surgery

- Bleeding.
- ECG changes.
- Hypothermia.
- Cerebral dysfunction.
- Haemolysis.
- Hyperglycaemia.
- Electrolyte disturbances.
- Renal dysfunction.

Nursing care

The patient is initially nursed in the intensive care unit.

- Ventilation, sedation scoring, and pain control.
- Monitor vital signs—heart rate, ECG, central venous pressure (CVP), temperature, and mean arterial pressure (MAP).
- Chest drains.
- Fluid balance—fluids with or without medication.
- Urine output.
- Blood tests: U&E, clotting, full blood count.
- Psychological care.

Further reading

Chikwe J, Cooke D and Weiss A. *Cardiothoracic Surgery*, 2nd edn. Oxford University Press: Oxford, 2013.

Mitral, pulmonary, and tricuspid valve disease and surgical procedures

There are two types of valve disease, which are known as stenosis and regurgitation.
- Stenosis occurs when the valve opening is smaller than normal, due to stiff or fused valves, which means that the heart has to work harder to pump blood through it.
- Regurgitation occurs when the valve does not close completely, which means that blood leaks backwards across the valve, causing hypertrophy and dilatation.

Causes of mitral stenosis
- Rheumatic fever is the major cause.
- Congenital abnormalities.
- Endocarditis.

Causes of mitral regurgitation
- Mitral valve prolapse due to myxomatous degeneration.
- Ischaemic heart disease.
- Rheumatic fever.
- Marfan syndrome—a genetic disorder of the connective tissue.
- Dilated cardiomyopathy.
- Endocarditis.

Causes of pulmonary stenosis
- Endocarditis.
- Congenital abnormality.

Causes of pulmonary regurgitation
- Pulmonary hypertension.
- Endocarditis.
- Congenital abnormality (e.g. tetralogy of Fallot).

Causes of tricuspid stenosis
- Rheumatic fever.
- Endocarditis.
- Carcinoid syndrome.
- Right atrial myxoma.
- Congenital tricuspid atresia.

Causes of tricuspid regurgitation
- Right ventricular dilatation due to left ventricular failure, inferior myocardial infarction, or cor pulmonale.
- Endocarditis.

Valve repair
Valve repair is used to treat mitral valve defects and congenital valve defects. The two main techniques used are annuloplasty and commissurotomy.

Annuloplasty

The aim of this technique is to repair the annulus at the base of the valve. This can be done by using sutures to make the valve opening smaller. The surgeon may also need to implant an annuloplasty ring to provide support for the valve.

Commissurotomy

This technique is used to treat regurgitation when the leaflets of the valve have been stiff or may have fused together at the base. The fused leaflets (commissures) may need to be cut with a scalpel, or alternatively a balloon catheter is inserted into the valve and inflated, causing the commissures to split.

Valve replacement

Valve replacement involves the use of either mechanical or biological valves.

Mechanical valves

These are made from plastic, carbon, or metal, which means that the patient requires lifelong anticoagulants due to the risk of thrombus formation on the mechanical valve. The main advantage of mechanical valves is that they do not undergo degenerative changes, and consequently have a lifespan that generally exceeds the patient's life expectancy.

Biological valves

Biological valves are either xenografts derived from animal (porcine or bovine) tissue, or less frequently allografts derived from the human tissue of a donated heart. The main advantage of biological valves is the low risk of thrombus formation, so long-term anticoagulant therapy is not required.

Further reading

hikwe J, Cooke D and Weiss A. *Cardiothoracic Surgery*, 2nd edn. Oxford University Press: Oxford, 2013.

Aortic valve and aortic root disease

Causes of aortic stenosis
- Calcific disease due to atherosclerosis or end-stage renal disease.
- Congenital abnormality (e.g. bicuspid valve).
- Endocarditis.

Causes of aortic regurgitation
- Endocarditis.
- Congenital abnormality.
- Rheumatic fever.
- Marfan syndrome, which causes abnormal widening of the base of the aorta.

Surgical interventions for aortic regurgitation and aortic stenosis
Aortic valve repair is a possible treatment for aortic regurgitation, but not for aortic stenosis. This is because debridement of aortic valve calcification leads to post-operative regurgitation due to leaflet fibrosis and retraction.

Aortic valve replacement involves the use of either a mechanical or biological valve. A homograft valve may be used while also performing a homograft aortic root replacement, for a diseased aortic root, or if endocarditis is present.

Thoracic aortic aneurysm and aortic dissection
Thoracic aortic aneurysm is the dilatation of the aorta by 50% or more. A true aneurysm involves all three layers of the aortic wall, and affects different parts of the thoracic aorta, which consists of:
- the ascending aorta
- the aortic arch
- the descending aorta.

Most thoracic aortic aneurysms are asymptomatic and are diagnosed incidentally.

Aortic dissection occurs when there is a tear in the intima of the aortic lining, allowing blood to enter the aortic wall under pressure and form a haematoma. This is usually preceded by an aortic aneurysm, and the majority of cases present with severe abrupt chest pain after the initial bleed has stopped. In the event of rupture the patient will collapse suddenly and death will follow.

Causes of aortic aneurysm and aortic dissection
- Atherosclerosis.
- Connective tissue disorders (e.g. Marfan syndrome).
- Trauma.
- Infection (e.g. syphilis).
- Hypertension.

Endovascular repair

Depending on the size and location of the aneurysm, it may be possible to perform an endovascular repair, which is a minimally invasive procedure. Under X-ray guidance a stent graft is inserted, via the femoral artery, into the site of the thoracic aneurysm.

Surgical repair

This involves replacing the weakened portion of the aorta with a Dacron® or Gore-Tex® graft. Aneurysms involving an extensive area of the aorta are repaired using a Dacron® elephant trunk graft. The surgical procedure involves placing the patient on cardiopulmonary bypass, and there may also be a period of hypothermic circulatory arrest.

Coarctation of the aorta

This is a type of birth defect which results in a narrowing of part of the aorta, and it is generally an isolated defect. It occurs in approximately 1 in 10 000 people, and is usually diagnosed in childhood, or in adults below the age of 40 years.

Depending on the severity of the narrowing and its position, it will be treated with balloon angioplasty or surgery. Surgery involves removing the narrowed section of the aorta, and may require a Dacron® graft to bridge the gap in the aorta.

Further reading

Chikwe J, Cooke D and Weiss A. *Cardiothoracic Surgery*, 2nd edn. Oxford University Press: Oxford, 2013.

Intra-aortic balloon pump

The intra-aortic balloon pump (IABP) is the most widely used cardiac assist device. Its primary functions are to decrease cardiac workload, increase coronary perfusion, and provide haemodynamic stability (see Figure 26.3).

Indications for use
- Acute myocardial infarction.
- Unstable angina.
- Cardiogenic shock.
- Acute mitral regurgitation.
- Weaning from cardiac bypass.
- Pre-cardiac surgery in unstable patients.
- Mechanical bridge to other assist devices or transplant.
- Support during coronary angiogram or angioplasty for high-risk patients.

Contraindications
- Aortic valve incompetence.
- Severe peripheral vascular disease.
- Abdominal or aortic aneurysm.
- Aortic dissection.
- Prosthetic graft in thoracic aorta.

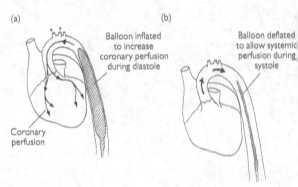

(a)

Balloon inflated to increase coronary perfusion during diastole

(b)

Balloon deflated to allow systemic perfusion during systole

Coronary perfusion

Figure 26.3 IABP. (a) Cardiac diastole. (b) Cardiac systole. Reproduced from PS Ramrakha, KP Moore and A Sam, *Oxford Handbook of Acute Medicine*, 3rd edition, 2010, with permission from Oxford University Press.

Insertion

The IABP catheter is usually inserted percutaneously through the femoral artery. Alternative routes of access include the brachial, subclavian, or iliac artery. The balloon is positioned in the descending aorta inferior to the left subclavian artery.

The balloon catheter is connected to a pump console which is responsible for inflating and then deflating the balloon with a predetermined volume of helium gas (30–40 mL) at a set interval.

Triggering and timing

This set interval is based on the cardiac cycle and needs to be timed to perfection.

- Inflation should start at the beginning of diastole.
- Deflation should start prior to the ejection phase of systole.

The console's 'trigger event' is often used to refer to the start of the cardiac cycle.

- When using an ECG trigger, the 'trigger event' is marked by the R wave.
- Deflation is set to occur just before the QRS complex, and inflation is set to occur during the T wave.
- When using a blood pressure trigger, the 'trigger event' is the upstroke in blood pressure.
- Deflation occurs just before the upstroke, and inflation occurs at the dicrotic notch which marks the start of diastole (aortic valve closure).

Complications

Numerous complications can occur, relating to either the insertion of the device, its dwelling within the aorta, or its removal from the body. These include:

- haemorrhage
- puncture or dissection of the aorta
- embolism due to rupture of the balloon
- incorrect positioning
- limb ischaemia
- sepsis
- renal failure
- aortic dissection
- timing problems
- thrombocytopenia
- thrombus formation.

Ventricular assist devices

Ventricular assist devices (VADs) are mechanical devices that suppor heart function. They are not artificial hearts, which generally require th removal of the patient's heart. The VAD decreases the cardiac workloa of the ventricles, which allows the heart time to rest and recover. Th pump and its connections are implanted during open heart surgery. A electronic controller, a power pack, and a reserve power pack are a external.

Indications for use
- Difficulty in weaning after coronary artery bypass surgery.
- Post myocardial infarction and STEMI.
- Decompensated coronary heart failure.
- End-stage cardiomyopathy.
- Awaiting cardiac transplant.
- Destination therapy.

Types of device
- The left ventricular assist device (LVAD) receives blood from the left ventricle and delivers it to the aorta.
- The right ventricular assist device (RVAD) receives blood from the right atrium or ventricle and delivers it to the pulmonary artery.
- The biventricular assist device (BVAD) assists both the right and left ventricles. It consists of three parts:
  - pump
  - power pack
  - electronic controller.

Advances in pump technology
First-generation pumps
- Pulsatile volume pumps.
- Problems with the size of the pump.
- Large surgical incision required.
- Prone to infection.

Second-generation pumps
- Axial flow pump.
- Smaller in size.
- Continuous flow.
- Much quieter and more durable.

Third-generation pumps
- Bearing less continuous flow pump.
- No mechanical wear and tear.
- Easy to implant as much smaller.

Complications

- Mechanical failure.
- Problems with clotting.
- Infection.
- Pulmonary embolism.
- Renal failure.
- Respiratory failure.

Pacemaker implantation

Pacemakers are devices that supply the myocardium (the muscle of th heart) with electrical impulses that stimulate contraction of the heart Pacemakers can be useful in clinical situations in which the heart is no beating correctly, as they can take over the role of the sinoatrial nod (the heart's natural pacemaker) and help the heart to beat at the appro priate rhythm and rate.

Components of a pacemaker

Pacemakers consist of:
- a central unit containing the battery and the pulse generator, weighir 20–50 g
- a number of electrode leads.

The pulse generator contains an electrical circuit that is responsibl for generating the electrical impulses. These electrical impulses can b generated and discharged at a fixed rate (asynchronous pacing) or on demand-only basis (synchronous pacing). Most modern pacemakers us the synchronous pacing mode.

Pulse generators can be either internal or external. External pace makers are often used for more acute indications, and are temporar whereas internal pacemakers are often permanent.

Indications for a permanent (internal) pacemaker

- Symptomatic bradycardia (heart rate < 40 beats/min) that is resistan to drug therapy.
- Drug-resistant tachyarrhythmias (heart rate > 100 beats/min).
- Complete heart block.
- Mobitz type II AV block.

Indications for a temporary (external) pacemaker

- Arrhythmias following an acute myocardial infarction.
- Acute onset of symptomatic bradycardia, leading to haemodynamic compromise, that is not responsive to drug therapy.
- Drug-resistant tachyarrhythmias.
- To help to treat the arrhythmias associated with drug overdose.
- During the peri-operative or post-operative periods.

Permanent pacemaker insertion

The central unit of permanent pacemakers is commonly located subcut neously on the upper part of the patient's chest. The leads that conne the pacemaker to the heart can be inserted in either of two ways.

Transvenous implantation (the commonest method)

The leads are inserted into the heart by threading them through t patient's veins, starting in the subclavian vein (which sits beneath the co lar bone). The procedure is performed using X-ray guidance to visuali whether or not the leads are in the correct position.

Epicardial implantation

The leads are fixed to the epicardium (the outer layer of the heart) while the patient's chest is open (i.e. following cardiothoracic surgery). When this method is used, the central unit is often located subcutaneously on the patient's abdomen rather than on their chest.

Pacemaker coding

Although all pacemakers have the same basic components, they can all operate in a variety of different modes. The way in which a pacemaker is functioning can be described by a simple three-letter code, the most widely used mode being VVI.

The first letter of the code refers to the chamber in the heart that is being paced, where V = ventricles, A = atria, and D = dual (i.e. both the atria and the ventricles are being paced).

The second letter refers to the chamber that is being sensed, and the letters V, A, and D are used in addition to O (= none).

The third letter denotes the pacemaker response to a signal being sensed, where I = inhibited, T = triggered, D = dual (must be a pacemaker in DDD mode), and R = reverse.

Heart transplantation

Advanced heart failure has a terrible prognosis, resulting in a poor qua ity of life for the patient. Heart transplantation provides an effectiv treatment for some of these patients. However, it should only be under taken when other maximal medical and surgical therapies have failed This is because heart transplantation commits the patient to a lifelon programme of treatment, including pharmacological immunosuppres sion treatment which is required to prevent the recipient's body from rejecting the transplanted heart.

The most common indications for heart transplantation are dilate cardiomyopathy and ischaemic heart disease.

Indications for heart transplantation
- End-stage heart failure with a life expectancy of 12–18 months.
- New York Heart Association (NYHA) functional classification of heart failure, class III or IV.
- Progressive symptoms with maximal therapy.
- Cardiogenic shock requiring mechanical assistance (e.g. ventricular assist device).
- Life-threatening ventricular arrhythmias despite medical and device interventions, such as implantable cardioverter defibrillator (ICD).

Absolute contraindications to heart transplantation
- Chronic systemic infection, including endocarditis.
- Active peptic ulcer.
- Continued alcohol or drug abuse.
- A mental health history that is likely to result in non-concordance with medical therapy.
- Severe peripheral or cerebrovascular disease.
- Malignancy.
- Any other life-threatening condition that is likely to cause death within 5 years.

Surgical procedure
The orthotopic procedure is used in the majority of heart tran plants, and involves putting the recipient on a cardiopulmonary bypa machine. The patient's diseased heart is excised except for the ba part of the atria. The donor heart is trimmed so that the front of the atri can be sutured onto the back part of the recipient's atria, and also on the recipient's great vessels.

Denervation of the transplanted heart
The transplanted heart does not have a nerve supply. This is known denervation, and it means that direct sympathetic and parasympathe innervation is absent.

The denervated heart will have a higher than normal heart rate 90–110 beats/min. There will be a delayed response to exercise, possi taking 10 min to respond to increased adrenaline levels, and the don heart will take longer to return to a resting heart rate after exercise.

Another problem associated with denervation is that the patient will not feel chest pain if they develop coronary artery disease in their new heart.

Complications

- Rejection of the transplanted heart due to autoimmune response.
- Infection due to the suppression of the immune system by immunosuppressant drugs.
- Allograft vasculopathy or transplant coronary artery disease.
- Malignant disease due to Epstein–Barr virus or immunosuppressant therapy.
- Hypertension due to immunosuppressant therapy or pre-existing disease.
- Dyslipidaemia due to immunosuppressant therapy.

Breast surgery

Anatomy of the breast and axilla

Gross anatomical topography

- The breasts, or mammary glands, are the specialized milk-producing tissues located on the chest, one on each side of the sternum. They lie over the pectoralis major muscle, and extend above as far as the second rib and below to the level of the sixth rib (see Figure 27.1).
- The base of this conically shaped mound, which measures on average around 10–12 cm, extends obliquely and laterally from the medial margin of the sternum to the midline of the axilla via a tongue of tissue called the tail of Spence. The bulk of breast tissue is therefore typically located in the upper outer quadrant of the breast, which is why this area is most commonly implicated in most benign and malignant breast lesions.
- The breasts of a nulliparous woman (one who has not borne children) are hemispherical in shape, whereas those of multiparous women tend to be broader and pendulous. A lactating breast can more than double in weight, from approximately 150 g to in excess of 500 g.
- The nipple–areola complex lies in the centre of the breast. It consists of two elements.
  - The nipple, or apex of the cone, is the small projection of skin that lies in the centre of the areola (and is approximately 10 mm in length), through which milk is delivered to the infant during lactation. It is the ultimate part of the 10–20 lactiferous ducts from the lobes.
  - The areola is the slightly raised pigmented circular area, of variable size, that surrounds the nipple. The surface of the areola presents small protrusions, known as the Montgomery glands, which are sebaceous glands that lubricate and protect the nipple during lactation.

Breast structures beneath the skin

- The breast is composed of fibrous, glandular, and fatty tissue. Thin filaments of fibrous fascia (found throughout the breast) form the suspensory ligaments of Cooper, which support and suspend the breast, maintaining its normal shape and contour. Tightening of this tissue by malignant infiltration results in the distinctive dimpling over carcinoma of the breast.
- The fibrous bands separate the glandular tissue into 15–20 lobes, which contain up to 40 lobules that are composed of the alveoli, or acini, which are the structures that produce and secrete milk. The milk is collected by distal lactiferous ducts or acini that amalgamate into minor and then major lactiferous ducts, which are lined with epithelial cells. The milk is propelled along the ductal system and ultimately empties into the ampulla, the reservoir where milk may be stored, before opening out onto the surface of the nipple.

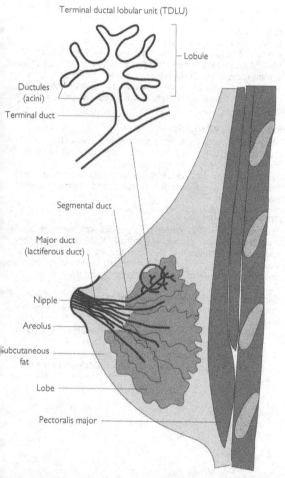

Figure 27.1 Cross section of the female breast. Reproduced with permission from *Training in Surgery: the essential curriculum for the MRCS*, edited by Matthew Gardiner and Neil Borley, © 2009, Oxford University Press.

- The glandular tissue of the breast is surrounded by adipose tissue. In younger women, especially those who are premenopausal, the breast tissue is dense, and the high ratio of ductal and glandular breast tissue to fatty and fibrous tissue makes detection of any irregularity during clinical breast examination and mammography more difficult. With age, the fat content of the breast tissue increases, the breast sags or droops (ptosis), but the increased fat content of the breast in older adults accounts for the superior quality of their mammographic images, as increased fat content is associated with improved image quality.

Blood and nerve supply

- The blood supply is from the perforating branches of the axillary, internal thoracic, and intercostal arteries, accompanied by the corresponding venous drainage vessels.
- The sensitivity of the breast nipple–areola complex results mainly from branches of the thoracic, intercostal, and intercostobrachial nerves.

Lymphatic drainage

- The breasts have an extensive lymphatic network. However, there is an apparent predominance of lymphatic drainage to the axillary nodes, which accounts for 75% of the mammary lymphatic drainage. Fluid from the lateral aspects of each breast flows into the ipsilateral axillary nodes, and the rest passes primarily into the internal thoracic nodes.
- Clinicians and histopathologists conventionally classify and define metastatic spread to the axillary lymph nodes according to three levels:
  - level I—the lymph nodes are inferior to (i.e. below) the lower edge of the pectoralis minor muscle
  - level II—the lymph nodes lie behind the pectoralis minor muscle
  - level III—the lymph nodes lie above the pectoralis minor muscle.

Further reading

Dixon JM (ed.). *Breast Surgery: a companion to specialist surgical practice*, 5th edn. Saunders, London, 2014.

Breast screening

In medicine, screening is a public health policy used in a population to detect a disease in individuals without any clinical signs or symptoms of that disease, with the intention that early diagnosis will enable earlier therapeutic interventions, so that morbidity and mortality can be minimized.

The first screening mammogram as part of the English national programme was performed in 1988. Currently, all women aged 50–70 years in the UK are offered a routine breast screening mammogram every 3 years, and more than 1.5 million women are screened annually in the UK.

The benefits of breast cancer screening

There is an overall decrease in mortality.

It has been estimated that early detection of breast cancer at screening in England each year saves the lives of up to 1400 women. Improved early detection of breast cancer has led to more breast-conserving treatment, thereby contributing to a reduction in psychological morbidity.

The harms of breast cancer screening

Over-diagnosis leading to unnecessary treatment.

Procedure-related pain and discomfort, and psychological distress.

False-positive mammograms leading to superfluous investigations.

False reassurance if the mammogram fails to detect the cancer and an incorrect diagnosis is made.

Undue radiation exposure, which may increase the risk of breast cancer.

Breast cancer screening procedures

Invitation to attend—informed consent.

X-ray imaging using two views:

- cranio-caudal projection (head to tail, through the top of the breast to the bottom surface)
- medio-lateral oblique projection, which angles the X-ray at 45° from the upper inner quadrant of the breast through to the lower outer quadrant.

Both projections involve compression of the breast between plate and film to reduce movement and radiation dose, and improve X-ray penetration and potential visualization of abnormalities.

Magnetic resonance imaging (MRI) may be advised if there is a family history of breast cancer, or known genetic predisposition.

Further reading

Vert P and Huffaker C. Breast cancer screening in women: an integrative literature review. *Journal of the American Academy of Nurse Practitioners* 2010; 22: 668–73.

Benign breast diseases

Benign breast diseases are far more common than malignant breast cancers. Benign breast diseases include a diverse group of conditions that range from developmental defects to inflammation and infection, with correspondingly disparate range of presenting features. The prevalence of benign breast diseases differs from that of malignant disorders in that the incidence begins to rise in the second decade of life and peaks in middle age, whereas the frequency of malignant disease continues to increase after the menopause.

Mastalgia
- Mastalgia, or breast pain, is a symptom rather than a discrete disease, but it may indicate underlying pathology, which is usually benign.
- It can be cyclical (related to the menstrual cycle) or non-cyclical.
- It may be treated with lifestyle measures (e.g. reducing caffeine intake), complementary therapies (e.g. evening primrose oil), non-steroidal anti-inflammatory drugs, or hormone-suppressing agents (e.g. danazol).
- Surgery is only performed in extreme intractable cases.

Mastitis
- Inflammation or infection of the breast.
- Management involves treating the cause—for example, breast emptying with frequent nursing, and manual breast pumping and empirical antibiotic management if lactation mastitis has developed as a consequence of breastfeeding.

Breast abscess
- Relatively common during breastfeeding.
- Treatment consists of antibiotics, aspiration and, if necessary, surgical drainage.

Cysts
- Cysts are fluid-filled discrete round or ovoid sacs, often associated with pain, that affect as many as one-third of women in the third to fifth decades of life. They present as smooth lumps in one or both breasts, and are often recurrent.
- Cysts are investigated by triple assessment.
- In general no treatment or follow-up is required, although cysts can be aspirated to relieve discomfort, and they usually disappear as a result.

Fibroadenoma

- Fibroadenomas are, on palpation, highly mobile rubbery lumps 1–3 cm in diameter, caused by a proliferation of the tissue around the breast lobule.
- They are common, most frequently presenting in young women aged 15–25 years.
- Fibroadenomas can be identified by triple assessment (using ultrasound instead of mammography if the patient is under 35 years of age, because of the higher breast density).
- They can be left in the breast, or if the patient wishes they may be surgically removed. If they are removed, the normal breast tissue will compensate and fill the void.

Further reading

uray M and Sahin A. Benign breast diseases: classification, diagnosis, and management. *The Oncologist* 2006; 11: 435–49.

Common forms of breast cancer

Epidemiology
Breast cancer is the most common cancer in the UK, with almost 48 000
new cases diagnosed each year, the vast majority (over 99%) of which
are in women. It has been estimated that the lifetime risk, or probability
of developing breast cancer is 1 in 1014 for men and 1 in 8 for women
in the UK.[1]

Risk factors
- Female gender.
- Age. Breast cancer is uncommon under the age of 35 years. Around
  75% of cases occur in women over 50 years of age.
- Family history. A woman with one affected first-degree relative
  (mother or sister) has approximately double the risk of breast cancer
  of a woman with no family history of the disease.
- Genetic predisposition. Inheritance of mutations in the breast cancer
  susceptibility genes BRCA1 and BRCA2 increases the lifetime risk of
  breast cancer, and genetic susceptibility accounts for 5–10% of cases.
- Reproductive factors, including age at menarche, age at first birth,
  parity, breastfeeding, and age at menopause.
- Exposure to hormones. As well as the increased risk of unopposed
  circulating oestrogen associated with nulliparity and late
  menopause, both hormone replacement therapy (HRT) and the oral
  contraceptive pill are associated with increased risk.
- Lifestyle factors. These include exposure to ionizing radiation,
  obesity, and alcohol consumption.

Clinical features
- There is commonly a painless breast lump.
- Involvement and invasion of the overlying skin leads to skin dimpling
  and tethering.
- Nipple inversion, elevation, deformation, ulceration, or bloody
  discharge.
- Axillary node involvement.
- In a late presentation, features of metastases.

Pathology
Breast cancer is a histologically heterogeneous disease, incorporating
number of distinctly dissimilar biological features that require different
treatment modalities. The vast majority of breast carcinomas begin
develop in the ducts, with greater numbers of these being invasive form
of the disease.

In-situ disease refers to carcinoma that has not invaded through th
epithelial basement membrane. There are two major types.
- Ductal carcinoma *in situ* is a pre-invasive form of malignant cancer
  that is confined to the ducts of the breasts. Treatment consists of
  breast-conserving surgery and adjuvant radiotherapy, although some
  women preferentially undergo mastectomy. Hormonal treatment (with
  tamoxifen) is recommended if the carcinoma is oestrogen-positive.

- Lobular carcinoma *in situ* (also known as lobular neoplasia) can predispose some women to later invasive disease, typically within two decades after initial diagnosis. Therefore regular monitoring is undertaken by biannual clinical examination and annual mammography. Preventative hormonal treatment may be recommended.

Invasive carcinoma can also be classified into two major types, which account for the majority of cases.

- Invasive ductal carcinoma originates in the ductal epithelium and invades through breast tissue into the vascular compartment and wider systemic circulation, and the lymphatic system. It accounts for around 75% of breast cancers. Surgery is commonly the initial treatment, although neoadjuvant chemotherapy, radiotherapy, or hormonal treatment may be used.
- Invasive lobular carcinoma is less common (10–15% of cases). It is characterized by often more diffuse, indistinct masses that are not easily diagnosed by palpation or mammography, which can make early diagnosis difficult and breast conservation approaches more complicated. It is also associated with uncommon metastatic spread, including spread to the gastrointestinal tract.

Other, less common, and rare breast cancers include medullary carcinoma, mucinous (colloid) carcinoma, tubular carcinoma, papillary carcinoma, inflammatory carcinoma, metaplastic breast cancer, Paget's disease, and sarcomas.

Routes of spread

- Local invasion involving the lymphatic regional nodes.
- Spread via the circulatory system, most commonly to bone, brain, lung, or liver.

Reference

Cancer Research UK. *Breast Cancer Statistics*. ℳ www.cancerresearchuk.org/health-professional/cancer-statistics/statistics-by-cancer-type/breast-cancer

Further reading

armer V (ed.). *Breast Cancer Nursing: care and management*, 2nd edn. Wiley-Blackwell: Chichester, 2011.

enkus E et al. Primary breast cancer: ESMO Clinical Practice Guidelines for diagnosis, treatment and follow-up. *Annals of Oncology* 2015; 26 (Suppl. 5): v8–30.

Staging and grading of breast cancer

Staging of breast cancer

Staging describes the size of the tumour and the extent of spread, and uses the TNM classification system, in which:

- T stages numbered from 1 to 4 describe the size of the tumour
- N stages numbered from 0 to 3 describe the extent of lymph node involvement, if any
- M stages, recorded as M0 or M1, indicate whether there is evidence of distant metastatic disease.

Grading of breast cancer

Tumour grading classifies cancer according to how closely the tumour cells resemble normal cells of the same tissue type—cellular differentiation, the size and shape of the tumour cell nucleus, and the percentage of tumour cells that are dividing. Breast cancer is graded as follows:

- Grade 1 describes a well-differentiated slow-growing tumour.
- Grade 2 describes a moderately differentiated tumour and intermediate rates of cell growth.
- Grade 3 describes a poorly differentiated high-grade aggressive tumour in which the cells no longer resemble the cells of their tissue of origin. A grade 3 tumour has a much worse prognosis.

Further reading
Cancer Research UK. *TNM Breast Cancer Staging*. www.cancerresearchuk.org/about-cancer/type/breast-cancer/treatment/tnm-breast-cancer-staging

Male breast cancer

Epidemiology

This is a rare disease, accounting for less than 1% of all malignancies in men and less than 1% of all invasive breast cancers in the UK, with approximately 340 cases per year.[2] There is an increasing global incidence, with a median age at diagnosis of 60–70 years, which is 10 years older than the median age in women.

Risk factors

- Genetic factors:
  - in a similar way to female breast cancer, a positive family history is associated with increased risk
  - inheritance of highly penetrant susceptibility genes, such as mutations in the *BRCA2* gene (*BRCA1* mutations are rarer)
  - Klinefelter syndrome.
- Disorders and treatments that cause elevated oestrogen levels:
  - obesity
  - liver cirrhosis
  - treatment for transsexualism that includes castration and administration of oestrogen
  - case reports suggest that castration and oestrogen treatment for prostate cancer could increase the risk.
- Testicular disorders, such as:
  - undescended testes
  - mumps orchitis
  - orchiectomy
  - testicular injury
  - congenital inguinal hernia
  - infertility.
- Exposure to ionizing radiation.

Clinical features

- The majority of men (75–85%) present with breast cancer under the nipple and areola. Other presenting complaints commonly include:
  - local pain
  - nipple discharge, bleeding, ulceration, or pain.
- Men are more likely to have delays in diagnosis than women.
- Presentation is often late, with over 40% of individuals having stage III or IV disease at diagnosis.

Pathology

Most cases (over 85%) of male breast cancer are invasive or infiltrating ductal carcinoma. Cases of invasive lobular carcinoma are extremely rare (1–2%, compared with an incidence of 15% in women). A higher percentage of male breast cancers are oestrogen-receptor positive (90%, compared with 75% of female breast cancers).

Treatment and prognosis

- Treatment is similar to that for women, and most commonly involves modified radical mastectomy.
- Post-operative radiotherapy of the chest wall improves local control and progression-free survival.
- Men benefit from adjuvant systemic therapy for breast carcinoma. Because the majority of tumours are oestrogen-receptor positive, hormonal therapy (e.g. tamoxifen) or selective aromatase inhibition is standard adjuvant therapy.
- Some individuals may also benefit from chemotherapy, particularly as palliation.
- About 70 men die of breast cancer each year in the UK.

Reference

2 Cancer Research UK. *Breast Cancer in Men*. ♫ www.cancerresearchuk.org/about-cancer type/rare-cancers/rare-cancers-name/breast-cancer-in-men

Further reading

Cancer Research UK. *Breast Cancer Mortality Statistics*. ♫ www.cancerresearchuk.org/health professional/cancer-statistics/statistics-by-cancer-type/breast-cancer/mortality
Fentiman I, Fourquet A and Hortobagyi G. Male breast cancer. *The Lancet* 2006; **367**: 595–60

Diagnostic procedures

A diagnosis of breast cancer typically follows one of two discrete pathways—those patients whose disease is found at screening, and those who present symptomatically. Patients who present to their general medical practitioner (GP) should be referred to, and seen by, a specialist breast unit within 2 weeks of referral. Specialist breast care units offer a three-stage process called *triple examination* or *triple assessment* to diagnose breast lumps. The three stages are history and clinical examination, imaging, and biopsy.

History and clinical examination

A detailed medical history is taken, including:
- age, past medical history, family history, age at menarche, age at menopause, and date of last menstrual period
- drug/medication history, especially use of the combined oral contraceptive pill and hormone replacement therapy
- age at the birth of the woman's first child, number of births, breastfeeding history, and history of presenting complaint.

The clinical examination consists of two elements—inspection and palpation—which may reveal evidence of:
- skin dimpling, hardening, pinching, eczema or erosion, erythema or increased vascularity or vascular distension, or peau d'orange
- nipple discharge, inversion, or retraction
- masses (obvious or invisible)
- asymmetry with regard to breast size and shape, and any recent changes.

Imaging

- Mammography—this involves taking a low-energy X-ray of the breast tissue. It is not usually performed on patients younger than 35 years, due to the increased breast density in this age group.
- Ultrasound scan—imaging using sound waves has the advantages of being relatively safe, inexpensive, and quick. It is useful for discriminating between solid tumours and benign cysts.
- Magnetic resonance imaging (MRI)—this is not routinely used except in patients with a high-risk family history and gene mutations, in younger women with denser breast tissue, or where multiple foci are suspected in more diffuse tumours (e.g. lobular carcinoma).

Biopsy

- Fine-needle aspiration cytology involves using a narrow-gauge (25–22G) needle to obtain a sample of a lesion for microscopic evaluation. The procedure, which can be performed freehand by the clinician in the outpatient department, allows minimally invasive and rapid diagnosis of tissue, but does not conserve its histological architecture.
- Core biopsies can also be taken freehand. A biopsy gun is used to remove a small coherent core of breast tissue, which is then sent for histological examination. It is quick, effective, and also useful when breast microcalcification is seen on mammography.

Further reading

Harmer V (ed.). *Breast Cancer Nursing: care and management*, 2nd edn. Wiley-Blackw
Chichester, 2011.

Surgical treatment of breast cancer

Multiprofessional teamworking is the cornerstone of modern breast cancer management, although surgical intervention remains the primary (and often only) treatment modality. The past 30 years have seen a shift towards breast-conserving surgery, which is appropriate for the majority of patients. However, one-third of patients presenting with breast cancer will require a mastectomy, and for many women this can be preferable in the sense that the cancer has been completely removed, or it may possibly obviate the need for adjuvant radiotherapy.

Breast-conserving surgery

- Removal of the breast tumour and microscopically clear radial margins (at least 2 mm has been recommended) to reduce local recurrence rate.
- Wide local excision—this is not routinely offered if the tumour is more than 4 cm in diameter, due to poor cosmetic outcomes. There is no upper age limit. Post-operative radiotherapy is strongly recommended. Survival outcomes are similar to those for mastectomy.
- Oncoplastic resection (volume displacement technique)—when the cancer is removed, the resected area is reconstructed by the rearrangement of the remaining breast tissue itself. Pedicles, or parenchymal flaps, are moved into the space left behind after resection, resulting in a net decrease in breast size and volume, so it is common to perform a mirror-image procedure on the contralateral breast. This procedure is more appropriate for patients with medium to large heavy ptotic breasts.
- Oncoplastic resection (volume replacement techniques)—when the cancer is removed, following a technique such as quadrantectomy, the resected area is reconstructed, usually with autologous tissue from outside the breast, such as a mini-flap reconstruction. Breast tissue volume is conserved and a contralateral procedure is not required.

Mastectomy

- Total mastectomy—this is the most common technique. Breast tissue is isolated from the skin and muscle and removed along with the nipple and the areola. Staging axillary lymph node biopsy is also performed.
- Modified radical mastectomy—the entire breast is removed, and removal or division of the pectoralis major allows axillary lymph node dissection.
- Subcutaneous mastectomy —the entire breast is removed, but the nipple and areola are left in situ. As this approach may leave some breast tissue under the nipple, this treatment is not recommended for most patients with breast cancer.

- Risk-reducing mastectomy—prophylactic bilateral mastectomy and reconstruction, which is offered to women at high risk of breast cancer, such as those with BRCA1 or BRCA2 gene mutations, or at risk of contralateral disease. Surgery does not completely eradicate the risk.
- Mastectomy is usually the recommended treatment for male breast cancer.
- Post-mastectomy radiotherapy may be required for large aggressive tumours with vascular involvement.

Axillary staging and clearance

- There are 20–30 axillary lymph nodes that drain fluid from the breast, chest wall, neck, and upper limb.
- Positive lymph node status remains a significant determinant of treatment and prognosis.
- Sentinel lymph node biopsy—the sentinel lymph node is the first node to drain lymph from the breast. Biopsy rather than full nodal clearance is now the accepted standard of care, because it is associated with lower morbidity and reduced hospital stay.
- Evidence of macrometastatic spread in the sentinel node conventionally directs treatment to axillary node clearance, which is associated with the development of lymphoedema.
- Research is continuing regarding the best treatment for micrometastatic spread and isolated tumour cells.

Surgery for in-situ malignancy (intra-epithelial neoplasia)

- Ductal intra-epithelial neoplasia can be treated with breast-conserving surgery, provided that an adequate margin is achieved.
- Total mastectomy with uninvolved margins in ductal intra-epithelial neoplasia is considered curative.
- Lobular neoplasia is regarded as a 'marker' of future risk of breast cancer. Accordingly, some women will opt for risk-reducing bilateral mastectomy.
- Axillary node evaluation is not required for in-situ disease.

Complications of breast surgery

- Seroma—serous fluid commonly collects at the post-operative wound site. This is sometimes uncomfortable (depending on the volume of fluid), and it may become infected. It can easily be drained.
- Infection—this is possible, although in practice it is rare.
- Cording—after lymph node surgery, scar tissue can develop in the axilla, forming a tight band. This is called 'cording', and it has been described as feeling taut, like a guitar string. It can be quite painful initially, but improves over time through massage and exercise.
- Flap necrosis—this is rare, although it is more common in smokers. It often resolves, but sometimes requires excision and skin grafting.
- Severe pain after a mastectomy is rare, and analgesia requirements should follow WHO guidelines[3] and individual need. However, some patients may develop prolonged post-mastectomy pain syndrome (PMPS), and will require specific advice from pain specialist teams.

Reference

World Health Organization. *Cancer Pain Relief.* 2nd edn. World Health Organization: Geneva, 1996.

Further reading

hen JJ and Wu J. Management strategy of early-stage breast cancer patients with a positive sentinel lymph node: with or without axillary node dissection. *Critical Reviews in Oncology/Hematology* 2011; 79: 293–301.

Chemotherapy and other systemic treatment

Neoadjuvant systemic therapy
This therapy is indicated for large operable or inflammatory breast tumours, prior to the primary surgery, in order to reduce the size of the tumour and so make it more amenable to breast-conserving techniques

Adjuvant systemic therapy
- Systemic treatment given after surgery includes combination cytotoxic chemotherapy, hormone therapy, and targeted (biological) therapy.
- Treatment is recommended if the reduction in the risk of recurrence and death can be achieved with a tolerable level of treatment-related adverse events.
- It is often regarded as a 'belt and braces' approach to treatment.
- Oestrogen receptor (ER) and human epidermal growth factor receptor-2 (HER2) status are the most influential factors with regard to the choice of treatment modality.

Adjuvant chemotherapy
- Recommended for patients with oestrogen-receptor-poor breast cancer or patients with HER2-overexpressing or amplified tumours.
- Various agents are active against breast cancer and used in combination or multi-agent regimens, including anthracycline agents (doxorubicin or epirubicin), which are recommended for most patients:
  - AC or EC (doxorubicin or epirubicin, fluorouracil); Epi-CMF (epirubicin followed by CMF); FEC (fluorouracil, epirubicin, cyclophosphamide); FEC–T (FEC followed by docetaxel).
- Use of prophylactic granulocyte colony-stimulating factor, to prevent or minimize the risk associated with low white blood cell count.
- As high-dose chemotherapy requiring bone marrow stem cell rescue shows no appreciable survival benefit, and is associated with unacceptable adverse events, its use is not recommended.

Adjuvant endocrine therapy
- Many breast cancers are stimulated to develop and progress by the female sex hormones oestrogen and progesterone. The vast majority (75%) of breast cancers are oestrogen receptor positive (ER positive), which means that the cancer is stimulated to grow by the female sex hormone oestrogen.
- Anti-oestrogen treatments may be considered less toxic than cytotoxic chemotherapy. However, menopausal symptoms can be acute and distressing.

Tamoxifen

- This is an anti-oestrogen drug.
- In premenopausal patients, tamoxifen alone (20 mg daily for 5 years), or after chemotherapy, improves survival and reduces the risk of contralateral cancer and osteoporosis, but is associated with an increased risk of thromboembolic disease and endometrial cancer.

Aromatase inhibitors

- In postmenopausal patients, aromatase inhibitors (AIs), including anastrozole, exemestane, and letrozole, can be prescribed sequentially for 2–3 years, after 2 years of tamoxifen treatment, but may also be used as an up-front treatment for 5 years.
- They reduce recurrence rates, with a reduced risk of thromboembolic disease and endometrial cancer, but are associated with various adverse events, including bone effects (decreased bone density, osteoporosis, and fractures), joint pain, fatigue, nausea, weight loss, vaginal irritation, pain in the extremities, and raised cholesterol levels.
- A dual-energy X-ray absorptiometry (DXA) scan is recommended to evaluate bone density and risk of osteoporosis prior to treatment.
- Women who are treated with aromatase inhibitors are advised about the need to preserve bone integrity (e.g. by undertaking regular low-impact exercise, and ensuring adequate dietary intake of calcium and vitamin D), and may be prescribed dietary supplements.
- Bisphosphonates are often prescribed to prevent further bone loss.

Trastuzumab

- HER2 is an oncogene that encodes a transmembrane tyrosine kinase receptor, which is overexpressed and amplified in up to one-third of invasive breast cancers. This gene amplification has been associated with aggressive disease and a poorer prognosis due to increased cell growth and motility, tumour invasiveness and metastases, accelerated angiogenesis, and reduced apoptosis (programmed cell death).
- Trastuzumab is a humanized monoclonal antibody that binds to the HER2 cell-surface receptors, blocking their action (i.e. the start of the signalling processes by which the cell is instructed to divide).
- As with all monoclonal antibodies, the targeted treatment is more elegant than chemotherapy, as it does not have a significant effect on healthy cells.
- Trastuzumab is administered every 3 weeks for 1 year upon completion of anthracycline-based treatment.
- Cardiac function should be routinely monitored.

Lapatinib

- Lapatinib is small molecule dual-targeted therapy that inhibits the action of both HER2 and HER1. Lapatinib differs from trastuzumab (which acts on the cell surface receptors) in that it blocks the intracellular tyrosine kinase signalling pathways for cell growth.
- Lapatinib is licensed but not approved by NICE as a treatment for secondary or metastatic breast cancer.[4] It is available as an oral tablet, which is taken once a day.

Reference

4 National Institute for Health and Care Excellence (NICE). *Lapatinib or trastuzumab in combination with an aromatase inhibitor for first-line treatment of metastatic hormone-receptor-positive breast cancer that overexpresses HER2*. Technology appraisal guidance 257. NICE: London 2012.

Further reading

Azim HA Jr et al. Long-term toxic effects of adjuvant chemotherapy in breast cancer. *Annals Oncology* 2011; 22: 1939–47.
Ross J et al. The HER-2 receptor and breast cancer: ten years of targeted anti-HER-2 therapy and personalized medicine. *The Oncologist* 2009; 14: 320–68.

Radiotherapy

Introduction

- Radiotherapy, sometimes referred to as radiation oncology, is the use of ionizing radiation to kill cancer cells.
- Radiotherapy damages DNA either directly or indirectly, by the ionization of water which forms free radicals that subsequently irreparably damage the DNA, resulting in cell death.
- There are two main forms of radiotherapy:
  - External beam radiotherapy—treatment with radiation sources such as the megavoltage X-rays produced by linear accelerators. Treatment is delivered in divided doses called fractions, and conventionally commences around 1 month after the completion of surgery or chemotherapy.
  - Brachytherapy—the use of radiation sources that are placed within or near to the tumour. It is now used only in breast cancer clinical trials.

Radiation therapy for invasive carcinoma

After breast-conserving surgery

- Whole-breast radiotherapy after breast-conserving surgery is recommended for reducing the risk of local recurrence. Additional irradiation is indicated in older patients, but may be considered discretionary in patients with presumed low risk (i.e. with a wide surgical margin, no nodal involvement, and no evidence of vessel invasion).
- Radiotherapy may be omitted without compromising survival in patients over 70 years of age with early-stage oestrogen-receptor-positive disease and clear surgical margins.

After mastectomy

- Post-mastectomy radiotherapy is always recommended for patients with ≥ 4 positive axillary lymph nodes, and is indicated for patients with T3–T4 tumours, regardless of nodal status.

Non-invasive carcinoma (intra-epithelial neoplasia)

- Adjuvant whole-breast irradiation after breast-conserving surgery for ductal carcinoma *in situ* (DCIS) reduces the risk of local recurrence, but has no effect on survival. It may be omitted in some patients with a low risk of recurrent DCIS.
- Total mastectomy with clear margins in DCIS is curative. Therefore radiotherapy is not recommended.
- Radiotherapy is not necessary in most cases of lobular neoplasia.

Recurrent and metastatic breast cancer

- External beam radiotherapy is useful in the palliative treatment of:
  - loco-regional disease
  - fungating lesions
  - painful bone disease
  - other metastatic disease (e.g. secondary brain lesions)
  - oncological emergencies (e.g. spinal cord compression), as an adjunct to steroids.

Further reading

Beaumont T and Leadbeater M. Treatment and care of patients with metastatic breast cancer. *Nursing Standard* 2011; 25: 49–56.

Hopwood P et al. Comparison of patient-reported breast, arm, and shoulder symptoms and body image after radiotherapy for early breast cancer: 5-year follow-up in the randomised Standardisation of Breast Radiotherapy (START) trials. *The Lancet: Oncology* 2010; 11: 231–40.

Reconstructive breast surgery

Breast reconstruction refers to the surgical interventions that are used to restore breast shape after removal of the breast (mastectomy) or removal of some breast tissue (lumpectomy or wide local excision). All suitable patients should be offered breast reconstruction because of the recognized benefits of improved quality of life when the impact of altered body image is reduced. The timing of reconstructive surgery is dependent upon treatment. The need for adjuvant radiotherapy may preclude certain types of implant-based immediate reconstruction, due to increased complication rates and poorer cosmetic results.

Aims of breast reconstruction

- To replace lost breast tissue volume and reconstruct a breast mound, to provide symmetry of size, volume, and contour, and remove the need for an external prosthesis.
- To restore self-esteem, appearance, and sense of attractiveness and wholeness.

Types of reconstructive surgery

Tissue expanders and implants

Expanders are inserted under the pectoralis major muscle to enlarge space when there is not enough skin to cover an implant. They are removed, if temporary, when the skin has stretched to accommodate a permanent silicone implant, which is placed under the pectoralis major muscle. This is a less invasive procedure than flap reconstruction, but it may be associated with infection, implant leakage, or contracture as fibrous tissue forms around the implant.

Latissimus dorsi flap reconstruction

This involves dissection and rotation from the back of the latissimus dorsi muscle and associated blood supply and skin, under the arm, and onto the front of the chest wall where the breast tissue was detached. It is suitable for larger-breasted women, but less appropriate for patients whose activities or lifestyle require use of the latissimus dorsi muscle, such as racket sports players.

Transverse rectus abdominis muscle flap

This involves the movement of muscle and overlying fat and skin from the abdomen through a subcutaneous channel onto the chest wall, where it is fashioned into a breast mound. It is suitable for larger-breasted women, but not for smokers (in whom delayed healing and failure are more likely) or obese women. This major surgery is associated with a longer recovery time, prominent abdominal scarring, and post-operative complications such as abdominal hernia and flap necrosis.

Deep inferior epigastric perforator

This uses fat and skin from the abdomen only, sparing the muscle and therefore minimizing the risk of herniation.

Nipple–areola reconstructive surgery

Mastectomy usually involves removal of the areola and nipple to reduce the risk of disease recurrence. After the reconstructed breast has healed and settled into its final shape, skin tissue can be removed from the remaining breast nipple, or the inner thigh, and formed into a nipple.

Lymphoedema

Definition, incidence, and impact

Lymphoedema after breast cancer is characterized by the accumulation of protein-rich lymph fluid in the ipsilateral at-risk limb and chest because of irreversible impaired lymphatic transport capacity. Approximately 20% of treated women develop lymphoedema. It is incapacitating, incurable, and progressive. It is also reputedly the most feared complication of breast cancer treatment. Lymphoedema is associated with:

- feelings of discomfort and disfigurement
- arm swelling and pain
- diminished quality of life
- anxiety
- depression
- psychological distress that undermines body image and affects social relationships
- functional limitation
- an increased risk of infection.

Risk factors for developing lymphoedema

- Higher staging of breast cancer and associated type of breast cancer treatment, including surgery such as modified radical mastectomy, axillary lymph node dissection, and radiotherapy to the axilla.
- Post-operative events, including:
  - infection
  - post-surgical drainage and seroma formation
  - cording
  - venepuncture in the affected limb.
- Older age (≥ 50 years) is associated with increased risk.
- Sedentary lifestyle.

Physical effects of lymphoedema

- Visible swelling, heaviness, and fullness of the limb affect function.
- Difficulty wearing clothing, rings, and jewellery.
- Skin changes due to lymph stasis—firm, dry, pigmented thickening (hyperkeratosis) develops as the limb tissues harden, ultimately giving rise to skin folds and a warty appearance (papillomatosis), due to fibrosis over dilated lymphatic vessels.
- Increased risk of infection, including fungal infections in skin folds, and bacterial cellulitis.
- Lymphorrhoea (leakage of lymph fluid through the skin surface).

Management of lymphoedema

- Accurate and full assessment, including vigilant examination of the arms of patients with breast cancer, is vital. Realistic patient-focused goal setting is of fundamental importance.
- Circumference measurement using a tape measure remains the gold standard for routine diagnosis and examination of arm swelling.
- Meticulous skin care is needed to promote skin integrity and prevent infection:

- daily inspection, and moisturization with unperfumed emollient
- avoidance of trauma (including injury such as venepuncture, cannulation, and blood pressure recording), and extremes of temperature
- prompt treatment of infection
- use of non-adherent dressings and short-term light compression for lymphorrhoea.
- Current recommendations limit activity of the arm affected by lymphoedema. However, some evidence suggests that there does not appear to be an increase in the incidence of lymphoedema or worsening of symptoms when progressive weight training or resistance exercises are employed post-operatively. Controlled individualized isotonic exercises, such as tensing the biceps (as it involves muscle contractions that stimulate the passive and active phases of lymph drainage within lymphatic vessels), can be planned.
- Manual lymph drainage gently massages the skin. Evidence to support its use is limited. However, some reports suggest that it does have some effect when used in conjunction with compression bandaging.
- Simple lymph drainage, which the patient or their carers can be taught, aims to massage fluid away from the congested limb, and has the benefit of increasing self-care and locus of control, as well as being easily applied by the patient's partner or relatives. This has the advantage of possibly increasing and improving their sense of involvement and intimacy by means of touch.
- Compression therapy:
  - This complements exercise by augmenting the muscle-pump effect. Lymphoedema bandaging is used extensively (and appreciated by patients) to reduce limb size and restore shape. It may also improve hyperkeratosis and papillomatosis. It should only be undertaken by a specialist nurse or therapist.
  - Compression garments. Elastic hosiery garments are used for patients with mild to moderate lymphoedema, and with lymphoedema bandaging in patients with severe lymphoedema. These garments are not suitable for patients with lymphorrhoea. Assessment and fitting should be undertaken by a specialist practitioner.

Further reading

Cavanaugh K. Effects of early exercise on the development of lymphedema in patients wi breast cancer treated with axillary lymph node dissection. *Journal of Oncology Practice* 20 7: 89–93.

Fleysher LA. Keeping breast cancer survivors lymphoedema-free. *British Journal of Nursing* 20 19: 826–30.

Honnor A. Understanding the management of lymphoedema for patients with advanced c ease. *International Journal of Palliative Nursing* 2009; 15: 162–9.

Psychological aspects of care

Cancer is often the most feared of all serious illnesses in the UK. Over a third of people are more worried about developing cancer than they are about developing any other life-threatening condition. Despite improvements in treatment and survival, for many individuals a diagnosis of cancer is still synonymous with a death sentence.

The prevalence of significant physical, functional, psychological, social, and sexual problems as a result of the diagnosis and treatment of cancer is well documented. Breasts may be regarded as a representation of womanhood, femininity, beauty, desirability, sexuality, and the woman's role as a mother.

Malignant disease of the breast and any form of treatment may be associated with considerable fear, anxiety, depression, and distress, affecting:
- body image
- the woman's sense of self-worth, self-esteem, and confidence
- feelings of attraction, intimacy, and sexuality
- sexual functioning and fertility
- survivorship, and living with uncertainty and fear of recurrence.

Factors that influence the psychosocial impact of breast cancer

Psychosocial factors
- Age (younger women reportedly have significantly poorer quality of life in terms of physical and emotional well-being), personality, and self-concept.
- Available and applied coping strategies.
- Previous experience—of life, illness, association with cancer, and association with breast cancer.
- Type and degree of disruption to life.
- Expectations of treatment.
- Previous history of psychiatric illness and depressive symptoms.
- Availability of psychological and social support.

Disease-related factors
- Type and stage of cancer.
- Treatment modality and adverse events, including symptom experience and chemotherapy-related cognitive difficulties (e.g. speed of information processing).
- Psychosocial support provided by healthcare professionals.

Psychosocial interventions
- All healthcare professionals should be able to provide essential psychological support. This includes listening and compassionate communication, responding effectively to distress, information giving, and assessment of psychological and psychiatric morbidity.
- Women with breast cancer have a high level of information needs. Individual and group peer support has been shown to be a valuable resource, with the non-statutory sector providing face-to-face and Internet group support.

- Increasing levels of psychological support require psychological techniques for problem solving, counselling, and anxiety management, and specialist mental health interventions such as psychotherapy, cognitive behavioural therapy, hypnosis, and stress management strategies.

Further reading

Galgut C. *The Psychological Impact of Breast Cancer: a psychologist's insights as a patient.* Radclif Publishing Ltd: London, 2010.
Saionen P et al. Changes in quality of life in patients with breast cancer. *Journal of Clinical Nurse* 2010; 20: 255–66.

Useful websites

Breast Cancer Care. 🔊 www.breastcancercare.org.uk
Cancer Advice. 🔊 www.canceradvice.co.uk

End-of-life care

- Survival rates for breast cancer have been steadily improving over the past few decades, and the current 5-year relative survival is 82%. Nevertheless, breast cancer accounts for almost 12 000 deaths annually in the UK, and nearly 20% of all female cancer mortality.[5]
- 'End-of-life care' could be considered to refer principally to the care of the dying.
- Palliative care is an approach that focuses on preventing and relieving the suffering of patients, and their families, associated with life-threatening illness, and is appropriate for all patients in all disease stages, not necessarily strictly and solely the terminal phases.
- Compassionate end-of-life care is a matter of significance for all nurses, not only the specialist practitioners.
- Discussing and delivering high-quality end-of-life care improves not only the quality of life and subsequent death of the patient, but also bereavement outcomes.

Preferred priorities for care

- Choice and control of end-of-life care should be available to all. However, the majority of patients do not die in their preferred place of care, and this may be in part because the majority of nurses who are concerned with end-of-life care were not trained in communication beyond a basic level, and initiating such discussions can be difficult. As a result, 'the elephant in the room', or the obvious truth of the patient's impending death, is never acknowledged or effectively addressed.[6]
- There are numerous resources to help the nurse, including the Royal College of Nursing publication *Route to Success: the key contribution of nursing to end of life care*,[7] which provides a useful and comprehensive account of assessment tools and clinical guidelines, including clinical management plans from the Liverpool Care Pathway and Gold Standards Framework.
- Prognostication is intricate and imprecise, so the 'surprise' question—'Would I be surprised if the patient died within the next 6–12 months?'—can be a helpful tool for guiding practitioners to make prompt and effective early referral to appropriate support services.

Advanced disease and symptom management

- Advanced breast cancer can present as local recurrence or widespread metastases. Local recurrence may be considered to herald the presence of distant metastases.
- Patients with advanced disease may live for several years, with their symptoms adequately controlled.
- The metastatic disease of primary breast cancer commonly presents in the bones, brain, lungs, and liver, and is often associated with a shortened survival.

References

5 Cancer Research UK. *Breast Cancer Mortality Statistics*. ℅ www.cancerresearchuk.org/
  health-professional/cancer-statistics/statistics-by-cancer-type/breast-cancer/mortality
6 Quill TE. Initiating end-of-life discussions with seriously ill patients: addressing the "elepha
  in the room." *Journal of the American Medical Association* 2000; **284**: 2502–7.
7 Royal College of Nursing. *Route to Success: the key contribution of nursing to end of life ca
  Royal College of Nursing: London, 2011.

Further reading

Marie Curie Palliative Care Institute. *The Liverpool Care Pathway for the Dying Patient (LCP): pock
  guide*. Marie Curie Palliative Care Institute: Liverpool, 2010.
National Cancer Intelligence Network (NCIN). *One, Five and Ten Year Cancer Prevalenc*
  NCIN: London, 2010.
Thomas K and Lobo B (eds). *Advance Care Planning in End of Life Care*. Oxford Univers
  Press: Oxford, 2011.

Useful websites

Gold Standards Framework. ℅ www.goldstandardsframework.org.uk
National End of Life Care Programme, *Planning for your Future Care; a guide*. ℅ www.nhs.u
  planners/end-of-life-care/documents/planning-for-your-future-care.pdf

Gynaecological surgery

Anatomy of the female reproductive system

The female reproductive system (see Figures 28.1 and 28.2) is usuall divided into internal and external organs.

Internal organs

These consist of the ovaries, the Fallopian tubes, the uterus (womb and the vagina.

Ovaries

These are the female sex glands, which produce oestrogen and proges terone. They are situated in the peritoneal cavity near the fimbriate ends of the Fallopian tubes. During a woman's fertile years the ovarie produce a mature ovum during each menstrual cycle.

Fallopian tubes

These are two muscular tubes connected to the uterus. At the dist ends are finger-like structures called fimbriae which lie near the ovarie The Fallopian tubes convey ova from the ovary to the uterus, and con vey sperm cells upwards to meet the ova. Fertilization takes place in th Fallopian tube.

Uterus (womb)

This pear-shaped organ is approximately the size of a fist, and consists three parts—the fundus, the body, and the cervix.

The uterus lining is called the endometrium, and the muscle fibres ar called the myometrium. The blood supply to the uterus is from the ute ine arteries, a branch of the internal iliac artery, and the uterine vei drain into the internal iliac veins.

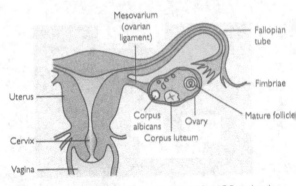

Figure 28.1 Female reproductive system. Adapted from G Pocock and C Richards, *Human Physiology: the basis of medicine*, 2nd edition, 2004, by permission of Oxford University Press.

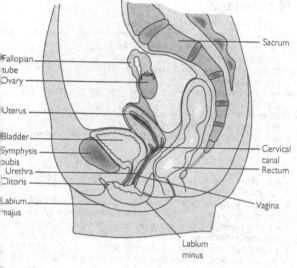

Figure 28.2 Side view of female reproductive system. Adapted from G Pocock and C Richards, *Human Physiology: the basis of medicine*, 2nd edition, 2004, by permission of Oxford University Press.

The functions of the uterus are menstruation, maintenance of pregnancy, and initiation of labour.

Vagina

The vagina is a fibromuscular channel extending from the cervix (internally) to the labia (externally), and thus connecting the internal and external reproductive organs. It is capable of great distension, and is composed of smooth muscle lined with mucous membrane, which is arranged in folds.

The functions of the vagina are to receive sperm, to act as a birth canal, and to provide an excretory duct for uterine secretions and menstrual flow.

External organs

These consist of the following:
- mons pubis
- labia majora
- labia minora
- clitoris
- urethral orifice
- vaginal orifice
- Bartholin's glands.

Miscarriage

Miscarriage is the loss of a pregnancy before 24 weeks' gestation. Women may present with vaginal bleeding and pain, although some will have few or no symptoms. Diagnosis is made on the basis of an ultrasound scan. There are several different types of miscarriage:

- missed miscarriage—in which the fetal heartbeat stops some time before diagnosis
- anembryonic pregnancy—in which the gestation sac grows but is devoid of contents
- incomplete miscarriage—in which the pregnancy tissue is not completely expelled from the uterus
- complete miscarriage—in which the uterus has completely expelled the pregnancy.

Treatment

Treatment of first-trimester miscarriage (less than 12 weeks) can include

- natural miscarriage
- medical management—misoprostol is given orally, sublingually, vaginally, or rectally in order to induce the miscarriage. Misoprostol is a prostaglandin analogue that can cause uterine contractions and ripening of the cervix
- surgical management—this is normally performed under a general or local anaesthetic, and the uterus is emptied using suction curettage.

Second-trimester miscarriage occurs between 12 and 24 weeks, sometimes with spontaneous expulsion of the fetus, or where the fetal heartbeat has stopped, and will require treatment to induce the miscarriage.

Complications

- Excessive vaginal bleeding and haemorrhage requiring hospital admission and further intervention such as surgical evacuation of the uterus and blood transfusion.
- Severe abdominal pains and cramping not controlled with simple analgesia.
- Psychological trauma from both the physical effects and grieving for the pregnancy loss. The severity of these effects varies. Some women cope well with minimal support from family, friends, and miscarriage nurse specialists, whereas others will require more formal counselling. The Miscarriage Association provides useful information on its website, and a range of leaflets.

Further reading

Miscarriage Association. ℰ www.miscarriageassociation.org.uk

Menstrual disorders

One in five women experience heavy menstrual bleeding; this is one of the most common gynaecological complaints. Many women begin to experience heavy and/or irregular bleeding in their thirties and forties, as they start to get closer to the menopause.

Types of menstrual disturbance

- Menorrhagia—heavy menstrual bleeding.
- Intermenstrual bleeding—bleeding between periods.
- Dysmenorrhoea—painful periods.
- Oligomenorrhoea—irregular or infrequent menstrual periods.
- Amenorrhoea—absence of menstrual periods in a woman of reproductive age.
- Post-coital bleeding—bleeding after intercourse.
- Post-menopausal bleeding—bleeding after periods have stopped for more than 1 year. In this situation the patient will be referred to outpatients on a 2-week wait pathway.

Investigations

- Ultrasound scan to identify uterine anomalies, measure the uterus, and look for fibroids, polyps, adenomyosis, and cysts.
- Cervical examination to identify any abnormality of the cervix.
- High vaginal and chlamydia swabs to look for vaginal infections.
- Endometrial sampling in women over 40 years of age with menorrhagia, to check for endometrial cancer.

Pathology

- Polyps (cervical or endometrial) are abnormal growths of tissue projecting from a mucous membrane.
- Fibroids are non-cancerous growths arising from the smooth muscle cells of the womb.
- Cervical extortion (or cervical erosion) is a condition in which the central (endocervical) columnar epithelium protrudes out through the external os of the cervix.

A period occurs when the endometrium is shed at regular intervals, leaving a layer of cells from which a new lining will grow after each period. In around 50% of cases there is no obvious reason why heavy periods have occurred. In other cases there may be an abnormality or hormonal imbalance.

Management

Often patients will start with first-line treatment and will pursue further treatments if medication fails.

- Medication frequently involves hormones such as the combined oestrogen and progestogen pill and norethisterone. Non-hormone treatments include tranexamic acid and mefenamic acid.
- The Mirena® intrauterine system is a small plastic T-shaped device containing the progesterone hormone levonorgestrel.
- Endometrial ablation is the surgical destruction of the lining of the uterus.
- Hysterectomy is the surgical removal of the uterus.

Sexually transmitted infections

Sexually transmitted infections (STIs) are diseases that are passed from one person to another through unprotected vaginal, anal, or oral sex. They may be contracted by genital contact or sharing sex toys.

Patients should be advised to attend the local sexual health clinic, genitourinary medicine (GUM) clinic, or GP surgery for a full sexual health screen, and it is important that their present and past partners are traced and treated as necessary.

It is important to treat all STIs, as if left untreated some of these infections may cause more serious health problems and infertility. These complications include pelvic inflammatory disease (PID), which is a condition that causes inflammation of the pelvis and usually presents as pain. It is generally caused by STIs. Treatment is with antibiotics, which are given either intravenously or orally, depending on the severity, and analgesia.

The following are the most common STIs:

- Chlamydia is one of the most common STIs in the UK. Symptoms may include pain, vaginal discharge, or bleeding between periods or after sexual intercourse. Most people are asymptomatic and unaware that they have the infection. Diagnosis is done by urine test or vaginal swab. Treatment is with antibiotics, and failure to treat can lead to serious long-term health problems, including infertility.
- Genital warts are a viral skin infection caused by the human papilloma virus (HPV), and spread by skin-to-skin contact, so penetrative sex is not necessary. They present as small fleshy growths or skin changes around the genital or anal area. Treatment is with antiviral creams or cryotherapy.
- Genital herpes is a long-term condition caused by the herpes simplex virus (HSV). Once a person has become infected, the virus remains dormant for most of the time, but certain triggers can activate it, causing outbreaks of painful blisters around the genital area. These outbreaks are treated with antiviral medication (topically or orally). Acute severe episodes may require admission for analgesia and catheterization until the symptoms settle.
- Gonorrhoea is a bacterial infection that can cause unusual vaginal discharge and/or pain when urinating. It is diagnosed by swab and treated with antibiotics.
- Syphilis is a bacterial infection that causes painless but highly infectious sores in the genital area or sometimes the mouth. The sores last for 2–6 weeks, after which secondary symptoms such as a skin rash and sore throat may develop. These may then disappear and the patient is asymptomatic. Treatment is with penicillin. If left untreated, syphilis can lead to stroke, paralysis, blindness, or death.
- Trichomoniasis is a condition caused by the parasite *Trichomonas vaginalis*. Women may present with soreness or itching around the vagina, and a change in vaginal discharge. Treatment is with antibiotics.

- Pubic lice (crabs) are tiny bloodsucking insects that live in coarse human body hair, and are most commonly found in pubic hair. They present with itching and redness to the genital area. Treatment is with insecticide medications.
- Scabies is a contagious skin condition caused by tiny mites that burrow into the skin. It presents with severe itching. It is spread by skin-to-skin contact with an infected person, so is not necessarily sexually transmitted. Treatment is with insecticide creams.

Benign ovarian tumours

Aetiology and pathology
- Around 94% of ovarian tumours are benign, and they are usually cystic.
- Around 24% of ovarian tumours are functional, and will usually resolve naturally within two to three menstrual cycles.
- Endometriotic (chocolate) cysts (5%).
- Epithelial cell tumours (serous and mucinous cystadenomas) (40%) are usually surgically removed.
- Germ-cell tumours (dermoids/teratomas) (20%) are surgically removed if they are large, but if there is no growth then no intervention is required.
- Fibromas (solid tumours) (5%) do not require any intervention unless they are symptomatic.

Investigations
- Pelvic ultrasound scans (transabdominal and transvaginal).

Management
- If they are small, asymptomatic, and persistent, no intervention is required.
- If they are large or symptomatic, laparoscopic ovarian cystectomy or laparotomy may be required. Some cysts can be drained under ultrasound guidance as an outpatient procedure. Occasionally an oophorectomy may be necessary.

Endometriosis

Endometriosis is a chronic oestrogen-dependent condition character-ized by the growth of endometrial tissue elsewhere in the body (usually, but not always, in the pelvis).

Symptoms

- Chronic pelvic pain, dysmenorrhoea, and dyspareunia (painful sexual intercourse).

Investigations

- Laparoscopy is required to diagnose the disease, although experienced transvaginal ultrasound is suitable for diagnosing an endometrioma.

Management

- Management may include hormone analogues, such as the combined oral contraceptive pill or the levonorgestrel intrauterine system (IUS).
- Surgical ablation of endometriotic spots can be effective in patients with minimal disease.
- Large endometriomas are surgically removed.
- Hysterectomy with bilateral salpingo-oophorectomy is performed in severe cases.
- Complications include an increased risk of ovarian cancer, adhesion formation, infertility, and increased risk of ectopic pregnancy.
- There is a high risk of relapse (20–50%) following treatment.

Endometrial cancer

Endometrial cancer is the fourth most common cancer in women, and the most common of the gynaecological cancers. In the UK there were 8475 cases in 2011, and 1930 deaths from the disease in that year.[1]

Aetiology and risk factors

Endometrial cancer is predominantly a disease of post-menopausal women, with a peak incidence among those aged 60–75 years.

Any factor that increases oestrogen exposure will increase the risk of endometrial cancer. This includes:

- early menarche
- delayed menopause
- obesity
- nulliparity
- use of unopposed oestrogens (e.g. some types of HRT)
- polycystic ovarian disease
- use of tamoxifen
- diabetes
- endometrial hyperplasia.

There is also an increased risk of developing endometrial cancer associated with hereditary non-polyposis colorectal cancer (HNPCC).

Investigations

- Transvaginal ultrasound scan is useful in the first instance to assess endometrial thickness. This should be less than 5 mm in post-menopausal women and less than 20 mm in pre-menopausal women.
- Endometrial biopsy is required in order to obtain a tissue diagnosis. This may be obtained by pipelle or hysteroscopy and curettage. Endometrial cancers are predominantly endometrioid adenocarcinomas. Rarer cancers of the endometrium/uterus include adenosquamous, serous papillary, and clear cell carcinomas, and sarcomas.
- Either MRI or CT scan (depending on the histological type of the cancer) is often requested in order to assess the extent of disease.
- Chest X-ray is required to rule out lung involvement.

Treatment

For most endometrial cancers, surgery is the preferred initial treatment even if it is anticipated that adjuvant treatment will be required. Surgery would usually involve hysterectomy, bilateral salpingo-oophorectomy, lymph node assessment and dissection, and peritoneal washings. This may be performed by a laparoscopic or open procedure.

A simple hysterectomy may be considered even in late-stage disease for palliation. Treatments that may be recommended in addition to surgery include external beam radiotherapy, brachytherapy, chemotherapy, hormone therapy, or any combination of these.

Post-surgical care

- Vaginal blood loss should be assessed every time vital signs are checked, in order to ensure that haemorrhage is not excessive.
- Pelvic surgery may result in inadvertent damage to the bladder or bowel. Therefore in the immediate post-operative period this should be considered if the patient is unwell.
- HRT is not usually recommended for patients who have had endometrial carcinoma.
- Follow-up may be undertaken in the oncology or surgical setting, and is usually continued until 5 years after the initial diagnosis.
- The overall 5-year survival for endometrial cancer is 80%, although the outlook is determined by the type, grade, and stage of cancer at diagnosis.

Reference

Cancer Research UK. *Uterine Womb Cancer: key facts.* Cancer Research UK: London, 2014.

Further reading

Cancer Research UK. *Uterine Cancer Incidence Statistics.* ℘ www.cancerresearchuk.org/cancer-info/cancerstats/types/uterus/incidence/uk-uterus-cancer-incidence-statistics

Cervical cancer

In the UK in 2011, a total of 3064 cases of cervical cancer were diagnosed, and there were 972 deaths from this disease.[2] Cervical cancer is the most common cancer in women under 35 years of age. There are two peaks in age-specific incidence—in the 30–34 years age group, and in those aged ≥ 75 years.

Aetiology and risk factors

Human papilloma virus (HPV) is present in virtually all cases (99.7%) of cervical cancer. Most women will have been exposed to and infected with HPV at some point in their life, although they may not necessarily be aware of this. HPV is usually cleared by the body's own immune system. There are over 100 types of HPV, of which 40 types affect the genitals. HPV types 16 and 18 pose the highest risk for developing a cervical malignancy. Increased risk of developing cervical cancer is generally associated with exposure to HPV and a weakened immune system. This includes:

- early age at first sexual intercourse
- number of lifetime partners
- high parity
- oral contraceptive pill use
- cigarette smoking
- HIV infection.

Cervical screening

The cervical screening programme invites women aged 25–49 years for 3-yearly cervical smears, and women aged 50–64 years for 5-yearly smears. This screening programme aims to detect pre-cancerous cells which can be treated in order to prevent cancer from developing. Treatment usually involves a colposcopy examination with or without loop excision of the cervix.

HPV vaccine

A vaccine to prevent infection by HPV was introduced in 2008 for girls aged 12–13 years. It is given to girls of this age because it is most effective if given before the first sexual contact occurs.

Investigations

- Biopsy is required for tissue diagnosis. This may be either a punch biopsy or loop excision.
- Two-thirds of cervical cancers are squamous-cell carcinomas, and 15% are adenocarcinomas. Rarer cancers of the cervix include adenosquamous carcinomas, small-cell carcinomas, and neuroendocrine tumours.
- An MRI scan of the pelvis is requested once cervical cancer has been diagnosed, to assess the extent of spread of the disease and to ensure that the appropriate treatment is offered.
- Chest X-ray is required to rule out lung involvement.

Treatment

Surgery is preferred for younger patients with a tumour of FIGO Ib (disease confined to the cervix < 4 cm) or less, as it conserves ovarian function and has fewer bladder- and bowel-related side effects. Surgical options include knife cone biopsy with or without pelvic lymph node dissection, radical trachelectomy (complete removal of the cervix), or radical hysterectomy.

Histological assessment will sometimes indicate that additional treatment is required following surgery. This may consist of radiotherapy and/or chemotherapy. For patients who are not suitable candidates for surgery, a combination of chemotherapy and radiotherapy is usually given.

Post-surgical care

Vaginal blood loss should be assessed every time vital signs are checked, to ensure that haemorrhage is not excessive. Pelvic surgery may result in inadvertent damage to the bladder or bowel. Therefore in the immediate post-operative period this should be considered if the patient is unwell.

During radical trachelectomy or hysterectomy, the nerves to the bladder may be disturbed and this can result in loss of bladder sensation. It is therefore important to monitor the ability to pass urine and to fully empty the bladder following initial removal of the urinary catheter. If a patient is unable to pass urine or fully empty her bladder, she may be taught intermittent self-catheterization while allowing the nerve supply to repair. Damage to the nerve supply during surgery may also result in a numb area in the thighs. This usually fully recovers within 6–12 months.

There is a small risk of developing lymphoedema of the legs due to pelvic node dissection. The patient should be educated about preventative measures which can be taken to reduce the risk of developing lymphoedema in the future.

For patients who have had fertility-preserving surgery (knife cone biopsy or trachelectomy), the ability to conceive is not usually affected. However, the risk of miscarriage or premature labour is increased. For those who have undergone a trachelectomy, a cerclage is usually required to maintain the pregnancy. Antenatal care must therefore be tailored accordingly, and patients must be counselled about the risks.

Follow-up may be undertaken in the oncology or colposcopy setting, and is usually continued until 5 years after the initial diagnosis. The overall 5-year survival for cervical cancer is 66.6%, although the outlook is determined by the grade, type, and stage of cancer at diagnosis.

Reference

Cancer Research UK. *Cervical Cancer: key facts*. Cancer Research UK: London, 2014.

Further reading

Cancer Research UK. *Cervical Cancer Statistics*. ℜ www.cancerresearchuk.org/cancer-info/cancerstats/types/cervix

Emergency gynaecology

Emergency gynaecology refers to acute problems relating to the femal
reproductive system, or problems in the early stages of pregnancy. The
main conditions that present within emergency gynaecology will b
summarized here.

Abdominal pain

Patients can present with abdominal pain ranging from mild to sever
in intensity. It can be unilateral, affecting one side of the abdomen, o
bilateral, affecting both sides. The most common causes of abdomina
pain within emergency gynaecology include the following:

- Pelvic inflammatory disease (PID)—this condition causes
  inflammation of the pelvis, and is generally due to an STI.
- Miscarriage—this is the loss of a pregnancy before 24 weeks'
  gestation. These patients will often present with abdominal pain and
  vaginal bleeding.
- Ovarian cysts—approximately 95% of these cysts will be harmless,
  and many women may only become symptomatic if the cyst ruptures
  becomes torted, or is very large.
- Ectopic pregnancy—the implantation of a fertilized egg anywhere
  outside the lining of the womb.

Vaginal bleeding

Patients can present with vaginal bleeding ranging from light flow t
heavy flow. They will present for a number of reasons, and the mos
common causes include the following:

- Miscarriage—the patient will often present with abdominal pain
  and vaginal bleeding. Not all bleeding in pregnancy will result in a
  miscarriage.
- Menorrhagia—prolonged and extremely heavy periods that occur
  at regular intervals. Most women can manage these symptoms at
  home, but at times may present to hospital if the bleeding becomes
  excessive.
- Post-menopausal bleeding—bleeding that occurs more than 1 year
  after the menopause. Sometimes it is excessive and requires
  treatment.
- Trauma to the female genitalia (vagina, vulva, and cervix). This can b
  caused by violent intercourse and/or foreign objects being inserted
  into the vagina. It can result in excessive vaginal bleeding, and severe
  trauma may require surgery.
- Heavy periods—if a woman's normal monthly periods (which
  occur due to shedding of the lining of the womb, known as the
  endometrium) become increasingly heavy, they may need treatment

Hyperemesis gravidarum

This is a severe form of nausea and vomiting in pregnancy that m
require admission of the patient due to dehydration. Treatment m
consist of an intravenous infusion (IVI) and anti-emetics.

Bartholin's abscess

The two Bartholin's glands lie next to the opening of the vagina, and are not usually noticeable. If the glands become blocked they will fill with fluid, and this can then cause an abscess. There are two ways to treat an abscess if antibiotics are not effective. A surgical incision (marsupialization) can be performed under a general anaesthetic to allow the pus to drain freely. An alternative treatment is a Word catheter. This is a small catheter that is inserted into the abscess and left for up to 4 weeks to allow free drainage.

Ectopic pregnancy

An ectopic pregnancy occurs when a fertilized egg implants anywhere outside the lining (endometrium) of the womb. It affects approximately 1 in 100 pregnancies, and most commonly occurs in the Fallopian tube, although it can also occur in the ovary, cervix, or abdominal cavity. A ectopic pregnancy cannot be successful, but may continue to grow for number of weeks. The Fallopian tube is not large enough to accommodate a pregnancy and will therefore stretch, causing pain in the abdomen. Vaginal bleeding may occur as the lining of the womb becomes thickened. *Ectopic pregnancies must be treated*, otherwise they can rupture, causing internal haemorrhage which can be fatal. In rare cases there may be two fertilized eggs, one outside the uterus and the other inside. This is known as a heterotopic pregnancy.

Causes

There are a number of risk factors for ectopic pregnancies, including:
- pelvic inflammatory disease
- chlamydia
- previous ectopic pregnancy
- infertility or use of assisted conception
- previous pelvic surgery.

Symptoms

- Pain is the most common symptom, and can range from mild to severe abdominal pain. The pain can also occur in the shoulder, which is due to blood leaking into the diaphragm.
- Vaginal bleeding—there may be no or minimal vaginal bleeding, and can often be watery and dark brown.

Management

- Surgery—this is usually performed by keyhole surgery, and often involves removal of the Fallopian tube (salpingectomy). An alternative may be to make an incision in the tube and remove the pregnancy, leaving the tube intact (salpingostomy). If rupture has occurred it may be necessary to perform a laparotomy.
- Medical treatment—a dose of intramuscular methotrexate (a cytotoxic drug) is administered in some cases. However, there are criteria for its use. This will cause the ectopic to dissolve, and close follow-up monitoring of the pregnancy hormone is required until it resolves. Conservative, minimal ectopics can be managed in this way and would require close monitoring of the patient's hormone level.

Complications

The most common complication is rupture of an ectopic, causing internal haemorrhage, which in rare cases can be fatal.

Prognosis

The risk of having another ectopic pregnancy is around 10–20%. Patients are advised to have an early ultrasound scan in subsequent pregnancies.

Ovarian cancer

Ovarian cancer is the fifth most common cancer in women in the UK. In 2011, around 7100 women were diagnosed with ovarian cancer.[3]

Types of ovarian cancer

Most ovarian cancers are of a type called epithelial cancer. Epithelial ovarian cancer means that the cancer originated in the cells that cover the surface of the ovary. There are several types of epithelial cancers of the ovary. The most common types are:

- serous
- endometrioid.

Less common types of epithelial ovarian cancer include:

- mucinous
- clear cell
- undifferentiated or unclassifiable.

The rare forms include:

- dysgerminoma
- endodermal sinus tumours
- teratoma, immature, mature, or mixed
- embryonal carcinoma
- choriocarcinoma
- sex cord-stromal tumours (5–8%)
- granulosa cell tumours
- Sertoli–Leydig tumours
- sarcomas.

Borderline tumours

Borderline tumours are growths composed of cells that are abnormal and may become cancerous if not treated.

Primary peritoneal cancer

Primary peritoneal cancer (PPC) is a rare cancer that behaves much like epithelial ovarian cancer, and is treated in the same way. It starts in the peritoneum. PPC can occur in men, although this is very rare.

Causes

The exact cause of ovarian cancer is not known. However, several factors may increase the risk:

- a family history of ovarian, breast, or colorectal cancer
- a personal history of breast cancer
- reproductive history—women who started their periods early or reached the menopause late may be at slightly increased risk of developing cancer, as may those who have never been pregnant
- infertility—stimulation of the ovary by drugs used during infertility treatment can slightly increase the risk of developing ovarian cancer
- being obese or overweight
- using HRT
- smoking.

Symptoms of ovarian cancer

- Loss of appetite.
- Swelling in the abdomen—this may be due to the accumulation of ascites.
- Changes in bowel or bladder habits.
- Indigestion, nausea, and a bloated, full feeling.
- Unexplained weight gain or an increased waist size.
- Shortness of breath.
- Pain in the lower abdomen.
- Lower back pain.
- Pain during sex.
- Abnormal vaginal bleeding, although this is rare.

Investigations

- Ultrasound scan.
- CT scan (thorax, abdomen, and pelvis).
- CA125 blood test (tumour marker).
- Abdominal fluid and/or lung fluid aspiration.
- Laparoscopy and biopsy.
- Laparotomy.

Treatment

Nearly all women who have ovarian cancer will require surgery. Sometimes it is not possible to confirm the stage of the cancer until the surgery is being performed. This would usually involve laparotomy, total abdominal hysterectomy, bilateral salpingo-oophorectomy, and omentectomy. Samples from other tissues may be taken, such as the lymph glands, diaphragm, and peritoneum. In some cases, bowel surgery may be required and colostomy performed. Chemotherapy may be recommended in addition to surgery. For some patients, neoadjuvant chemotherapy is required followed by interval debulking surgery.

Post-surgical care

- Vaginal blood loss should be assessed every time vital signs are checked, in order to ensure that haemorrhage is not excessive.
- Pelvic surgery may result in inadvertent damage to the bladder or bowel. Therefore in the immediate post-operative period this should be considered if the patient is unwell.
- Post-operative paralytic ileus may occur. Observe the patient for signs of vomiting, abdominal fullness and distension, and diarrhoea.
- Observe for signs of deep vein thrombosis and pulmonary embolism.
- HRT is not usually recommended for patients who have been diagnosed with ovarian cancer.
- Follow-up may be undertaken in the oncology or surgical setting, and is usually continued until 5 years after the initial diagnosis.

Reference

3 Cancer Research UK. *Ovarian Cancer: key facts.* Cancer Research UK: London, 2014.

Further reading

Cancer Research UK. *Stages of Ovarian Cancer.* ℑ www.cancerresearchuk.org/about-cancer-type/ovarian-cancer/treatment/stages-of-ovarian-cancer

Vulval cancer

Vulval cancer is a rare cancer in the UK. In 2011, a total of 1203 women in the UK were diagnosed with cancer of the vulva.[4]

Types of vulval cancer
- Squamous-cell carcinoma.
- Vulval melanoma.
- Adenocarcinoma.
- Basal-cell carcinoma.
- Verrucous carcinoma.

Causes
The exact cause of vulval cancer is not yet known, but several risk factors have been suggested, including:
- human papilloma virus (HPV) infection—this is thought to be responsible for approximately 40% of vulval cancers. HPV is passed from one person to another during sexual contact
- vulval intra-epithelial neoplasia (VIN)—pre-cancerous changes in the skin cells of the vulva. There is a risk that these may go on to develop into vulvar cancer
- benign inflammatory skin conditions
- smoking
- weakened immune system due to autoimmune conditions such as HIV or drugs that can lower immunity.

Symptoms
- A lump or swelling in the vulva.
- Persistent itching.
- Vaginal discharge or bleeding.
- Pain or soreness.
- Pain during intercourse.
- Changes in skin colour—areas that are red, irritated, white, or dark coloured.

Investigations
- Vulval, groin, and pelvic examination.
- Biopsy.
- CT, MRI, and PET-CT.

Treatment
The main treatment for vulval cancer is surgery.
- Wide local excision—removal of the area containing the cancer, along with a border of healthy tissue around it.
- Radical local excision—removal of the cancer and a larger area of the normal tissue all around the cancer. The lymph nodes in the groin may also be removed.
- Partial vulvectomy—removal of part of the vulva.

- Radical vulvectomy—removal of the entire vulva, including the inner and outer labia and sometimes also the clitoris. In addition, the lymph nodes are removed from both groins.
- Sentinel lymph node biopsy (SLNB)—a sentinel lymph node is the first lymph node (or nodes) to which cancer cells are most likely to spread from the primary tumour. It can be used to help to determine the spread, or stage, of vulvar cancer. Because SLNB involves less extensive surgery and the removal of fewer lymph nodes than standard lymph node surgery, potential side effects are reduced.

Treatments that may be recommended in addition to surgery are radio therapy and/or chemotherapy. They may be used before surgery, t reduce the size of the cancer, or after surgery, to ensure that any remain ing cancer cells are destroyed, or to reduce the likelihood of a futur recurrence.

Post-surgical care
- Vaginal blood loss should be assessed every time vital signs are checked, in order to ensure that haemorrhage is not excessive.
- Damage to the nerve supply during surgery may also result in numb areas in the thighs. This usually fully or partially recovers within 6–12 months.
- Observe for signs of bladder infection.
- Observe for signs of wound infection or breakdown, particularly in the groin.
- Lymphocyst—observe for signs of localized swelling (golf ball size or larger) in the groin and upper thigh. If the swelling is small and not infected, it is usually monitored but left to reabsorb spontaneously with no medical or surgical intervention. If the patient has a temperature and the lymphocyst is large and infected, antibiotic treatment and fine-needle aspiration may be required.
- Lymphoedema—observe for signs of accumulation of fluid (in wome who have had their lymph nodes removed) in one or both legs or in the genital area. Lymphoedema may remain as a lifelong problem, and the patient may need to be referred to the lymphoedema nurse specialist.

Reference
4 Cancer Research UK. *Vulval Cancer: key facts*. Cancer Research UK: London, 2014.

Further reading
Cancer Research UK. *Stages of Vulval Cancer*. ℘ www.cancerresearchuk.org/about-cance type/vulval-cancer/treatment/stages-of-vulval-cancer

Vaginal cancer

Cancer of the vagina is a rare cancer. In 2011, a total of 256 women in the UK were diagnosed with vaginal cancer.[5]

Types of vaginal cancer
- Squamous-cell carcinoma.
- Adenocarcinoma.
- Malignant melanoma.
- Leiomyosarcoma.
- Rhabdomyosarcoma.

Causes
- Age—almost 50% of cases occur in women aged 70 years or older at the time of diagnosis.
- Exposure to diethylstilbestrol (DES) as a fetus (i.e. the patient's mother took DES during pregnancy).
- History of cervical cancer.
- History of cervical precancerous conditions.
- Human papilloma virus (HPV) infection.
- HIV infection.
- Vaginal adenosis.
- Vaginal irritation.
- Smoking.

Symptoms
Bleeding or discharge not related to menstrual periods.
Difficult or painful urination.
Pain during intercourse.
Pain in the pelvic area.
Constipation.
A mass that can be felt.

Investigations
Pelvic examination of the vagina—colposcopy.
CT, MRI, and PET-CT.
Biopsy.

Treatment
Removal of small tumours or lesions
Cancer that is confined to the surface of the vagina may be cut away, together with a small margin of surrounding healthy tissue to ensure that all of the cancer cells have been removed.

Removal of the vagina (vaginectomy)
Removal of part of the vagina (partial vaginectomy) or the entire vagina (radical vaginectomy) may be necessary in order to remove all of the cancer. Depending on the extent of the cancer, the surgeon may recommend surgery to remove the uterus and ovaries (hysterectomy) and nearby lymph nodes (lymphadenectomy) at the same time as the vaginectomy.

Removal of the majority of the pelvic organs (pelvic exenteration)
This extensive surgery may be an option if cancer has spread throughout the pelvic area, or if the vaginal cancer has recurred. During pelvic exenteration, the surgeon removes many of the organs in the pelvic area including the bladder, ovaries, uterus, vagina, rectum, and lower portion of the colon. Openings are created in the abdomen to allow urine (via a urostomy) and waste (via a colostomy) to exit the body and collect in ostomy bags.

Treatments that may be recommended in addition to surgery are radiotherapy and/or chemotherapy.

Post-surgical care
- Vaginal blood loss should be assessed every time vital signs are checked, in order to ensure that haemorrhage is not excessive.
- Damage to the nerve supply during surgery may also result in numb areas in the thighs. This usually fully recovers within 6–12 months.
- Observe for signs of bladder infection.
- Observe for signs of wound infection or breakdown, particularly in the groin.
- Lymphocyst— observe for signs of localized swelling (golf ball size) in the groin and upper thigh. If the swelling is small and not infected, it is usually monitored but left to reabsorb spontaneously with no medical or surgical intervention. If the patient has a temperature and the lymphocyst is large and infected, antibiotic treatment and fine-needle aspiration may be required.
- Lymphoedema—observe for signs of accumulation of fluid (in women who have had their lymph nodes removed) in one or both legs or in the genital area. Lymphoedema will generally resolve over a period of 2–12 months, and the patient may need to be referred to the lymphoedema clinic.

Reference
5 Cancer Research UK. *Vaginal Cancer: key facts.* Cancer Research UK: London, 2014.

Further reading
Cancer Research UK. *The Stages of Cancer of the Vagina.* ℘ www.cancerresearchuk.org/about-cancer/type/vaginal-cancer/treatment/the-stages-of-cancer-of-the-vagina

Index

Tables, figures, and boxes are indicated by an italic *t*, *f*, and *b* following the page number.